Jose Costa

D0858142

OTHER MONOGRAPHS IN THE SERIES,
MAJOR PROBLEMS IN PATHOLOGY

Published

Forthcoming

JOHN G. AZZOPARDI, BSc, MD, MRCPath

Professor of Oncology, The Royal Postgraduate Medical School,
University of London
Honorary Consultant Pathologist,
Hammersmith Hospital, London

with contributions by

ALI AHMED, MD (Manchester)

Senior Lecturer in Pathology,
University of Manchester

and

ROSEMARY R. MILLIS, MB, BS, MRCPath

Consultant Pathologist to Guy's Health District and to the Imperial
Cancer Research Fund Breast Unit at Guy's Hospital, London
Honorary Research Consultant to the Breast Unit, The Royal Marsden
Hospital, London

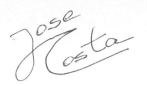

PROBLEMS IN BREAST PATHOLOGY

Volume 11 in the Series
MAJOR PROBLEMS IN PATHOLOGY
JAMES L. BENNINGTON, MD, *Consulting Editor*

Chairman, Department of Pathology
Children's Hospital of San Francisco
San Francisco, California

1979
W. B. Saunders Company Ltd   London · Philadelphia · Toronto

W. B. Saunders Company Ltd: 1 St Anne's Road
Eastbourne, East Sussex BN21 3UN

West Washington Square
Philadelphia, PA 19105

1 Goldthorne Avenue
Toronto, Ontario M8Z 5T9

Library of Congress Cataloging in Publication Data
Azzopardi, John G.
   Problems in breast pathology.

   1. Breast—Diseases—Diagnosis. 2. Breast—Cancer—Diagnosis.
   3. Histology, Pathological.
I. Ahmed, Ali, joint author.
II. Millis, Rosemary R., joint author.
III. Title. [DNLM: 1. Breast diseases—Pathology.   WP840 A999p]
RG493.A99   1979   618.1'9'07   79-1523

ISBN 0–7216–1463–9

© 1979 by W. B. Saunders Company Ltd. All rights reserved. This book is protected by copyright. No part of it may be reproduced, stored in a retrieval system, or transmitted in any form or by any means, electronic, mechanical, photocopying, recording, or otherwise, without written permission from the publisher.

Printed at T. & A. Constable Ltd, Edinburgh

Print No: 9   8   7   6   5   4   3   2   1

FOREWORD

There are few areas in the practice of surgical pathology where the pathologist is as frequently 'under the gun' to make a diagnosis which so completely and unalterably affects the surgical therapy of a patient as with tumours of the breast. Breast tumours are relatively common and a large percentage are biopsied. Fortunately, making the key distinctions of benign versus malignant and in situ versus invasive is not difficult for the experienced pathologist in the majority of cases.

Those cases in which the diagnosis is not clear cut are not common but are important out of proportion to their numbers in terms of their difficulty of diagnosis and the devastating consequences of their misdiagnosis. It is these 'problem lesions' of the breast which this book is all about: how to recognize subtle but important variations in breast pathology and in particular benign masquerading as malignant and vice versa.

Professor John G. Azzopardi has managed to impart in this monograph his logical, systematic and morphologically sound approach to the diagnosis of breast lesions. He is well known for his many important contributions to the literature in the field of surgical pathology, but he has surpassed himself with *Problems in Breast Pathology*, which should become an indispensable and timeless reference for all those who are interested in the surgical pathological diagnosis of breast tumours.

James L. Bennington, MD

PREFACE

This book is essentially concerned with diagnostic problems encountered in breast pathology. The surgical pathologist has a very formidable task and shoulders a great weight of responsibility. He can only hope to undertake it with reasonable confidence if he works in close collaboration with clinicians, radiologists and workers in other disciplines. No apology is made for the repeated stress on the need for such collaboration.

It may appear naive to write about the place of naked-eye examination and of objectivity in describing specimens, had not the experience of the last 20 years shown otherwise. Nevertheless, I decided not to include photographs of gross specimens for a number of reasons. Black and white illustrations of gross specimens convey very little additional information which cannot be put into words and the cost of colour illustrations is prohibitive. Furthermore, good colour illustrations are already available in a number of well-known works. On the other hand, there is a great deal of histopathology which cannot be accurately described and the nature of which can only be conveyed by illustration. I believe this to be particularly applicable to the 'difficult' or 'early' in situ carcinomas, and the various hyperplasias with which they can be confused. It has been necessary, therefore, to illustrate certain sections profusely, and I have been especially liberal in this respect in Chapters Seven and Ten, and fairly liberal in Chapters Five and Nine. The illustrations in these four chapters account for more than half of the total in Chapters One to Sixteen. I wish I could have been even more liberal, because I believe that it is impossible to begin to understand the problems involved without a vast array of histological illustrations.

On the other hand, I have had to cut down drastically on illustrations in areas in which they are not absolutely essential; for example, it seems pointless to illustrate Paget's disease of the nipple at the light microscopic level when it is already so well illustrated in numerous works. But there are other fields in which I have also had to be short on illustrations where more would have been very desirable, to say the least.

There has been no deliberate attempt to be comprehensive. The emphasis throughout is on the more common and the more difficult problems encountered in practice, and especially on those aspects which are not fully dealt with in generally available texts. There is an unavoidable element of repetition in different chapters, both because the topics dealt with overlap to some extent, and because it seemed desirable to emphasize important points, if only from a slightly different view-point.

The value and dangers of frozen section diagnosis constitute such an important topic that they are dealt with first. The basic facts of normal histology and anatomy are considered inasmuch as they are relevant to pathological processes. It is also of some importance to have a working knowledge of breast function. The problems of nomenclature as they apply to the normal structures become correspondingly more complex and confusing when pathological processes are considered. The major emphasis is on the distinction between benign and malignant lesions, to which

Chapters Seven to Ten are exclusively devoted. This is far and away the most crucial practical problem for the surgical pathologist and a distinction which is of obvious importance to the patient.

I have deliberately selected references mainly from the last 10 to 20 years and have included only those which have made a significant contribution. The reader of the literature has been confronted with several thousand papers on breast pathology in major journals in the last 10 years alone and it is a quite impossible task for a general pathologist to wade through even a small fraction of this material. I have therefore been very selective, and out of about 3000 original papers and review articles consulted have extracted those which appeared to me to be the most valuable. References in the older literature have been included only when they are acknowledged classics or of outstanding merit, or when they were considered necessary to put a problem in a historical perspective. In this way I have managed to keep the references below the 500 mark. All the references, unless otherwise stated, have been read in their entirety, many of them more times than I care to remember.

Ultrastructural and histochemical studies are incorporated where they have contributed to a better understanding of disease processes at either a practical or a theoretical level. Ultrastructural studies have become increasingly valuable in clarifying problems that have remained unsolved or at least contentious at light microscopic level and I have been very fortunate in having Dr A. Ahmed contribute Chapter Seventeen to cover those ultrastructural aspects which are essential to a proper and more complete understanding of breast disease.

Similarly, Dr R. R. Millis has bridged the gap between the radiologist and the pathologist, a role of great importance in the management of patients with breast disease as well as of women seen at screening clinics. Both contributors have been allowed to express their views uninhibitedly. Nowhere is there any disagreement of substance between us and, if there was any initially, it must have been stifled at the embryo stage. It has been a great pleasure working with both my collaborators and I trust that they were not overwhelmed by my, at times, inordinate demands.

I wish to thank my clinical colleagues for all they have taught me over the years, and in particular Dr B. E. Nathan for his valuable discussion of mammographic problems.

I am enormously in the debt of the many pathologists whose cases and material I have been permitted to use, either by way of mention in the text or by illustration. I am especially grateful to Dr A. Alessi (Ravenna), Dr S. M. Ali (Kuwait), Dr J. T. Anim (Accra), Dr I. D. Ansell (Nottingham), Professor A. Arrigoni (Treviso), Dr T. G. Ashworth (Salisbury, Rhodesia), Dr B. Azadeh (Shiraz), Dr M. H. Bennett (Northwood), Dr J. L. Bennington (San Francisco), Dr W. K. Blenkinsopp (London), Professor G. Bussolati (Turin), Dr Barbara Callanan (London), Dr Cynthia Cohen (Johannesburg), Dr M. G. Cook (Adelaide), Dr R. A. Cooke (Brisbane), Professor B. N. Datta (Chandigarh), Dr J. Deguara (Malta), Dr F. Dowling (Mansfield), Dr Jennifer Dyson (London), Dr J. Eide (Bergen), the late Professor H. Hamperl (Bonn), Dr M. D. Lagios (San Francisco), Dr L. T. Hou (Hong Kong), Dr D. T. Janigan (Halifax, Nova Scotia), Professor P. Lampertico (Milan), Dr R. N. Laurini (Glasgow), Dr P. W. Leedham (Shrewsbury), Dr Dorothy Lewis (Johannesburg), Dr C. A. Liveris (Nicosia), Dr Jane Lomax-Smith (Adelaide), Dr J. W. Magner (Cork), Professor E. Magni (Ravenna), Dr V. Mambelli (Ancona), Professor A. M. Mancini (Bologna), Professor G. M. Mariuzzi (Ancona), Dr Virginia Martinez (Santiago), Dr M. Millard (Miami), Dr A. Mills (Bulawayo, Rhodesia), Dr Elizabeth Molland (London), Professor D. O'B. Hourihane (Dublin), Dr Minnie Pang (Singapore), Dr R. Pisa (Verona), Dr D. J. Pollock (London), Dr S. Rao (Glasgow), Dr Chula Seneviratne (Zambia), Professor H. Schornagel (Rotterdam), Dr C. P. Schwinn (Los Angeles), Dr E. A. Sweeney (Dublin), Dr A. Talerman (Rotterdam), Dr V. Tison (Faenza) and Dr G. Tremblay (Montreal).

I wish to thank Professor R. E. Cotton and Blackwell Scientific Publications Ltd for the use of Figures 10–32 and 10–33 reproduced from *Histopathology*, Dr J. E. Rhoads and the American Cancer Society for Figures 15–2 to 15–5 and Figure 15–7 reproduced from *Cancer*, and Professor W. G. Spector for Figures 9–7 to 9–10 and Figures 9–13 and 9–14 reproduced from the *Journal of Pathology*.

I am deeply indebted to Mr E. G. Hamilton, Miss Yvonne Madison, Mr K. J. Dawwas and their staff for their technical prowess, to Mr W. Hinkes for his inordinate care and much tried patience over the illustrations and to Mr D. Simmonds for his advice with the schematic diagrams.

For seemingly endless typing and for her help in the preparation of the manuscript I am greatly indebted to Mrs Sally Azzopardi. Miss Eileen M. Read and her staff in the Wellcome Library have given invaluable and willing assistance at all times.

I am particularly grateful to Dr V. Eusebi, Mrs Christine Betts-Eusebi and Dr R. Salm, whose ever-willing help in countless tasks has been of incalculable value.

It is a great pleasure to thank Dr James L. Bennington for his invitation to contribute a monograph to his series and the W. B. Saunders Company for their courtesy and co-operation, in particular Mr David Inglis for his valuable assistance and consideration at all times. To Dr James L. Bennington goes the credit for having egged me on when the spirit was flagging.

My only regret is that for a long period I have been unable to devote more than a small fraction of my time to the training of our junior staff in surgical pathology, a task which is usually a source of great pleasure and which has of necessity been neglected. To them I can only extend my apologies.

No words can express the understanding of my family who have forgone many pleasures and put up with intolerable conditions at home, where the littered floors were more reminiscent of a battlefield than of a domicile.

November, 1978   JOHN G. AZZOPARDI

CONTENTS

Chapter Five

Chapter Six

Chapter Seven

Chapter Eight

Chapter Nine

Chapter Ten

Chapter Eleven

Chapter Twelve

Chapter Eighteen

TO MY WIFE, SALLY

Chapter One

Macroscopic Examination and Frozen Section Diagnosis: General Principles and Major Pitfalls

MACROSCOPIC EXAMINATION

The naked-eye examination of a surgical specimen is just as important as the microscopic and must not be divorced from it. It would be unnecessary to say this were it not for the fact that the macroscopic examination is sometimes left largely or entirely to a junior or inexperienced pathologist while the consultant opinion is reserved for histological examination. Experience has taught the writer that this warning is not sufficiently heeded. With frozen sections, attention to naked-eye appearances is, if it were possible, even more vital.

Objectivity in Descriptions. There is no necessity to detail here the parameters of a breast lump that must be measured, described or assessed. It is necessary, however, to stress a few points of both academic and practical importance. Pathologists must always attempt to be objective in their macroscopic descriptions. This sounds self-evident, but it is remarkable how often descriptions are marred by subjective interpretations. The subjective interpretations are frequently derived from other workers' interpretations, and these are not all necessarily correct.

To take two concrete illustrations: rounded and ovoid spaces visible to the naked eye are frequently referred to as 'dilated ducts' merely because they are large. The pathologist, knowing that the largest parenchymal structures in the breast are ducts, sometimes assumes that a 'large' space is a diseased duct, but this is far from being always the case. He is comforted in his subjective interpretation by the fact that all too frequently workers use terms like 'cyst', 'cystically dilated duct' and 'dilated duct' interchangeably. Some authors go so far as to state, and many certainly imply, that cysts are frequently of ductal origin. For this reason cysts are commonly referred to as dilated ducts on gross examination. At the microscopic level the reverse error, of referring to dilated ducts as cysts, is the more frequent one. These types of error are, as will be shown later, one of the many reasons why cystic disease and duct ectasia are so frequently confused with each other and why duct ectasia in its many forms has not achieved the recognition it deserves. What the pathologist should describe is the size and shape of the spaces, the nature of their lining and contents, their relationship to the nipple, their relationship to one another, e.g. in a segmental distribution in the breast, and so on. But even then there is considerable room for error. In describing the contents of a space, words like 'blood-stained', 'pus', 'milky', etc., are sometimes used when amber, brownish, greenish, opaque and white would be more accurate and non-committal. The reason for the amber colour of the thin liquid content of a true cyst of the breast is not known. Even if the colour of the cyst fluid were due to haemosiderin, 'blood-stained' would be as inappropriate as to apply this label to the liver in haemochromatosis. But there is not even any good evidence that the colour of the cyst fluid is attributable to haemosiderin. There is, as will be shown later, considerable controversy relating to the structures present in the epithelial lining of breast cysts. The contents of the cysts, however, have been the subject of far fewer investigations, though there has recently been a surge of interest (Haagensen et al, 1977).

A second example of the importance of objectivity in description can be seen in the names applied to the yellow streaks and flecks that are seen in typical examples of the common 'scirrhous' carcinoma of the breast. For the last three decades especially, these have been generally referred to as 'necrotic foci' or 'chalky streaks'. Had they been described as yellow or yellow-white streaks with a sharply defined edge, a careful observer might also have noticed that they frequently contain a central slit or space. The yellow flecks are in fact foci of elastosis affecting periductal tissues and the walls of blood vessels. Had they been described objectively in the first place, the idea that they represented necrotic foci or chalky streaks would probably not have become so firmly entrenched in the literature. This represents a good example of how an erroneous subjective interpretation of a pathological appearance, repeated often enough, can become consolidated into so-called 'experience'. These two examples of the importance of objectivity in description should convince one that no apologia is needed for mentioning this apparent truism.

Specimen Radiography. Macroscopic examination may entail specimen radiography. How often this is carried out will depend on whether the examination is a purely diagnostic one or part of a research programme in addition. It will also depend on the facilities and resources available to individual departments. This will be discussed more fully in the section on mammography and calcification.

FROZEN SECTION DIAGNOSIS

It is important at this juncture to consider the specific problems of frozen section diagnosis, which is being utilized increasingly in most surgical departments.

OVERDIAGNOSIS

Epithelial Hyperplasia in a Fibroadenoma. Great importance should be attached to the degree of circumscription of a given nodule. A fibroadenoma can occasionally be difficult to distinguish from a medullary carcinoma on gross examination, though careful examination with a hand lens or other magnifier will enable a distinction to be made in practically all cases; histologically, the two lesions are so distinct that all doubt is removed. There is at least one situation in which attention to circumscription will obviate important errors. Florid epithelial hyperplasia in a fibroadenoma can be mistaken for either in situ or even for infiltrative carcinoma. This error is especially likely to occur when one is dealing with a small piece of tissue or with a frozen section which does not include adjacent normal tissue. The curve on the edge of the section should immediately focus one's attention on the circumscribed nature of the lesion. The problem can be accentuated if a block is cut from the centre of the lesion and the curved edge is not included, but there are very few circumstances, if any, in which a block would be taken *only* in this position. Inexperienced pathologists have been known to diagnose florid epithelial hyperplasia in a fibroadenoma as carcinoma because they were not aware that they were dealing with a fibroadenoma in the first place. Errors of this kind are more likely to occur with small lesions: the larger fibroadenoma has a distinct cleavage plane and the compressed tissue around it often appears smooth and glistening to the extent that it mimics, and is often (usually erroneously) referred to as, a capsule. This larger variety of fibroadenoma is usually easily recognized by the surgeon, is rarely sent for frozen section and is hardly likely to escape gross identification even by a very junior pathologist. It is the smaller lesion with a marked epithelial proliferation which can cause very occasional difficulty.

The Edge of a Tension Cyst may be difficult to recognize on frozen section. Compressed fibrous tissue with deeply staining plump fibroblasts and/or inflammatory cells as a result of rupture of the cyst can give rise to anxiety about the correct diagnosis. This is particularly likely to happen if the cyst has collapsed because of complete rupture occurring spontaneously or as a result of surgical trauma: in these circumstances even a very careful pathologist may be unaware that he is including a cyst wall, or usually only a small part of it, in the blocks selected. The main clue lies in recognizing that the cellular part in the section (fibroblasts or inflammatory cells) is arranged in band-like fashion along a fibrous wall, an appearance hardly ever seen in a malignant lesion. If, in addition, the fibrous wall shows some metachromatic staining with methylene blue, the nature of the lesion is more easily established. Naturally, any shreds of apocrine epithelium that still remain will draw attention to the fact that one is dealing with a cyst wall. But in tension cysts apocrine epithelium is often grossly attenuated, and it is frequently detached and lost in the course of cutting or processing the tissue; in ruptured tension cysts these obscuring phenomena are even more pronounced. For these reasons it is necessary to identify such cysts in the absence of recognizable apocrine epithelium and, indeed, in the complete absence of any epithelial lining whatever. It is therefore essential that pathologists should familiarize themselves thoroughly with the appearances of tension cysts, at various stages of their natural history, as seen in paraffin sections. Only then is it possible to appreciate fully the significance of all the possible variations that are encountered and to interpret correctly their appearance on frozen section.

A Chronic Inflammatory Mass, of any derivation, can occasionally give rise to difficulty, especially with a less than perfect section. The absence of a trabecular arrangement of the cells is an important negative point in excluding malignancy. The recognition of foci of plasma cells is useful, though, of course, their presence does not rule out a malignant lesion by any means. In general, the cellular infiltrate in an inflammatory mass is more pleomorphic. Often help is obtained from the clinical history, e.g. a history of a lactational abscess which was treated with antibiotics, with improvement in the acute symptomatology, but leaving a residual lump. The macroscopic appearances can also be extremely useful in such cases, a reminder that microscopic and naked-eye pathology are separated at one's peril. The differential diagnosis between an inflammatory mass and an infiltrating lobular carcinoma or, for that matter, any type of dissociated-cell cancer, can still be problematical. If there is any serious doubt about the diagnosis, it is safer to await the paraffin sections.

A Papilloma or Papillary 'Cystadenoma' is by no means easy to distinguish from papillary carcinoma on frozen section. The cytological appearances often look 'worse than they really are' on an unfixed cryostat section stained with methylene blue. In general, methylene blue preparations can be trusted for the architecture of the lesion, but haemalum–eosin is safer for the interpretation of cellular changes. Difficulty is experienced more frequently with the so-called papillary cystadenoma than with the less complex and more obviously fronded papilloma, though there is no sharp dividing line between the two. The problem with the 'cystadenoma' is that it may be a predominantly solid lesion and its situation within the duct, or other pre-existing epithelium-lined space, may be missed on frozen section. Indeed the relationship to a duct is not always very obvious even in paraffin sections, especially if one does not make use of stains for elastica. When, on frozen section, no papillae are seen, the lesion which appears cellular and compact can be misdiagnosed as infiltrating carcinoma. The two-layered structure characteristic of this lesion is not always easy to discern. Apocrine epithelium may not be present in the section examined and, even when it is, its identity can be missed, especially in a methylene blue preparation. This emphasizes again the necessity of not relying on methylene blue preparations alone for cytological study. But the papillary cystadenoma is well circumscribed in a manner which is hardly ever seen in the well-differentiated infiltrating carcinoma, with which it can be confused even by experienced pathologists. It is essential that such a lesion is examined with *a very low power objective* of a good microscope, if mistakes are to be avoided.

The distinction between a benign papillary tumour and infiltrating carcinoma can and should be made on frozen section. On the other hand, the distinction between papilloma and papillary carcinoma is sometimes very difficult on a frozen section and occasionally well-nigh impossible. In case of doubt one should always wait for paraffin sections before proceeding to a mastectomy. Indeed some workers refuse to go further than the diagnosis of a papillary neoplasm on a frozen section.

The reader will have noticed that the lesions discussed so far as potential candidates for frozen section misdiagnosis have been placed, more or less, in order of increasing inherent difficulty: fibroadenoma, ruptured cyst, chronic inflammatory mass, papilloma, papillary 'cystadenoma'.

Sclerosing Adenosis. This is the lesion which is most commonly overdiagnosed on frozen section. It is fair to say that, for experienced pathologists, the majority of cases of overdiagnosis can be attributed to this one condition. These errors can be very substantially reduced and almost eliminated by scrupulous attention to macroscopical appearances. There are generally differences, often subtle, in the gross appearance of sclerosing adenosis and carcinoma. But there is no denying that on rare occasions sclerosing adenosis can mimic infiltrating carcinoma closely in the gross specimen. Even yellow streaks of elastosis (so-called 'chalky streaks') may be present in sclerosing adenosis, increasing the mimicry of a cancer. Sclerosing adenosis is the commonest breast disease that can be confused with cancer grossly even by careful and experienced observers. This is especially true of the variety of sclerosing adenosis referred to later as 'infiltrating epitheliosis'. Nevertheless the macroscopic examination is frequently important in making the distinction between the benign and malignant conditions. On the few occasions in which I have seen this error of overdiagnosis of sclerosing adenosis committed by able and experienced pathologists, *the naked-eye appearance usually did not suggest malignancy.* Combined macroscopic and microscopic examination, use of the very low power objectives of a good microscope and knowledge of all relevant clinical data can practically eliminate such errors of overdiagnosis. The use of a good microscope is not as obvious as it seems because there is still a distinct tendency, at any rate outside North America, for some laboratories to use a rather antiquated and dilapidated microscope for frozen section diagnosis while concealing their better microscopes in the cleaner and often less-used corners of a comfortable pathologist's sanctuary. While the practical reasons for these habits can be appreciated, this tradition would not be regarded sympathetically by those women who have been mutilated for a perfectly benign condition.

Overdiagnosis in the Presence of a Macroscopic Appearance of Cancer. There are two conditions in which circumstances will combine to deceive at times even the very experienced pathologist. In these situations, the macroscopic appearances usually suggest malignancy. The commoner one is the variety of sclerosing adenosis described in Chapter Nine under the heading of '*infiltrating epitheliosis*'. This type of lesion is relatively common and yet it received little or no attention in the literature prior to 1974. It is easily mistaken mammographically and surgically for a cancer and the pathologist must beware of making an erroneous diagnosis at frozen section. The importance of this lesion will probably increase further as radiologists refine their methods of detection of small stellate disturbances in the breast architecture which are sufficiently suspicious as to warrant biopsy on mammographic grounds.

The second, much less common but important, lesion to remember is the so-called *granular-cell 'myoblastoma'.* This is more commonly situated in the skin or subcutaneous tissue overlying the breast than in the breast parenchyma proper but, when the pathologist is faced with an isolated lump, the distinction as to the precise site is not usually made clear to him, since in many of these cases the clinical signs are those of a breast cancer. If the pathologist bears this lesion in mind, it should not be difficult to make the correct diagnosis even on frozen section.

UNDERDIAGNOSIS

So far only overdiagnosis of lesions has been discussed. *Overdiagnosis is commoner* than underdiagnosis *in frozen section studies* of breast disease. Diagnostic accuracy on paraffin sections, on the other hand, has reached the stage where the pendulum is swinging the other way and I believe that now, among the more experienced pathologists, *underdiagnosis is probably as common an error as overdiagnosis on paraffin sections*. Of course this varies enormously in different institutes and hospitals and from country to country. This underdiagnosis applies particularly to the in situ lesion.

In Situ Carcinoma

Carcinoma Lobulare In Situ, conveniently abbreviated to CLIS by Hamperl (1972), is very difficult to diagnose with any reliability on frozen section. Except with extensive and rather obvious cases, it is doubtful whether a definitive diagnosis of CLIS should even be attempted by the less experienced. Benfield, Jacobson and Warner (1965) also believe that the role of the frozen section in the management of patients with lobular carcinoma in situ is minimal. Ashikari, Huvos and Snyder (1977) were able to diagnose correctly only 18 per cent of cases of CLIS on frozen section.

Whenever there is any doubt at all it is essential to wait for paraffin sections before proceeding to any major ablative surgery. This is even truer when one considers the present position in relation to the prognosis of patients with CLIS treated by only local excision, and the controversy currently raging about the correct treatment of this condition.

Ductal Carcinoma In Situ. In comparison with CLIS, most in situ ductal carcinomas are more easily diagnosed on frozen section. This is particularly true of the comedocarcinoma with its pleomorphic cytology, and of the cribriform carcinoma with its characteristic structural pattern. The solid and 'clinging' forms of in situ cancer are somewhat more difficult to assess. The 'clinging' variety is, in the opinion of the writer, frequently missed even on paraffin section, a problem that will be discussed in Chapter Ten. If a categorical diagnosis of malignancy can be made, this will save a second operation, especially since there is little argument about the correct treatment of in situ ductal, as opposed to lobular, carcinoma. If there is any doubt, as there may well be with the 'clinging' variety and, to a lesser extent, with the solid, cribriform and other varieties, it is mandatory to await the result of paraffin sections. There is no reason to believe that there is any increased risk to the patient and the drawback of a second operation must be balanced against the unnecessary sacrifice of the breast in other cases. Ashikari, Huvos and Snyder (1977) were able to diagnose correctly 55 per cent of cases of intraductal carcinoma at the time of frozen section.

Underdiagnosis is not the only possibility with in situ carcinoma. In cases of duct ectasia, the epithelium can appear worrying on frozen section. The overall appearance of the lesion is of far greater importance than an isolated microscopic field. Whenever there is any doubt it is essential to wait for paraffin sections, for the reasons already stated.

Infiltrating carcinoma

Infiltrating lobular carcinoma is one of the tumours most commonly underdiagnosed on frozen section examination. There are at least two major reasons for this occurrence. Firstly, in the gross specimen, the pathologist may miss the presence of the lesion completely, for this type of carcinoma has a tendency to produce an ill-defined induration rather than a distinct lump and, moreover, an induration which frequently merges imperceptibly with the normal tissues so that no definite 'lump' may be apparent. An inexperienced pathologist can easily fall into this trap and may sample the wrong area altogether. Of course, this does not apply only to frozen section diagnosis; it is even more true of a mastectomy specimen if no clinical or mammographic indication is given as to the position of the 'lump'. The writer has seen a very conscientious pathologist completely miss such an area of induration partly because his attention was diverted by other, more grossly obvious but benign pathology in the breast. Secondly, at the microscopic level, an infiltrating lobular carcinoma lacks most of the features which make the ordinary infiltrating ductal carcinoma easily identifiable in the vast majority of cases. Nevertheless, the classical bull's-eye, dartboard or Indian-file appearance is generally recognizable. If a block is taken from an area of 'sparse cell carcinoma', or if there is any significant degree of squeeze or other artefact, the diagnosis is made correspondingly more difficult. Further blocks of tissue for frozen section may be necessary to arrive at a definitive diagnosis.

A Tubular Carcinoma, especially when small, may give rise to similar problems on frozen section. The problem here is the differentiation from sclerosing adenosis and the same principles apply as govern the differential diagnosis with paraffin sections.

CLINICAL DATA

Both for practical reasons and because of theoretical considerations clinical data are of paramount importance. The patient's age, the precise site of the lesion, the symptoms and signs (the presence of nipple inversion or a discharge, the size of any lump, its mobility or attachment and its consistency), any history of trauma, whether the patient is or has recently been pregnant, previous surgery to the same or to the contralateral breast: all such information must be made available to the pathologist. Without it, at best, the pathologist's job is made duller: at worst, he is liable to make serious mistakes. The value of such correlation cannot be overemphasized. It will ensure that sampling of a specimen is correct and adequate and that attention is focused on all significant parts.

A few simple dicta are here in order as their observance would eliminate a substantial number of errors. Like all generalizations they must be treated as such and exceptions allowed for.

1. **Never report on a frozen section when you are mentally or physically preoccupied with something else. Never use a microscope without a very low power objective. Never report without examining the gross specimen.**
2. **If the microscopic pathology does not fit the macroscopic description or the clinical history, you may be missing something vital. The alternative is dual (or multiple) pathology.**
3. **Overdiagnosis is commoner than underdiagnosis, especially with pathologists of less than 10 years' experience and especially with infiltrating (as opposed to in situ) malignancy.**
   Underdiagnosis of in situ lesions on frozen section is not too serious.
   Overdiagnosis of infiltrating carcinoma is a mutilating error. If in doubt, await paraffin sections.
4. **If the macroscopic appearance is benign, beware of diagnosing carcinoma. Think again. The microscopic interpretation is probably wrong. (Certain in situ carcinomas are the exception.)**

Points 1 and 2 are partially applicable to paraffin as well as to frozen sections.

A few specific examples of erroneous diagnoses will emphasize these points.

(a) *Severe epithelial hyperplasia in a fibroadenoma* was diagnosed by an inexperienced pathologist as infiltrating carcinoma. Insufficient attention had been paid to the circumscribed margin of the lesion, and the fact that it was a fibroadenoma had been completely missed. In this instance the hyperplasia was unusually exuberant but benign.

(b) *Papillary 'cystadenoma'.* An extremely able pathologist diagnosed a lesion as infiltrating carcinoma. Macroscopically it looked perfectly benign to him and to me. He called it malignant because he was too busy, because he was using a poor microscope without a scanning lens and had relied too much, perhaps, on the impression derived from the methylene blue preparation. Because of this combination of errors he failed to recognize a papillary 'cystadenoma'. The two-layered lining in parts of the lesion was hardly discernible with the optical apparatus available. Even more important, in the absence of a scanning view, it was difficult to appreciate the very well delineated outline of the lesion. The small focus of apocrine epithelium could be recognized with some difficulty in the H and E preparation and with much greater difficulty in the methylene blue preparation. All these points were clarified when a good microscope with a scanning lens was used. Personally I was only really suspicious of the erroneous diagnosis of malignancy because of Dictum 4: both of us had regarded the macroscopic appearances as *unequivocally* benign. In this situation, with experienced pathologists, I have yet to come across an instance of infiltrating carcinoma, though doubtless, extremely rarely, one of microscopic size will produce just such a situation.

(c) *Sclerosing adenosis with apocrine metaplasia* can mimic the pleomorphism and atypia of malignancy even on paraffin section, if one is unaware of the problem. I have seen this error committed by a group of consultants, including a surgical pathologist with an international reputation. On frozen section, the problem can be even more difficult. Again, a good microscope, a scanning view of the lesion and examining H and E sections for the identification of apocrine metaplasia are all-important. Knowledge of the existence of this type of lesion and remembering Dictum 3 can be crucial.

(d) *Sclerosing adenosis in pregnancy.* An excellent pathologist, with a first-class reputation on both sides of the Atlantic, was just about to label a lesion carcinoma when specific enquiry elicited the information that the patient was pregnant. Failure of the surgeon to appreciate that this data might constitute vital information nearly led to a mastectomy in another patient with sclerosing adenosis.

(e) *Sclerosing adenosis.* One of the best pathologists I have known and the present writer were shown sections of a difficult case which the senior registrar (senior resident or chief resident) regarded as probably malignant. We both concurred and another patient with sclerosing adenosis lost a breast. We were both preoccupied with another problem and made the cardinal error of not examining the macroscopic specimen. This case also illustrates the important point that an erroneous diagnosis is not any more correct for having been replicated by several observers. **Multiplication of the same erroneous diagnosis does not make that diagnosis correct!** Also neither of the two consultants involved in this case was the consultant 'on call'. In these circumstances I believe that there is probably an unconscious tendency to feel less personal responsibility for the diagnosis.

The last two circumstances which led to an error in this case could be prevented by attention to what could be called the **'principle of divided and diminished responsibility'.** Just as a patient should have a single clinician who acts as the final pathway for diagnosis and treatment, the patient should have a single consultant who, in the final analysis, takes the sole responsibility for a histopathological opinion.

References

Ashikari, R., Huvos, A. G. and Snyder, R.E. (1977) Prospective study of non-infiltrating carcinoma of the breast. *Cancer,* **39,** 435-439.

Benfield, J. R., Jacobson, M. and Warner, N. E. (1965) In situ lobular carcinoma of the breast. *Archives of Surgery,* **91,** 130-135.

Haagensen, D. E., Jr, Mazoujian, G., Holder, W. D., Jr, Kister, S. J. and Wells, S. A., Jr (1977) Evaluation of a breast cyst fluid protein detectable in the plasma of breast carcinoma patients. *Annals of Surgery,* **185,** 279-285.

Hamperl, H. (1972) Zur Kenntnis des sog. Carcinoma lobuläre in situ der Mamma. Beiträge zur pathologischen Histologie der Mamma V. *Zeitschrift für Krebsforschung,* **77,** 231-246.

Chapter Two

Nomenclature of the Microanatomy of the Breast: Parts Affected in Different Diseases: Normal Structure and Involution

All pathologists accept that it is essential to have a thorough knowledge of the normal structure of, say, the kidney or the liver before studying and reporting on the pathology of that organ. Yet some are happy to delve into the pathology of the breast with a much less thorough knowledge of the normal structure and its variations. The reader is referred to Bonser, Dossett and Jull (1961) or other comprehensive monographs for a detailed account of the structure and function of the human breast, but it must be stressed that there is no substitute for one's own detailed study of its architecture and cytology.

In this chapter only those features of the normal structure which are relevant to pathological processes and to pathogenesis will be emphasized. Variants of the normal mature breast as well as of the involuting breast that can be misconstrued as abnormal will also be considered.

NOMENCLATURE OF THE MICROANATOMY

The terminology used by different authors varies quite considerably. This matters less if the terms employed are clearly defined. However, the 'terminal duct' of one author, which refers to the smallest epithelial unit in the lobule, may be confused with the 'terminal duct' of another author, which refers to the largest duct that opens on to the surface of the nipple. It is not entirely clear whether logically 'terminal duct' should be applied to the largest or the smallest duct. From a practical point of view it would be adequate to refer to: major ducts of the nipple region, large and medium-sized ducts, ductules and the smallest epithelial units contained within a lobule. With such a simplified nomenclature, only the term 'ductule' is not self-explanatory. This term should be reserved for a special part of the ductal system, for reasons which will become clear. For purposes of convenience the epithelial system is labelled in Figure 2–1 in the following order from the nipple opening: collecting duct, lactiferous sinus, segmental duct, subsegmental (large and medium-sized) duct, ductule and lobule (lobular epithelial units or acini) (Figure 2–6A). Whether the non-lactating human breast contains acini in the lobules is highly controversial. It is partly because many

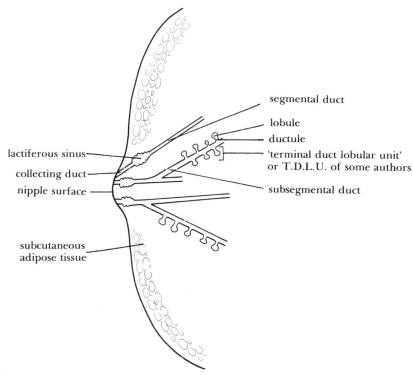

segmental duct

lobule

ductule

'terminal duct lobular unit'
or T.D.L.U. of some authors

subsegmental duct

lactiferous sinus

collecting duct

nipple surface

subcutaneous
adipose tissue

Figure 2–1 The nomenclature
of the main anatomical parts of
the breast.

Figure 2–1

workers believe that it does not, that the term 'terminal ductule' is used by many to describe the lobular epithelial units (Figure 2–6B). Because the matter is not conclusively resolved, the term 'acinus' is used here for convenience since it is at least obvious that it refers to the smallest epithelial structure which is situated within the lobule, and has, moreover, the merit of distinguishing it from the ductule ('terminal duct' of many authors), most of which is usually situated outside the lobule (Figure 2–6).

PARTS AFFECTED IN DIFFERENT DISEASES

From the pathologist's point of view, a clear understanding of the normal anatomical relationships is essential to an understanding of diseases of the breast. Certain diseases affect certain parts of the duct–lobule system dominantly or even exclusively (Figure 2–2). The clinically commonest benign breast lesions, fibroadenoma and cystic disease, are both diseases of the lobules. This fact explains

the specialized nature of the connective tissue component of a fibroadenoma in its actively growing phase. It also explains why fibroadenomas develop only after puberty and usually before the menopause, i.e. during the time that most breasts are well endowed with lobules and are subjected to certain hormonal influences which affect the lobule. Of course, a fibroadenoma present before the menopause will persist and may, on rare occasions, present clinically in later years or be found incidentally by the pathologist when he is examining an amputated breast; but such fibroadenomas are almost always of the quiescent and often hyalinized variety. The fact that a fibroadenoma is a lobular neoplasm explains why it can become cancerized via the 'feeding' ductules in the same way as normal lobules become cancerized (page 325). It also explains the convincing evidence, collected in recent years, that most examples of carcinoma that have a definite origin solely within the fibroadenoma are instances of lobular carcinoma (lobular neoplasia). That pure cystic disease of the breast without any significant hyperplasia is also a disorder of lobules is not generally recognized, but the evidence for this

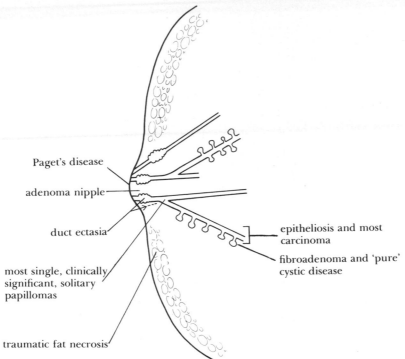

Paget's disease

adenoma nipple

duct ectasia

epitheliosis and most
carcinoma

fibroadenoma and 'pure'
cystic disease

most single, clinically
significant, solitary
papillomas

traumatic fat necrosis

Figure 2–2   Diagram to show the
anatomical sites affected by different diseases.

Figure 2–2 Diagram to show the anatomical sites
affected by different diseases.

is just as conclusive (Figure 2–2). It is essential
to appreciate this histogenetic mechanism in
order to understand the clinicopathological
distinctions between cystic disease and duct
ectasia, discussed in Chapter Five. The fact
that breast cysts are of lobular origin is vital to
the understanding of the concept of a 'tension
cyst'. Such a cyst, though it may measure
several millimetres or even several centimetres in diameter, originates in a lobule after
the lobule has undergone apocrine transformation. There is only one exit, the ductule,
and if this becomes blocked, for whatever
reason, a 'tension cyst' results with all the
potential complications to which this is liable.

By contrast, there are diseases which affect
ducts as well as lobules and others which affect
the ducts dominantly or selectively. Carcinoma may affect any part of the ductal system,
although there is growing evidence that the
smaller ductal ramifications including the
intralobular ones are more often involved
than the larger ducts (Figure 2–2). But the
largest ducts, including those which open on
to the nipple, may also be involved by
carcinoma, for example in Paget's disease.
Epitheliosis affects most parts of the ductal

system, with the important exception of the
largest ducts (Figure 2–2). Lobules may be
affected by either carcinoma or by epitheliosis,
though perhaps relatively more commonly by
carcinoma. Macroscopically visible papillary
tumours, benign and malignant, may affect
any part of the ductal system with a preference
for the larger ducts (Figure 2–2); rarely they
may even originate in breast cysts. Duct
ectasia, as the name implies, is primarily a
disease of the ducts, with the breast lobules
showing only secondary changes (Figure 2–2).
This distinguishes duct ectasia from traumatic
fat necrosis, with which it can on occasion be
confused. Traumatic fat necrosis affects the
subcutaneous adipose tissue and involves the
breast parenchyma proper only to a limited
degree, if at all (Figure 2–2).

The breast is composed of about 15 to 20
segments or sectors which converge on the
nipple in radial fashion. Even the number of
segments is in dispute. Hartmann (1975) cites
the catheter studies of Sartorius as showing
that there are only five to nine ductal openings
and not the 15 to 20 usually stated. According
to Sartorius the rest of the openings on the
nipple are merely pits which end blindly.

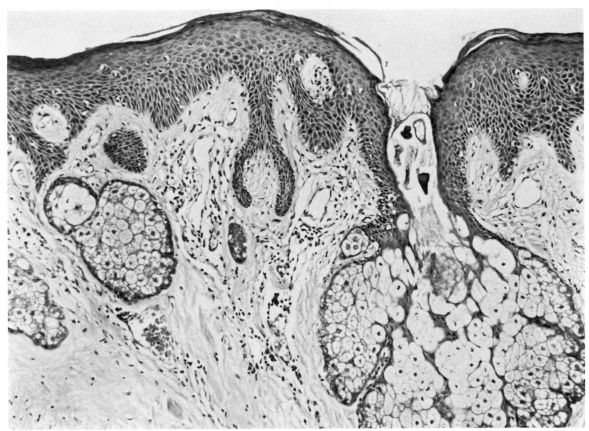

Figure 2–3 Sebaceous gland of nipple opening on to surface independently of hair follicle. H and E. ×150.

Though there is no visible or palpable anatomical separation of the segments, their ductal and lobular systems are distinct. Each segment opens at the nipple by a separate duct, hence enabling the segmental localization of breast pathology in the case of a nipple discharge. In duct ectasia, anything between one and all segments of the breast may be involved. If a given segment is severely involved, the whole ductal system of that segment is affected and its lobules involute secondarily while, in contrast, adjacent segments may remain completely unaffected. Duct ectasia is the prime example of a truly segmental breast disease.

NORMAL STRUCTURE

The nipple and areola have such a specialized and distinctive structure that a block of tissue taken from this region can be readily identified from its histological appear-ance. Numerous sebaceous glands are present superficially close to the surface and open independently of hair follicles (Figure 2–3). The stroma consists of dense collagen in which abundant smooth muscle tissue is embedded; these are the erectile muscles of the nipple. Cutaneous leiomyomas occur most commonly in the genital areas, including the nipple. Leiomyoma of the nipple arises from this smooth muscle. Apocrine glands are also embedded in the nipple stroma. These glands are physiological structures unrelated to the apocrine metaplasia observed in the lobules as part of cystic disease. The apocrine glands of the nipple are indistinguishable from those seen in the skin of the genital areas, the axilla and elsewhere. Presumably they can very rarely be affected by pathological processes but there is little, if any, evidence to support the statement that the rare 'adenoma of the nipple' is derived from these glands (Symmers, 1966). All the evidence indicates that this uncommon tumour arises in the largest mammary ducts. The nipple region

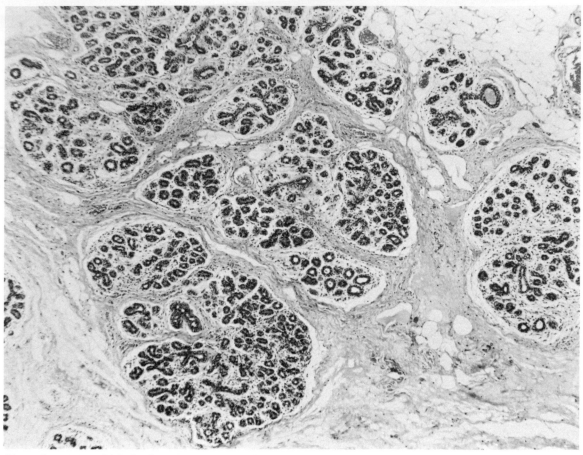

Figure 2–4   Normal lobules from 28-year-old nulliparous woman. H and E. ×60.

contains the converging segmental ducts, each of these opening into an irregular corrugated space, the lactiferous sinus, which is a characteristic feature of the nipple (Figures 13–1 and 15–5). Because of its irregular contour in the contracted state, the beginner may mistake the lactiferous sinus for a pathological condition. This is more likely in a tangential cut than with longitudinal or transverse sections; in these circumstances, 'papillomatoid hyperplasia' may be suspected. The sinus communicates with the surface of the nipple via the collecting duct or galactophore. In its proximal portion this duct is lined by epithelium similar to that of the rest of the ductal system, but its superficial portion is sealed by keratinizing stratified squamous epithelium continuous with the nipple surface. The junction between the glandular and the squamous epithelium is abrupt.

A knowledge of the structure of the periductal and lobular stroma is important because of its bearing on the understanding of many disease processes. The periductal connective tissue differs from the ordinary interlobular and intersegmental supporting tissues in many respects. There is a cuff of specialized stroma around the ducts, specialized in the sense of being looser, slightly more cellular and more vascular than ordinary connective tissue. The periductal lymphatics run in this zone. The stroma is even more highly specialized in the lobule (Figure 2–4). It contains fine collagen fibres and abundant reticulin and is highly vascular. It is much more cellular than the interlobular stroma and this cellularity can be gauged from the number of fibrocytic nuclei. Apart from being more loosely textured and more cellular than the periductal stroma, the lobular stroma is also more abundant, so that it constitutes a major part of the actual bulk of the lobule (Figure 2–4). These quantitative and qualitative differences are responsible for the fact

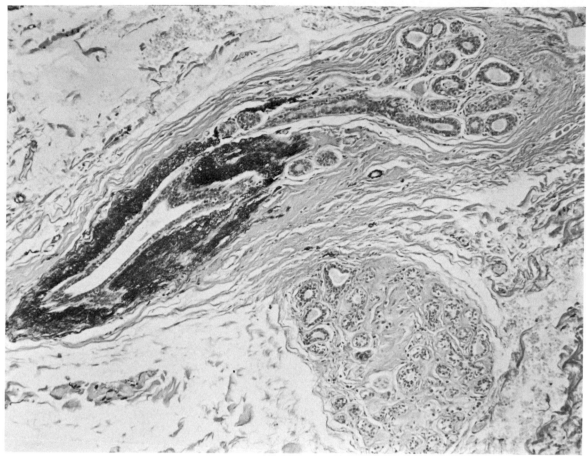

Figure 2–5 Two lobules and a duct. The duct is connected to one of the lobules by a ductule. The duct wall has an abundant content of elastic tissue. There is a little elastica in the ductule but none within the lobules. Weigert elastin stain and haematoxylin Van Gieson. ×120.

that the lobular stroma is much more distinctive than the periductal tissue. A little-recognized but important feature is the mucoid character of the lobular connective tissue. An alcian blue or similar stain will amaze anyone who has not made a conscious note of the quality of the lobular stroma. In such stains the lobules are very clearly delineated from the banal interlobular stroma.

The study of the distribution of elastic tissue in the ductal–lobular system of the breast has been very much neglected in the past. Study of the elastic tissue can be as important in breast disease as it is in arterial disease. In general, the ducts are invested by elastic tissue while the lobules are completely devoid of it (Figure 2–5). In the mature breast of a young woman the ductal system contains at least some elastic fibres in the cuff of the specialized connective tissue which invests it. The amount of elastic fibre varies considerably and some of the

factors that affect it are known. The breast of an older woman, up to the menopause at any rate, tends to contain more elastic tissue. There is very good evidence that parous women have more elastic tissue in the duct walls than non-parous women, at least as far as the major ducts of the nipple are concerned (Davies, 1973). This increase of elastic tissue with parity probably applies to the whole of the ductal system. It is not clear whether age, per se, has a direct influence on the amount of elastic tissue to be found after full development of the virginal breast has taken place, by about the age of 25 years. The increase in elastic tissue with increasing age is largely attributable to the effect of pregnancy. Age, per se, is probably associated with some increase of elastic tissue in the major ducts of the nipple, but whether this is strictly physiological or the result of mild disease, which is very common at this site in older age groups, is not known.

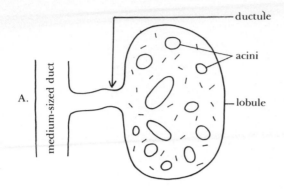

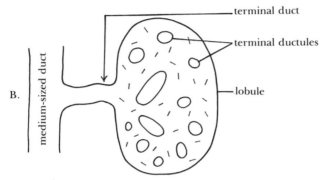

Figure 2–6 A. The nomenclature of the ductule–lobule system used here compared with B, the alternative nomenclature used by many workers.

Figure 2–6

It has been suggested that in the later decades there is some decrease of elastic tissue, even amounting to complete loss, in the smaller ducts as part of the involutionary process. This point requires further investigation.

Newly formed ducts lack elastic tissue, as is shown, for example, by the newly sprouted ducts in the breast in pregnancy. There is little information on the length of time it takes for ducts to acquire an elastic coat in different circumstances. In gynaecomastia the ducts lack any elastic tissue and the writer has failed to find any, even in a man who was known to have had the condition for five years, but one cannot infer from this that the same time-lag necessarily applies to women. This is a problem awaiting further investigation and clarification.

At the nipple end of the ductal system, elastic tissue extends to the site where the duct pierces the epidermis. In fact, there is a focal increase at this point, anchoring the duct, as it were, by an elastic tendon. At the peripheral end, elastic tissue ends at about the level of the ductule. Here the elastic tissue becomes thinner and splays out into the collagenous tissue (Figure 2–5). At the point where the

ductule enters the lobule the elastic tissue is absent.

This is a convenient place to define the concept of the 'ductule' as used here. Ductules are the smallest ducts that arise from the subsegmental ducts (large, medium-sized and small). They branch off the ducts more or less at right angles and are generally but short structures, approximately equal in length to the diameter of a breast lobule (Figure 2–5). Their length and, to a lesser extent, the angles they make with the ducts from which they spring are subject to considerable variation. Their investing connective tissue is continuous with that of the duct on the one hand and that of the lobule on the other. As already stated, the ductule is the cut-off point for the elastic coat of the ductal system. For these and other reasons, it is desirable that it should have a specific name and the term 'ductule' (literally small duct) is as appropriate as any (Figure 2–6A). It should be pointed out, however, that many authors use the term 'ductule' or 'terminal ductule' to signify the smallest lobular epithelial unit, while 'terminal duct' is used to describe the structure called here a ductule (Figure 2–6B).

Knowledge of these normal findings and

their variations is essential to an understanding of breast pathology. Thus, for practical purposes, there is no elastic tissue in a fibroadenoma. Similarly, cysts and apocrine cysts do not contain elastic fibres in their wall as they are derived from lobules which do not contain any elastic tissue. In duct ectasia elastic tissue may be altered in various ways, as is the specialized periductal collagenous tissue (page 77). The value of elastic tissue stains in general, and in malignant disease in particular, will be considered in Chapter Fifteen.

Another feature vital to the understanding of pathological changes is the specialized two-cell-type lining of the whole of the ductal–lobular epithelial system of the breast. The number of cell layers in different parts of the system and their precise arrangement have been debated for decades. Even with light microscopy it is abundantly clear that there are two cell types and that they are arranged as shown in Figure 2–7. The outer cell is smaller and wedged between the bases of two adjacent inner-type cells. The inner cell is larger and taller, rests on the basement membrane but extends inwards to the luminal space. The lumen is lined entirely by inner-type cells. This particular arrangement of epithelial cells is characteristic of the breast and is suited to the needs of gross distension during lactation. It is not strictly speaking 'stratified' and it is confusing to describe it merely as 'pseudostratified', since this could imply that there is only one cell type with nuclei situated at different levels, as seen in the proliferative phase endometrium. The writer is unaware of any term which describes this type of structure accurately and clearly. Until an acceptable term is found and adopted, it is better to illustrate it (Figure 2–7).

The tall cells that line the lumen are clearly epithelial by any structural, ultrastructural or functional criterion. In the past the nature of the outer cell type has been controversial. Some workers have regarded it as also epithelial and others as of unproven nature. Many have regarded the outer cell type as a myoepithelial cell, but, even so, there has been dispute as to whether myoepithelial cells are present only in some ducts, or in all ducts, or in the lobules as well. Species differences have added to the problem. It seemed likely by analogy with apocrine and eccrine sweat glands and with the salivary glands that some of the outer cell type in the breast represented myoepithelium, but traditional methods like phosphotungstic acid–haematoxylin and

Masson trichrome, though suggestive, did not conclusively settle the issue. Ultrastructural studies have now shown conclusively that the outer cell type shows at least some myofibrillar differentiation and should thus be regarded as a myoepithelial cell. The reader is referred to the elegant work of Ozzello (1971) for a detailed study of this problem.

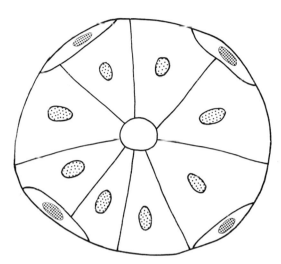

Figure 2–7 The arrangement of epithelial and myoepithelial cells in the acini or 'terminal units' ('terminal ductules' of many workers) of the lobule of the human breast.

Appreciation of the two-cell-type structure is extremely important in distinguishing between benign diseases or tumours and malignant tumours. In sclerosing adenosis, in most of its variant forms, two cell types are a distinctive feature. In papillomas and papillary 'cystadenomas', a two-cell type structure in some parts of the lesion is a very important criterion in distinguishing the lesions from papillary carcinoma. Again, the two-cell type structure is important in the recognition of the 'adenoma of the nipple'. By contrast, the well-differentiated 'tubular carcinoma' can be distinguished from benign conditions partly by the lack of two cell types in its glands and tubules.

The myoepithelial nature and qualities of the outer cell type are markedly accentuated in certain pathological conditions. Thus full-blown myoid cells are sometimes seen in sclerosing adenosis. They may be present in papillomas and, rarely, can even be found in fibroadenomas. Hamperl (1939) was one of the first authors to stress such myoid differentiation. It is as if the potential for myoepithelial differentiation finds its full expression in diseased states, culminating in the production of fully differentiated smooth muscle cells. This is a good example of pathology illuminating normal histology and cytology, just as in other instances the reverse is true.

Of course problems arise in the definition of what is strictly normal. Haagensen (1977) included 'microcysts', 'apocrine metaplasia' and 'blunt duct adenosis' among the microscopical lesions 'normally seen in the breasts of modern women'. Although this point of view may not commend itself to the purist, and quantitative factors have also to be considered, there is much to be said in favour of Haagensen's (1977) contention.

The cellularity of the specialized connective tissue of the lobule has already been stressed (Figure 2–4). It is mainly due to the large number of fibrocyte nuclei. However, a few lymphocytes are usually also present, as well as the very occasional histiocyte. Lymphocytes are said to be most numerous between five and ten days after the onset of menstruation (Foote and Stewart, 1945), but since Haagensen (1971) has denied that such changes in the breast can be correlated with the phase of the menstrual cycle, the question needs reinvestigation. There is some doubt whether plasma cells should be regarded as a normal constituent. They are not usually present in normal lobules, but an occasional plasma cell may be seen in otherwise normal lobules. The problem is the definition of what is strictly normal. Surgical and necropsy material is either abnormal or, at any rate, its strict normality is usually impossible to prove. Probably forensic necropsies on accident cases could answer this problem adequately. The writer has seen plasma cells in the apparently normal lobules of women in pregnancy and in non-pregnant women, both when taking anti-ovulatory agents and when taking no medication. But the problem is the acquisition of material from strictly normal women and preferably ones in whom the date of the menstrual cycle is known. Necropsies on accidental deaths are the best source, and, since a menstrual history is very unlikely to be available in such cases, a comparison with the state of the endometrium needs to be undertaken. In practice, occasional plasma

cells in the lobule should be regarded as normal. This only applies, of course, in the absence of any other changes which indicate an abnormality. With experience every pathologist develops his own criteria and, in the presence of conspicuous numbers of plasma cells, he has a duty to exclude other more definite evidence of disease. The periductal stroma contains a few lymphocytes in addition to the obvious fibrocyte nuclei but plasma cells are usually absent or very sparse. Plasma cells are more likely to indicate the presence of disease when in the periductal stroma than when situated in the lobular stroma.

Functional Activity

The whole of the lobular–ductal system is capable of secretion and absorption. That secretion occurs during lactation is self-evident but the breast parenchyma is also secreting in its resting state. This secretion does not normally appear at the nipple because the exit of the major ducts is occluded by a keratinous plug. The neutral and acidic mucosubstances secreted in the resting state were described by Ozzello and Speer (1958) and more recently by Cooper (1974).

The fact that absorption also occurs throughout the lobular–ductal system is supported by circumstantial evidence in the human and by direct evidence in animals after injection of non-physiological substances into lactiferous ducts. Evidence of absorption of less artificial substances, e.g. diphtherial antitoxin, has been provided by Bonser, Dossett and Jull (1961). Here we are concerned solely with the relevance of these functions to pathological processes, a subject which will be discussed further in Chapter Five. For example, the apocrine tension cyst develops because secretion and absorption do not proceed at the same pace. The apocrine epithelium secretes fluid and this accumulates slowly since the cyst outlet is blocked. If absorption of fluid occurs in this cyst at all, it occurs at a slower rate than the secretion, and fluid accumulates under pressure.

In most breast carcinomas mucin secretion is altered quantitatively and perhaps qualitatively. Spicer et al (1962) found sialomucin predominantly in mucoid carcinoma though Norris and Taylor (1965) suggested that it was a poorly sulphated mucopolysaccharide. Cooper (1974) confirmed the dominance of sialidase-labile sialomucin but suggested that abundant neutral mucin was also present. Medullary carcinoma is one of the few common types of breast cancer in which mucin secretion is conspicuous by its absence. Differentiation in this tumour is possibly towards epithelial cells of absorptive type, while the secretory function is completely in abeyance.

NORMAL INVOLUTION

Knowledge of the involutionary process is essential in order to distinguish the physiological from the pathological, and also in order to understand the complexities of certain disease processes when these are superimposed on, or complicated by, involution. Lack of understanding of the normal involutionary process is one of the many reasons why normal variations are misconstrued as pathological, and is the major reason for diagnoses which imply that 'fibrosis' of the breast can occur as a primary disease entity. Involution takes place after pregnancy and lactation, and around the time of the menopause. As might be expected, most of the information available concerns perimenopausal involution. The precise duration of the process is not known but it appears to be of the order of three to five years. This information is derived from sequential biopsies on near-normal breasts, and from necropsy studies of breasts of 'normal' women around the time of the menopause. It can be considered, for convenience, under the headings of lobular, ductal and stromal involution.

LOBULAR INVOLUTION

Both epithelium and specialized stroma are involved. The basement membrane of the acini becomes thickened and the double-layered epithelium shrinks and becomes flattened while the luminal space narrows and becomes almost obliterated and epithelial secretion ceases. At the same time, the specialized mucoid loose connective tissue of the lobule gradually becomes converted into dense, hyaline collagen, which blends to varying degrees with the thickened acinar

basement membranes (Figures 2–8 and 2–9). The specialized connective tissue of the lobule is lost and comes to resemble ordinary connective tissue. Because of this, it merges with and 'sinks into' its background so that the original lobular outline is lost without trace: in these circumstances, only remnants of the epithelial tissue will indicate where the lobule has been: when the epithelial remnants vanish, the lobule disappears as completely as the Inca civilization. The conversion of the lobular to ordinary stroma sometimes proceeds to the extent that it becomes actually denser and less cellular than the adjacent interlobular stroma (Figure 2–8). Where this happens the lobule is represented by an ovoid structureless hyaline mass which sometimes shows slight artefactual separation from the interlobular stroma, a feature which helps with its identification. Eventually it presumably merges into surrounding stroma as described above. At no stage does this process indicate 'fibrosis' in a pathological sense — it is to be regarded as an involutionary process.

Cystic Lobular Involution. There is a little-known variant of lobular involution which is less common than the more usual process just described. It may be termed 'cystic lobular involution' (Figures 2–10 and 2–11) and is easily mistaken for cystic disease: it is sometimes a precursor of one variety of cystic disease (Hayward and Parks, 1958). We are partly indebted to a surgeon for accurately defining this condition. In cystic lobular involution, acini join up to form microcysts, which have rounded or serpentine outlines, depending on the stage of the process (Figures 2–10 and 2–11). The lobular stroma is still of the specialized variety (Figure 2–11) and this is the essential distinction between cystic lobular involution (physiological) and non-apocrine cystic disease (pathological). The cystic type of involution probably involutes further in the manner described for the more common type of involution. In any case, as long as there is any specialized connective tissue, the microscopic epithelial cysts can involute normally and the lobule disappears. It is a curious and ill-understood fact that specialized stroma is necessary for involution to proceed normally. In the absence of specialized stroma, cysts are pathological but only in the sense that they do not involute further and remain as permanent structures into old age.

The distinction between the two types of lobular involution must not be taken to

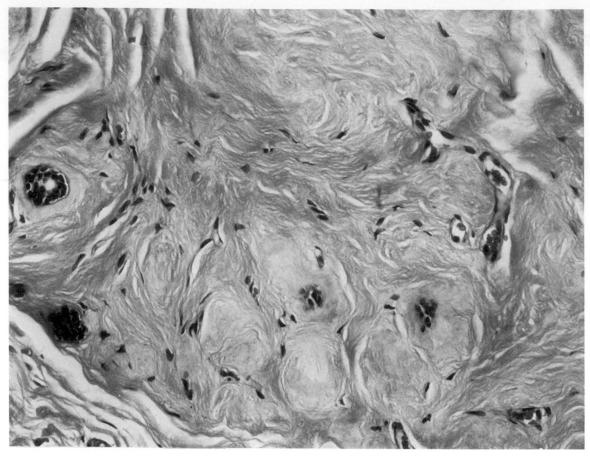

Figure 2–8 The common form of lobular·involution. The lobular stroma is hyalinized and the collagen has become even denser than that between the lobules. This may result in an artefactual cleavage, as seen here, between the involuted lobule and the ordinary breast stroma. Four remnants of acini (terminal ductules) are identifiable: two are distinct while two are barely discernible. H and E. ×300.

indicate that the more usual and the cystic types of lobular involution are mutually exclusive; both may be found together in the same breast in varying proportions.

DUCTAL INVOLUTION

Very little is known about the disappearance of the ductules and small ducts in the older age groups. The increase of elastic tissue around the larger ducts with age is probably

not involutionary but related to disease, as previously discussed.

STROMAL INVOLUTION

With involution, changes in the supporting stroma are as profound as, though less complex than, the changes in the parenchyma. The banal connective tissue partly or largely disappears by a process which is far from clear and is, to varying degrees, replaced

Figure 2–9 (*Opposite, above.*) Same tissue as shown in Figure 2–8. This is stained for elastic tissue, which is absent. Six epithelial structures persist and four of these have distinct lumina, compared with four and one respectively in Figure 2–8. The stromal hyalinization is even more evident than in the H and E preparation. Weigert elastic and HVG. ×300.

Figure 2–10 (*Opposite, below.*) Two lobules showing cystic involution. This is physiological and does not constitute cystic disease. H and E. ×150.

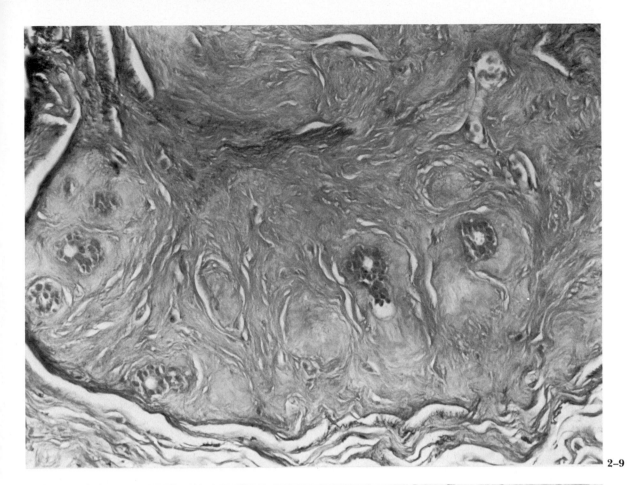

2–9

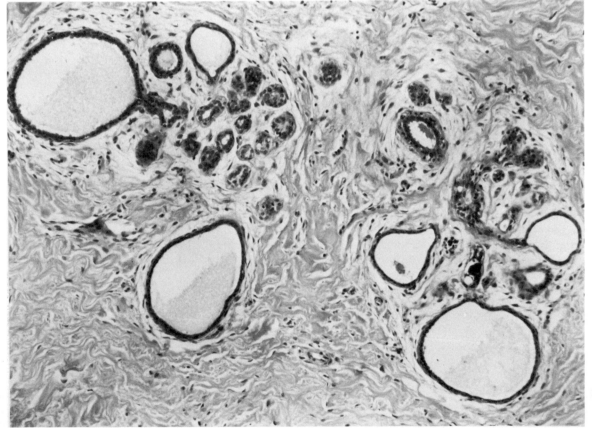

2–10

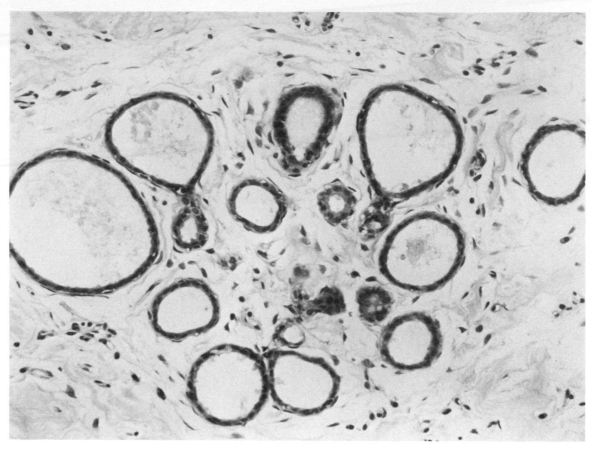

Figure 2–11   Cystic lobular involution. This is normal and not to be confused with pathological conditions. Specialized lobular stroma is still present. H and E. ×375.

by adipose tissue. This leads to either a small atrophic and flabby breast or, at the other extreme, to a voluminous and pendulous breast, of the type beloved by the seaside postcard artist, which consists very largely of adipose tissue in which there are widely dispersed ductal remnants of the parenchyma and any lobules that have escaped involution. In most involuting and involuted breasts there is both loss of connective tissue supporting structures and adipose tissue replacement.

The stromal involution is not uniform in time throughout the breast or even in adjacent parts. This can give rise to marked differences in consistency in different areas depending chiefly on the amount of adipose tissue. Adipose metaplasia is frequently patchy in distribution and thus small areas of pre-existing fibrous tissue may alternate with newly developed adipose areas, resulting in a slightly granular consistency on palpation. Very occasionally adipose metaplasia may partially isolate a large area of fibrous stroma:

this will produce a palpable firm lump against the soft background of adipose tissue and carcinoma may be suspected. It is likely that such a clinically obvious lump will be surgically excised and the pathologist may be tempted to furnish a diagnosis of 'fibrosis'. As will be explained in the following chapter, there is probably no disease of the breast in which fibrosis can be regarded as the primary phenomenon. The condition described here is not even pathological; it is merely an unusual manifestation of normal stromal involution. It is the adipose tissue which is newly formed while the fibrous tissue, which may present as a 'lump', is an area of pre-existing normal stroma.

Adipose metaplasia of the stroma with increasing age is of great importance in mammographic work. It accounts for the increased radiological lucency which makes mammography of increasing value after the age of about 40 or 45 years.

The frequency of adipose stromal metaplasia in normal circumstances may also explain the frequency of adipose metaplasia in cystosarcoma phyllodes, with the occasional development of frankly liposarcomatous areas. The tumour may be reflecting, at the neoplastic level, the latent potential of the breast stroma to undergo adipose metaplasia.

Both lobular and stromal involution take place in patchy fashion. Lobules may be in an advanced state of involution in one part of the breast and appear normal in another part. In addition, parenchymal and stromal involution do not necessarily commence at the same time or proceed at the same rate. Stromal involution may appear advanced when there is little change in the lobules or the reverse may be true. When there is extensive adipose tissue in the stroma with little or no significant lobular change, it is possible that the breast stroma has been fatty ab initio and that its abundant adipose component does not represent an involutional change. However, involution remains the chief cause of an extensively adipose stroma.

With involution, fatty tissue replaces much of the interlobular stroma and occasionally it can also replace the lobular stroma, producing appearances which can be misconstrued. In these circumstances, the lobular acini rest on and are separated by adipose tissue, an appearance which can be mistaken for neoplastic infiltration. The lobular grouping is, however, still maintained to some extent, even though it may be a little distorted by the presence of abundant fatty tissue. Malignancy can also be excluded by the demonstration of a two-layered epithelial structure, though when the epithelium is low or flattened this feature may be obscured and needs to be searched for diligently.

NORMAL ULTRASTRUCTURE

The ultrastructure of the normal human mammary 'ductule' (terminal ductule) was described in detail by Tannenbaum, Weiss and Marx (1969). These workers pointed out that most previous studies dealt with 'so-called normal regions of glands that contain abnormalities elsewhere' and did not deal with completely normal breast tissue; they pointed out the dangers of such a practice. By contrast, their study was carried out on tissue taken for biopsy because of the presence of 'vague

breast masses' only and which showed perfectly normal mammary parenchyma histologically. Breast biopsies were obtained from three patients aged 33, 40 and 43 years. The patients were menstruating regularly, were parous but none had been pregnant in the preceding year.

The terminal ductule (or acinus) of the truly normal resting female mammary gland is composed of an inner continuous layer of columnar or cuboidal epithelial cells and an outer discontinuous layer of myoepithelial cells. The epithelial cells have their long axes and those of their nuclei arranged radial to the lumen, corresponding to the orientation visible on light microscopy. They may extend to the basement membrane or be separated from it by myoepithelial cells. The luminal surfaces may have a profusion of microvilli while their other surfaces have fewer, or, alternatively, there may be few microvilli on the luminal surfaces with none on the other surfaces. The nucleus varies in outline between oval and deeply invaginated. The nucleolus is large and is often situated near the centre.

Elongated mitochondria are present in all parts of the cytoplasm. The Golgi apparatus is usually situated between the nucleus and the luminal surface.

Epithelial cells are connected by terminal bars, desmosomes and invaginations of cell membranes which resemble microvilli and may be related to them.

The myoepithelial cells are aligned with their long axes at right angles to the long axes of the epithelial cells. The plasma membrane bordering the basement membrane is irregularly undulating. Hemidesmosomes are present on the peripheral cell membrane. The myofibrils, which characterize the cell, are frequently marked with patches of greater density. The mitochondria tend to be smaller than those of the epithelial cells.

Tannenbaum, Weiss and Marx (1969) stress the similarities as well as the differences between the two cell types. Thus, the nucleus is similar in dimension, in its component parts and its appearance. They disagree with those workers who found that the nuclei of the myoepithelial cells are smaller and denser. Such a finding was not consistent in their material. The Golgi apparatus and endoplasmic reticulum of the two cell types are similar in appearance. Microvilli are a feature of both cell types. Basement membrane ensheathes not only the myoepithelial cells but also the epithelial cells which extend to the periphery of the ductule. Even a characteristic cilium was identified in a myoepithelial cell. Light and dark variants of both cell types were found.

Tannenbaum, Weiss and Marx (1969) questioned the 'normality' of many of the 'controls' studied in previous reports, because of the method of collection of the material. The more reliable reports were regarded by them as too brief to be really informative. They reject the identification by Toker (1967) of five cell categories on the basis of the study of a single case. In particular they do not regard the 'light' and 'dark' cells as distinct categories since they found gradations among the cells of many ductules, indicating that they are different stages of a single cell type.

They regard the only useful division of cell types as that which distinguishes between epithelial and myoepithelial. They stress, moreover, that it is probable that these two cell types are genetically related. They emphasize that 'basement membrane, which is now believed to be an epithelial product, forms around both cell types'.

The work of Tannenbaum, Weiss and Marx (1969) was essentially confirmed by the more encyclopaedic study of Ozzello (1971), which constitutes essential reading.

More recently, the fine structure of the resting breast has been described by Stirling and Chandler (1976, 1977) and a detailed account has been supplied by Ahmed (1978). Ahmed described and illustrated copiously the ultrastructure of the resting breast, the breast in pregnancy and lactation and the changes occurring at different phases of the menstrual cycle. As Ahmed pointed out, the latter are in need of further ultrastructural study, as indeed they are even at light microscopic level. Ahmed (1978) is a valuable source of references.

References

Ahmed, A. (1978) *Atlas of the Ultrastructure of Human Breast Diseases*. pp. 1–25. Edinburgh, London and New York: Churchill Livingstone.

Bonser, G. M., Dossett, J. A. and Jull, J. W. (1961) *Human and Experimental Breast Cancer*. London: Pitman Medical.

Cooper, D. J. (1974) Mucin histochemistry of mucous carcinomas of breast and colon and non-neoplastic breast epithelium. *Journal of Clinical Pathology*, **27**, 311–314.

Davies, J. D. (1973) Hyperelastosis, obliteration and fibrous plaques in major ducts of the human breast. *Journal of Pathology*, **110**, 13–26.

Foote, F. W. and Stewart, F. W. (1945) Comparative studies of cancerous versus noncancerous breast. I. Basic morphologic characteristics. *Annals of Surgery*, **121**, 6–53.

Haagensen, C. D. (1971) *Diseases of the Breast*. Second edition — Revised reprint, p. 60. Philadelphia, London, Toronto: W. B. Saunders.

Haagensen, C. D. (1977) The relationship of gross cystic disease of the breast and carcinoma (Editorial). *Annals of Surgery*, **185**, 375–376.

Hamperl, H. (1939) Über die Myothelien (myoepithelialen Elemente) der Brustdrüse. *Virchows Archiv für pathologische Anatomie und Physiologie und für klinische Medizin*, **305**, 171–215.

Hartmann, W. H. (1975) Pathologic anatomy and classification of cancer of the breast. *American Journal of Clinical Pathology*, **64**, 718–719.

Hayward, J. L. and Parks, A. G. (1958) Alterations in the microanatomy of the breast as a result of changes in the hormonal environment. In *Endocrine Aspects of Breast Cancer* (Ed.) Currie, A. R. pp. 133–134. Edinburgh and London: E. & S. Livingstone.

Norris, H. J. and Taylor, H. B. (1965) Prognosis of mucinous (gelatinous) carcinoma of the breast. *Cancer*, **18**, 879–885.

Ozzello, L. (1971) Ultrastructure of the human mammary gland. In *Pathology Annual* (Ed.) Sommers, S. C. Vol. 6, pp. 1–59. London: Butterworth.

Ozzello, L. and Speer, F. D. (1958) The mucopolysaccharides in the normal and diseased breast. *American Journal of Pathology*, **34**, 993–1009.

Spicer, S. S., Neubecker, R. D., Warren, L. and Henson, J. G. (1962) Epithelial mucins in lesions of the human breast. *Journal of the National Cancer Institute*, **29**, 963–970.

Stirling, J. W. and Chandler, J. A. (1976) The fine structure of the normal resting terminal ductal-lobular unit in the female breast. *Virchows Archiv A: Pathological Anatomy and Histology*, **373**, 205–226.

Stirling, J. W. and Chandler, J. A. (1977) The fine structure of ducts and subareolar ducts in the resting gland of the female breast. *Virchows Archiv A: Pathological Anatomy and Histology*, **373**, 119–132.

Symmers, W. St. C. (1966) The breasts. In *Systemic Pathology* (Ed.) Payling Wright, G. and Symmers, W. St. C. Ch. 28, Vol. 1, p. 986. London: Longmans, Green.

Tannenbaum, M., Weiss, M. and Marx, A. J. (1969) Ultrastructure of the human mammary ductule. *Cancer*, **23**, 958–978.

Toker, C. (1967) Observations on the ultrastructure of a mammary ductule. *Journal of Ultrastructure Research*, **21**, 9–25.

Chapter Three

Terminology of Benign Diseases and the Benign Epithelial Hyperplasias

DEFINITION OF PATHOLOGICAL TERMS (NAMES USED AND ABUSED)

The nomenclature of diseases of the breast is far from standardized, perhaps less so than in most organs in the body. The reasons for this lie largely in the complexity of the pathology and the pathogenesis of breast diseases and the dearth of knowledge about their aetiology. The variations in the normal histology and the variations occurring at different times of life add to the problems of terminology. If in addition one considers the variations in space and time of the involutionary process, both epithelial and stromal, the problems of terminology will begin to be appreciated.

GENERAL HEADINGS

CYSTIC DISEASE

Mazoplasia. Some of the terms used, both past and present, have confused more than they have clarified. Terms like 'mazoplasia', used by some pathologists, have no generally accepted definition; mazoplasia means different things to different pathologists. The pathologist sometimes uses mazoplasia to describe minor abnormalities which he feels unable to label or, worse, as a face-saving device to describe normal breast in one of its variant forms, in a misguided effort to make the surgeon believe that he has removed pathological tissue, when it was in fact normal. In the long term such a practice renders a disservice to the clinician, his patients and to the pathologist himself. The use of the term mazoplasia should be discontinued.

Mastopathy. The term 'mastopathy' is slightly better but, in practice, unless qualified by the prefix 'cystic', it is all too often used to include virtually all non-malignant disease of the breast, with the exception of fibroadenoma.

'*Mammary Dysplasia*' is perhaps one of the most objectionable and ill-defined terms in common use. This term has the disadvantages of 'mastopathy' with the additional implication of changes of unspecified type and severity, which may or may not have a 'precancerous' connotation. The term includes cases of cystic disease with little or no hyperplasia as well as cases of florid epithelial hyperplasia with few or no cysts. It includes cases which a pathologist may consider atypical but benign, cases of 'borderline malignancy' and even cases which are probably malignant. It is in practice an umbrella term or wastebasket to disguise ignorance and has contributed a great deal to confuse further an intrinsically very complex subject. Unfortunately the disease 'duct ectasia', as a clinical and pathological entity, has become obscured and submerged by the use of terms like 'mammary dysplasia'. Its use cannot be sufficiently deprecated.

'*Fibroadenosis*' does not suffer from the disadvantages and the objectionable connotations of 'dysplasia' but it is not an ideal name for cystic disease. Fibrosis is not an essential ingredient of cystic disease, though it is a major part of the response to rupture of a 'tension cyst' with slow leakage or sudden extrusion of its contents. The omission of any indication that the lesion contains cysts adds to the poverty of this name.

Cystic Disease, Cystic Mastopathy and Cystic Hyperplasia. In choosing names for diseases, it is highly desirable to use terms which are as objective and self-explanatory as possible. It is logical to call '*cystic disease*' exactly that, and to use the term 'cystic hyperplasia' when it is accompanied, as it frequently is, by significant benign epithelial proliferation of any form. These terms do not suffer from the disadvantage of the alternatives already considered. Historically, 'cystic hyperplasia' meant a hyperplasia which was followed by cystic excavation of the solid hyperplastic mass leading to cyst formation. Since nobody would now claim that cysts form in this way, the term can legitimately be used in the sense defined here. The alternative to cystic hyperplasia is '*cystic disease and epithelial hyperplasia*' but this is too cumbersome for everyday use. 'Cystic mastopathy' is a perfectly valid alternative to cystic disease. Terms like '*chronic mastitis*' and '*cystic mastitis*' suffer from some obvious disadvantages but their use has lingered on for traditional reasons.

FIBROUS DISEASE OF THE BREAST

'Fibrosis of the breast' as a diagnosis lacks real meaning and such diagnoses are generally attributable to a lack of understanding of both normal involutional and pathological processes. Terms like '*fibrous disease of the breast*', '*fibrous mastopathy*' and '*chronic indurative mastitis*' are used to describe a clinical 'lump' in the breast which consists of bland interlobular connective tissue. This is certainly not a mastitis in any sense of the term and there is no real evidence that it even represents a pathological process. It usually reflects the patchiness of the physiological involutionary process as it affects the stroma, as described in the last chapter. Chemical and histochemical analyses of these 'lesions' show them to be composed of apparently normal collagen (Vassar and Culling, 1959). It is true that the 'lump' consists dominantly of fibrous tissue but it is generally normal pre-existing fibrous tissue, more or less isolated by adipose metaplasia, which affects the stroma in a more patchy fashion than is seen in most women. One cannot doubt that this condition represents a clinical entity but the writer can find no good evidence that it represents a pathological entity.

FIBROADENOMA

In the case of '*fibroadenoma*' there are practically no terminological problems, though one could argue over its nosological status. There is slight difficulty over the inclusion by some authors of '*fibroadenomatoid hyperplasia*' in the cystic disease/cystic hyperplasia group of diseases. In general, it is best to consider fibroadenoma as a completely distinct entity, while admitting that very rarely it may appear to form part of the cystic hyperplasia complex.

The term '*giant fibroadenoma*' should mean just that, a lesion identical with fibroadenoma histologically and differing from it only in size. The dividing line between the two forms is, of course, somewhat arbitrary. It is important not to use 'giant fibroadenoma' as synonymous with '*cystosarcoma phyllodes*'. Essentially, the latter differs from the former in the character and cellularity of its connective tissue component, as discussed in Chapter Fourteen. Size, though in the vast majority of cases a distinguishing point between cystosarcoma and fibroadenoma, is not *the* essential and overriding criterion for making the distinction. There are clinical and pathological differences between giant fibroadenoma and cystosarcoma phyllodes, as here defined, which makes the distinction between them a pragmatic one as well. An attempt is made in Chapter Fourteen to suggest alternatives to replace the unwholesome designation of 'benign cystosarcoma' applied to many tumours in the cystosarcoma group.

THE BENIGN EPITHELIAL HYPERPLASIAS AND THEIR INTERRELATIONSHIPS

BENIGN EPITHELIAL HYPERPLASIAS

EPITHELIOSIS ('PAPILLOMATOSIS')

There is just as little, if not less, agreement about the terms used to describe the various types of epithelial hyperplasia and hypertrophy. The term 'epitheliosis' has gained much wider acceptance in Britain than it has in North America. It is an eminently satisfactory name for the solid and quasi-solid benign epithelial proliferation which is found predominantly in small ducts, ductules and lobules. Epitheliosis is best known as a component of cystic hyperplasia but it can less often be found on its own. There is unfortunately a very frequent tendency to refer to epitheliosis as a papillary proliferation or papillomatosis because of the way it forms tongue-like projections into epithelial lumina. It does not have connective tissue cores in papillae in the sense that this term is used in other organs and there is therefore no good reason to continue using the term 'papillary' in this context.

Epitheliosis is the condition which has to be distinguished from in situ ductal cancer (and cancerization of lobules, q.v.). Even when the condition is less solid and contains numerous luminal spaces, the structure and cytology of the solid parts is indistinguishable from that seen in the more solid forms, and the term 'epitheliosis' is equally applicable. It is true that a focus of epitheliosis sometimes merges with a microscopic papilloma or, much less frequently, even with a papillary 'cyst-adenoma', but that surely does not justify the designation 'papillary' for the non-papillary component. It merely means that different forms of epithelial hyperplasia frequently co-exist in the same breast and, perhaps not unexpectedly, these sometimes even merge with one another.

ADENOSIS

The term 'adenosis', if not further qualified, is such a comprehensive one that it may legitimately be used to include all the non-neoplastic glandular hyperplasias. In this sense it could encompass even the physiological adenosis of pregnancy. At least two reasonably distinct varieties of major importance are recognized: 'blunt duct adenosis' and 'sclerosing adenosis'.

Blunt Duct Adenosis

Blunt duct adenosis (BDA) is the condition usually referred to when 'adenosis', unspecified further, is used in a pathological sense (Figures 3–1 and 3–2). It is one of the commonest types of benign epithelial hypertrophy and hyperplasia. At one end of the spectrum, the mildest degrees merge into the appearances of normal lobules and are frequently not noted or recognized, while, at the other end of the spectrum, blunt duct adenosis has an easily recognizable structure. Although the term is used very frequently, there have been hardly any adequate descriptions of the appearance of the condition since the classical work of Foote and Stewart (1945). Lobules are probably the main structures involved or, at any rate, it is here that the most distinctive appearances are seen (Figures 3–1 and 3–2).

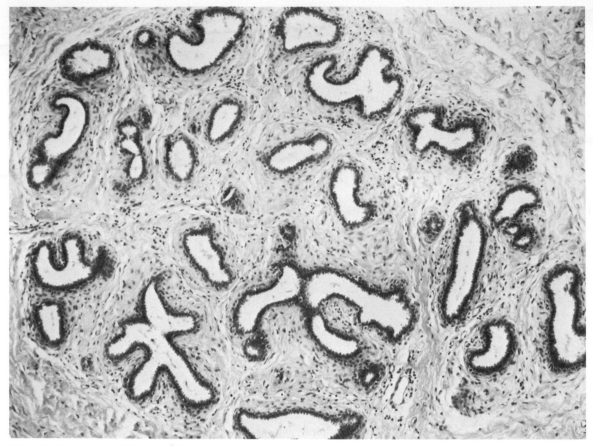

Figure 3–1   An organoid type of blunt duct adenosis (BDA). H and E. ×120.

BDA is a convenient descriptive term for all the pathological hyperplasias and hypertrophic processes affecting the parenchyma of the breast which give rise to two-layered epithelial structures with blunt lateral outlines and blunt endings and which are associated with a specialized type of stroma identical with or akin to the specialized stroma of the lobular and periductal tissue (Figures 3–1 to 3–6). In this sense, BDA covers all types of pathological adenosis, with the exception of sclerosing adenosis in its variant forms. In a well-developed case one finds marked enlargement of all the epithelial units of the lobule with hypertrophy of both cell layers, enlargement of lumina and consequently a greatly increased diameter of the individual epithelial units. In addition there may be an increase of the specialized connective tissue of the lobules. The process has the appearance of an *organoid hypertrophy* involving all the elements of the lobules. There is little or no actual increase in the number of terminal lobular units, a feature which is only easily appreciated when normal lobules in the adjacent tissues are available for comparison. Nor is there any convincing evidence that the increased size of the epithelial units is attributable to a

Figure 3–2   (*Opposite, above.*)   Blunt duct adenosis (BDA) with hypertrophy of all elements. Two-cell-type epithelial differentiation is very conspicuous. Apical snouts or cytoplasmic blebs are prominent here. H and E. ×400.

Figure 3–3   (*Opposite, below.*)   BDA. Organoid hypertrophy and hyperplasia of all lobular elements with two distinct epithelial types and an increase of specialized laminated connective tissue. Luminal cell edges are convex but without blebbing. H and E. ×150.

26

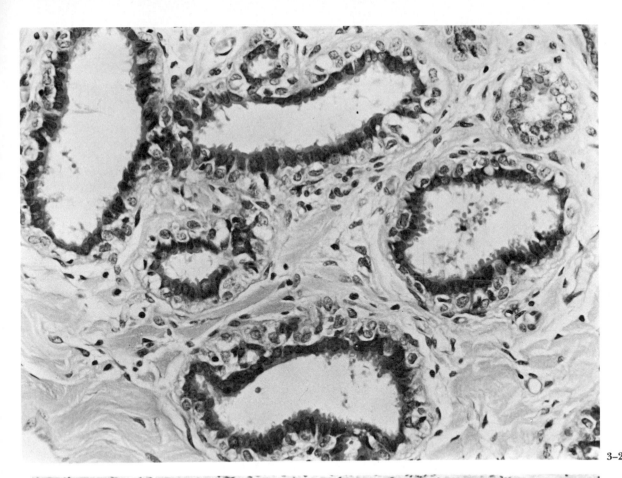

3-2

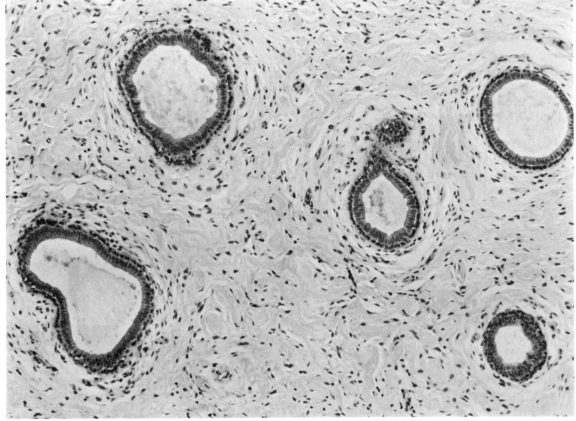

3-3

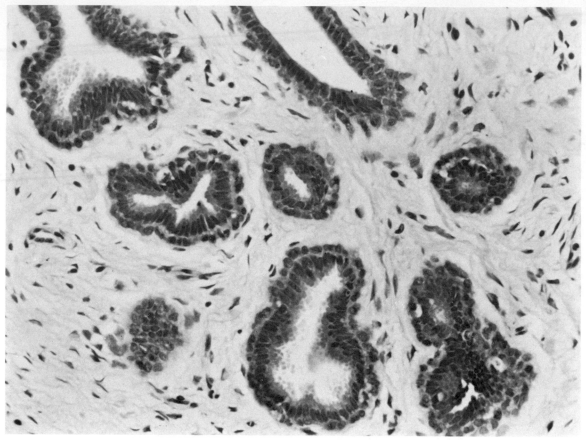

Figure 3–4 Adenosis with two very distinct cell types around the glandular lumina. There is an increase also of the specialized lobular connective tissue. H and E. ×400.

significant degree of hyperplasia. It is cell hypertrophy, occurring in a highly organized fashion, which is the conspicuous feature.

No name coined to date really does justice to or adequately describes this curious and very frequent component of mammary hyperplasia. BDA is a very good descriptive term which has stood the test of time. It is not clear from many descriptions whether BDA represents an alteration in pre-existing normal lobules or whether it represents, as those who coined the name apparently believed, a new formation of abnormal structures derived from the ducts. Nor does one mechanism necessarily exclude the other. The term 'columnar metaplasia', used by Bonser, Dossett and Jull (1961), refers apparently to the same condition. Though this name is not in general use, it has the merit of recognizing that epithelial hypertrophy is one of the main features of the disorder; it also implies that the alteration is in a pre-existing normal structure, which is probably true of the vast majority of cases. Columnar metaplasia affects ductules and ducts as well, but it is less common and somewhat less easy to recognize in these structures unless it is gross.

The morphological changes of BDA are mirrored in the altered response to hormonal stimulation in pregnancy. This takes the form of a lessened or absent secretory response by the epithelium.

Figure 3–5 (*Opposite, above.*) BDA. The curved structure represents a giant organoid hypertrophy of a lobule. There is gross hypertrophy of all epithelial and connective tissue elements. Compare with normal lobules at the edge. H and E. ×60.

Figure 3–6 (*Opposite, below.*) Same tissue as shown in Figure 3–5. Adenosis is of lobular origin and contains no elastic tissue. There is a cuff of elastic tissue in the duct wall. Weigert elastic and HVG. ×60.

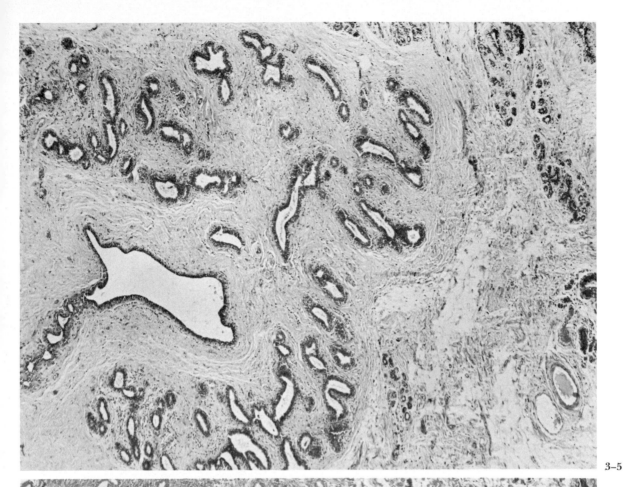

3–5

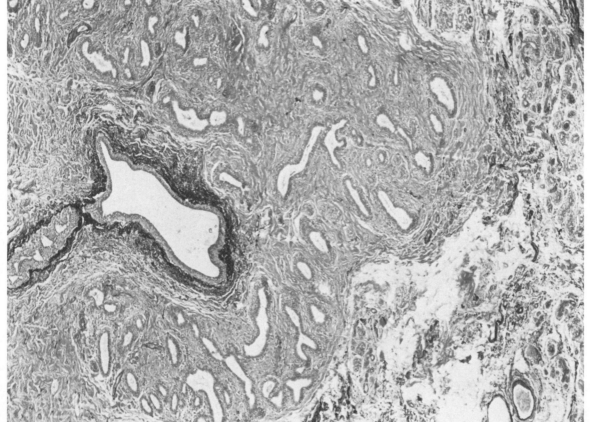

3–6

BDA is a benign condition and there is nothing to suggest that it carries any increased risk of malignancy (Black et al, 1972). On the other hand, Bonser, Dossett and Jull (1961) suggested that a spectrum of changes links columnar metaplasia with in situ malignancy. Both these apparently contradictory and irreconcilable views are probably correct. BDA as defined here, and as used by most authors, excludes any cytological or nuclear atypia and there is nothing to indicate an increased risk of cancer in such cases. Rarely, 'columnar metaplasia', in the sense of Bonser, Dossett and Jull (1961), merges with atypical epithelium, which in turn merges with 'early' in situ carcinoma. But the appearances of typical adenosis hardly ever merge with those of in situ carcinoma. Convincing evidence of transitional forms between adenosis and in situ malignancy is very difficult to find. The two forms of hyperplasia, benign and malignant, part company at an early phase in their respective developments. This very important question is discussed fully in Chapters Six and Ten.

Foci of BDA occasionally show changes of epitheliosis at the same site. This is to be expected; it is perhaps a little remarkable that transitions are not more common than they are.

The changes of BDA described so far could be regarded as the most highly organized form of benign hypertrophy and hyperplasia. In this form, the epithelium and the stroma of the lobule participate about equally. The degree of change in any given lobule is highly variable, ranging from the minimal and barely detectable degrees to the more obvious forms. These changes can be more striking when only part of the lobule is affected, and the larger epithelial units can then be contrasted with the unaffected part of the same lobule.

In most cases, BDA does not affect the epithelial and stromal components of the lobule equally; the epithelial hypertrophy is usually dominant and the stroma is relatively less bulky so that it accounts for a smaller percentage of the volume of the lobule. In BDA there are many lobules with a diameter which is only moderately or slightly increased, or is even normal, while the epithelial units are markedly hypertrophic. It would appear that the stimulus to the epithelium and its response is usually greater than that of the stroma. In this form of BDA the lesion is also sharply circumscribed and there is always some specialized connective tissue in the abnormal lobules. But the proportions of epithelium to specialized stroma vary greatly from case to case and in different lobules in the same breast. The description given so far applies to the simpler forms of BDA. In these there is hypertrophy of epithelial units with hypertrophy of individual cells, without any very convincing evidence of epithelial hyperplasia.

Microcystic Blunt Duct Adenosis

The variety of types of adenosis and the difficulties of terminology become more obvious when one considers other appearances that are encompassed by the term BDA. Cysts sometimes undergo changes in the epithelium similar to those seen in BDA and this applies particularly to the cysts which have not undergone apocrine metaplasia. Since these pre-existing cysts have already lost the specialized lobular connective tissue, this may be regarded as a form of BDA in which the connective tissue component is not involved. Microscopic papillomas lined by similar epithelium may project into these altered cysts, complicating the appearances and again reflecting the mixed types of hyperplasia that are frequently encountered in practice. When it is recalled that cysts may, to varying degrees, appear to have lost their lobular grouping, it will be readily appreciated that in this situation the BDA appears to be less organoid. Adjacent cystic lobules affected by BDA give the appearance of somewhat poorly circumscribed nodules of hyperplastic tissue, as the margins of the lobules have become a little blurred because of the pathological processes previously affecting them. The number of epithelial units is often actually diminished because the hypertrophic and hyperplastic changes affect a lobule which has already become cystic, i.e. it has been converted into fewer but much larger epithelial structures.

Nodules of adenosis, in which the number of units may be normal or less than normal, but in which the units are large enough to be considered cystic, are not only the result of changes in pre-existing cysts (Figure 3–7): the cystic change may occur pari passu with the hyperplasia. The mechanism of cyst formation is debatable. Since the epithelium in these cases is not only usually very hypertrophic but also shows a noticeable increase in mitotic activity, it is almost certain that there is hyperplasia as well as hypertrophy of the epithelium (Figure 3–7). The hyperplasia

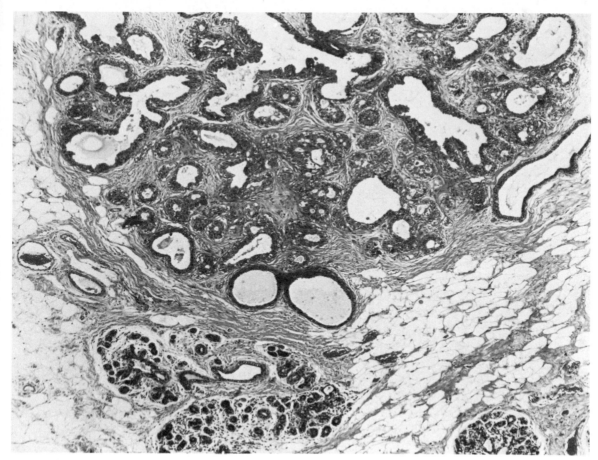

Figure 3–7   Microcystic BDA. Organoid hypertrophy and hyperplasia of all elements of lobule including the connective tissue. There is some cystic dilatation of the glandular spaces. Compare with normal lobules in the same field. H and E. ×60.

could well be the major factor causing microcyst formation but it is possible that 'unfolding' of the units may also play a part in the production of larger units. Whatever the mechanism, this type of BDA is microcystic. As with most other forms of blunt duct adenosis, it is associated with some specialized connective tissue but this is usually not very abundant and not as mucoid as the normal lobular connective tissue (Figure 3–7).

The simpler forms of BDA show clear evidence of origin in pre-existing lobules, witness the lobules that show only partial involvement by BDA. Most microcystic BDA is merely a variant of the simpler form of BDA and is likewise of lobular origin (Figure 3–7). It is possible, however, that some types of microcystic BDA represent neoformations arising from ducts or ductules rather than alterations in pre-existing lobules. This

possibility needs to be considered, especially when the foci of adenosis consist of a very few large units. It is difficult to visualize how alterations in pre-existing lobules could bring this about, unless the unfolding mechanism already hinted at is operative.

Non-organoid Blunt Duct Adenosis

The types of BDA described so far are all more or less organoid, though the lobular grouping is not as obvious when BDA arises in pre-existing cysts. But some variants of BDA are not organoid. Epithelial structures similar to those described in the preceding paragraphs are sometimes only irregularly grouped (Figure 3–8) and very occasionally they appear randomly scattered. Descriptively, one could call this a non-organoid BDA.

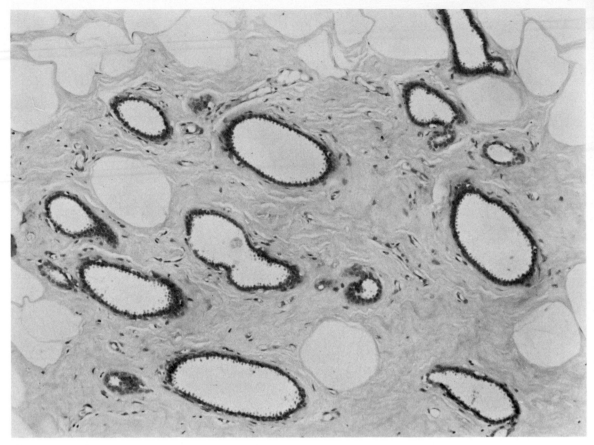

Figure 3–8 Adenosis without obvious organoid pattern. It is not always clear in cases of this type whether adenosis has originated from a pre-existing lobule or de novo. H and E. ×150.

This type of lesion raises the possibility of a ductal origin in addition to a lobular origin even more cogently, for there is little to suggest an origin in pre-existing lobules in such cases. This non-organoid type of BDA may rarely infiltrate the walls of veins in the same manner as is seen in sclerosing adenosis (Figures 9–13 and 9–14) and, in this sense, it constitutes a link with sclerosing adenosis.

Nodular Adenosis

There is another variety of adenosis related to BDA. It is a type of florid adenosis which forms a link between BDA on the one hand and sclerosing adenosis on the other. It is usually found in only small foci but occasionally it is a conspicuous or even a dominant component of breast hyperplasia. The adenosis takes the form of more or less nodular foci of proliferating epithelial tissue, hence the descriptive label 'nodular adenosis' (Figures 3–9 to 3–11). These nodules are frequently associated with a cellular but collagenous tissue, which may appear slightly compressed by the often expansile mode of growth. Both epithelial and myoepithelial cells participate in the proliferation but nodular adenosis differs from typical BDA in that there is less contrast between the two cell types. The epithelial cells lining small glandular lumina are not as tall as in BDA and they do not show the opaque eosinophilic or

Figure 3–9 (*Opposite, above.*) 'Nodular adenosis', a variant of sclerosing adenosis, originating in small ducts. H and E. ×60.

Figure 3–10 (*Opposite, below.*) Higher magnification of part of field shown in Figure 3–9. There is florid hyperplasia of both epithelial and myoepithelial cell types. H and E. ×150.

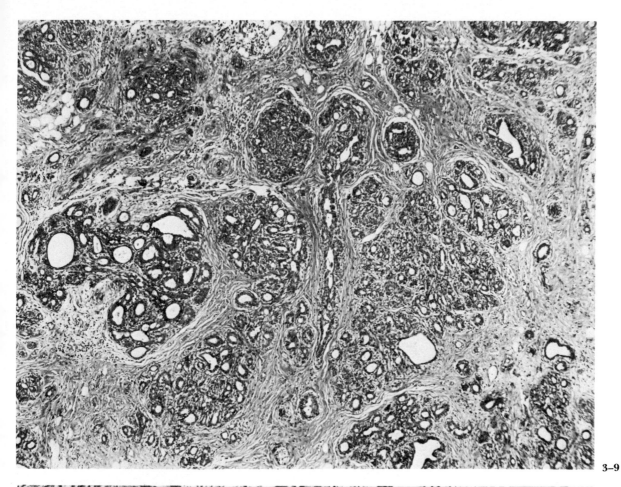

3–9

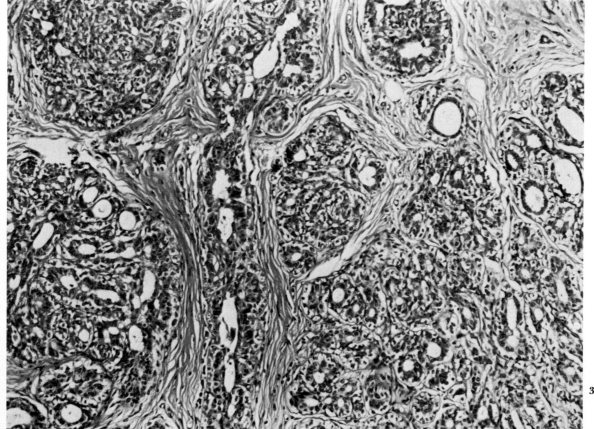

3–10

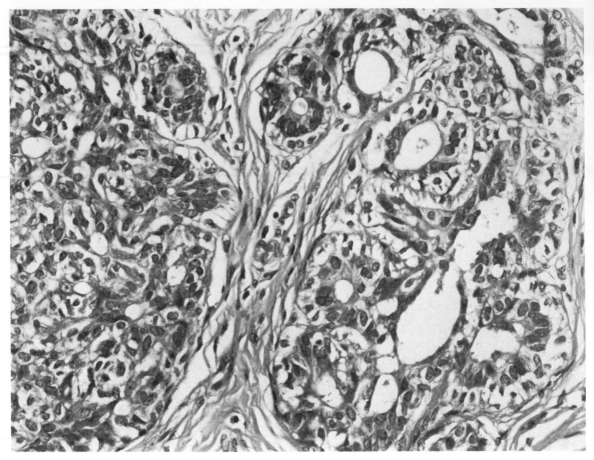

Figure 3–11 Nodular adenosis. There is differentiation of both epithelial and myoepithelial cells though many cells appear transitional between the two or are indeterminate in type. There was extensive venous wall and some neural infiltration in this benign disease. H and E. ×400.

amphophilic deep staining quality of the cytoplasm seen in BDA (Figures 3–10 and 3–11). They usually lack significant snout formation or cytoplasmic 'blebbing' at the luminal margin. For these reasons the epithelial cells do not appear very different from the clear outer myoepithelial cell layer. The other way in which nodular adenosis differs from BDA is in the extent of hyperplasia of the outer cell type in relation to the inner. There is a moderate to marked overgrowth of myoepithelial cells, so that the nodules consist of small glandular spaces set in a background of more solid, somewhat spindled and pale-staining myoepithelial cells.

Mitoses are easily found in nodular adenosis in both epithelial and myoepithelial cells.

Nodular adenosis differs from classical sclerosing adenosis in not showing the distortion and sclerosis exhibited by the latter. It could be argued that nodular adenosis represents an early non-sclerotic phase of sclerosing adenosis; this is probably true of some instances at least. Also nodular adenosis infiltrates into the intima of blood vessels (Figures 9–7 to 9–12) in the manner of sclerosing adenosis. All the benign hyperplasias which infiltrate neurovascular bundles in this way are probably closely related. But, in general, nodular adenosis lacks the striking

Figure 3–12 (*Opposite, above.*) Another type of adenosis with evidence of an origin from ducts rather than lobules. 'Infiltrating epitheliosis' with perineural invasion was present in other fields. H and E. ×150.

Figure 3–13 (*Opposite, below.*) Higher magnification of part of field shown in Figure 3–12. A form of microglandular adenosis based on a central duct. H and E. ×400.

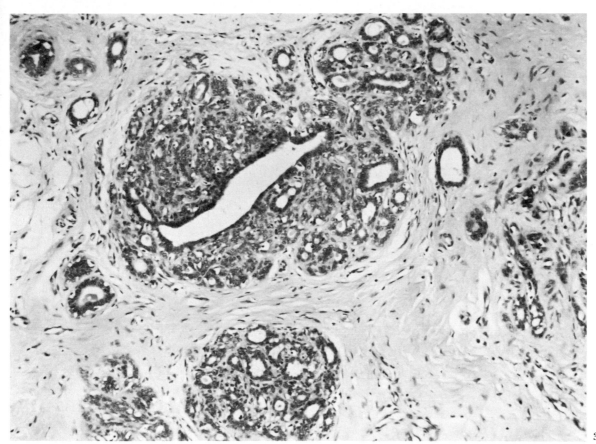

3–12

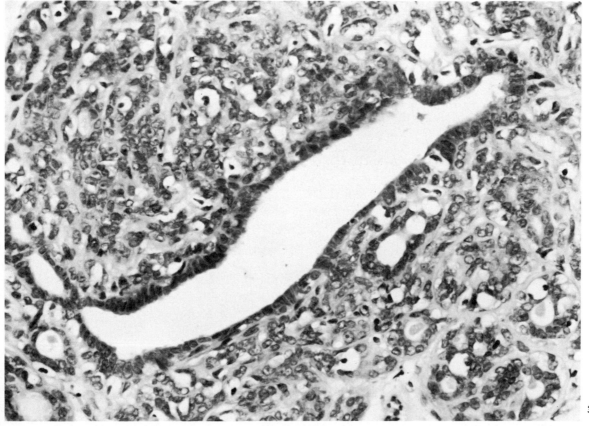

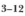

3–13

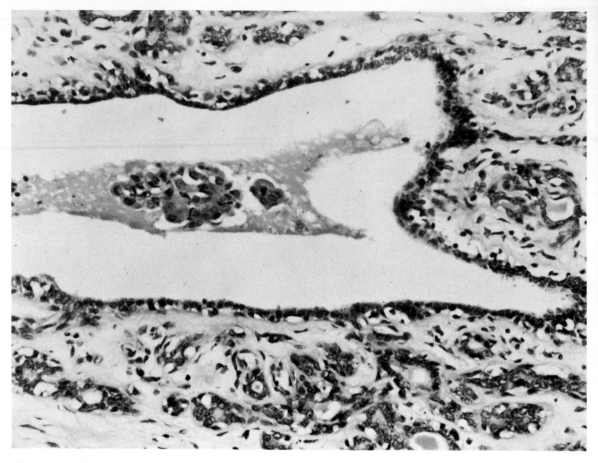

Figure 3–14   Same tissue as preceding two illustrations. Note tail-like connections in at least two foci between the adenosis and the central duct. H and E. ×375.

stromal hyperplasia which is so characteristic of sclerosing adenosis. Furthermore, while typical sclerosing adenosis has a lobular origin, nodular adenosis arises sometimes in small ducts, and thus has a somewhat different histogenesis.

Nodular adenosis can be regarded as *a microglandular adenosis in which myoepithelial differentiation outstrips epithelial differentiation* (Figures 3–9 to 3–11). There is little hypertrophy of epithelial cells as seen in BDA, and epithelial differentiation is rudimentary. Hyperplasia is the dominant feature and, perhaps because of this, epithelial cells do not show appreciable degrees of specialization. The appearances are sufficiently distinctive to require separate recognition.

An adenosis which is basically indistinguishable from that just described except that it forms more diffuse cuffs of proliferating tissue, rather than nodular outgrowths, also originates from the small ducts rather than from the lobules (Figures 3–12 to 3–14). This conclusion is based on a serial study of two cases by the writer. Tanaka and Oota (1970) reached similar conclusions about sclerosing adenosis in general and likened the proliferation to bundles of noodles twisted around the ducts of origin. The writer agrees with Tanaka and Oota (1970) that these forms of nodular and more diffuse adenosis do have a ductal origin in some cases, though it is too early to say that none originates from lobules also. Still less can one say, as Tanaka and Oota (1970) maintained, that *all* sclerosing adenosis has its origin in ducts to the exclusion of a lobular origin. It is generally held that sclerosing adenosis of the classical variety originates in lobules and the writer shares this view.

In conclusion, one can say that in *classical BDA* hypertrophy of epithelium is the dominant finding, in *microcystic BDA* there is both hypertrophy and hyperplasia of the epithelium, whereas in *nodular adenosis* there is predominant hyperplasia manifesting itself as a florid microadenosis. Nodular adenosis represents a bridging link between BDA and sclerosing adenosis.

Adenosis with Involution of the Connective Tissue Element

The descriptions of adenosis given here by no means exhaust all the appearances commonly encountered. Thus, for instance, the characteristic changes are sometimes superimposed on lobules which have undergone partial involution. The residual epithelium in these lobules is apparently not immune to the influences which induce hypertrophy in non-involuting tissue. Because of stromal involution, the specialized lobular connective tissue is sclerosed and thus this BDA is not associated with any specialized stroma. BDA may also lack a specialized stroma when stromal involution occurs after the lesion has developed, whilst the epithelial lesion persists. Changes of this type are called 'mazoplasia' in some modern texts. Terms like mazoplasia serve only to confuse; they are usually undefined and, indeed, probably indefinable in any meaningful sense. Rather than label minor variations in appearance by artificial names, we should attempt to describe the appearances accurately and to think in terms of disease processes, their interrelationships and the appearances they produce when they co-exist or are complicated by involutional changes. Since so little is known about the aetiology of breast disorders, one must try all the harder to unravel the complex pathology and to probe into pathogenetic mechanisms.

Sclerosing Adenosis

Sclerosing adenosis is the other major variety of adenosis that has received specific recognition and been given a distinctive label. Foote and Stewart (1945) wrote a precise description of this condition which has never been bettered. Dawson (1954) also wrote a definitive paper on the subject over two decades ago, referring to it as a 'little known mammary picture'. The classical form of sclerosing adenosis is too well known to need any description here. Apart from the classical form, however, there are *two variants or related*

conditions to be considered. One has already been described under the non-committal designation of *'nodular adenosis'*. The other, more important one, which is sometimes referred to as 'sclerosing adenosis with pseudo-infiltration', is best termed '*infiltrating epitheliosis*'. This forms a bridging link between epitheliosis and sclerosing adenosis. It is fully described on page 174 ff.

Mixed and Transitional Forms of Adenosis

The foregoing is not meant to imply that the different types of adenosis or BDA are distinct entities. They are usually found in association with one another, although one type may be dominant in a given case or in some areas of the breast. It must be stressed that mixed forms abound and that transitions between one type and another may be present. Because of such transitions it is perfectly possible for the same section to be labelled BDA by one observer and sclerosing adenosis by another, equally skilled, pathologist. The purpose of describing the variants of adenosis in some detail is to draw attention to the complexity of the disorders and attempt to analyse objectively the major types of change that are seen. By so doing it is hoped that the complex pathology can be more clearly defined, an aim which requires the use of a definable and reasonably standardized terminology.

INTERRELATIONSHIPS OF BENIGN EPITHELIAL HYPERPLASIAS

Figure 3–15 is a schematic representation of the various types of adenosis and epitheliosis and of their interrelationships. The primary division into *organoid* and *non-organoid* lesions is a useful one, especially when combined with the division into *non-infiltrative* and *infiltrative* lesions. Organoid refers to the lobular origin of some forms and their micronodular configuration, with significant participation of both epithelial and myoepithelial elements and association with a specialized stroma. It can be seen that epitheliosis and infiltrating epitheliosis are non-organoid, while sclerosing adenosis occupies an intermediate position, some forms having an organoid

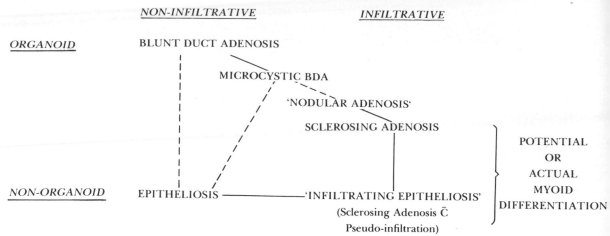

Figure 3–15   Benign epithelial hyperplasias.

structure while some lack it or lose it, because of the indistinctness of the nodular outlines and because of collagenous sclerosis. It is precisely because of this partial lack of an organoid pattern that sclerosing adenosis can be confused with malignant disease. This applies even more to the variant known as 'infiltrating epitheliosis'. Thus the non-organoid, non-infiltrative lesion (epitheliosis) has to be distinguished from in situ carcinoma, while the non-organoid infiltrative lesions (infiltrating epitheliosis and some types of sclerosing adenosis) have to be distinguished from infiltrating carcinoma. The continuous lines in Figure 3–15 are meant to indicate the close relationship between many of the disorders represented in the diagram, while the interrupted lines indicate affinities which are not as close.

References

Black, M. M., Barclay, T. H. C., Cutler, S. J., Hankey, B. F. and Asire, A. J. (1972) Association of atypical characteristics of benign breast lesions with subsequent risk of breast cancer. *Cancer*, **29**, 338–343.

Bonser, G. M., Dossett, J. A. and Jull, J. W. (1961) *Human and Experimental Breast Cancer*. London: Pitman Medical.

Dawson, E. K. (1954) Fibrosing adenosis: a little recognized mammary picture. *Edinburgh Medical Journal*, **61**, 391–401.

Foote, F. W. and Stewart, F. W. (1945) Comparative studies of cancerous versus noncancerous breast. I. Basic morphologic characteristics. *Annals of Surgery*, **121**, 6–53.

Tanaka, Y. and Oota, K. (1970) A stereomicroscopic study of the mastopathic human breast. I. Three-dimensional structures of abnormal duct evolution and their histologic entity. *Virchows Archiv A: Pathology*, **349**, 195–214.

Vassar, P. S. and Culling, C. F. A. (1959) Fibrosis of the breast. *Archives of Pathology*, **67**, 128–133.

Chapter Four

Fibroadenoma

Modifications or variations of the characteristic structure of a fibroadenoma may give rise to problems of interpretation. These are mostly of academic interest; at other times they are of more practical importance. In any case they must be recognized inasmuch as they reflect on an understanding of breast disease in general.

METAPLASIA AND ITS IMPLICATIONS

EPITHELIAL CHANGES

Apocrine Metaplasia. Apocrine epithelium is a fairly frequent component of a fibroadenoma although its presence is not often mentioned in the literature. In routine examination it has been found by the writer in no fewer than 14 per cent of 100 consecutive tumours and no doubt more extensive sampling would reveal its presence even more frequently. Usually it is present only in small foci and hence it often escapes recognition; only when the apocrine change is more extensive is it readily identified, and then its presence does attract attention. It is of no practical significance; its presence merely reflects the fact that, in general, apocrine metaplasia is more frequent in lobular diseases than it is in diseases which affect the ducts.

In addition to apocrine metaplasia within the substance of the tumour, apocrine cysts are not infrequently congregated in a crescent along the edge of the tumour, but it is doubtful whether the latter should be regarded as an integral part of the tumour. Their position and orientation suggest rather that they represent a modification of adjacent lobules, induced secondarily by the presence of the tumour. Apocrine metaplasia within the tumour or adjacent to it, as just described, may be partly responsible for the view sometimes expressed that fibroadenoma and cystic disease are part of the same disease process. However, in general, they should be regarded as quite distinct entities, even though very occasionally a fibroadenomatoid hyperplasia does appear to form part of the cystic mastopathy complex. This is the exception that proves the rule.

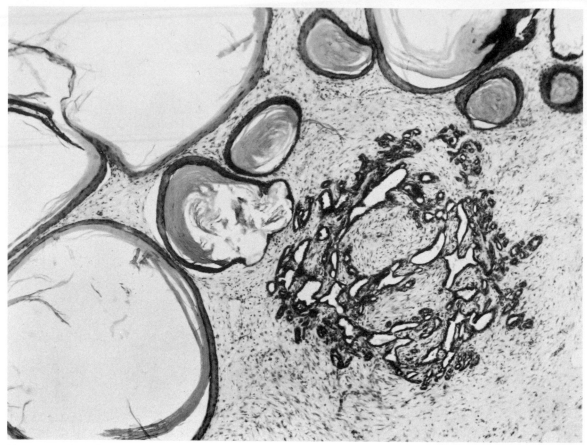

Figure 4–1   Keratinous squamous cysts in a giant fibroadenoma. A focus of sclerosing adenosis is also present. H and E. ×60. (By courtesy of Dr R. Salm.)

Squamous Metaplasia in fibroadenomas is rare. The writer has seen a case in which squamous cysts containing keratin were the dominant epithelial component of the tumour (Figure 4–1). Squamous metaplasia in a fibroadenoma was described by Salm (1957). It is worth noting at this point that squamous metaplasia is rare in benign breast disease of all types. The writer has occasionally seen it affecting a very small part of an otherwise normal duct, but this has been largely in selected material seen in consultation. On a solitary occasion I have even seen it affecting a single lobule. Evans (1966) mentioned its occurrence in benign ductal papillomas and the writer has also seen it rarely in this situation. Squamous metaplasia is distinctly more common in cystosarcoma phyllodes (q.v.).

Florid Epithelial Hyperplasia. Carcinoma arising primarily within a fibroadenoma generally takes the form of lobular carcinoma in situ (CLIS) (page 327). The epithelium lining the crevices of a fibroadenoma usually gives rise to little or no concern. Very occasionally there is a florid epithelial hyperplasia, sometimes with many mitoses. In practice this 'dubious' hyperplasia can be safely ignored and regarded as benign. Of course this applies only to exuberant hyperplasia restricted to the tumour itself, not to cancerization (page 325), which may affect the tumour as well as the surrounding tissue in continuity. The diagnostic problem is somewhat analogous to an exuberant hyperplasia in gynaecomastia, which is virtually always benign in practice. Why such an epithelial hyperplasia in a fibroadenoma can be safely ignored is not entirely clear, nor is it entirely certain that it never progresses to carcinoma. Nevertheless, it is a good working rule that, in the absence of cancerization or the specific features of CLIS, an unusually florid epithelial hyperplasia in a fibroadenoma has no sinister connotation.

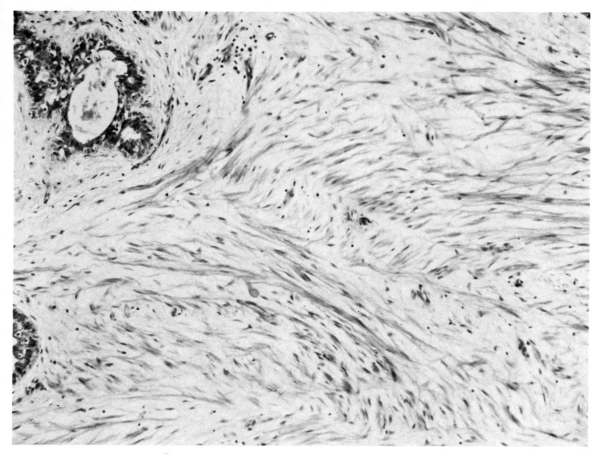

Figure 4–2 Smooth muscle differentiation in an otherwise typical fibroadenoma. H and E. ×150.

CONNECTIVE TISSUE CHANGES

Variations in the types of stromal element are less frequent than variations of the epithelial component. The connective tissue component is usually exclusively fibroblastic. There are, of course, the well-known marked variations in the cellularity, mucinous nature or hyalinization of the connective tissue element. Adipose tissue may be found in a fibroadenoma but it is rare. This may come about in one of two ways. Firstly, it may represent incorporated or 'included' inter-lobular stroma containing adipose tissue, since most fibroadenomas grow both by expansion and by the accretion of new foci which develop from neighbouring lobules. Secondly, adipose tissue may be the result of metaplasia in the connective tissue of the fibroadenoma itself, but this is apparently extremely rare (Willis, 1967). Calcification is common enough and a well-recognized feature of the quiescent hyalinized tumour. Cartilaginous and osseous metaplasia are rare (Willis, 1967) though common in the bitch. Smooth muscle metaplasia is one of the rarest changes encountered (Figure 4–2) (Mackenzie, 1968; Riddell and Davies, 1973). The writer has seen two instances of smooth muscle in fibro-adenomas, one in our own and one in referred material. Riddell and Davies (1973) considered their two cases to be hamartomat-ous lesions rather than fibroadenomas, a view which was entertained and considered likely in one of a total of three personally studied cases. Nevertheless, since the other two lesions were essentially similar to each other and showed the definite structure of a fibroaden-oma in part of the lesion, it is considered that some of these lesions represent fibroadenomas in which small, or more rarely large, foci of muscular metaplasia have developed.

Elastic Tissue. Negative findings can be as significant as positive ones. Thus, for example, elastic tissue is not usually found in fibroadenomas. This tallies well with the fact that fibroadenomas are lobular tumours and that elastic tissue is hardly ever seen within the lobule. The virtual absence of elastic tissue in fibroadenomas reflects the normal structure of the breast and also confirms the lobular origin of this tumour, a view which is based on independent evidence. As always, exceptions will be found. A little elastic fibre is sometimes found in a fibroadenoma and can usually be traced to the compressed interlobular tissue between the aggregates of lobular tumour, a finding which again reflects on the mode of origin and growth of fibroadenomas.

MODIFICATIONS OF BOTH EPITHELIUM
AND CONNECTIVE TISSUE

Myoid Differentiation. This is the best place to mention structural modifications that involve both the epithelium and the connective tissue element, and also alterations that involve that curiously versatile cell, the myoepithelial cell. In fibroadenomas, the latter is usually recognizable, at the light microscope level, merely as the distinct, outer, smaller cell type wedged between the bases of the epithelial cells, with a cytoplasm which is tinctorially different and which has a distinctive nuclear appearance. In pathological circumstances, the myoepithelial cell can become more prominent and can assume an elongated frankly myoid appearance, with an eosinophilic cytoplasm, an elongated rod-like nucleus and longitudinal fibrils which are easily demonstrable with phosphotungstic acid–haematoxylin, iron haematoxylin and other appropriate stains (Ahmed, 1974). This myoid differentiation is most frequently seen in sclerosing adenosis and in the larger types of ductal papilloma; myoid differentiation is characteristic of benign disease and is, for practical purposes, never seen in carcinoma of the breast. Myoid differentiation may also occur in fibroadenomas, though it is rarely a prominent finding. It is not, strictly speaking, a metaplasia in the sense of the metaplasias already described, but is rather an expression of the myoepithelial cell developing its full potential and turning into an easily recognizable myoid or, dare one say it, smooth muscle cell. One hesitates to say 'smooth muscle cell' because, to some pathologists, the concept of the conversion of a cell of epithelial origin into a connective tissue cell still has explosive

connotations, but the evidence that this can happen is so overwhelming that reluctant pathologists should abandon their scepticism. The best oncological evidence for this conversion derives from the study of benign 'mixed' tumours of the salivary gland and other sites. Myoepithelial cells show every transition to chondroid tissue and even to true cartilage, sufficiently like cartilage for the host to treat it as such in the sense that it can, and does, undergo osseous transformation by a process of endochondral ossification. This is seen most frequently in the 'mixed' salivary-type tumour of the skin or chondroid syringoma but also, very rarely, in the 'mixed' tumour of the salivary glands.

Sclerosing Adenosis. Another change in fibroadenomas that can give rise to puzzling appearances and even difficulties in diagnosis is sclerosing adenosis (Figure 4–1). The writer has found this change in less than 10 per cent of a consecutive series of 100 tumours and it was conspicuous in only 6 per cent of cases. Sclerosing adenosis affects both the epithelial and connective tissue elements of the tumour. In the involved part the changes are the same as those seen in sclerosing adenosis as it affects non-neoplastic breast tissue. Myoid differentiation may be present in the foci of sclerosing adenosis in the same way as it occurs in sclerosing adenosis in general. The presence of sclerosing adenosis in fibroadenoma does not correlate with other histological features or with any special clinical data, apart from its tendency to affect patients who are somewhat older than the mean age for fibroadenoma. It is not known whether, in such cases, there is a greater likelihood of sclerosing adenosis being present also in the non-neoplastic breast tissue, since the tumours are generally shelled out without significant amounts of the surrounding non-neoplastic tissue.

SECRETORY ACTIVITY

Effects of Pregnancy and Hormone Administration. In pregnancy, changes that affect the normal breast can also, to a variable degree, affect a fibroadenoma. The secretory changes of pregnancy are frequently reflected, at least in part, in the tumour. It has become apparent that exogenous hormone therapy, as with the contraceptive pill, can have the same effect.

The writer has seen these changes when large doses of hormone have been used, and especially in patients on Depo-Provera (medroxyprogesterone acetate).

INFARCTION OF FIBROADENOMA

A phenomenon which deserves wider recognition and attention than it has received hitherto is infarction of a fibroadenoma and the whole question of spontaneous mammary infarction, whether in a fibroadenoma or not. Infarction of a fibroadenoma was first described by Delarue and Redon (1949). In three of their six patients the clinical suspicion of carcinoma was sufficiently great to have led to a mastectomy without prior biopsy: a fourth patient had a partial mastectomy.

Despite this early reference, no mention is made of it in standard textbooks of pathology and it was a surgeon who first drew our attention to it in a textbook (Haagensen, 1971). Haagensen found five cases of infarcted fibroadenoma in a series of about 1000 tumours, an incidence of one in 200 tumours.

Pambakian and Tighe (1971) focused attention on this condition and made a number of important observations. They found no fewer than three patients with mammary infarction during an 18-month period at one large hospital: two had infarction of fibroadenomas, while the third had no apparent underlying tumour. They drew attention to the danger of misdiagnosis on frozen section expecially if the condition is not well known and the possibility not even considered. Two of their three patients were Negresses. The presentation was usually with a slightly tender lump in the breast. Of their two patients with infarction in fibroadenomas, one was postpartum, the other a 59-year-old postmenopausal woman.

All 10 of the patients described by Wilkinson and Green (1964) with mammary infarction were pregnant or lactating. It is not clear how many of these patients had an underlying fibroadenoma, and this paper is sometimes referred to as illustrating mammary infarction in the absence of an underlying tumour. However, Wilkinson and Green (1964) described an underlying fibroadenoma in two of their patients and an 'adenoma' of lactation as the background lesion in six further cases, while in the remaining two only 'lobular hyperplasia' was present. Thus, it seems probable that no fewer than eight of their 10 patients had an underlying fibroadenoma or a related tumour which underwent infarction.

Newman and Kahn (1973) reported on five patients with infarcted fibroadenomas; in contrast with the findings of most recent workers, only one case was associated with pregnancy and lactation. Two further instances associated with pregnancy were reported by Majmudar and Rosales-Quintana (1975).

Infarction of bilateral, and bilateral and multiple, tumours was recorded by Pambakian and Tighe (1971) and by Majmudar and Rosales-Quintana (1975) respectively.

Infarction of a fibroadenoma can be partial, subtotal or even total (Figures 4–3 and 4–4). Pregnancy and lactation are the main known predisposing factors and the more extensive instances of infarction have mostly been observed in such patients (Figure 4–3). Case 1 of Pambakian and Tighe (1971) in a postmenopausal woman and no fewer than four cases of Newman and Kahn (1973) are notable exceptions. The writer has studied four cases of infarction, three of them in pregnant or lactating women; in two patients there was a history of tenderness or pain. Pain, tenderness or transient pain was present in at least three of the five cases of Newman and Kahn (1973). On the other hand, no symptoms attributable to infarction were noted by Haagensen (1971).

The pathogenesis of this condition is obscure. It has been attributed to a relative vascular insufficiency brought about by the increased proliferative, secretory and general metabolic activity in the breast, and this seems a very plausible explanation for the phenomenon when it occurs in pregnant and lactating women. It is very difficult to understand the mechanism in the very rare cases found postmenopausally (Case 1 of Pambakian and Tighe, 1971), especially since fibroadenomas at this period of life are generally dormant quiescent lesions. Evidence of vascular disease has not been noted in most specimens but was seen in two of the five cases of Newman and Kahn (1973). However, because of the relatively small size of the thrombosed vessels, they could not be certain that the thrombosis was not the result of the infarction rather than its cause. The pathogenesis of infarction in fibroadenomas requires further study.

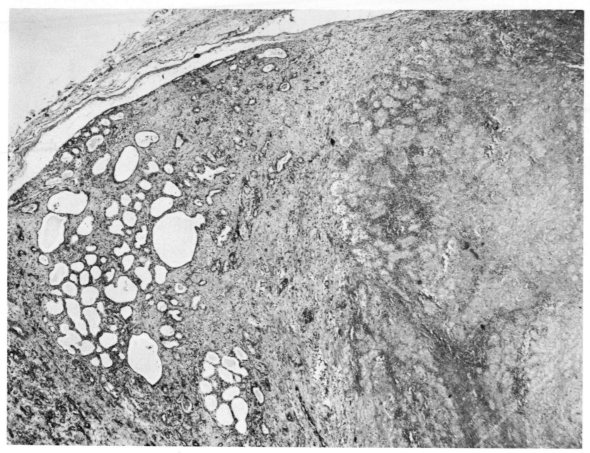

Figure 4–3 Subtotal infarction of a fibroadenoma during pregnancy. H and E. ×40.

Other instances of this phenomenon have probably been missed in the past, since the condition appears to be commoner than the scanty literature on the subject would suggest. The condition may be mistaken for infarction of non-neoplastic mammary tissue and the presence of an underlying fibroadenoma go completely unnoticed. When necrosis is very extensive, careful examination and adequate sampling of the periphery of the lesion is essential, for it is here that a rim of surviving tissue may provide a clue to the presence of an underlying tumour. Reticulin silver impregnation is invaluable for outlining ghost structures in the necrotic tissue and the trichrome stains are superior to haemalum–eosin for this purpose.

INFARCTION UNRELATED TO FIBROADENOMA

Infarction of a fibroadenoma must be distinguished from spontaneous infarction of non-neoplastic breast tissue occurring in late pregnancy or in the puerperium. These patients present with a palpable, usually painless, lump. Although transient tenderness is sometimes experienced, the mass may be mistaken clinically for a malignant tumour. The possibility of confusion with carcinoma is even greater in frozen sections. Knowledge of the existence of this entity should assist the pathologist in avoiding an erroneous diagnosis of carcinoma. It cannot be emphasized too strongly that full clinical data must be supplied to the pathologist to help eliminate the possibility of error.

The true incidence of spontaneous infarction is difficult to determine: Lucey (1975) expressed the view that many cases reported as infarction in 'adenoma' or 'lactation adenoma' represent mistaken diagnoses and actually represent instances of spontaneous infarction of normal mammary tissue. Hasson and Pope (1961) were apparently the first to draw attention to the condition of spontane-

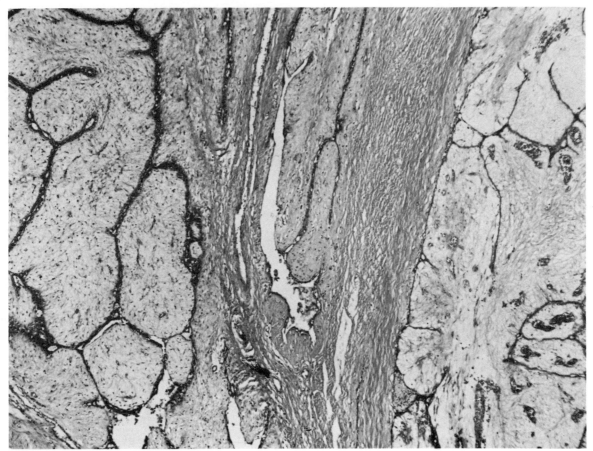

Figure 4–4   Partial infarction of a fibroadenoma in a non-pregnant woman. There is early necrosis of tumour tissue to the right. H and E. ×40.

ous infarction of non neoplastic breast tissue and described three such cases. Further instances have been documented by Wilkinson and Green (1964) and Pambakian and Tighe (1971) and are cited in the literature as documented by Rickert and Rajan (1974). However, only two of the 10 reported on by Wilkinson and Green (1964) and only one of the three cases of Pambakian and Tighe (1971) did not involve an underlying tumour. Also, Rickert and Rajan (1974) in fact reported on two adolescent pregnant girls of 19 and 17 years, each of whom had two distinct infarcted fibroadenomas. They even stressed the necessity of reticulin impregnations in order to demonstrate the architectural features of the necrotic zones. From an analysis of the literature and personal observations, I suspect that the more usual error is in the reverse direction from that postulated by Lucey (1975).

RACIAL DIFFERENCES: MULTIPLE, GIANT AND 'JUVENILE' FIBROADENOMAS

Race. According to Haagensen (1971) fibroadenomas are said to be more common in Negroes than in Caucasians, though he had no personal data to confirm this. Haagensen (1971) was under the impression that fibroadenomas are more often multiple in Negroes than in other races, but actual analysis of the data showed that the incidence of multiplicity was around 20 per cent in both racial groups.

Giant Fibroadenoma and Multiple Fibro-adenomas. The massive or giant fibroadenoma of the adolescent female should be regarded as a more or less distinct clinicopathological entity (Nambiar and Kannan Kutty, 1974). Haagensen (1971) had seven patients in this category, of whom five were Negro and only two Caucasian. The truly giant fibroadenoma is commoner in Negroes and occurs predominantly in young patients between the ages of 10 and 20 years. This is as distinct from cystosarcoma phyllodes, which is commoner in the succeeding decades: this difference in age incidence is one of the distinctions to emerge between giant fibroadenoma and cystosarcoma phyllodes. Of Haagensen's seven massive tumours, five were solitary while two were multiple and bilateral, filling both breasts more or less completely.

Fibroadenoma in Adolescents. Nambiar and Kannan Kutty (1974) reported on a series of 25 patients with giant fibroadenoma in adolescent females. They reviewed the literature extensively and found 61 other cases, making a total of 86 patients. Their patients ranged in age from 11 to 20 years, with seven of the 25 under 15 years of age. In three patients the lump was noticed before the menarche, in another three in the same year as menarche. The children under 15 years of age showed a rapid increase in the size of the swelling from the onset to clinical presentation, within six months. In the patients between 18 and 20 years, there was a two- to three-year history of a lump with recent enlargement. The average size of the tumours was 12 cm and six were as large as 18 cm.

Dilated veins in the skin of the breast were noted in 20 of 25 patients, with ulceration of the skin in three.

Although bilateral tumours of this type were reported in nine of the cases tabulated by Nambiar and Kannan Kutty (1974), none of their own 25 patients presented in this way: three had an ordinary small fibroadenoma in the opposite breast.

Of their 25 patients, 15 were Chinese, eight were Malays and the remaining two were Indian. They concluded that Chinese women may share with Negroes a greater propensity to develop this disease than some other races, although adolescent Chinese girls, unlike Negroes, have much smaller breasts.

These lesions were all treated by local excision only and there were no recurrences or distant metastases. Twelve patients had been followed for between five and eight years and six patients between two and five years, with the rest observed for shorter periods only. Normal breast development ensued in all patients following local excision with careful suturing together of the conserved

normal breast tissue. These workers strongly supported the view of Ashikari, Farrow and O'Hara (1971) that local excision is the treatment of choice. They stressed that mastectomy had frequently been performed in the past in the treatment of this condition; yet, in the 61 collected cases from the literature and tabulated by them, there was not a single instance of malignant behaviour.

Mastectomy is clearly unnecessary in the treatment of this condition and is particularly to be condemned in this age group. Nambiar and Kannan Kutty (1974) rightly stressed that the term 'cystosarcoma phyllodes' with its potentially ominous implications to the surgeon should be used with great caution in patients under 20 years of age.

Three of the 25 tumours of Nambiar and Kannan Kutty (1974) were regarded as fibrosarcomatous histologically and were classified as 'borderline' cystosarcoma phyllodes. These tumours, however, were not associated with a sinister outlook and the authors found a discrepancy in this age group between the histological findings and the clinical behaviour of the tumours. This is a discrepancy which is also seen in adult patients to some extent (Norris and Taylor, 1967), hence the necessity for retaining a 'borderline' category of tumours according to most workers. It would appear that, in the younger age groups, greater latitude should probably be allowed for the inclusion of tumours in the fibroadenoma as opposed to the cystosarcoma category. Even in the rare event of one making a diagnosis of cystosarcoma, this should always be prefaced by the qualification 'benign', unless there is extremely strong evidence for doing otherwise. In this way the tragedy of a mastectomy in a young girl can be avoided. The cautionary tale of these workers is a very important one. The term cystosarcoma, especially unqualified by the prefix 'benign', should never be used in a pathological report unless one is certain that the surgeon concerned knows exactly what this signifies. And this applies also, of course, to adult patients.

'Juvenile type' of Fibroadenoma. Ashikari, Farrow and O'Hara (1971) studied 181 fibroadenomas in adolescent female patients. Of these, 169 were classified microscopically as 'adult' in type, while 12 belonged to a 'juvenile' category of fibroadenoma. Thus almost 93 per cent of these fibroadenomas found in adolescence were of the conventional

type seen in adult women while 7 per cent were of the so-called 'juvenile' variety. These workers identified six additional juvenile-type tumours from the years preceding those of their main study group: 18 juvenile-type fibroadenomas were thus available for study.

These 'juvenile fibroadenomas' were apparently more floridly glandular than the conventional variety and their stroma rather more cellular. This was the primary means of identification of this microscopic variant.

There were nine Negro and nine Caucasian girls (the latter including one of mixed white and Japanese parentage). The juvenile type of fibroadenoma is said to be relatively commoner in Negroes, with a 1/1 ratio of Negro to Caucasian patients, while the adult type was commoner in whites, with a ratio of 103 whites to 63 Negroes.

The juvenile type of fibroadenoma is usually larger than the adult type, with the largest tumour in this series measuring 19 cm. Some of the tumours reported on by these workers would obviously fall, therefore, into the giant fibroadenoma category, which is one of the main reasons for including them here.

Ashikari, Farrow and O'Hara (1971) considered and illustrated the differences between the juvenile fibroadenoma, on the one hand, and the adult type of fibroadenoma and benign cystosarcoma phyllodes, on the other. The latter is very rare in the adolescent age group. They also pointed out important clinical differences from virginal hypertrophy of the breast, with which juvenile fibroadenoma can be confused clinically.

Treatment of the juvenile fibroadenoma consists of simple excision only.

It remains to be ascertained how distinct the juvenile type of fibroadenoma is at the microscopic level. Most of these lesions appear to qualify as giant fibroadenomas.

'Cystosarcoma' in Adolescents. There were only three cases of cystosarcoma phyllodes in girls under 20 years of age in the series of McDivitt, Urban and Farrow (1967) and a further three among the 94 patients reported on by Norris and Taylor (1967). Amerson (1970) reported on seven adolescent patients with cystosarcoma phyllodes. They were all Negroes. All seven were classified histologically as benign. While the consideration of cystosarcoma phyllodes belongs properly in another place (Chapter Fourteen), Amerson (1970) stressed the relatively benign be-

haviour of these tumours in adolescents. Amerson (1970) strongly supported the contention of Wulsin (1960) that cystosarcoma phyllodes in the adolescent age group behaves rather differently from the same tumours when they occur in adults and that they should generally be treated as if they were only large fibroadenomas. Judging by the illustrations of Amerson (1970) some, at least, of his tumours would indeed seem to qualify for the cystosarcoma category, albeit the benign one. Amerson (1970) reviewed a total of 20 cases of cystosarcoma phyllodes in prepubertal and adolescent females reported in the American literature: 18 were classified as benign and two as malignant. Amerson (1970) stressed that, at that time, there had been no reported instances of distant metastasis or deaths from cystosarcoma in this age group. This remained true up to 1977 with the solitary exception of a fatal cystosarcoma in a 14-year-old girl (see Chapter Fourteen).

Cystosarcoma phyllodes in children is extremely rare; it is possibly commoner in Negroes. When it occurs, it is almost always of the benign variety. Malignant cystosarcoma in adolescence is an extremely rare tumour and such a diagnosis should be entertained only after extensive and appropriate consultation. Only in this way can these girls and young women be saved from unnecessarily extensive surgery.

FIBROADENOMA VARIANT

During the last 10 years the writer has collected more than 20 benign breast tumours which are essentially related to fibroadenomas in structure and composition but which show sufficient difference to raise problems in diagnosis and precise classification. When these lesions were shown to other pathologists similar difficulties were experienced, though they have usually, but by no means invariably, been recognized as lesions with varying degrees of affinity to fibroadenomas. Indeed, a number of these cases have only come to light in consultation with experienced pathologists who were puzzled by certain odd features in these fibroadenoma-like lesions. The combination of certain special features establishes these tumours as a reasonably well-delineated entity.

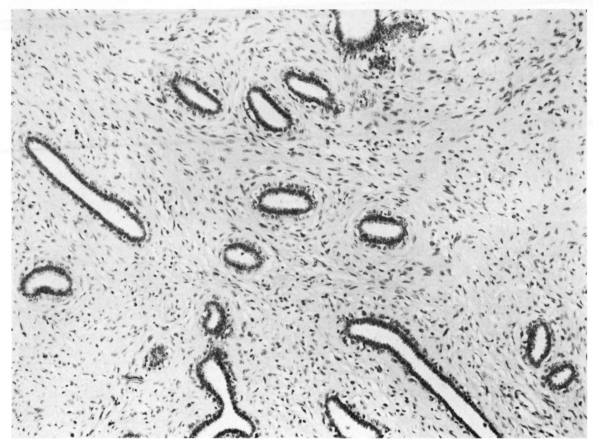

Figure 4–5 Fibroadenoma variant measuring 1.5 cm in diameter. The tumour has a very cellular yet collagenous connective tissue component. H and E. ×150.

Connective Tissue. The tumours possess an unusual type of connective tissue, often associated with a somewhat unusual epithelial element also (Figures 4–5 and 4–6). They are circumscribed and well delineated as with conventional fibroadenomas. The stroma is, at one and the same time, highly collagenous and cellular, this being one of the main features which gives these lesions their distinctive appearance. Conventional fibroadenomas usually have a mucoid cellular connective tissue component or a more fibrous or even hyalinized one, depending on the state of activity of a particular tumour — whether it is in an actively growing phase or in a relatively dormant or quiescent phase of its life cycle. In the lesions under consideration the connective tissue is highly collagenous but also cellular with abundant fibroblasts, the interstitial and cellular components frequently having a somewhat laminated appearance (Figures 4–5 and 4–6). In addition, lymphocytes, diffusely distributed or focally arranged, are usually more numerous and conspicuous than in a typical fibroadenoma. In some cases plasma cells form an appreciable proportion of this infiltrate.

Epithelial Tissue. It is the nature and general appearance of the connective tissue which first drew attention to this type of lesion. But closer inspection, and careful comparison with typical fibroadenomas, led to the recognition of subtle differences in the epithelial component also. This has the usual two-layered arrangement but there is sometimes an increase of the N/C ratio and an increased vesicularity of the nuclei of the epithelial cells. There is no appreciable difference in the amount of mitotic activity.

Relationship to Conventional Fibroadenoma. It is possible that this type of lesion represents merely a special type of pericanalicular fibroadenoma in a particular growth phase,

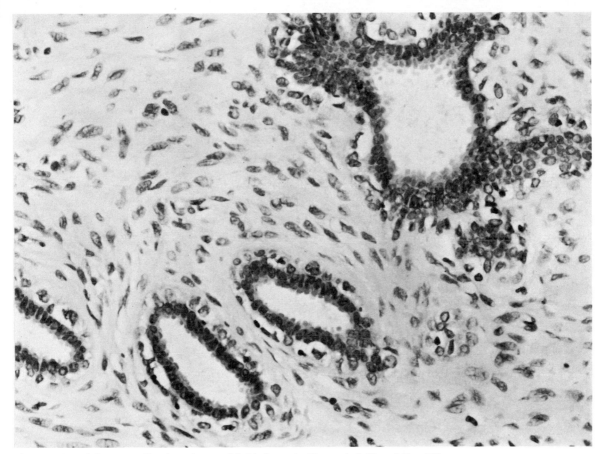

Figure 4–6 . Higher magnification of part of field shown in Figure 4–5. H and E. ×400.

but this would seem to be an oversimplification. Perhaps it is best classified provisionally as a variant of fibroadenoma until more has been learnt about it. Clinical data do not so far suggest any significant differences between it and the ordinary fibroadenoma. Specifically, there is nothing to suggest that treatment with the contraceptive pill is in any way responsible for its development. Having initially segregated this small group of distinctive tumours, study of all cases coded as fibroadenoma revealed that about 5 per cent showed some features of the segregated group. This suggests that the group under discussion does probably represent one one end of a spectrum and that it has close links with fibroadenoma. Nevertheless the end of the spectrum, if such it be, requires separate recognition because of its distinctive appearance, highlighted by the problems of diagnosis and classification experienced by pathologists who have seen these tumours.

Relationship to Benign Cystosarcoma Phyllodes. This group of tumours may also have affinities with the benign cystosarcoma phyllodes. In a few of the tumours a reasonable case could be made for classifying them in this way. Nevertheless, their connective tissue component is generally less cellular than the connective tissue component of the benign cystosarcoma phyllodes. If, in a particular case, there is difficulty in distinguishing between the fibroadenoma variant and benign cystosarcoma phyllodes, the lesion should be regarded as a fibroadenoma and treated as such. The average age of the patients with the fibroadenoma variant is the same as for fibroadenoma in general, and the size of the tumours is also similar. At this stage, however, it would be unwise to deny that there might be an overlap between the fibroadenoma variant and benign cystosarcoma. This is of some importance when one comes to consider the relative frequency of benign and malignant

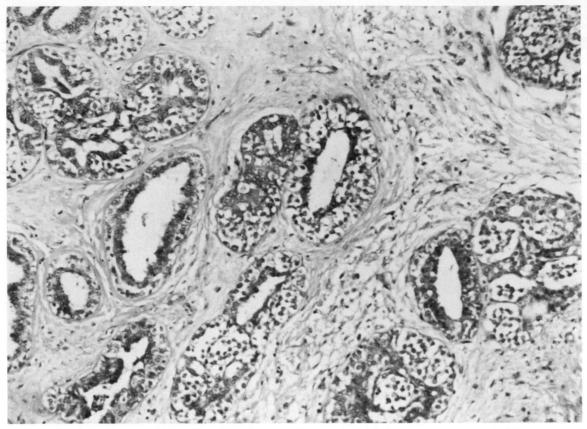

Figure 4–7 Fibroadenoma with proliferation of outer cell type of glandular spaces as nests and diffuse zones of argyrophilic cells. This is easily confused with lobular carcinoma in situ. H and E. ×150.

cystosarcomas. If some of the cases described here as fibroadenoma variant are classified as benign cystosarcoma, the number of tumours diagnosed as benign cystosarcoma becomes greater and the proportion of benign to malignant cystosarcomas rises accordingly. This is one of the many reasons why it is so difficult to state precisely what the ratio is between benign and malignant cystosarcoma (page 357). But there are other, more important reasons also.

ARGYROPHILIC CELLS IN FIBROADENOMAS

One of this curious group of tumours ('fibroadenoma variant') showed a very unusual feature (Figures 4–7 to 4–9). The outer cell layer showed such an unusual degree of proliferation that it overshadowed the inner epithelial layer in parts of the tumour. The outer layer sometimes lined the

Figure 4–8 (*Opposite, above.*) Same tissue as shown in Figure 4–7. The contrast between the cells in the buds and ordinary epithelial cells is well shown. One of the two elongated clumps in this field consists almost exclusively of cells of the type which constitute discrete buds in other areas. H and E. ×400.

Figure 4–9 (*Opposite, below.*) Same tissue as the two preceding illustrations. Here the proliferation takes the form of nearly solid clumps with little evidence of epithelial cells of the type ordinarily seen in fibroadenomas. H and E. ×400.

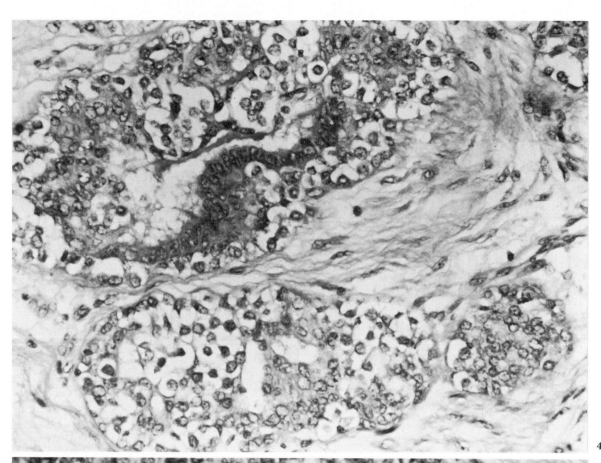

4–8

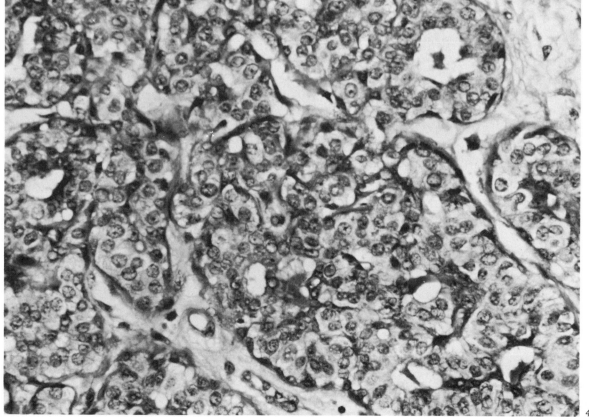

4–9

51

epithelial lumina because the inner layer was completely absent in these areas. But the main proliferative activity of the outer cell layer took the form of solid sprouts and buds that projected away from the lumina towards the adjacent connective tissue. These cells had large vesicular nuclei that contrasted sharply with the smaller darker nuclei of the epithelial cells (Figures 4–7 and 4–8). The most surprising feature was the fact that these proliferating outer cells were argyrophilic with the Bodian silver impregnation method. To my knowledge, this unique finding of argyrophilic cells in a benign breast tumour has not been recorded previously. Apart from the intrinsic interest of this finding, it also illustrates that the outer cell layer of the epithelial component of a fibroadenoma, which usually consists of myoepithelial cells, can at times differentiate in other directions. It has previously been pointed out that it can develop into easily recognizable myoid cells. The differentiation into argyrophil (? endocrine-type) cells suggests that the differentiating potentialities of the generative epithelium of the breast are not yet fully appreciated.

Very recently a second case of fibroadenoma containing argyrophil cells has been seen in consultation. This particular tumour is inportant for a number of reasons. Firstly, its identity as a fibroadenoma was not very evident to some pathologists. Secondly it showed an even greater degree of solid compact budding of the outer cell type than in the first case. It was for this reason considered by the contributor to contain a lobular carcinoma in situ (CLIS). By the generally accepted criteria this appeared to be CLIS in a fibroadenoma or a fibroadenoma variant, as here defined. On careful study, the neoplastic buds appeared slightly more cohesive than is usual in CLIS and the neoplastic cells had, in parts, a slightly more granular cytoplasm; the overall appearance suggested the possibility of an endocrine tumour, especially one of the carcinoid variety. Bodian silver impregnation showed argyrophilia of these cell buds and Grimelius silver impregnation a much weaker argyrophilia. This appears to confirm the probable endocrine nature of the neoplasm. No argentaffin cells are demonstrable by the conventional methods used to detect them. In the literal sense this case shows 'lobular neoplasia' in situ. Haagensen (1971) preferred this term to CLIS because of his firm belief that the designation 'carcinoma' should not be

applied to it in view of its behaviour (Chapter Ten). Since it would now appear that lobular epithelial tumours can take a form other than that of orthodox carcinoma (or adenoma), the value of the term 'lobular neoplasia' may be even greater than has been appreciated hitherto.

Lobular Endocrine Tumour. It appears that 'lobular neoplasia' includes not only the tumour that is usually called CLIS or LCIS but also an endocrine-type tumour which is argyrophilic. The two examples studied have both been situated within fibroadenomas and, probably fortuitously, one was in a 'fibroadenoma variant'. At the time of writing, a third case has just been studied and this was situated in a conventional fibroadenoma. These three tumours have been seen during the last four years and it is almost certain that they cannot be as rare as would appear currently. Tumours of this type could doubtless be easily missed and regarded as examples of an unusually florid epithelial hyperplasia in a fibroadenoma or else they could masquerade in the guise of an ordinary lobular carcinoma in situ.

The relationship of this lobular endocrine tumour (? carcinoid) to CLIS remains to be explored. If intermediate forms are discovered, one might be dealing with a position analogous to that seen in the large bowel, vermiform appendix and even the prostate, in which tumours exist which are at one and the same time mucin-secreting epithelial tumours and carcinoid (Azzopardi and Evans, 1971). That such a relationship probably exists in the breast is suggested by a case of bilateral infiltrating carcinoma in my collection, in which parts of the in situ lesions on both sides show argyrophilic cells detected only by the Grimelius method. This is a field wide open to investigation by light microscopic, histochemical, silver impregnation and ultrastructural techniques.

TUBULAR ADENOMA AND 'LACTATING ADENOMA'

The existence as a separate entity of a 'pure adenoma' of the breast has, until recently, been the subject of much argument. There is little doubt that many, if not most, of the cases so labelled in the older literature were merely

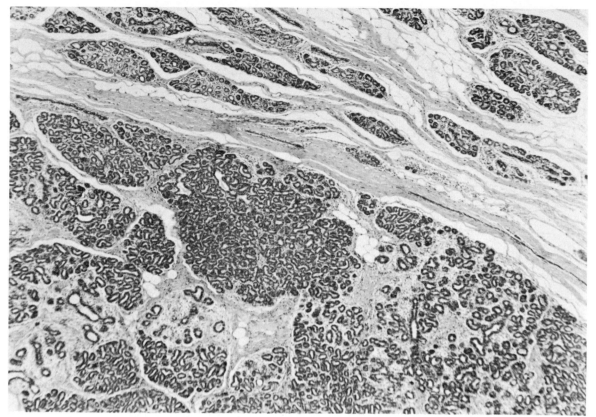

Figure 4–10   The edge of a pure or tubular adenoma. The junction with normal tissue is shown. H and E. ×45.

variants of fibroadenoma. Persaud, Talerman and Jordan (1968) accepted only two cases from the entire literature as authentic examples of pure adenoma of the breast and added a third well-documented case of their own.

That a 'pure adenoma' of the breast exists as a distinct entity has been fully established by Hertel, Zaloudek and Kempson (1976). In this rare type of tumour, the amount of connective tissue is very scanty and no more than one would expect as a supporting scaffolding (Figures 4–10 and 4–11). There is nothing to suggest that the trivial amount of stroma present is an integral part of the tumour in the sense that the fibroadenoma is a genuinely fibroepithelial tumour: the epithelial element is the sole neoplastic ingredient. The tubular adenomas or pure adenomas are sharply demarcated nodules without a true capsule. They are homogeneous and characterized by uniform, closely approximated, small tubular structures (averaging 30 to 50 μm) lined by a prominent epithelial-cell layer and an attenuated, inconspicuous and sometimes barely visible myoepithelial-cell layer. These tubules are almost indistinguishable from the smallest units of the normal breast lobule. Cellular atypia is conspicuous by its absence. A few larger epithelial structures cut at various angles are also present. As indicated, the stroma is scanty and consists of a delicate fibrovascular network. Some diffuse lymphocytic infiltration is commonly present.

'Lactating adenoma' is a debatable entity which was regarded by Hertel, Zaloudek and Kempson (1976) as very closely related to tubular adenoma. They regarded the two tumours, on very reasonable evidence, as 'the same biologic process examined during different physiologic states'. Persaud, Talerman and Jordan (1968), on the other hand, regarded 'lactating adenoma' as a mere fibroadenoma affected by pregnancy changes.

Both tubular adenoma and lactating adenoma are benign tumours, though three

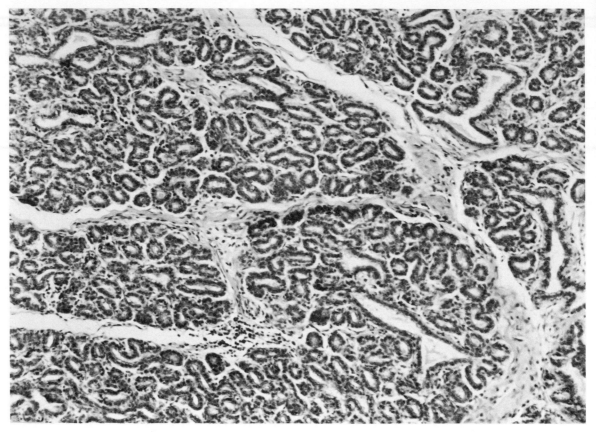

Figure 4–11   A tubular adenoma of the breast. H and E. ×150.

cases of carcinoma in association with adenoma have now been reported (Hertel, Zaloudek and Kempson, 1976).

There is no association between tubular adenomas and the administration of oral contraceptive hormones, and none is said to exist for lactating adenomas either.

Ultrastructural Studies showed that tubular adenomas retain a normal epithelial–stromal junction (ESJ). This contrasts with the disruption found in the ESJ in fibroadenomas (Hertel, Zaloudek and Kempson, 1976). This important finding, if confirmed, adds another criterion in the separation of tubular adenoma from fibroadenoma. The one is not simply a variant of the other. Further data are clearly essential before it can be stated with any confidence that intermediate forms do not occur. But, even if they do, the identity of the tubular adenoma is now well established.

In the three cases of tubular adenoma in the writer's collection the features are essentially as described by Hertel, Zaloudek and Kempson (1976). In two cases there were very small foci of clear-cell change in the epithelial cells, which may represent secretory activity (material for frozen sections for fat stains was not available). This clear-cell change could not be attributed to the presence of glycogen or of mucin.

Now that a pure or tubular adenoma has been shown to exist, there is a danger of the condition being overdiagnosed, as there is a natural inclination to make a diagnosis of something exotic, unusual or new rather than of a more mundane lesion. It must be stressed that this is a very rare type of lesion, witnessed by the fact that all the writer's cases were seen in referred material. If the term is to retain any significance, the criteria for making the diagnosis should be very strict and, before new cases are reported, very extensive sampling of any given tumour is necessary. Indeed Hertel, Zaloudek and Kempson (1976) made the point that tumours exist which consist of a combination of a fibroadenoma and a tubular adenoma (Figure 4–12).

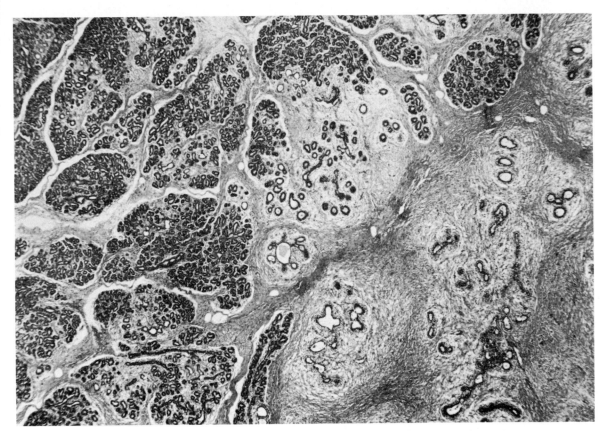

Figure 4–12 A tumour composed partly of fibroadenoma and partly of tubular adenoma. The junction of the two components is illustrated.

Other Adenomas

Hertel's (1976) paper puts forward a good working basis for the classification of all types of breast adenoma. The sweat-gland types of adenoma are considered in Chapter Thirteen.

Unclassified Adenomas

That individual tumours will disobey the rules is illustrated by a recently studied case which had features of a tubular adenoma, of a fibroadenoma, and of a salivary-gland type of tumour of the breast. This peculiar tumour contained moderately large amounts of elastic tissue between the epithelial elements, serving as a link with the sweat-gland and salivary-type tumours (Azzopardi and Zayid, 1972). It will be recalled that the fibroadenoma lacks elastic tissue. This extraordinary type of tumour virtually defies classification, a fact which must be allowed for in any classification.

MALIGNANCY IN FIBROADENOMA

This is discussed in Chapter Twelve.

References

Ahmed, A. (1974) The myoepithelium in human breast fibroadenoma. *Journal of Pathology,* **114,** 135–138.

Amerson, J. R. (1970) Cystosarcoma phyllodes in adolescent females: a report of seven patients. *Annals of Surgery,* **171,** 849–858.

Ashikari, R., Farrow, J. H. and O'Hara, J. (1971) Fibroadenomas in the breast of juveniles. *Journal of Surgery, Gynecology and Obstetrics,* **132,** 259-262.

Azzopardi, J. G. and Evans, D. J. (1971) Argentaffin cells in prostatic carcinoma. *Journal of Pathology,* **104,** 247–251.

Azzopardi, J. G. and Zayid, I. (1972) Elastic tissue in tumours of salivary glands. *Journal of Pathology,* **107,** 149–156.

Delarue, J. and Redon, H. (1949) Les infarctus des fibro-adénomes mammaires: problème clinique et pathogénique. *Semaine des Hôpitaux de Paris,* **25,** 2991–2996.

Evans, R. W. (1966) *Histological Appearances of Tumours.* Second edition. London: E. & S. Livingstone.

Haagensen, C. D. (1971) *Diseases of the Breast,* Second edition — Revised reprint. pp. 213, 215. Philadelphia, London, Toronto: W. B. Saunders.

Hasson, J. and Pope, C. H. (1961) Mammary infarcts associated with pregnancy presenting as breast tumors. *Surgery,* **49,** 313–316.

Hertel, B. F., Zaloudek, C. and Kempson, R. L. (1976) Breast adenomas. *Cancer,* **37,** 2891–2905.

Lucey, J. J. (1975) Spontaneous infarction of the breast. *Journal of Clinical Pathology,* **28,** 937–943.

Mackenzie, D. H. (1968) A fibro-adenoma of the breast with smooth muscle. *Journal of Pathology and Bacteriology,* **96,** 231–232.

Majmudar, B. and Rosales-Quintana, S. (1975) Infarction of breast fibroadenomas during pregnancy. *Journal of the American Medical Association,* **231,** 963–964.

McDivitt, R. W., Urban, J. A. and Farrow, J. H. (1967) Cystosarcoma phyllodes. *Johns Hopkins Medical Journal,* **120,** 33–45.

Nambiar, R. and Kannan Kutty, M. (1974) Giant fibro-adenoma (cystosarcoma phyllodes) in adolescent females — a clinicopathological study. *British Journal of Surgery,* **61,** 113–117.

Newman, J. and Kahn, L. B. (1973) Infarction of fibro-adenoma of the breast. *British Journal of Surgery,* **60,** 738–740.

Norris, H. J. and Taylor, H. B. (1967) Relationship of histologic features to behavior of cystosarcoma phyllodes. Analysis of ninety-four cases. *Cancer,* **20,** 2090–2099.

Pambakian, H. and Tighe, J. R. (1971) Mammary infarction. *British Journal of Surgery,* **58,** 601–602.

Persaud, V., Talerman, A. and Jordan, R. (1968) Pure adenoma of the breast. *Archives of Pathology,* **86,** 481–483.

Rickert, R. R. and Rajan, S. (1974) Localised breast infarcts associated with pregnancy. *Archives of Pathology,* **97,** 159–161.

Riddell, R. H. and Davies, J. D. (1973) Muscular hamartomas of the breast. *Journal of Pathology,* **111,** 209–211.

Salm, R. (1957) Epidermoid metaplasia in mammary fibro-adenoma with formation of keratin cysts. *Journal of Pathology and Bacteriology,* **74,** 221–222.

Wilkinson, L. and Green, W. O. Jr (1964) Infarction of breast lesions during pregnancy and lactation. *Cancer,* **17,** 1567–1572.

Willis, R. A. (1967) *The Pathology of Tumours.* Fourth edition. p. 215. London: Butterworth.

Wulsin, J. H. (1960) Large breast tumors in adolescent females. *Annals of Surgery,* **152,** 151–159.

Chapter Five

Cystic Disease: Duct Ectasia: Fat Necrosis: 'Fibrous Disease of the Breast'

CYSTIC DISEASE AND DUCT ECTASIA

The major problems that will be considered in this section are:

1. The differentiation of cystic disease from duct ectasia,
2. The pathogenesis of cysts and 'tension cysts', and
3. The identification of cysts when their epithelium is grossly altered.

It is possibly more clear to the reader to start with some simple conclusions about these problems and then to expound on them. Cystic disease is a disease of lobules and not of ducts; even large macroscopically visible cysts are of lobular derivation. It is wrong and very confusing to use the terms 'cyst' and 'dilated duct' as if they were interchangeable. Lobules do not contain elastic tissue, and hence elastic tissue is not involved in pure cystic disease. Apocrine metaplasia is, of course, a very common finding in cystic disease. Cysts, except in their very early formative stages, are ovoid or globular structures.

By contrast, duct ectasia is mainly a disease of ducts, i.e. of extralobular structures, which may be large, medium-sized or even small, but it is always ducts which are primarily involved. Because, with a few exceptions, ducts are endowed with elastic tissue they can be distinguished from altered or cystic lobules on this basis; in addition, the elastic tissue is often involved in the pathological process and the changes in the elastic tissue are frequently so characteristic that a diagnosis of duct ectasia can be made by virtue of these alterations. Apocrine metaplasia is hardly ever seen in duct ectasia — a negative point of some importance. When the ducts become dilated, they tend to have irregular tube-like contours rather than neatly ovoid or rounded ones, as seen characteristically in cystic disease. The reader might well be excused for wondering why, if the distinction appears to be as simple as this, there is room for so much confusion. In practice, the problems are often much greater than would appear at first sight and one has to remember that the simple conclusions and distinctions drawn here represent a distillation of the detailed work of many pathologists over many decades.

Table 5–1 The major distinctions between cystic disease and duct ectasia

Cystic disease	Periductal mastitis or duct ectasia
1. Lobular disease: in cystic hyperplasia, the hyperplasia affects ducts as well	Ductal disease: lobules affected mainly by involution
2. Affects any part of breast	Major, subareolar ducts mostly. Spreads centrifugally. Often segmental
3. No nipple discharge	Nipple discharge in about 20 per cent of those with clinical disease
4. No nipple inversion	Nipple inversion common because of periductal fibrosis with traction on nipple summit
5. Disorder of involution with cyst formation, ± epithelial hyperplasia. No inflammatory disease except with ruptured tension cysts	Inflammatory disease duct walls, usually chronic. No epithelial hyperplasia
6. Cysts rounded or ovoid with thin, yellow to brown contents (may be opaque white with ruptured cyst with acute inflammation)	Irregular dilatation ducts with thin contents initially, followed by creamy or pultaceous contents. Other ducts obliterated partially or completely by fibrous plug
7. Rarely mammographic calcification. More 'amorphous', scattered and not in line of ducts	Calcification common in periductal fibrosis producing tubular, annular and linear shadows on mammogram
8. No elastica in cyst walls because they arise in structure lacking elastic, viz. lobule, and no stimulus to elastic formation ordinarily	Irregularly cylindrical, dilated ducts usually have elastic in wall. Often focally damaged by inflammation and sometimes focally increased
	Amount found depends on (i) amount present initially in duct wall (ii) how affected by inflammatory process
9. Epithelial lining usually apocrine	Apocrine metaplasia very rare
In large cysts *often absent* either because destroyed or, more usually, because 'shed' during cutting or processing. Parts may be found *free in cyst*. Epithelium attached to wall may be *extremely attenuated* and barely recognizable as epithelium	As long as lumen persists, lining epithelium persists. Epithelium not found free in lumen. Remains recognizable as epithelium
Specific granules can help definitive identification	No 'specific' granules
When epithelial lining not present, recognition based on finding smooth zone of compressed connective tissue or broader zone of inflamed fibrous tissue in case of ruptured cyst	*Epithelium absent only if lumen obliterated* by fibrous plug
	Ectatic ducts have periductal fibrosis outside normal epithelium
10. Lumen empty or contains small amount pale grey or blue-staining stringy or homogeneous material. Foamy macrophages sometimes	Lumen contains foamy macrophages, cell debris, ceroid-containing cells
	Later *granular, deeply eosinophilic inspissated debris*

Table 5–1—*continued*

Cystic disease	Periductal mastitis or duct ectasia
11. 'Mazoplasia' indefinable 'Dysplasia' bad term 'Fibroadenosis' not ideal name Fibrosis not essential ingredient Adenosis not essential but very frequent '*Cystic disease*' (or mastopathy) or 'cystic hyperplasia' (when accompanied by hyperplasia) are descriptively accurate 'Fibrous disease of the breast' is a clinical but probably not a pathological entity. In any case it is quite unrelated to cystic disease. 'Fibrous mastopathy' and similar terms must not be used as if these conditions formed part of the spectrum of cystic disease	'Plasma cell mastitis' poor name which has not contributed to understanding. Refers only to inflammatory phase; plasma cells are not always conspicuous and they are present also in damaged tension cysts and in traumatic fat necrosis '*Duct ectasia*' good name emphasizing result most obvious to surgeon and pathologist. It masks the other end of the spectrum, however, represented by obliterated ducts ('mastitis obliterans'). The obliterative form has acquired a new importance. '*Periductal mastitis*' is probably the best name

Terminological Difficulties

Terminological problems have contributed greatly to the blurring of these important distinctions. The term 'mammary dysplasia', apart from its inherently sinister connotation, has served to obscure the understanding of non-neoplastic diseases. Its use cannot be condemned too strongly. 'Mazoplasia' and 'chronic mastitis' are almost as objectionable and, for reasons already given (Chapter Three), 'fibroadenosis' is not an ideal name either. 'Plasma cell mastitis' is an unhelpful term as a synonym for periductal mastitis (duct ectasia).

Pathological Difficulties

Derivation of Cysts. It is not by any means generally appreciated that 'pure' cystic disease, i.e. cystic disease without significant epithelial hyperplasia, is exclusively a disease of lobules and not of ducts. The increased diameter of lobular epithelial structures in disease has led frequently to their being confused with ducts; this is true of both non-neoplastic diseases, e.g. cysts, and of neoplasms (cf. cancerization of lobules, which was regularly confused with ductal carcinoma

until work in the last few years greatly clarified the issue, see page 105). Cysts have frequently been assumed to arise from extralobular ducts, or at least this erroneous inference can be drawn from much of the literature, unless the opposite is categorically stated. It is paradoxical but true that cysts derive from the smallest epithelial units of the breast, i.e. intralobular structures. This concept of the origin of cysts, including apocrine cysts, from lobules is absolutely crucial to an understanding of cystic disease. Only after appreciating the correctness of this statement regarding cysts of microscopical size can one make the conceptual leap necessary to realize that the same pathogenesis applies to larger cysts, which may measure several millimetres or even centimetres in diameter.

Analysis of the Shape and Contours of epithelium-lined spaces, in the attempt to differentiate between cystic disease and duct ectasia, must clearly take into account the plane of sectioning of individual spaces, but, with this proviso, it is a very helpful point.

Alterations in Elastic Tissue are a valuable pointer both to the seat of disease and to its nature, but elastic tissue involvement can only be properly assessed with elastic tissue stains. Such stains are as essential to a proper understanding of breast pathology as they are in the study of vascular disease. It is extraordinary, therefore, that elastic tissue stains do not even achieve a mention in many of the best-known publications on the subject.

Apocrine Metaplasia, so common in cystic disease and virtually never seen in duct ectasia, should be a very valuable distinguishing point, and this it is. But, again, one must remember that apocrine epithelium in cysts is often grossly altered and identifiable only with difficulty, for reasons to be considered later. It is also true that there are some cysts which do not undergo apocrine metaplasia.

Cystic Disease and Duct Ectasia in Combination

In practice, cystic disease and duct ectasia are not infrequently seen together in the same breast; they are common diseases that affect similar age groups. Indeed, it is not at all uncommon to find both diseases in the same block of tissue. One or the other disease process may dominate at the pathological level, or both may be of significant severity. In such cases, unravelling the two disease processes can be difficult, although it is generally possible to do so provided one understands the different basic pathology and pathogenesis of the disorders. It is also important to determine which disease is responsible for the clinical presentation. This obviously requires close clinicopathological correlation. Some of the major distinctions between cystic disease and duct ectasia are listed in Table 5–1.

CYSTIC DISEASE

The smaller cysts in cystic disease represent the pathological equivalent of 'cystic lobular involution' (Hayward and Parks, 1958). Cystic disease is probably best regarded as a disorder of involution, though its occasional occurrence in young post-pubertal girls who have never been pregnant makes it difficult to rule out the possibility that some cases may have a different mode of development. In the simplest form of cystic disease, groups of small cysts are lined by a more or less normal

A

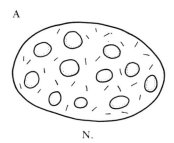

N.

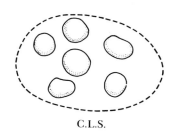

C.L.S.

B

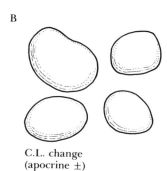

C.L. change
(apocrine ±)

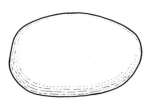

Single cyst replacing
lobule (usually apocrine)

Figure 5–1 A. A normal lobule compared with 'cystic lobular sclerosis', which represents the pathological equivalent of cystic lobular involution: in cystic lobular sclerosis the specialized connective tissue has become sclerosed. B. The commoner and clinically more important form of cystic disease. A few larger cysts are derived from the lobule with a concomitant disappearance of the specialized connective tissue. Apocrine metaplasia is usual in this type of cyst.

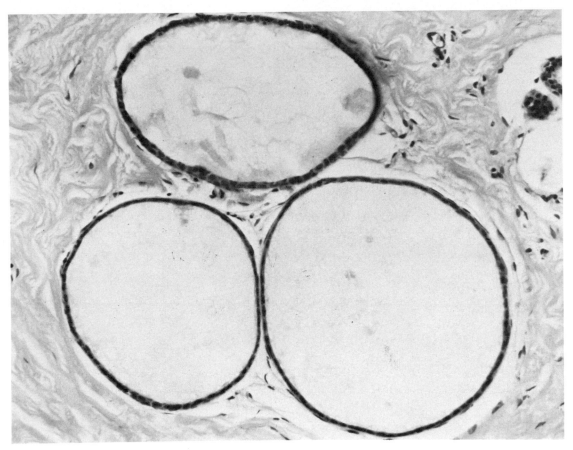

Figure 5-2   Cystic change in a lobule. No residual specialized connective tissue is present. H and E. ×525.

two-tiered slightly flattened epithelium (Figure 5-1A). The specialized lobular connective tissue has undergone sclerosis and become indistinguishable from the surrounding ordinary interlobular stroma. If this happens when the lobular 'units' are still cystic and the epithelium has not yet involuted, the cystic condition remains permanent and this represents cystic disease in its simplest form — as opposed to cystic lobular involution (physiological), in which some specialized lobular connective tissue is still present around the cystic spaces.

A more advanced and much more complex form of cystic disease is seen when the whole of a lobule is converted into fewer but larger cysts, say only two or three as seen in two dimensions, instead of more numerous smaller ones (Figure 5-1B). These larger cysts, judging from the study of the formative stages, appear to develop by a 'running together' of tubules and acini with a concomitant disappearance, rather than

sclerosis, of the specialized lobular stroma by a mechanism which is not understood (Figure 5-1B). This type of cyst is the commonest form in patients with cystic disease. Such cysts may be lined by ordinary mammary epithelium (Figure 5-2) but, for unknown reasons, they are more frequently lined by apocrine-type epithelium, with or without the additional formation of small apocrine papillae (Figures 5-3 and 5-4). Myoepithelial cells are inconspicuous, though usually still identifiable, in such cysts. It needs emphasizing that, except in neoplastic disease, apocrine metaplasia is uncommon in the ducts though it does occur, and rarely may be found even in the lactiferous sinuses (Figure 5-5). It is a good working rule that all spaces lined by apocrine epithelium should be regarded as having a lobular origin, unless proved otherwise.

At very low scanning magnifications, apocrine cysts can be seen lying grouped together (Figures 5-3 and 5-4) and showing a

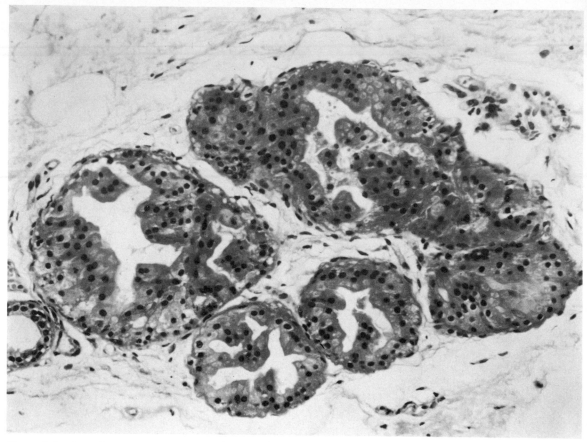

Figure 5–3 Apocrine metaplasia of a lobule. The lobular grouping is clearly evident. Small papillae are present. A little residual loose connective tissue is present centrally. Note ill-defined supranuclear vacuoles usually containing an eosinophilic rod-like structure (? nature). H and E. ×300.

relationship to ducts that characterizes their lobular origin (Figure 5–6). This point has been repeatedly proven by serial section, but it is not sufficiently appreciated and needs re-emphasizing. In addition, apocrine cysts lack any elastic tissue in their walls (with some exceptions, vide infra); in contrast, elastic tissue is almost always demonstrable in the walls of ducts of comparable diameter. Apocrine cysts may have a little elastica in their wall where they join the ductule, as one would expect. 'Tension cysts' in the breast also lack elastic fibre in their walls and this is generally also true of a ruptured tension cyst. When such a ruptured cyst shows marked mural

fibrosis, a little elastic fibre is occasionally found, but it is rarely present in sufficient amount to cause the cyst to be confused with a disease of the ducts. Presumably this rare finding of elastic fibre is a response of the stroma to the action of the extruded cyst contents.

APOCRINE METAPLASIA

At this point it is necessary to comment on the nature of what is generally referred to as apocrine epithelium. The earlier views that such glands represented developmentally

Figure 5–4 (*Opposite, above.*) The cluster of apocrine cysts is derived from a lobule. The neighbouring duct is affected by mild periductal mastitis and has a slightly irregular contour. Many of the apocrine cysts have a diameter which is larger than that of the duct even where the latter is slightly dilated. H and E. ×60.

Figure 5–5 (*Opposite, below.*) Apocrine metaplasia affecting a large duct as well as ductules or sessile lobules opening into it. H and E. ×150.

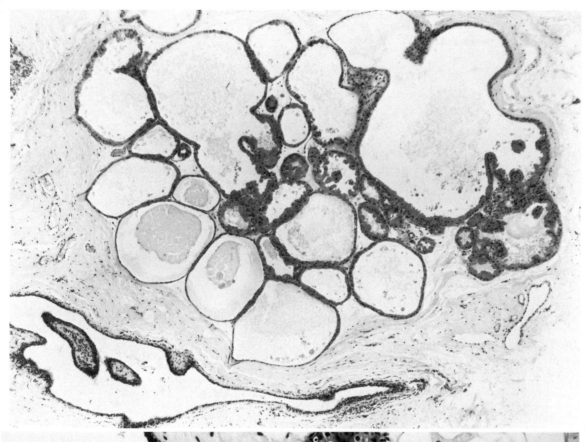

5–4

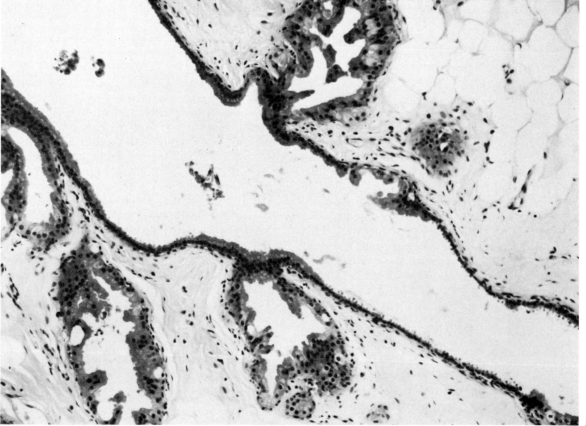

5–5

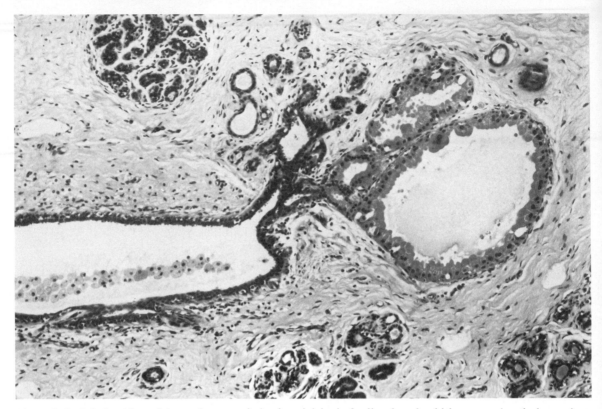

Figure 5–6   Lobule with partial apocrine metaplasia where it joins its feeding ductule which connects it to the larger duct. Note that the diameter of the apocrine structures is much greater than that of the ductule. H and E. ×150.

aberrant apocrine glands, or even that apocrine glands are normally present deep in the breast tissue, are of historical interest only. If the areolar region is excluded, apocrine glands are not seen in *strictly* normal breast tissue (but see Haagensen, 1977, cited in Chapter Two). Modern authors, almost without exception, regard the 'pale cells' of Dawson (1932) and the 'pink cells' of Bonser, Dossett and Jull (1961) as a metaplastic alteration of mammary epithelium. The remaining controversy is largely over whether or not the alteration represents a metaplasia to an apocrine sweat gland-type of epithelium as suggested by Lendrum (1945). The evidence that it does represent a metaplasia to an epithelium at least closely related to apocrine epithelium is very strong and it is not always easy to follow the arguments of those who reject it. The light microscope resemblances are too well known to need reiteration. Though not by itself conclusive, this resemblance strongly suggests the *possibility* of close affinity.

Supranuclear Vacuoles and Haemosiderin. The frequent presence of an ill-defined vacuole, occasionally associated with a pale yellow-brown pigment, in the supranuclear position is shared with apocrine glands as found in the skin of the axilla and anogenital region (Figure 5–3). Iron pigment has been identified by some workers in this vacuole (Bonser, Dossett and Jull, 1961). The present writer has found iron to be inconstant in the breast epithelium in question and has found that, when present, its localization varies. It is sometimes present among the glycolipid granules, which characterize this epithelium and are a distinctive feature of it. In rare cases I have found haemosiderin on the free luminal margin of the cell beyond the zone of the glycolipid granules, while it was absent in other parts of the cytoplasm. The whole question of the incidence, quantity, localization, and significance of stainable iron in this epithelium is wide open to investigation.

Lipofuscin. Not all the pigment present is

necessarily haemosiderin. On rare occasions, the writer has observed lipofuscin among the glycolipid granules. This is another field requiring investigation.

Glycolipid Granules. More important than these pigments in characterizing this epithelium is the regular presence of glycolipid granules (Figures 5–7 and 5–8) of the type described on page 70. These granules are also present in and characteristic of the apocrine glands of the skin. These granules correspond exactly in their site, size, number and other characters to the dense osmiophilic structures beautifully illustrated by Pier, Garancis and Kuzma (1970), and confirmed by Ahmed (1975) and Fisher (1976). These granules had already, in fact, been demonstrated by Lendrum (1945) with the use of a special staining technique, but his paper did not receive the attention it deserved. Archer and Omar (1969) suggested that Lendrum's granules were in fact mitochondria but this is obviously incorrect

from an examination of his careful work. Lendrum's (1945) granules and mitochondria are quite distinct structures. Lendrum (1945) found that his staining method 'seems to show more granules than the test for iron, and has revealed, in all of twenty cases of cystic disease, that wherever there is "pale epithelium" some of it contains granules'. While Lendrum's method has been superseded by the PAS method as a more reliable stain for these granules, his paper should be read by all those interested in this problem.

Mitochondria. The number, size and shape of the mitochondria described and illustrated by Pier, Garancis and Kuzma (1970) is fully consistent with that found in apocrine sweat glands. Indeed, the number, size and distribution of these mitochondria can be well studied in phosphotungstic acid–haematoxylin preparations with a high dry objective lens or with an oil immersion lens. This type of study has the advantage that it can localize the cells with far greater speed

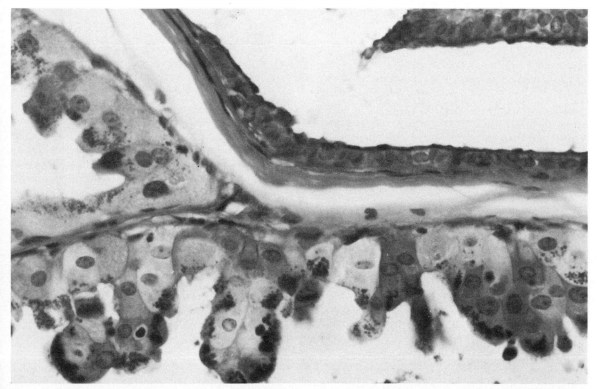

Figure 5–7 Apocrine epithelium contains a crescent of PAS-positive granules close to, but not quite reaching, the luminal margins. Compare with non-apocrine cells lining the third cyst included in the illustration. Apocrine cells frequently have prominent nucleoli. Diastase–PAS. ×600.

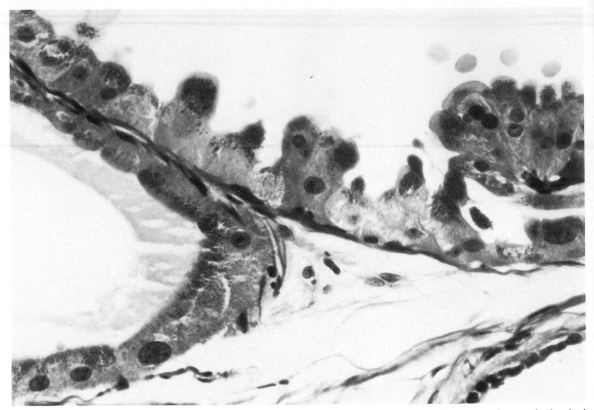

Figure 5–8 Apocrine epithelium with the specific glycolipid granules forming bands and crescents close to the luminal margins. Granules stained brilliant red in original. Masson trichrome. ×600.

than can ultrastructural studies and thus variations in different cells and different areas of tissue can be much more easily appreciated. Ultrastructural study has been invaluable for showing that the mitochondria of so-called 'pink cells' usually have few or incomplete cristae that do not extend into the central area (Archer and Omar, 1969; Pier, Garancis and Kuzma, 1970; Ahmed, 1975); this is not a feature of oncocytes, in which cristae are usually well developed and complete. The infolding of cell membranes, particularly at the base, seen in the abnormal breast epithelium is also a feature of apocrine epithelium revealed at ultrastructural level (Pier, Garancis and Kuzma, 1970). Archer and Omar concluded that the number and appearance of the mitochondria were inconsistent with apocrine epithelium, the cytoplasm being so tightly packed with mitochondria as to obscure other organelles; this has not been the experience of other workers. Ozzello (1971), in a detailed and beautifully illustrated description of these cells, concluded that they are 'ultrastructurally similar

to the secretory cells of normal apocrine sweat glands'. He also commented on the 'slender cristae' possessed by the mitochondria. Archer and Omar's view (1969) that 'the term oncocyte to describe the pink cells of the breast has the advantage of replacing a variety of misleading or non-specific terms' is untenable. This would replace the non-specific terms by a somewhat erroneous one. Apocrine and oncocytic epithelium are not identical; the granules originally described by Lendrum (1945) are a very good index of one important difference.

By analogy with the light and electron microscopic appearances of apocrine glands of the skin (Hashimoto, Gross and Lever, 1966) it is suggested by the present writer that the apocrine metaplastic cells in the breast contain the following structures:

1. An ill-defined 'supranuclear vacuole', which probably corresponds to the Golgi apparatus, though this tentative suggestion is in need of proof.

2. The characteristic glycolipid granules correspond to the dark osmiophilic granules and are probably lysosomal derivatives (Hashimoto, Gross and Lever, 1966).
3. The lighter ultrastructural granules are probably modified mitochondria (Hashimoto, Gross and Lever, 1966).
4. Inconstant pigments of at least two types: pale yellow to brown lipofuscin, present in the same site as the glycolipid granules and presumably also of lysosomal derivation; and, secondly, haemosiderin granules, with a variable localization.

Bonser, Dossett and Jull (1961) have some legitimate reservations about the apocrine nature of this metaplasia. One of their more cogent arguments is related to the fact that this epithelium in the breast is frequently hyperplastic and that even malignant disease has its origin in 'pink epithelium' in certain cases of breast cancer, while these changes are rare in the apocrine glands of the skin. Bonser, Dossett and Jull (1961) do admit that carcinogenic influences may affect the two tissues in a different way, but their argument is still a valid one. A pertinent, and possibly related, interesting observation is that of Izuo et al (1971), who found that while apocrine glands of the skin consistently have diploid nuclei, as assessed by nuclear DNA measurement, apocrine areas in the breast have a diploid to tetraploid population. Nevertheless, in my opinion, the resemblances greatly outweigh the differences and, while complete identity has not been proven and there may well be some other, more subtle and still unrecognized structural and functional differences, Lendrum's (1945) suggestion that we are dealing with apocrine metaplasia has been very largely, if not completely, vindicated.

CONCEPT OF THE 'TENSION CYST'

A 'tension cyst' is an apocrine cyst containing fluid under pressure as a result of obstruction of its outflow tract. Many of the lumps palpated by the clinician in cystic disease are tension cysts. Tension cysts expand gradually, reaching a size of several millimetres or even centimetres in diameter. The epithelial lining of the cyst is unable to reabsorb fluid at the rate at which it is secreted and, as a result, fluid accumulates slowly under pressure.

The Cause of the Obstruction to the Outflow Tract is variable and in the majority of cases very difficult or impossible to detect with any certainty. Benign epithelial hyperplasia, i.e. epitheliosis of ductules and of ducts, is a frequent cause of the obstruction (Figure 5–9). Apocrine proliferation, papillomatous, solid or both, is another important cause of obstruction at the neck of the cyst. Frequently, however, there is no evidence of any hyperplasia either in the ductal system or at the neck of the cyst. Another possible cause of obstruction is fibrous obliteration of the lumina of small ducts, which is the end result of the obliterative form, as opposed to the better-known ectatic form, of duct ectasia or 'periductal mastitis'. Such occluded and indeed obliterated ducts are scarcely visible at all in haemalum–eosin sections, though their 'ghost outlines' can be well defined by means of elastic tissue stains. A rare cause of ductal obstruction with tension cyst formation is so-called 'satellite duct' formation (page 88). These are four mechanical but non-neoplastic causes of tension cyst formation.

Rarely a tumour may be the cause of the obstruction and the writer has seen at least two cases of a clinically solitary tension cyst caused by in situ ductal carcinoma, in one case accompanied by a microscopic infiltrating cancer (Figure 7–34). A papilloma within the cyst itself, by causing obstruction at its neck, is another rare cause of outlet obstruction.

It is quite common, however, to fail to find even a potential cause of obstruction histologically, let alone to demonstrate it on serial section as the definitive cause. In these cases kinking of the outflow tract, i.e. the extralobular ductule, by stromal involutionary changes may play a part. Such kinking could produce a functional, as opposed to an organic, obstruction and the gradual accumulation of fluid would accentuate the kink and thus render the obstruction permanent and irreversible. Such a functional type of obstruction can be considered to have been the operative mechanism only when serial, or at least step, sections have failed to demonstrate any of the six known potential mechanical causes.

Treatment. The clinical argument as to whether tension cysts should be aspirated or excised continues unabated. The opponents of the policy of aspiration argue that an occult carcinoma might be 'lurking unsuspectedly' in the cyst. However, carcinoma in a tension cyst

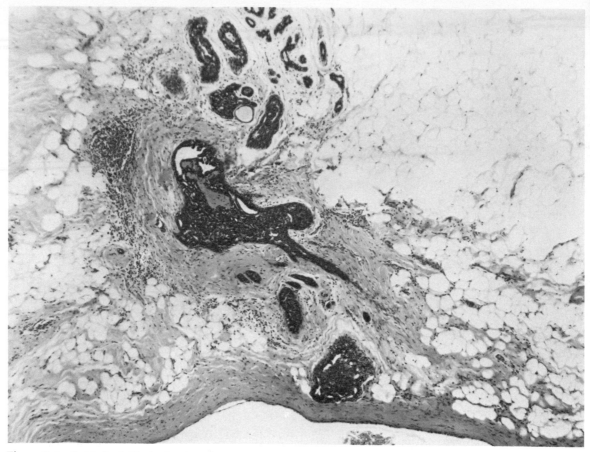

Figure 5–9 Epitheliosis blocks the ductule connecting with the tension cyst visible on the edge. H and E. ×60.

is a rare finding, so rare that most surgeons who regularly aspirate tension cysts are inclined not to worry unduly about this possibility, though they do take precautions to allow for it. The slightly greater risk, perhaps, is that the tension cyst itself may, on rare occasions, be the result of obstruction of the outflow tract by a carcinoma, but the writer has been able to identify this occurrence only twice amongst upwards of 500 cases of cystic disease studied.

Pathology. Tension cysts usually contain a clear yellow to brown liquid; the cause of the brown colour has not, to my knowledge, been identified. Microscopically, they are lined by apocrine epithelium showing varying degrees of attenuation and flattening (Figure 5–10). A variable, usually short, segment of the lining generally consists of cuboidal or columnar epithelium, which is easily recognizable as apocrine. Whether this part, which often corresponds to the neck rather than the dome

of the cyst, is identified depends on the plane of the sectioning.

RUPTURED CYST

A frequent complication of cysts coming to surgery is rupture, occurring either spontaneously or as the result of minor trauma. This leads to a brisk inflammatory response, which represents the only genuine inflammatory component found in cystic disease (Figure 5–11). In the presence of inflamed ruptured cysts the old-fashioned term 'mastitis' might be applicable, although, for historical reasons, it is best avoided. The ruptured cyst presents clinically as a painful and tender lump. Microscopically, in the compressed fibrous tissue around the cysts, there is an inflammatory infiltrate of lymphocytes, plasma cells, histiocytes and macrophages of various types, including foamy macrophages, and, not infrequently, significant numbers of poly-

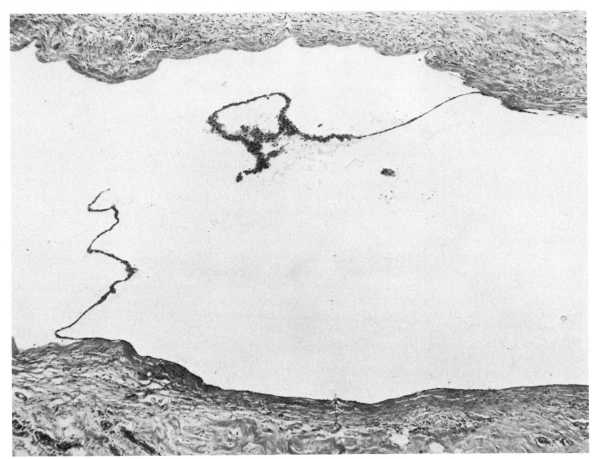

Figure 5–10   Tension cyst with highly attenuated, barely visible apocrine epithelial lining continuous with detached and folded apocrine epithelium in the lumen. H and E. ×60.

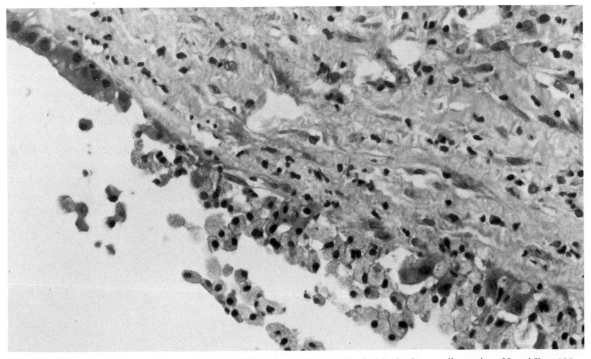

Figure 5–11   Ruptured apocrine cyst with three isolated apocrine cells buried in the foam cell reaction. H and E. ×400.

morphonuclear leucocytes. In the rare instances in which there is a heavy polymorphonuclear infiltrate, the cysts may show, on naked-eye examination, opaque white material adhering to their wall. This is the type of situation in which a *galactocoele is sometimes erroneously diagnosed.*

A galactocoele is excessively rare and more likely to be seen by the clinician than by the pathologist. It is described as a cyst containing inspissated milk, occurring in women whose lactation was terminated more or less abruptly within the few months preceding the appearance of a clinical mass, and usually situated in the central breast area. A galactocoele is usually treated by aspiration but, if the condition is not kept in mind by the surgeon, it may be unnecessarily operated upon (Haagensen, 1971). Any such case which is resected should be carefully studied pathologically to determine whether it is really a cyst or a dilated duct, and to identify the nature of the epithelial lining and any other features of interest. I have been unable to find any record of a microscopic description of the condition. A galactocoele is not part of the spectrum of cystic disease.

ATTENUATION, DETACHMENT, LOSS OR DESTRUCTION OF THE CYST LINING

The epithelium of tension cysts, and especially that of ruptured tension cysts, frequently becomes detached or destroyed and is often for the greater part lost. But segments of varying length are usually to be found either attached to the wall or, frequently, loose, folded and free within the cavity (Figure 5–10). When apocrine epithelium becomes detached from the stroma, it usually does so as long strips in which the cells remain adherent to one another, though their adhesion to the wall on which they previously rested is obviously tenuous. Because of this detachment, the strips are frequently lost, partially or even totally, in the course of sectioning or processing of the tissue (Figure 5–12). After rupture of a cyst the apocrine epithelium is usually destroyed by the inflammatory process, but, more rarely, segments of epithelium survive and become buried in granulation and fibrous tissue that grows in and tends to obliterate the cystic space (Figure

5–11). Even in the attenuated epithelium of apocrine cysts, the deep opaque eosinophilia of the cytoplasm, sometimes with a hint of a convex luminal margin, is often a good indicator of the apocrine nature of the epithelium (Figures 5–10 and 5–11).

Value of Glycolipid Granules in Identification of Altered Apocrine Epithelium. Many authors stress the presence of iron and of supranuclear vacuoles as a means of identifying apocrine epithelium. Whereas granules containing haemosiderin are an inconstant feature, ill-defined supranuclear vacuoles are regularly observed in virgin, unaltered apocrine epithelium, but they are not usually apparent in even slightly attenuated apocrine epithelium and are thus of little value in these circumstances. The most useful, and relatively little-known, feature in confirming the apocrine nature of a given piece of epithelium is the frequent presence of numerous eosinophilic refractile granules close to the free margin of the cells; these are the granules originally recognized by Lendrum (1945) (see page 65) and are not to be confused with mitochondria (Figures 5–7 and 5–8). They form a crescent or demilune of fine to moderately coarse, closely aggregated granules situated between the supranuclear vacuole and the free margin of the cell, which they do not quite reach (Figures 5–7 and 5–8). Their refractile quality is usually striking. These granules stain red with Masson's trichrome (Figure 5–8), they are positive with Sudan black B in paraffin sections and stain a deep red colour with PAS after diastase digestion, an indication of their glycolipid content (Figure 5–7). They largely persist even in attenuated epithelium and are very useful indicators of the true nature of even small residual shreds of apocrine epithelium, which is otherwise barely identifiable. PAS staining, after diastase digestion, is the most valuable method for demonstrating these granules.

Identification of Cysts in the Absence of Epithelium. Even when no epithelium is found, one should still be able to recognize the presence of a tension cyst (Figure 5–12). This is evident by virtue of the lining of compressed fibrous tissue with or without an inflammatory infiltrate. When only part of the cyst circumference is included for blocking, the wall of the cyst will, of course, appear on the

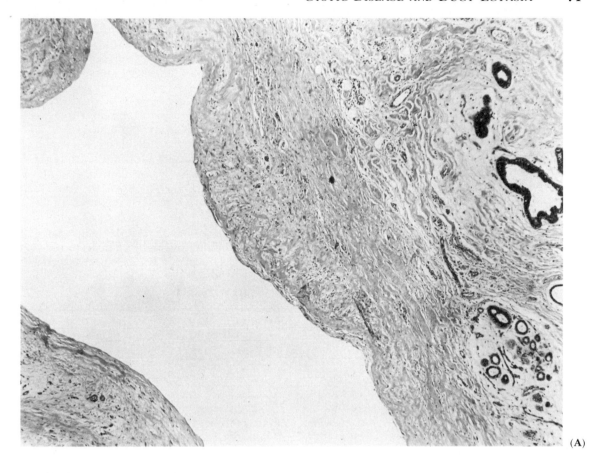

(A)

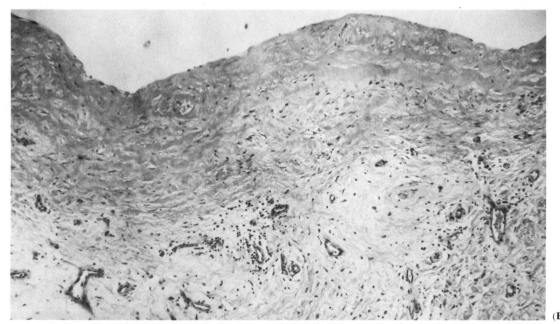

(B)

Figure 5–12 A. Collapsed cyst with a fibrous wall and no epithelial lining. The very existence of such a cyst is easily missed if the appearances are not correlated with the macroscopic findings. H and E. ×50. B. Part of cyst wall shown in Figure 5–12A. The fibrous wall lacks an epithelial lining. There is a mild inflammatory reaction to leaked or spilled contents. This should be identified as a tension cyst despite the absence of any epithelial lining. H and E. ×120.

edge of the block with a curved margin. It is surprising how frequently this cyst lining, denuded of all epithelium, is missed by the pathologist because of its nondescript appearance while he concentrates instead on more obvious and easily noted changes around the cyst wall, whether they be inflammatory 'spillage', accompanying hyperplasia or some other feature. This is especially likely to happen if the reporting pathologist has not himself examined the operation specimen and selected the blocks. The presence of such cysts will not be missed if a note has been made of the position in which tissue blocks have been taken and if greater attention is paid to low-power appearances; and provided also that the frequency with which attenuated epithelium is detached and lost is appreciated, the significance of a curvature on the edge of a block is understood and the pathologist has familiarized himself with the appearance of the fibrous wall of tension cysts.

The larger cysts and the ruptured cysts are the most easily missed at the microscopic level, and yet these are the ones that have the greatest clinical significance. Microscopic apocrine cysts, of little clinical importance, are easily appreciated even by the trainee pathologist, while the larger cysts, denuded of epithelium or otherwise altered, may go unnoticed histologically. *This is one of the frequent causes of a discrepancy between clinical findings and histopathological reports.* It is somewhat analogous to the situation encountered with endometriosis. In the symptomatic patient, the pathologist often has difficulty finding convincing endometrial tissue because of the destruction of the cystic functional tissue by extensive haemorrhage. These discrepancies between clinical findings and pathological reports can be abolished through proper and constant clinicopathological liaison. Both sides have much to learn through such contacts.

DUCT ECTASIA (PERIDUCTAL MASTITIS)

This frequent and important disease deserves greater recognition than it usually receives. The reasons for this relative neglect by some pathologists are many, prominent among them being the very complex pathology and pathogenesis of the various components of cystic disease, with which duct ectasia can be confused. The designations 'mammary dysplasia', 'fibroadenosis' and 'cystic mastopathy' are too often used even today as all-embracing terms to include practically all the common non-neoplastic diseases of the breast. Yet duct ectasia has been recognized for a long time and excellent descriptions of it are available.

Duct ectasia was fully described in the older literature by Ingier (1909), Bloodgood (1921, 1923), Adair (1933), Cutler (1933), Tice, Dockerty and Harrington (1948) and Haagensen (1951); the classical paper of Bloodgood (1923) and those of Tice, Dockerty and Harrington (1948) and of Haagensen (1951) are particularly valuable. The lesion was called 'comedo-mastitis' by Tice, Dockerty and Harrington (1948) and 'mammary-duct ectasia' by Haagensen (1951).

Sandison and Walker (1962) wrote that the condition of mammary duct ectasia was not as widely recognized as it might be and that some surgeons and pathologists were still not aware of the importance of this condition and of the protean ways in which it may manifest itself clinically. They noted that this state of affairs existed despite the persuasive writings of Haagensen (1951). There is a wealth of valuable data in this work of Sandison and Walker (1962). Suffice it to say that the relative ignorance about this condition, deprecated by Sandison and Walker in 1962, persists to some extent even today. The condition is best known in centres where there is close liaison between surgeons and pathologists. The advent of wide-scale mammography has also served to draw the attention of pathologists to the condition.

The papers of Sandison and Walker (1962) and Walker and Sandison (1964) deal extensively with both the pathological and clinical aspects of the disease and are very valuable sources of information. The works of Frantz et al (1951) and Sandison (1962) should be consulted for an analysis of the frequency of this condition and its pathology as seen in necropsy studies.

Terminology. Haagensen (1951) introduced the term 'mammary duct ectasia' but, although 'duct ectasia' is the name by which this condition is usually known and it covers many of the more important clinical features of the disease very adequately, it is not an entirely satisfactory name for a number of reasons. Firstly, it does not sufficiently emphasize the inflammatory nature of the disorder. Secondly, it does not cover the whole range of pathological changes since there is, as we shall see, an obliterative form of the disease which is the reverse of the implication of the term 'duct ectasia'. The term 'periductal mastitis' is probably the most appropriate, at least to the pathologist. But for historical and other reasons the term 'duct ectasia' is almost certain to remain the one in most common use.

Pathogenesis. The pathogenesis of the disorder is debatable. Most earlier workers, e.g. Tice, Dockerty and Harrington (1948) and Haagensen (1951), regarded ductal dilatation with stasis of ductal contents as the initial manifestation of the disorder. Inflammation was regarded as a secondary phenomenon, attributable to the irritant effect of the contents passing through the duct wall. Bonser, Dossett and Jull (1961) pointed out that this postulated sequence of events ignored the findings of most workers that inflammatory cases of the disease predominate in the younger age groups. Bonser, Dossett and Jull (1961) emphasized that periductal inflammation, and not ductal dilatation, is the initial and essential pathological manifestation of the disorder. The data supplied by them strongly support their concept of the sequence of events.

Those workers who regarded ductal dilatation as the initial phase of the disease searched for endocrine imbalance and abnormalities of development as possible causes of this dilatation. Inverted nipples, ill-fitting garments and benign breast tumours have all been suggested as aetiological agents but little or no convincing evidence has been produced in support of most of these factors as possible causative agents. A possible role for developmentally inverted nipples has been suggested again recently by Rees, Gravelle and Hughes (1977). Haagensen (1951) attributed duct ectasia to the changes of ageing and involution but Sandison and Walker (1962) demonstrated that this was not by any means an adequate explanation for all cases. Four out of 34 patients in the series of Walker and Sandison (1964) were virgins and two of these four were shown to be virgins by vaginal examination. This challenges the argument of some earlier workers that ductal dilatation occurs *only* in parous women.

Aetiology. The factors which appear to be most probably related to duct ectasia are pregnancy and perhaps lactation. Thus, in the series of Bonser, Dossett and Jull (1961), only 20 per cent of women with duct ectasia were nulliparous compared with 39 per cent of nulliparous women with other breast diseases and without duct ectasia. Of the parous women in the two groups, 72 per cent of those with duct ectasia had suckled their young compared with only 60 per cent of those without duct ectasia. Rees, Gravelle and Hughes (1977) have questioned the role of lactation in the aetiology of this disorder. The precise mechanism whereby pregnancy and perhaps lactation favour the development of the disease is not known. Damage to the major ducts during suckling is a possibility postulated by Bonser and her colleagues (1961). The contact between ductal contents and periductal tissues might initiate an inflammatory reaction, but this does not by itself explain why an active inflammatory process can be found in the tissues many years after the last pregnancy. Assuming that suckling is an important trigger mechanism, the perpetuation of the slow inflammatory process might perhaps be dependent on the establishment of an autoimmune process. This hypothesis is susceptible to experimental proof.

It will be apparent that the aetiology of this condition and its pathogenesis are by no means settled. The best evidence indicates that parity and perhaps lactation and suckling play an aetiological role, although even these factors have been questioned (Rees, Gravelle and Hughes, 1977). The pathogenetic mechanism postulated by Haagensen (1951), with a primary dilatation of ducts, has been very widely accepted, but the view put forward by Bonser, Dossett and Jull (1961) has much to commend it. Davies (1971) supported the concept of a primary inflammatory disease of the ducts, hence the designation 'periductal mastitis'. The writer's own observations are generally in accord with Bonser and her colleagues (1961) and with Davies (1971). It must, however, be admitted that in many cases with minor disease of some of the large ducts of the nipple, the ductal dilatation is unaccompanied by inflammatory reaction or any obvious residues of it. It may well be that, in such cases, the evidence of the postulated inflammatory reaction has disappeared without trace, while damaging the duct walls sufficiently to cause permanent dilatation. But the alternative possibility that more than one pathogenetic mechanism is involved has not been excluded.

More recently, there has been a revival of interest in the condition, mainly on the part of surgeons and radiologists. Milward and Gough (1970) drew attention to the dangers of clinical misdiagnosis of carcinoma in patients with duct ectasia and traumatic fat necrosis. Over an eight-year period, they found eight such patients (with a definite but incorrect clinical diagnosis of carcinoma) in whom the true diagnosis was duct ectasia or traumatic fat necrosis. These eight patients were seen over a period in which 691 patients underwent mastectomy for malignant disease. This indicates an incidence of just over one per cent of carcinoma, clinically diagnosed, in patients who would have had their breast sacrificed if pathological examination had not been undertaken before proceeding to mastectomy.

Rees, Gravelle and Hughes (1977) recently drew attention to the frequency of nipple abnormalities, retraction in particular, in duct ectasia. They found 30 patients over a three and one-half year period with nipple changes attributable to this disease. These workers stress that, although nipple retraction in this condition was first described in 1923, its frequency in duct ectasia is still not widely appreciated. They detail the nipple changes in this condition and discuss the clinical management of patients with nipple retraction who are deemed to have duct ectasia as the cause on both clinical and mammographic grounds.

Rees, Gravelle and Hughes (1977) suggested that there may well have been a true increase in the incidence of this disease in recent years, but the alternative suggestion, that this is more apparent than real, and accounted for by greater awareness of the condition and its pathology, seems more likely.

Tedeschi and McCarthy (1974) documented a case of mammary duct ectasia in a man aged 57 years.

Frequency. Duct ectasia is a frequent pathological finding in surgical material and at necropsy, since 30 to 40 per cent of women above the age of 50 years show some evidence of this abnormality. Clinically it is, of course, much less common. Nevertheless, approximately one case of clinically significant duct ectasia will be seen by the histopathologist for every 10 or 15 cases of cystic disease. The precise ratio will vary with a number of factors, especially the proportion of patients with cystic disease who are treated by excision as opposed to aspiration. The relative frequency of the disorders may also vary in different countries and at different times (Rees, Gravelle and Hughes, 1977). Duct ectasia is much commoner as a purely pathological finding, unrelated to any clinical symptoms. It is found particularly commonly in the nipple block taken from mastectomy specimens. In excision specimens cystic disease and duct ectasia often co-exist and it is not always easy to ascertain which of the two diseases is responsible for the patient's symptoms.

DIFFERENCES BETWEEN CYSTIC DISEASE AND DUCT ECTASIA

'Duct ectasia' is not an entirely satisfactory designation for this disease entity. Duct ectasia or 'periductal mastitis', as it could be more accurately called, differs from cystic disease clinically, pathologically, pathogenetically and probably also aetiologically. Some of the more important differences are tabulated (Table 5–1). Duct ectasia is essentially an inflammatory disorder of the ducts, usually affecting first the major ducts close to the nipple and tending to spread centrifugally in a segmental manner through the breast (Figures 5–13 and 5–14). In each of these respects it differs from cystic disease. It leads to periductal fibrosis with varying degrees of ductal dilatation (Figure 5–15). Because of the ductal dilatation, it has acquired the name of duct ectasia, but this is probably, in most cases at least, a relatively late phase of the disease. This name does not take account of the less obvious forms of the disease in which ductal lumina are narrowed or actually obliterated.

Discharge from the Nipple, unilateral or bilateral, is present in 15 to 20 per cent of cases that present to the clinician. The discharge may be straw-coloured, cream-coloured, greenish or it may have a brownish colour;

Figure 5–13   (*Opposite, above.*)   Inflammatory phase duct ectasia. H and E. ×150.

Figure 5–14   (*Opposite, below.*)   Same tissue as Figure 5–13. There is some disruption of the elastic coat. Weigert elastic and HVG. ×150.

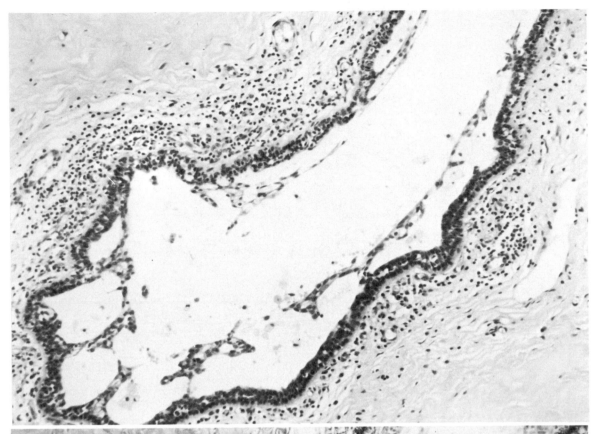

5–13

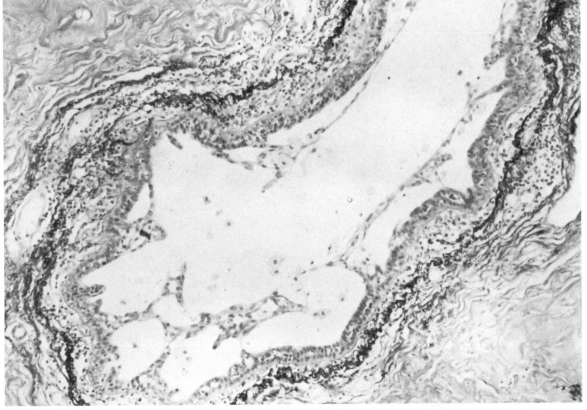

5–14

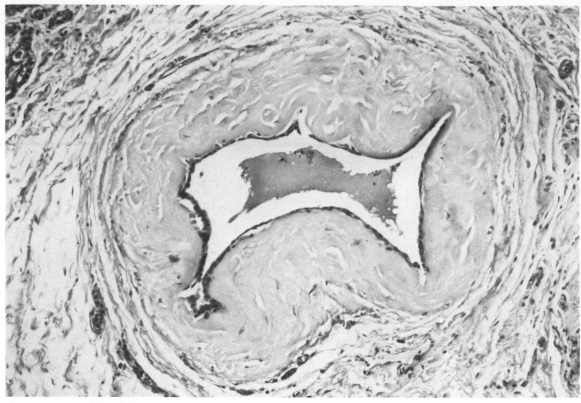

Figure 5–15   Periductal fibrosis of late stage periductal mastitis. H and E. ×225.

rarely will it be frankly blood-stained. By contrast, no nipple discharge occurs in cystic disease. This is related to the fact that cystic disease is a lobular disease and any secretion has to travel the length of the entire ductal system before appearing at the nipple. The ductal system is capable of absorbing physiological as well as other substances and hence any secretions associated with lobular disease have ample room and time for absorption to occur in the ductal conduit. The same is not true of duct ectasia, in which the brunt of the disease frequently falls on major ducts. *If the patient or clinician observes a discharge from the nipple and the pathologist makes a diagnosis of cystic disease only, one or other physician is probably in error* and consultation between the two is needed. Nipple discharge may lead to irritation of the nipple and the writer has seen three patients who presented with an eczematoid condition of the nipple apparently due solely to irritation from the nipple discharge. Obviously, in such cases, the pathologist has a paramount obligation to exclude Paget's disease. Two of these three patients were seen more than five years ago

and the third over three years ago, and in view of the very careful study to exclude Paget's disease conducted at the time, there can be little doubt now about the accuracy of the original interpretation.

Nipple Inversion. Duct ectasia, especially late in the disease process, frequently produces inversion of the nipple. It should be noted that the nipple frequently becomes inverted rather than retracted or distorted. Inversion is caused by periductal fibrosis (Figure 5–15), which contracts, exerting an increasing pull upon the galactophores which open at the summit of the nipple. This inward drag on the nipple leads to inversion, and sometimes both nipples are affected. By contrast, nipple inversion is not a feature of cystic disease — understandably, because in cystic disease there are no pathological changes affecting the major ducts. If the surgeon reports that there is a recently acquired nipple inversion and the pathologist merely furnishes a diagnosis of cystic disease, the diagnosis must be considered incomplete and consultation between pathologist and clinician is necessary.

PATHOLOGY

Periductal Fibrosis and Changes in Elastic Tissue. Accompanying the periductal fibrosis of duct ectasia there is usually patchy destruction of the elastic coat of the duct (Figure 5–14). Elastic tissue stains are invaluable in the study of this disorder; in cases of severe cystic disease accompanying duct ectasia, stains for elastic tissue will assist greatly in unravelling the complex pathology. As already pointed out, cysts do not usually have any elastic tissue in their walls. Ducts usually do, and the elastic coat is especially well developed in parous women (Davies, 1973). With duct ectasia of any severity, there is some disturbance and, later, usually destruction of this elastic tissue. The destruction is variable in degree but, even with almost total destruction, fragments of elastica almost invariably persist as tell-tale pointers to the anatomical structure involved and to the destructive nature of the disease process. At the other end of the scale — cases of the disease in which damage to the elastic coat has not been severe — there is hyperelastosis rather than destruction at the healed stage, accompanied by the more common, almost universal, periductal fibrosis. For this reason, the major ducts of the nipple frequently show fibrosis with increasing age as well as some degree of elastosis, though the latter does not reach statistical significance (Davies, 1973).

The Acute Type of Duct Ectasia presents clinically as an 'abscess' in the areolar region. Microscopically there is an intense polymorphonuclear infiltrate and oedema instead of the more usual dominant lymphocyte and plasma cell infiltrate. Even a granulomatous response can be found rarely with this acute type of presentation.

Foam Cells and Ochrocytes. There are two special features of the cellular infiltrate of periductal mastitis which must be mentioned (Figures 5–16 to 5–18). Lipid-filled foam cells are common in the ductal lumina. They are believed by most authors (e.g. Davies, 1974a) to represent altered macrophages, by others (e.g. Hamperl, 1970) to represent myoepithelial cells. The writer has, on rare occasions, found foam-cell change even in the duct-lining epithelial cells of patients with this disease. With severe ductal involvement, foam cells are also present in the tissues around the ducts (Figures 5–16 and 5–17). The precise origin, or origins, of these foam cells remains to be established. While a histiocytic origin appears very likely, for most of the foam cells at least, it is curious that they are not seen more frequently in the periductal stroma while they are so commonly present in ductal lumina. The same unresolved problem arises for the derivation of the foam cells frequently associated with epitheliosis.

Another cell type frequently found in periductal mastitis contains a ceroid pigment. These cells are found in the lumina, within the actual epithelial lining and in the periductal stroma. Hamperl (1970), who referred to these cells as 'fluorocytes' because of their yellow autofluorescence in ultraviolet light, regarded them also as of myoepithelial origin. Davies (1974b) called the same cells 'ochrocytes' and considered them to be phagocytic histiocytes. The writer is inclined to the latter view because of the known frequency with which auto-oxidation can occur in stagnant fatty material of the type found in the lumen in duct ectasia, resulting in the production of ceroid.

Severe and Late Stage Disease. Patchy destruction of elastic tissue, periductal fibrosis and irregular dilatation of varying lengths of ducts are the commoner features of duct ectasia which earned it this name. In a typical severe case, one is eventually left with a collection of irregularly dilated ducts containing inspissated, eosinophilic, proteinaceous and fatty material, the result of the degradation of cell products (Figures 5–19 and 5–20). This debris in the lumen is not absorbed because of the interruption of the normal lymphatic and other vascular pathways by the periductal fibrous tissue, which obliterates the specialized normal periductal stroma. Any inflammatory infiltrate still present at this stage is situated externally to the zone of periductal fibrosis. As the process becomes burned out in the major ducts close to the nipple, the inflammatory process may be fanning out segmentally into medium-sized and small ducts, so that an active inflammatory process may be present in the smaller ducts when it is no longer in evidence in the larger ducts.

Fibrous 'Cushions'. Other less well known features of duct ectasia also deserve mention. Instead of the more usual concentric periductal fibrosis, eccentric fibrous plaques or 'cushions' may be formed that bulge into

Text continues on page 82

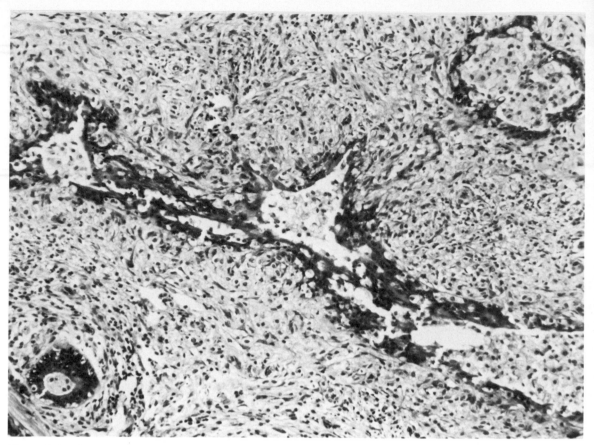

Figure 5–16 Severe periductal mastitis with an intense foam-cell reaction especially in the periductal tissue. The epithelial lining of the duct is hyperplastic, desquamated and focally missing. H and E. ×150.

Figure 5–17 (*Opposite, above.*) Part of field shown in Figure 5–16. In periductal mastitis of this severity, the epithelium is sometimes hyperplastic and it may be focally denuded. H and E. ×400.

Figure 5–18 (*Opposite, below.*) Severely damaged ducts in heavily inflamed fibrous tissue. Lipophages occupy the lumina and, in cases of severe disease, are also present in the periductal tissues. Must be distinguished from fat necrosis. H and E. ×75.

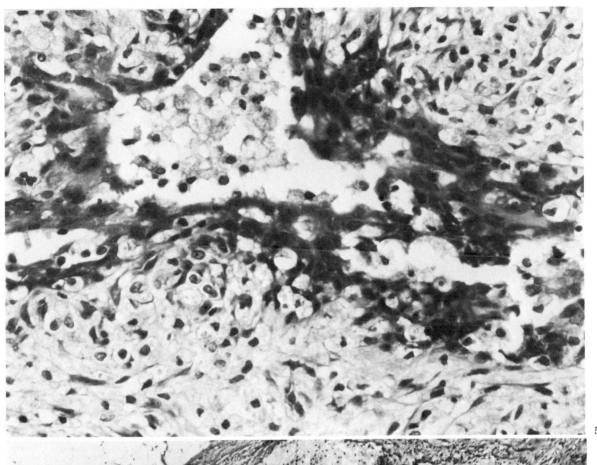

5–17

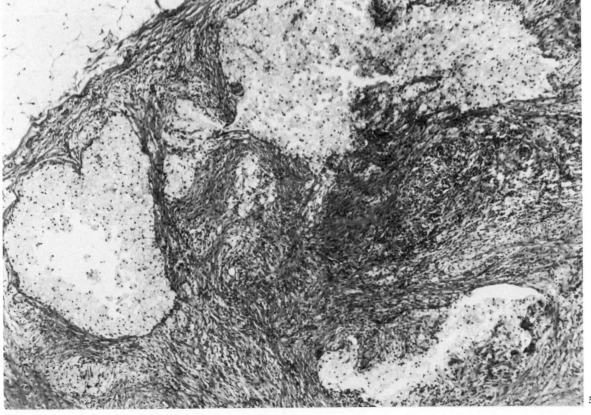

5–18

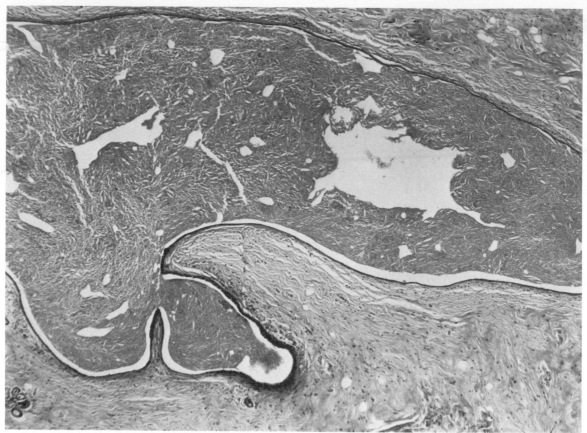

Figure 5–19 Late stage duct ectasia with irregularly dilated ducts. Inspissated contents with small needle-shaped clefts. H and E. ×60.

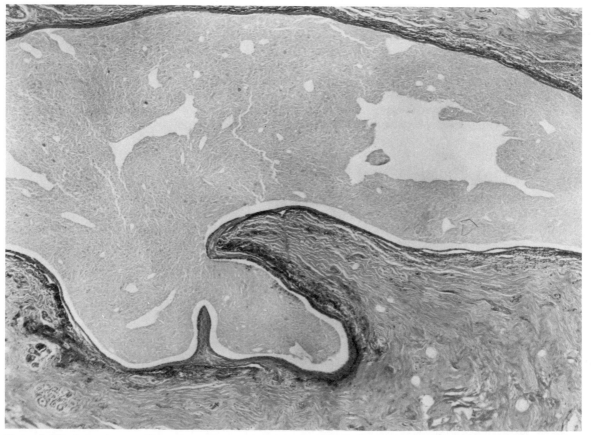

Figure 5–20 Same tissue as Figure 5–19. Remnants of disrupted elastic tissue in wall. Weigert elastic and HVG. ×60.

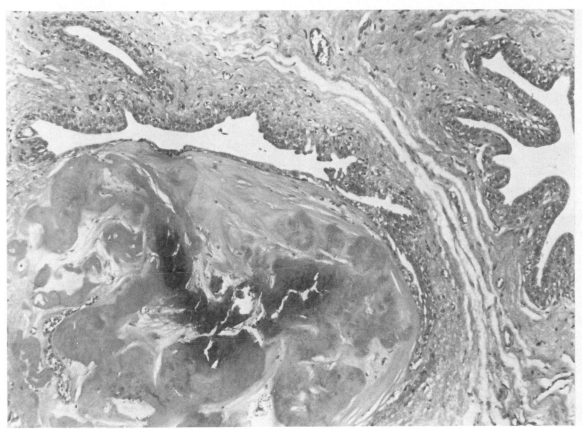

Figure 5–21 Fibrocalcareous cushion projecting eccentrically in wall of lactiferous sinus. The lumen is compressed into a slit. The overlying epithelium is attenuated but intact. H and E. ×120.

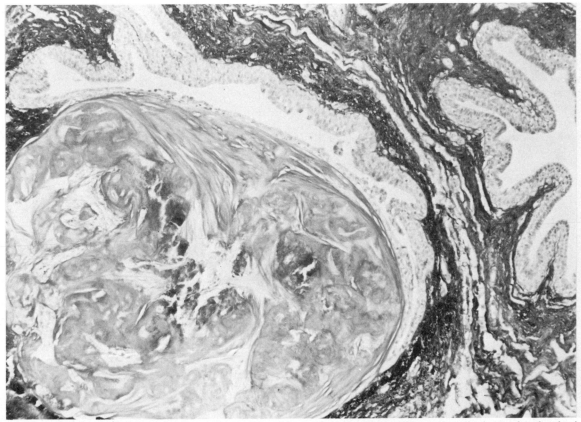

Figure 5–22 Same tissue as Figure 5–21. The mural cushion in the wall of the lactiferous sinus lies internal to the elastic tissue coat. Weigert elastic and HVG. ×120.

the lumen of a duct which may be dilated or of normal diameter (Figures 5–21 and 5–22). Several fibrous cushions may project into a short segment of a duct, producing a strikingly distorted pattern. Sometimes a large eccentric fibrous cushion will press the overlying lining epithelium to meet the other side, so that the ductal lumen is converted into a narrow crescentic slit (Figures 5–21 and 5–22). Only an elastic tissue stain can show the true state of affairs, demonstrating that the fibrous cushion is situated within the original elastic coat of the duct wall and that, by projecting from one side, it has grossly narrowed and distorted the lumen.

'Disappearing Ducts' of the Breast

It is not generally realized that the end stage of this disease process can be a total obliteration of the ductal lumen by fibrous tissue with complete disappearance of the epithelial lining. This is occasionally seen in the larger ducts but it is much more common in the medium-sized and small ducts. When there is total fibrous obliteration of ducts, this is the type of disease which can justifiably be called 'mastitis obliterans' (Ingier, 1909). As used by Ingier (1909) and later by Payne, Strauss and Glasser (1943), 'mastitis obliterans' apparently referred to only partial obliteration of ducts by a radial ingrowth of granulation and fibrous tissue. 'Mastitis obliterans' represents the other end of the spectrum of duct ectasia. This obliterating variant renders the ducts virtually invisible in routine haemalum–eosin preparations because, with the epithelium destroyed, the lumen obliterated by fibrous tissue and the inflammatory infiltrate long since disappeared, there is nothing to indicate the outline of the original duct.

Most of these obliterated ducts or disappearing ducts of the breast are missed in routine sections, even on careful scrutiny. Elastic tissue stains are essential to outline the original ductal contours. Having studied these, if the pathologist then returns to the H and E sections he is usually just able to make out the 'ghost' outlines of the obliterated ducts. Phagocytes containing yellowish ceroid pigment are often present in very small numbers in the fibrous plugs that occupy the ductal lumina. These are easily mistaken for siderophages but they give negative reactions for iron, while they are positive with PAS stains after diastase digestion and with Sudan

black B; they are acid-fast with the long Ziehl–Nielsen method and they react positively with other tests for lipofuscin or ceroid.

This obliterative form of the disease is one of the main reasons why the term 'duct ectasia' is not wholly appropriate, as it does not cover the entire spectrum of appearances which are encountered. On the contrary, the term 'duct ectasia' further lessens the chances of recognizing this obliterative variety, since in this variant the changes are diametrically opposed to the meaning of this term.

'Garland' and 'Recanalization' Variants

There are two somewhat rare forms of obliterative duct ectasia which produce most confusing patterns. In one form, the ductal lumen is occupied by fibrous tissue but the epithelium regenerates in such a way as to produce a double row of lining epithelial layers at the periphery of the fibrous tissue occupying the original lumen (Figures 5–23 and 5–24). Several lumina thus produce a 'garland' surrounding the fibrous plug. It is only by studying examples in an intermediate stage of development, and by the use of elastic tissue stains, that this unusual pattern of healing can be understood.

In the commoner, 'recanalization' variant, a fibrous plug fills the original lumen as with the preceding variety. As in the case of the completely obliterated or disappearing duct, the epithelium which originally lined the duct is destroyed but epithelial regeneration occurs from one or other end of the occluded duct. Thus a single channel, a few scattered or grouped channels or, rarely, even more than three or four epithelial channels penetrate longitudinally into, and sometimes right through, the fibrous plug. Each individual channel is lined by a fairly normal two-layered epithelium. If the epithelial channels are grouped, they closely mimic a small lobule (see Figures 4 and 5 of Davies, 1975), and are almost certain to be so interpreted without the benefit of an elastic tissue stain. The microscopic appearances can be most confusing in longitudinal and oblique cuts, which may reveal small islands and strands of epithelial cells in a dense core of connective tissue (Figures 5–25 and 5–26). Especially in frozen sections these can be deceptively alarming, and it is therefore important to acquaint oneself thoroughly with the appearance in paraffin sections. The analogy with recanalization of a thrombus is an apt one.

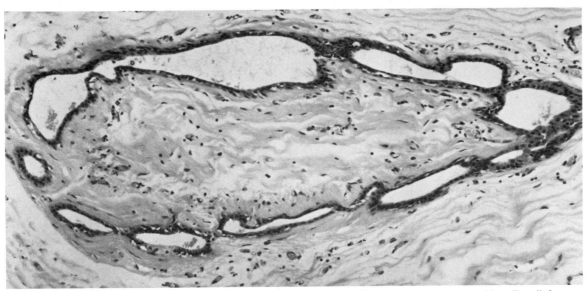

Figure 5–23 Obliterated duct in late stage periductal mastitis. The epithelium has regrown as a double collar all the way round the fibrous plug which has obliterated the original lumen. This produces a 'garland' effect. Ceroid-containing macrophages are present in the fibrous plug. The fact that this is a duct is clear only from elastic tissue stains. H and E. ×150.

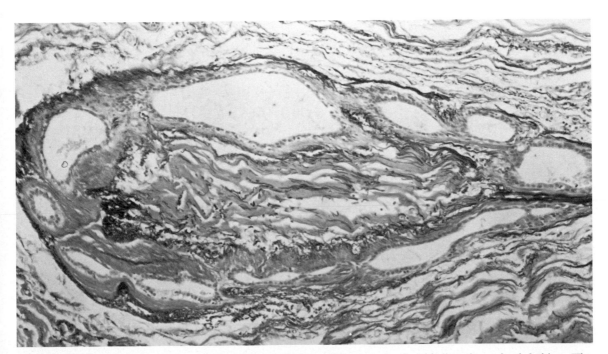

Figure 5–24 Same tissue as Figure 5–23. Obliterated duct with regrowth of epithelium in garland fashion. The designation duct ectasia is hardly applicable to this variant. Weigert elastic and HVG. ×150.

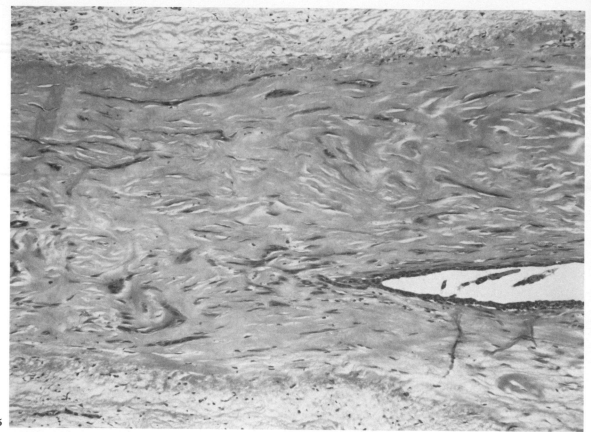

5–25

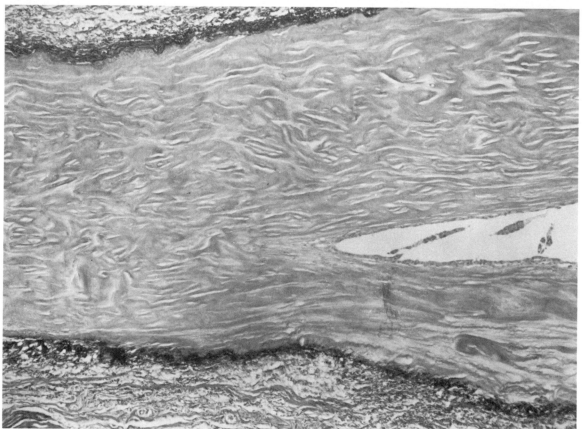

5–26

84

MAMMOGRAPHY AND DUCT ECTASIA

With the emphasis on mammography in the last 15 years, a thorough understanding of the pathology of duct ectasia has attained an even greater importance. In its classical form, duct ectasia may calcify in the periductal fibrous tissue, producing the characteristic 'ring' and 'tubular' shadows on mammography, the type depending on whether the ducts are viewed end-on or from the side; obviously, shadows of intermediate appearance will be seen in oblique views of the ducts. Less commonly, calcification is found in obliterated fibrous ducts, in which case the radiological opacities may be partly solid. Calcification is also present sometimes in the less common eccentric fibrous cushions described above, again producing solid rather than ring shadows (Figures 5–27 and 5–28).

Duct ectasia and its attendant calcification not infrequently accompany a breast carcinoma in mammographic studies, although there is no evidence that duct ectasia is associated with an increased frequency of malignant disease. There are two reasons, however, why it may appear to radiologists that it is associated with malignancy more frequently than would be expected by chance. Firstly, as it is predominantly a disease of older women, it is commonest in the age groups in which cancer has its highest incidence. Indeed, the advent of mammography and its increasing use has focused attention on the high radiological frequency of duct ectasia and has made pathologists take renewed interest in the condition. Secondly, the pathological process in duct ectasia leads to atrophy of the specialized parenchyma throughout the affected segment or segments of the breast. It will be recalled that the segmental lymphatics drain mainly periductally towards the areolar region. Possibly the periductal fibrosis, by obliterating the lymphatic pathways, may interfere with the nutrition of the lobular tissue and contribute to the involutionary process. Whatever the precise mechanism, there is total involution of the normal breast parenchyma in the affected segments and this may occur prematurely. There is adipose replacement of much of the stroma, as happens with normal breast involution. This results in increased radiological translucency, so that any neoplasm present stands out in stark relief against its surroundings. For these two reasons, mammographic studies may give a false impression of a relationship between duct ectasia and carcinoma (Young, 1968). But this impression is based merely on the common age incidences and the technical reasons stated. Certainly it is true that it is easier to detect a neoplasm mammographically if that breast has been previously affected by duct ectasia.

CONCLUSION ON CYSTIC DISEASE AND DUCT ECTASIA

Some of the important features of, and the contrasts between, cystic disease and duct ectasia can be summarized in the following rather categorical statements:

1. Cystic disease, with or without accompanying epithelial hyperplasia, is a very complex disease. At best, the nomenclature used to describe it is often unfortunate and sometimes downright confusing and misleading. 'Mammary dysplasia' and 'mazoplasia' are terms which should be abandoned. 'Chronic mastitis' and, to a lesser extent, 'fibroadenosis' are also undesirable.
2. Cysts, of whatever size, arise from lobules and not from ducts.
3. 'Tension cysts' are apocrine cysts containing fluid under pressure.
4. The apocrine epithelium in a tension cyst is often grossly attenuated. It is often detached from the stroma, lies loose in the cavity, or is partly or totally lost.

Figure 5–25 (*Opposite, above.*) Late stage periductal mastitis. This cylindrical rod of dense fibrous tissue was seen on frozen section examination. The epithelial strands in it were difficult to interpret until they were found to connect with the luminal lining of the duct. H and E. ×120.

Figure 5–26 (*Opposite, below.*) Same tissue as Figure 5–25. Black-appearing elastic tissue on margins of 'rod' outlines the extent of the periductal fibrosis. The patient had an acquired nipple inversion. Weigert elastic and HVG. ×120.

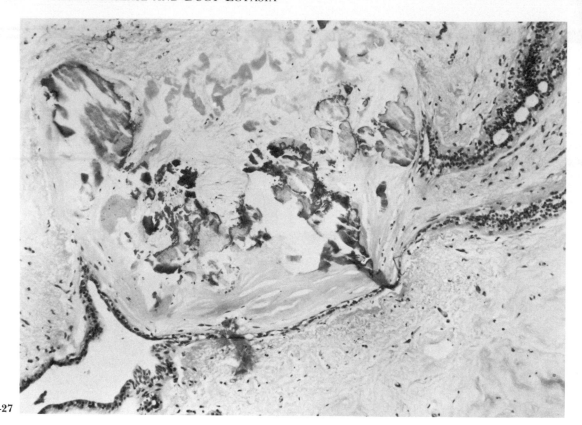

5–27

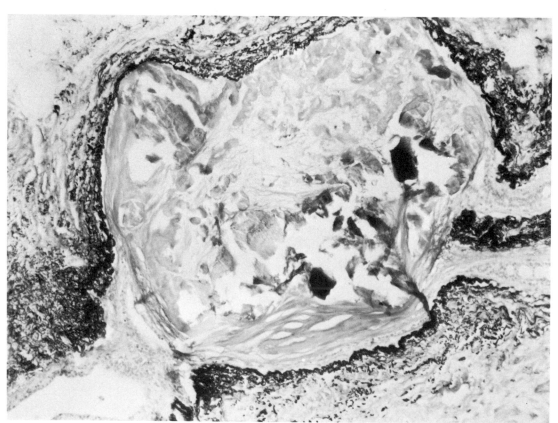

5–28

5. Haemosiderin is not a constant finding in apocrine epithelium. Supranuclear 'vacuoles' usually are, but cannot be detected in attenuated epithelium. An important feature of apocrine epithelium is the presence of a crescent of eosinophilic, highly refractile granules of glycolipid nature close to the luminal margin. These granules usually survive attenuation. They stain strongly with PAS, which is a useful aid for identifying this type of epithelium when it is severely modified and barely recognizable with conventional stains.

6. A 'leaking' or ruptured tension cyst excites an inflammatory reaction and productive fibrosis. This is the only truly inflammatory component of cystic disease and one which frequently produces the clinical symptoms which bring a woman to surgery.

7. A galactocoele in a surgically resected specimen is extremely rare; it is quite unrelated to cystic disease. Any possibly authentic case deserves thorough study.

8. Cysts do not involute further and, with few exceptions, persist indefinitely into old age.

9. Duct ectasia (periductal mastitis) is a very common condition at the subclinical, histopathological level.

10. Duct ectasia has a characteristic spatial (segmental) and temporal type of spread within the ductal system. It usually affects first the major ducts near the nipple.

11. Partly because of the localization of the lesions, nipple discharge is sometimes present with duct ectasia (none in cystic disease).

12. Periductal fibrosis in duct ectasia can lead to nipple inversion, unilateral or bilateral (not in cystic disease).

13. Elastic tissue stains are very useful in distinguishing most ducts from cysts, and in studying duct ectasia. Focal or even subtotal elastic tissue destruction is associated with severe involvement of a duct. In milder cases of duct ectasia the fibrosis may actually be accompanied by slight to moderate hyperelastosis.

14. Mammographic calcification is commoner and coarser in duct ectasia than in cystic disease. Ring and tubular calcifications are characteristic of duct ectasia, as are linear ones orientated in the line of the ducts.

15. If, in a histopathological laboratory, duct ectasia is a diagnosis which is seldom considered and rarely made, the diagnostic criteria should be revised. A good starting point is the study of elastic tissue stains on, perhaps, 200 consecutive breast specimens. This should go a long way towards mastering the features of both diseases in their variant forms.

TRAUMATIC FAT NECROSIS

Traumatic fat necrosis in the breast is identical with fat necrosis as seen in other parts of the body. It is frequently stated that a history of trauma is present in only about one-half or even fewer of the patients. This is mainly due to the confusion with other disease, in particular duct ectasia. There is no doubt that fat necrosis of the breast as a primary disease, unrelated to surgery, is a relatively rare condition and that it has been greatly overdiagnosed in the past. If it is strictly defined, a history of trauma can always be elicited, the traumatic episode being severe and usually easily remembered by the patient.

Figure 5–27 (*Opposite, above.*)   Eccentric compression of ductal lumen by bulbous fibrocalcific mass. Undecalcified section. It is impossible to envisage the state of affairs without a stain for elastica. H and E. ×120.

Figure 5–28 (*Opposite, below.*)   Same tissue as Figure 5–27. Elastic tissue of the duct wall outlines the duct, the calcific mass and the ductal bifurcation. The fibrocalcareous mass is situated within the elastic coat and hence represents an alteration of the duct wall. The ductal lumen is here reduced to a minute slit or potential lumen only with apposed epithelial linings, as seen in Figure 5–27. Weigert elastic and HVG. ×120.

The process affects the superficial subcutaneous tissue rather than the breast parenchyma proper, though the latter may be involved on the deep aspect of the lesion. Traumatic fat necrosis is frequently accompanied by an element of traumatic haematoma, sometimes one, sometimes the other predominating. The classical story is that of an injury, blunt but severe, to the breast of a woman who is often young and well endowed with fat. After about 7 to 14 days, an indurated area or a hard mass develops at the site. Skin tethering is frequent and the clinical resemblance to a carcinoma may be extremely close. Pathological examination establishes the benign nature of the lesion with ease.

Differentiation from Duct Ectasia

Unfortunately duct ectasia has been confused with traumatic fat necrosis, largely because of insufficient appreciation of the frequency and the very variable appearances of duct ectasia. The dilated saccular spaces of duct ectasia with their largely fatty contents have sometimes been misinterpreted as fat necrosis. On rare occasions the fatty contents can be extruded from the ducts and the resulting inflammatory mass in the areolar tissue is then microscopically indistinguishable from fat necrosis *in the area of extrusion*. But attention to the accompanying ductal changes and the fact that, in other areas, the fatty contents are situated largely in the lumina makes distinction easy. In severe periductal mastitis, with a marked inflammatory response, foam cells can be found in profusion in the stroma accompanied by inflammatory cells of all types, mostly lymphocytes and plasma cells. This type of reaction is, taken in isolation, indistinguishable from that seen in traumatic fat necrosis. There is no doubt that cases of this type have been confused with, and diagnosed as, fat necrosis in the past. If attention is paid to the ductal changes and to the relationship of the foam-cell deposits to the ducts, little difficulty should be experienced in distinguishing between the two conditions.

Though traumatic fat necrosis usually presents within two to three weeks after injury, detection of the lesion may, exceptionally, be long delayed. A confusing situation arises in which the mass is excised only many months or years later. The sequence of events is as follows: the patient receives an injury of the type already described but the resulting lesion is too small or otherwise unremarkable to draw attention to itself. Many years later, it presents as a small hard nodule which is painless and suspected clinically to be a cancer. Excision reveals an orange-brown lesion which consists microscopically of a siderotic fibrous nodule, occasionally even with some calcification. Presumably, in such cases, the softening of the breast with adipose replacement occurring with involution renders the nodule more conspicuous, and thus a mass may present clinically many years after the original injury. That this sequence is factual and not conjectural is based on two personally observed cases in which very reliable witnesses, both doctors' wives, gave a clear preoperative history of severe trauma to the site involved many years previously; in one case the injury was caused by a golf ball driven with such force as to make the woman lose consciousness for a few seconds.

FORMATION OF SATELLITE DUCTS

This curious condition has not, to my knowledge, been described outside the German literature (Hamperl, 1972). It is described here mainly for convenience and partly because it is sometimes associated with ductal obliteration. It is not in any way related to duct ectasia, but represents a proliferative epithelial reaction which, in the broadest sense, could be classified as an adenosis, though of highly distinctive appearance. New ducts bud off a duct wall and form a cuff of 'satellite ducts' around the parent duct (Figure 5–29). The satellite ducts are often numerous, numbering as many as 14, with an average of about six or seven. The subsidiary or satellite ducts may have a narrow but open luminal communication laterally with the main duct or may be joined to it but lack any luminal connection. In the latter case, they may be joined by means of both epithelial and myoepithelial layers, or merely by the myothelium or the basement membrane alone. Some satellites eventually lose the lateral connection with the parent duct and appear completely separated in transverse section. Satellite ducts may in turn generate second-order satellites, and even third-order satellites are present, still more rarely. The parent duct is usually narrowed when

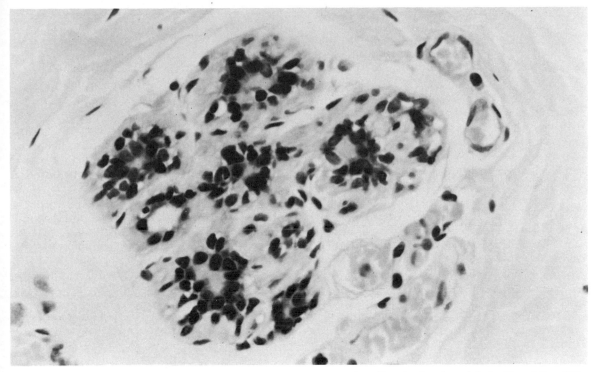

Figure 5–29 'Satellite duct' formation. This curious ductal alteration is easily mistaken for a lobule. H and E. ×675.

numerous satellites are present and, inexplicably, its lumen may become virtually obliterated (Figure 5–29). The satellite ducts originate from a normal duct, run parallel with it and surround it for a distance that may measure up to several millimetres, and then rejoin the duct. Satellites and their parent ducts have a strictly organoid relationship and, for this reason, there is no risk of confusing this ductal 'adenosis' with malignancy (Figure 5–29). This probably explains why this curious phenomenon has not been recognized previously. In its minor forms, it is likely to be missed altogether or mistaken perhaps for an artefact of contraction. In its more florid forms it is likely to be lumped together with other forms of 'adenosis' or even be mistaken for a lobule. However, silver impregnation methods will demonstrate the pathology of this condition very clearly. The proliferative process remains confined within the specialized periductal connective and elastic tissue sheath.

'FIBROSIS OF THE BREAST': 'FIBROUS DISEASE OF THE BREAST': 'CHRONIC INDURATIVE MASTITIS': 'FIBROUS MASTOPATHY'

These are the names chosen to describe what is essentially the same clinical entity by Vassar and Culling (1959), Haagensen (1971), Stewart (1950) and Minkowitz et al (1973). For reasons discussed in Chapter Two and touched on in Chapter Three, the writer seriously doubts whether this is a pathological entity. It is a very definite clinical entity, produced by variation in the involutionary process as it affects the stroma of the breast.

Stewart (1950) described it as a condition which simulates a tumour clinically and is found in older women. The only constant microscopic finding is apparently 'advanced parenchymatous atrophy'. Stewart remarked that 'only by microscopic examination can this lesion be distinguished from a very parvicellular mammary carcinoma'. McDivitt, Stewart and Berg (1968) did not refer to it.

Vassar and Culling (1959) described 20 lesions in patients aged 17 to 49 years. The average age was 33 years, .in contrast with Stewart's (1950) observation and Haagensen's (1971) mean age of 40.3 years. Vassar and Culling (1959) found no difference in the collagen and hydroxyproline content on chemical analysis of the cases with 'fibrosis of the breast' compared with normal controls. These workers indeed seem, from their description, to have recognized that the process is an involutional one (their Figure 2). It is not easy to follow their description of 'mazoplasia' and their Figure 4 would be regarded as normal by many pathologists. Their description of mazoplasia is at variance with some others; the term does not seem to have any accepted meaning, as indicated in Chapter Three, and it should be dropped from the pathologist's vocabulary. Vassar and Culling (1959) appear to have had serious doubts about whether or not the process was truly pathological, but concluded that 'the patient and the surgeon can feel a definite palpable mass in the breast ... leads us to believe that wider recognition of the process is necessary'. The writer agrees, but in a physiological rather than a pathological sense.

Minkowitz et al (1973) called the condition 'fibrous mastopathy' and reported on 51 patients. They recognized three types of disease based on the relative amounts of acinar tissue and stroma present, with a peak age incidence for the whole group between 25 and 40 years. Pertinently, the average ages of types I, II and III of this 'disease' were 27, 31 and 44 years respectively. The writer does not agree that their Figure 3 shows 'sclerosing adenosis': this represents lobular involution. These workers found no evidence of any predilection for a particular quadrant, in contrast with Vassar and Culling (1959) and Haagensen (1971), who found a predilection for the upper outer quadrant of the breast.

There is some difference of opinion about the clinical features of this disease but the striking feature is the lack of any agreement about the pathology of the condition. These inconsistencies and the absence of any consistent pathology, reproducible between different series, are explicable if one accepts that this clinical entity is dependent on a gross variation in the normal involutional process. It is the writer's contention that pathologists have strained themselves too far in the search for the pathology of this condition. The reason for failure is that they have been searching perhaps for a non-existent 'disease'. It is not easy to tell a surgeon that a 2 or 3 cm lump he has clearly palpated in the breast is 'normal'. The writer has tended to call this the 'fibrous lump of involution' and to regard it as the extreme of the normal spectrum. He has not found that surgeons mind the explanation offered. Any variable pathology which may be found in an individual case — and little has been described in the literature — would appear to be merely fortuitous. Excision of the lump is usually necessary in these cases and the pathologist's task is, as Stewart (1950) stressed, to exclude a sparse-cell carcinoma.

Nobody would doubt Haagensen's (1971) belief that this is a very real clinical entity. But the absence of any descriptions of convincing pathology in the last 25 years must make one seriously consider the alternative suggested here. Certainly it is wrong to lump this condition with fibrocystic disease as 'incurious pathologists and surgeons' have done in the past (Haagensen, 1971). 'Fibrocystic disease' should no more be used as a wastebasket than the even more embracing 'mammary dysplasia'. It is very refreshing to have a surgeon encourage pathologists to define their nomenclature accurately.

References

Adair, F. E. (1933) Plasma cell mastitis — a lesion simulating mammary carcinoma. *Archives of Surgery,* **26,** 735–749.

Ahmed, A. (1975) Apocrine metaplasia in cystic hyperplastic mastopathy. Histochemical and ultra-structural observations. *Journal of Pathology,* **115,** 211–214.

Archer, F. and Omar, M. (1969) The fine structure of fibroadenoma of the human breast. *Journal of Pathology,* **99,** 113–117.

Bloodgood, J. C. (1921) The pathology of chronic cystic mastitis of the female breast with special consideration of the blue-domed cyst. *Archives of Surgery,* **3,** 445–542.

Bloodgood, J. C. (1923) The clinical picture of dilated ducts beneath the nipple frequently to be palpated as a doughy worm-like mass; the varicocele tumor of the breast. *Surgery, Gynecology and Obstetrics,* **36,** 486–495.

Bonser, G. M., Dossett, J. A. and Jull, J. W. (1961) *Human and Experimental Breast Cancer.* London: Pitman Medical.

Cutler, M. (1933) Benign lesions of the female breast simulating cancer. *Journal of the American Medical Association,* **101,** 1217–1222.

Davies, J. D. (1971) *Periductal Mastitis*. Thesis presented for the degree of Doctor of Medicine in the University of London.

Davies, J. D. (1973) Hyperelastosis, obliteration and fibrous plaques in major ducts of the human breast. *Journal of Pathology,* **110,** 13–26.

Davies, J. D. (1974a) Human colostrum cells: their relation to periductal mononuclear inflammation. *Journal of Pathology,* **112,** 153–160.

Davies, J. D. (1974b) Pigmented periductal cells (ochrocytes) in mammary dysplasias: their nature and significance. *Journal of Pathology,* **114,** 205–216.

Davies, J. D. (1975) Inflammatory damage to ducts in mammary dysplasia: a cause of duct obliteration. *Journal of Pathology,* **117,** 47–54.

Dawson, E. K. (1932) Sweat gland carcinoma of the breast. A morpho-histological study. *Edinburgh Medical Journal,* **39,** 409–438.

Fisher, E. R. (1976) Ultrastructure of the human breast and its disorders. *American Journal of Clinical Pathology,* **66,** 291–375.

Frantz, V. K., Pickren, J. W., Melcher, G. W. and Auchincloss, H., Jr (1951) Incidence of chronic cystic disease in so-called 'normal breasts'. A study based on 225 postmortem examinations *Cancer,* **4,** 762–783.

Haagensen, C. D. (1951) Mammary duct ectasia: a disease that may simulate carcinoma. *Cancer,* **4,** 749–761.

Haagensen, C. D. (1971) *Diseases of the Breast*. Second edition — Revised reprint. pp. 76, 185–189. Philadelphia, London, Toronto: W. B. Saunders.

Hamperl, H. (1970) The myothelia (myoepithelial cells). In *Current Topics in Pathology,* Vol. 53. Berlin: Springer-Verlag.

Hamperl, H. (1972) Satellite ducts in the breast in cases of proliferating mastopathy. *Beiträge zur pathologischen Anatomie und zur allgemeinen Pathologie,* **146,** 339–350.

Hashimoto, K., Gross, B. G. and Lever, W. F. (1966) Electron microscopic study of apocrine secretion. *Journal of Investigative Dermatology,* **46,** 378–390.

Hayward, J. L. and Parks, A. G. (1958) Alterations in the microanatomy of the breast as a result of changes in the hormonal environment. In *Endocrine Aspects of Breast Cancer* (Ed.) Currie, A. R. pp. 133–134. Edinburgh and London: E. & S. Livingstone.

Ingier, A. (1909) Über obliterierende Mastitis. *Virchows Archiv für pathologische Anatomie und Physiologie und für klinische Medizin,* **198,** 338–345.

Izuo, M., Okagaki, T., Richart, R. M. and Lattes, R. (1971) DNA content in 'apocrine metaplasia' of fibrocystic disease of the breast. *Cancer,* **27,** 643–650.

Lendrum, A. C. (1945) On the 'pink' epithelium of the cystic breast and the staining of its granules. *Journal of Pathology and Bacteriology,* **57,** 267–270.

McDivitt, R. W., Stewart, F. W. and Berg, J. W. (1968) *Tumors of the Breast*. Atlas of Tumor Pathology, Second series, Fascicle 2. Washington, D.C.: Armed Forces Institute of Pathology.

Milward, T. M. and Gough, M. H. (1970) Granulomatous lesions in the breast presenting as carcinoma. *Surgery, Gynecology and Obstetrics,* **130,** 478–482.

Minkowitz, S., Hedayati, H., Miller, S. and Gardner, B. (1973) Fibrous mastopathy. A clinical histopathologic study. *Cancer,* **32,** 913–916.

Ozzello, L. (1971) Ultrastructure of the human mammary gland. In *Pathology Annual* (Ed.) Sommers, S. C. Vol. 6, pp. 1–59. London: Butterworth.

Payne, R. L., Strauss, A. F. and Glasser, R. D. (1943) Mastitis obliterans. *Surgery,* **14,** 719–727.

Pier, W. J., Garancis, J. C. and Kuzma, J. F. (1970) The ultrastructure of apocrine cells. In intracystic papilloma and fibrocystic disease of the breast. *Archives of Pathology,* **89,** 446–452.

Rees, B. I., Gravelle, I. H. and Hughes, L. E. (1977) Nipple retraction in duct ectasia. *British Journal of Surgery,* **64,** 577–580.

Sandison, A. T. (1962) *An Autopsy Study of the Adult Human Breast*. National Cancer Institute Monograph No. 8, pp. 1–145. Washington, D.C.: U.S. Department of Health, Education and Welfare.

Sandison, A. T. and Walker, J. C. (1962) Inflammatory mastitis, mammary duct ectasia, and mammillary fistula. *British Journal of Surgery,* **50,** 57–64.

Stewart, F. W. (1950) *Tumors of the Breast*. Atlas of Tumor Pathology, Section 9, Fascicle 34, p. 99. Washington D.C.: Armed Forces Institute of Pathology.

Tedeschi, L. G. and McCarthy, P. E. (1974) Involutional mammary duct ectasia and periductal mastitis in a male. *Human Pathology,* **5,** 232–236.

Tice, G. I., Dockerty, M. B. and Harrington, S. W. (1948) Comedomastitis. A clinical and pathologic study of data in 172 cases. *Surgery, Gynecology and Obstetrics,* **87,** 525–540.

Vassar, P. S. and Culling, C. F. A. (1959) Fibrosis of the breast. *Archives of Pathology,* **67,** 128–133.

Walker, J. C. and Sandison, A. T. (1964) Mammary-duct ectasia. A clinical study. *British Journal of Surgery,* **51,** 350–355.

Young, G. B. (1968) Mammography in carcinoma of the breast. *Journal of the Royal College of Surgeons of Edinburgh,* **13,** 12–33.

Chapter Six

The Histogenesis of 'Early' Carcinoma

THE RELATIONSHIP OF CYSTIC DISEASE AND BENIGN HYPERPLASIA TO CARCINOMA: FACT OR FANCY?

Views on this subject are often emotionally charged and do not always appear to be based on dispassionate analysis. They vary from the famous statement that 'any competent pathologist . . . will find it difficult to remain patient with those surgeons who deny the precancerous potentialities of cystic hyperplasia' (Willis, 1967) to the view of many surgeons and pathologists that the relationship, if any, is a tenuous one. As is so often the case when very competent and experienced authorities hold diametrically opposed views, the truth often lies somewhere in between. Unfortunately, a good deal of the literature does not help in solving this very difficult problem. Opposite views are put forward with equal vigour but the evidence presented lacks precision and cannot be expected to yield valuable information.

Buhl-Jørgensen et al (1968), in discussing the 'cancer risk in intraductal papilloma and papillomatosis', concluded that in both groups the incidence of breast cancer is significantly higher than would be expected by chance, but that patients with intraductal papilloma are at greater risk than those with intraductal papillomatosis. A great deal hinges on the correct diagnosis having been made in the first place, yet no pathologist was involved in this study nor are we assured that a pathologist had reviewed the material in order to check the original diagnosis. Twenty years ago such practice was more understandable, but there was no justification for it in 1968. At the other end of the scale, Devitt (1972) writes provocatively under the title 'Fibrocystic disease of the breast is not premalignant'. But the data presented in his Table 1 are not very relevant to the question he is attempting to answer, and his statement that 'indeed, in this series, the absence of a history of a previous benign biopsy was associated with a risk of finding cancer that was three times greater', while literally true, is grossly misleading in its implication.

THE EVIDENCE FOR AND AGAINST A RELATIONSHIP OF CYSTIC DISEASE TO CARCINOMA

The types of evidence recorded can be considered under six headings:

1. Relationship of Cystic Disease and Carcinoma to Parity

Cystic disease and carcinoma have a similar relationship to parity in the pre- and postmenopausal periods, with a higher than expected incidence of both diseases in the parous premenopausally, especially below the age of 40 years, and a lower incidence postmenopausally (Bonser, Dossett and Jull, 1961). This type of evidence can, at most, point to the possible sharing of aetiological agents; it cannot show that disease A predisposes to disease B.

2. Demonstration of the Initial Stages of Cancer in Pre-existing Cysts and in Foci of Epitheliosis or Other Benign Hyperplasias

Convincing transitions from epitheliosis to malignancy are extremely difficult to demonstrate, the problem being analogous to the relationship between papilloma and papillary carcinoma. Transitions are sufficiently rare to make some workers doubt whether they occur other than by chance. Similarly, an 'early' carcinoma restricted to a cyst with clear evidence of transitional changes from benign to malignant epithelium is a rare phenomenon. Carcinoma arising in a large tension cyst is a considerable rarity. Taking into account the frequency of cystic disease, it is perhaps surprising that such evidence is not more easily found. Nobody would deny that carcinoma can arise in a cyst, even in a large tension cyst, or from epitheliosis or other type of hyperplasia, just as it can arise in any breast disease (e.g. duct ectasia) and in any breast structure, but this tells us nothing about any putative increased frequency with which malignancy may supervene on cystic disease, compared with normal breast tissue.

The next three types of study are basically statistical but the data have been collected in such a way as to render their validity very variable.

3. Incidence of Cystic Disease in Patients with Carcinoma

Studies on the incidence of cystic disease in patients with carcinoma subjected to mastectomy have often led to the conclusion that there is a definite association between the two at the pathological level and that one disease leads to the other at the clinical level. These studies suffer badly from a paucity of data on control 'normal' populations. The data of Frantz et al (1951) and Sandison (1962) on 'control' populations are, however, notable exceptions. Nevertheless, most workers studying this problem have had to adopt as their 'normal' controls the findings of other workers, often obtained in a different country or at least in a different institute, and usually at a different period of time. These types of comparison may have diminished or exaggerated any association that might exist between cystic disease and malignancy.

The magnitude of the problem can be judged from a study of the paper by *Davis, Simons and Davis (1964)*. The pooled data of other workers who had used defined diagnostic terms showed that at necropsy no fewer than 21 per cent of 'normal' women had macroscopic breast cysts while 58.3 per cent had microscopic cysts. These figures are remarkably close to the accurate data of Frantz et al (1951), who gave values of 19 per cent and 53 per cent respectively. Davis, Simons and Davis (1964), in their own 327 cases of breast carcinoma, found microscopic cystic disease in 39.1 per cent, an 'incidence lower than that reported in the literature for autopsied women without clinical breast pathology'. Davis, Simons and Davis (1964) concluded that it would be illogical to use the fact that they had found cystic disease in the breasts operated upon for cancer to try and prove that cystic disease had predisposed to carcinoma.

Haagensen (1956) studied 713 specimens of breast carcinoma in conjunction with *Dr A. P. Stout*, and found an incidence of grossly visible cystic disease of 24.7 per cent, using the same criteria as Frantz et al (1951) in their necropsy study of women without a history of previous clinical cystic disease. Haagensen (1956) stated that 'when we compare a gross cystic disease incidence of 24.7 per cent in our carcinoma series with the 19 per cent incidence found by Frantz et al (1951) in their non-carcinomatous autopsy series, the difference is not very impressive'.

Indeed, *Foote and Stewart (1945)* found that macroscopic cysts are commoner in non-cancerous than in cancerous breasts, but this is such a partial quotation of their conclusions as virtually to constitute an untruth. The reader is advised to consult this classic paper in its entirety.

Bonser, Dossett and Jull (1961) examined the problem very critically and found that cancerous breasts did show an increased incidence of cystic disease and epithelial hyperplasia compared with 'normal' breasts (the series of Frantz et al (1951) was used to extract data for 'normal' controls). Cystic disease by itself occurred with an increased frequency of only ×1.7, while epithelial hyperplasia and cystic hyperplasia occurred with an increased frequency of ×3.3 and ×3.8 respectively.

While there are problems in the interpretation of these data, including the validity of using different workers' series as a control 'normal' group, Bonser, Dossett and Jull (1961) were probably the first to demonstrate reasonably convincingly that patients with breast cancer have an increased frequency of cystic disease and especially of cystic hyperplasia or pure hyperplasia in their breasts. This finding was confirmed by the more recent and extensive work of *Wellings, Jensen and Marcum (1975)* on the incidence of epithelial abnormalities of all types in other parts of the breasts in patients with breast cancer (page 105). But this does not necessarily imply that the benign hyperplastic lesions are precursors of malignancy in space and time. Nor, at the practical level, does it tell us anything about the future behaviour of patients *treated* for benign cystic disease.

The work of Kern and Brooks (1969) is inconclusive in the present context, although they made some interesting observations, and the same is true of the work of Tellem, Prive and Meranze (1962).

4. Retrospective Studies

Foote and Stewart (1945) studied the problem by a retrospective survey of patients with breast cancer and control patients with skin, uterine and other non-mammary types of cancer. They searched the records to establish how many patients had had a previous breast operation, other than for lactational abscess, prior to the operation for cancer. The

incidence as determined from the records of 1200 test cases was only 2.2 times that of the 1200 patients in the control group. In a small parallel series of breast cancer patients who were questioned directly, the incidence of previous breast operations was 4 per cent compared with 2.4 per cent as determined from the records: the figure of 2.4 per cent compares with 1.08 per cent for non-mammary carcinoma. These data have sometimes been interpreted as showing an increased cancer incidence in cystic disease of ×4 but this is unjustified, since the test and control series have to be compared by the same method of retrieval of information. This study suffers from the usual problems of a retrospective survey and some special factors which could either have masked or exaggerated a relationship with cystic disease. It is noteworthy that, in four of the 12 patients in the test series, the operation for 'benign' disease was carried out only zero to four years before the radical mastectomy for cancer; despite this obvious potential source of error, the increased incidence was merely of the order of ×2.2.

Steinhoff and Black (1970) carried out a special type of retrospective study to determine whether, in patients who subsequently developed breast cancer, the preceding breast biopsies for benign disease differed from those of patients who had not subsequently developed cancer. They claim to have found 'florid cystic disease' in 23 of the 30 test cases as opposed to only eight of the 30 age-matched control patients. Their data are unconvincing and their Figure 6 is not suitable to illustrate a convincing example of carcinoma.

5. Prospective Studies

Several prospective studies carried out between 1940 and 1960 reached the conclusion that the incidence of malignant disease of the breast in patients who have had previous operations for cystic disease is between 2.5 and 5 times the expected incidence. *Many of these studies can best be described as prospective observational studies done in retrospect*: women with benign biopsies performed x years previously were identified and their subsequent course over the ensuing years charted. Most of these studies were carried out long before the criteria for distinguishing epitheliosis from in situ carcinoma had become well defined and before CLIS had even been described, let alone become widely recognized. Also the follow-up information was often inadequate and the follow-up periods shorter than desirable.

Warren (1940) found an increased risk of ×4.5. Broken down by age groups, the increased risk was ×11.7 between the ages of 30 and 49 years and ×2.5 for those over 50 years of age.

Clagett, Plimpton and Root (1944) found an even greater risk of ×5. The same criticisms levied against the Warren (1940) study are applicable. The histological data are inadequate to allow for even partial reassessment in a modern context as attempted by McDivitt, Stewart and Berg (1968) with the Warren (1940) study. The major criticisms that can be raised against the Warren study (1940) are well outlined by McDivitt, Stewart and Berg (1968). For an updating of this series of patients see Monson et al (1976), whose work is discussed on page 97.

A very frequently quoted monograph on the subject is that of *Kiaer (1954)*. This encompasses 'simultaneous' studies of cystic disease and carcinoma, as well as prospective studies of cystic disease. This very comprehensive study suffers from the frequent absence of a dependable original diagnosis by present standards. It is important to remember that when this monograph was published, in 1954, lobular carcinoma in situ was rarely recognized and, more importantly, even the criteria for diagnosing duct carcinoma were by no means as well established as they are today. One has only to consider his Figures 50 to 59 to appreciate this. A student of breast pathology will recognize that Figures 50 to 52 are, in fact, typical in situ carcinoma and not 'grade 3 fibroadenomatosis' (the term used as a synonym for 'chronic mastitis'). Kiaer's (1954) Figures 53 and 54 probably represent lobular carcinoma in situ; Figure 55 (from the same case) shows epithelial hyperplasia or 'papillomatosis', while Figures 56 and 57 represent duct carcinoma, but there is nothing to indicate transition from the epitheliosis to the carcinoma. Figures 58 and 59 are very instructive: they are labelled 'grade 3 (grade 2?) fibroadenomatosis'. In the opinion of the writer, they are now identifiable structurally as well as cytologically as a malignant lesion. These are types of cancer that are sometimes being missed even today, but, fortunately, Kiaer's (1954) illustrations are sufficiently good to allow identification. In reading the literature, allowance has to be made for the diagnostic criteria in general use at the time of publication.

Two decades ago underdiagnosis of in situ lesions was a fairly frequent occurrence and some of the proliferative lesions identified by pathologists as potentially 'precancerous' were in fact already cancers at the time of initial diagnosis. This criticism applies equally to studies considered under section 4.

Davis, Simons and Davis (1964), pooling the data of six critical studies, found an increased incidence of 2.6 times that expected for women in general. In their own patients with cystic disease, however, breast carcinoma developed 1.73 times as often as in the general female population, a much lower proclivity to cancer than was generally cited at that time. Even their group with epithelial hyperplasia had an incidence only 2.5 times greater than the expected rate.

Many of the more recent studies have failed to present crisp and convincing evidence. Humphrey and Swerdlow (1968) purport to demonstrate the malignant potential of epithelial hyperplasia affecting large as opposed to small ducts, but the evidence presented is unconvincing.

Potter, Slimbaugh and Woodward (1968) were one of the first groups in more recent times to attempt a scientific analysis of the problem. They questioned 300 women who had undergone biopsy for benign lesions of the breast 16 to 20 years before a specified date. No other element of selection was involved. Follow-up information was obtained on only 110 patients, a poor response which could have biassed the results in either direction. Their series comprised 1930 patient-years at risk. The predicted incidence of carcinoma was 2.084 and the observed incidence was 10 patients, about 4.8 times the expected frequency. The mean time interval between biopsy and subsequent development of carcinoma was nine years. Interestingly, carcinoma developed in either breast with equal frequency. These workers divided their cases into pathological categories, which they illustrated. Rather unexpectedly, there was no difference in precancerous proclivity between cases characterized by epithelial hyperplasia, cases of fibroadenoma and cases with 'unremarkable or minimally inflamed breast parenchyma' (their groups A, C and E respectively and the three groups with the highest incidence of subsequent breast cancer). The absence of any cancers in their group with 'large cysts' in the presence of a low incidence with 'small cysts' is at variance with some data discussed later. Potter, Slimbaugh and Woodward (1968) were also apparently puzzled by some of their findings and concluded that the incidence of carcinoma 'appeared related to years at risk, but not to specific pathological processes in benign biopsies'. This work suffers from certain weaknesses but it did at least lay the foundation for subsequent research.

MacGillivray (1969) investigated the reasons why 'the incidence of breast cancer complicating "chronic mastitis" with epitheliosis has been reported to be as high as 45 per cent and as low as 6 per cent'. The 45 per cent figure was given by Kiaer (1954) on the basis of nine out of 20 women developing breast cancer while the 6 per cent figure given by Davis, Simons and Davis (1964) was based on their observation that only one of their 16 patients, with 'solid epithelial hyperplasia' on excision biopsy, subsequently developed cancer. MacGillivray's (1969) paper is a model of clarity with accurate definitions, an attempt at grading epitheliosis, superbly chosen illustrations and careful and accurate quotations of his sources. None of his series of 32 patients with epitheliosis developed cancer: 30 of these had been treated by local excision, including 10 patients with severe epitheliosis (defined), in eight of whom the follow-up period was over five years. The main shortcoming of this paper, as MacGillivray (1969) admits, is that the average follow-up period was only seven years. For reasons he discussed, very long periods of time of up to 20 years and more may have to elapse before the malignant potential of epitheliosis can be accurately assessed. On the other hand, the average follow-up period in the group of patients of Davis, Simons and Davis (1964) with 'solid epithelial hyperplasia' was 14 years, a figure comparable with the average 17-year follow-up in the series of Kiaer (1954). And yet these two series yielded the grossly discrepant results, already quoted, that stimulated the MacGillivray (1969) study. With investigations of this type, the possibility of initial underdiagnosis of malignancy, which would result in the erroneous demonstration of an apparently close relationship between epitheliosis and cancer, must be remembered. MacGillivray (1969) concluded that, on the available evidence, there was no justification for anything more radical than a local excision in the treatment of patients with even severe epitheliosis.

In the work of *Chardot, Varroy and Parache (1970)* an increased incidence of malignancy of ×7.5 was found in patients with fibrocystic mastopathy. Unfortunately as many as 122 out of the 206 test cases had aspiration of cysts only, as opposed to excision procedures. Six of their 206 patients with cystic disease developed breast cancer later: however, three of these six patients did so within three years of presentation. There are no details about the availability of biopsy material in the patients who subsequently developed cancer.

Another important paper is that of *Pellettiere (1971)*. He reported on 97 patients with 'papillomatous disease' treated by local excision, 57 of whom were followed for 10 to 18 years. He divided the papillary lesions into 'arborescent', 'solid' and 'mixed' types. The 'solid' papillary lesions correspond, as he rightly emphasized, to the British term 'epitheliosis' (see page 113). Four of the 97 patients subsequently developed invasive cancer, ipsilateral in two and contralateral in the other two. The two ipsilateral cancers developed within one to three years of the local excision. Pellettiere (1971) concluded that 'the risk of a woman's developing cancer following a biopsy in which papillomatous disease is found is 7.4 times greater than the expected risk . . .'. The main weakness of this work is the absence of detailed documentation of the four patients who developed invasive cancer; this would have been invaluable. It is also remarkable that all four cancers developed within four years, despite the fact that 57 women were followed for 10 to 18 years. Nevertheless, Pellettiere's (1971) work is a good deal more careful than many papers written on this topic. But it lacks the precision of MacGillivray (1969).

Hermann (1971) investigated the question of 'mammary cancer subsequent to aspiration of cysts in the breast'. Of 402 consecutive patients with cancer, 33 (8.2 per cent) had cysts of one or both breasts treated prior to the discovery of the neoplasm. Of the 33 patients, 17 had cancer developing on the same side and 10 on the opposite side (six had been treated for bilateral cysts). This evidence is suggestive of a relationship between 'gross' cystic disease and cancer which may not be fortuitous. On the positive side, Hermann (1971) established that the group of patients with preceding cystic disease did not have a significantly higher incidence of a family history of breast cancer than those without preceding cystic disease. This is an important point since few studies have taken account of this factor. For this type of evidence to be convincing, however, one needs to know what proportion of the general population in the drainage area concerned had aspirations for breast cysts. Without this information, we have nothing with which to compare the figure of 8.2 per cent. It also would have been very valuable to know what proportion of the patients with a 'cyst–carcinoma' interval of less than five, and perhaps 10 years, had developed ipsilateral rather than contralateral carcinoma. But Herrmann's (1971) evidence is suggestive and points in the same direction as the next paper to be considered.

Evidence has been marshalled by *Haagensen, Lane and Lattes (1972)* in support of a relationship between cystic disease and carcinoma. This must be given due weight both because of the reputation of the authors and the relatively recent date of their publication. In this article, dealing primarily with lobular 'neoplasia' but also discussing the whole topic of sclerosing adenosis ('adenosis'), they stated 'we have no evidence that the microscopical lesions, including adenosis, papillomatosis and microscopical cystic disease, are precancerous. But our data show very clearly that the women who have had multiple intraductal papilloma, subsequently develop carcinoma with an increased frequency.' *Haagensen (1971)*, after reviewing the numerous published studies, concluded that they all failed because they did not meet one or other of the two basic requirements of this kind of research. His two basic requirements are a clear definition of terms and the avoidance of statistical fallacy. Haagensen (1971) regarded the study of Davis and associates (1964) as about the best study he had found. In an extremely careful study, based on over two thousand patients with 'gross' cystic disease, Haagensen (1971) concluded that breast cancer developed with four times the expected incidence; his findings were statistically highly significant. There were 72 instead of the expected 17 cancers among 1693 patients followed for more than one year. Cancer developed just as often in the opposite breast as it did in the breast in which the initial cyst occurred; this finding has very important theoretical and practical implications. Haagensen (1971) in no way implies that the cancers develop in the cysts. Because of the bilateral distribution of the cancers that develop, those who would recommend prophylactic mastectomy would

be opting for a bilateral procedure. Haagensen (1971) himself disapproved of such mutilating surgery and adopts a much more conservative approach. He is a champion of the 'aspirators' and he demolishes any potential opponents of this therapy with great conviction.

One very interesting feature of Haagensen's (1971) work is that 'gross' cysts rather than epithelial proliferation are the pathological feature which is statistically associated with an increased cancer risk. *Veronesi and Pizzocaro (1968)* also found no difference in cancer incidence in patients with cystic disease depending on whether or not there were associated hyperplastic epithelial changes. This is at variance with most other authors, who stress the potential significance of epithelial hyperplasia rather than of cysts, e.g. Davis, Simons and Davis (1964). Haagensen's (1971) work should be read carefully by all those interested in this problem. It is very much more valuable than most that has been written on this complex topic.

Donnelly et al (1975) are among the more recent workers to examine this problem statistically. Their work indicates that in 'chronic cystic mastitis' there is an increased risk of cancer developing of the order of ×2.9. Like Haagensen (1971), they found that carcinoma developed in the contralateral as frequently as in the ipsilateral breast. Unfortunately the original microscopic slides could only be re-examined in 25 per cent of their cases, although they tried to circumvent this potential source of error by a method they explain carefully.

Monson et al (1976) provide us with one of the best studies to date, including an updating of the series of patients originally reported on by Warren in 1940. They concluded that there is an excess risk of dying from breast cancer in patients with 'chronic mastitis' but that it is only of the order of ×2.5, compared with the figure of ×4.5 suggested by Warren in 1940. They found that the highest 'standard mortality ratio' occurred in women followed up for less than 10 years; this suggests that some cases may have been wrongly diagnosed and partly explains the difference between the original factor of ×4.5 and the current, presumably more reliable, figure of ×2.5. It is pertinent to note that the increased risk of cancer, although small, persisted for at least 30 years after biopsy for benign disease. The authors justifiably point out that the very long latent period which may intervene between the diagnosis of benign disease and the appearance of clinical cancer fairly clearly rules out the possibility that the observed association results merely from incorrect diagnosis of the original lesion.

The timing of the paper by Monson et al (1976) was very appropriate since *Devitt (1976),* only a few months before, published the contrary view, also in *The Lancet.* There is a great deal to be said in support of Devitt's (1976) point of view that women with benign breast disease must not be frightened into thinking that the threat of breast cancer must be constantly with them. One sympathizes also with Devitt's impatience with the 'niceties of pathological classifications' and 'the statistical manipulations of those who try to calculate the number of breast cancers that they expect to find in their series': but the real answer is not in belittling other disciplines but in closer collaboration with good pathologists, statisticians, etc. Devitt (1976) has fallen into the same trap as he did in his 1972 work: he states, 'Of the 163 patients with a previous benign breast-biopsy specimen only 14 (9 per cent) had breast cancer compared with 13 per cent in women without such a history'. Surely there is a serious flaw in this reasoning.

Kodlin et al (1977) attempted an elaborate statistical follow-up study, which suffers from the usual disadvantages of a retrospective pathological analysis. The 'total' increased risk of patients with 'chronic mastopathy' was of the order of ×2.7, a figure in good agreement with the ×2.9 of Donnelly et al (1975) and the ×2.5 of Monson et al (1976). When their data are examined according to 'major histopathological groupings at first biopsy', some differences emerge. Very remarkably, the fibroadenoma group of patients had the highest increased risk of ×7, an extraordinary finding not commented on by the authors. The next highest risk groups, with an increased cancer incidence of ×5, were their 'adenosis or fibrosing adenosis' group and cases of intraduct papilloma. By contrast, the increased risk in their patients with fibrocystic disease and those with 'hyperplasia or metaplasia' was ×1.9 and 2.4 respectively. But the criticism levelled above, and some other statements made, reduce the value of this otherwise valuable work.

The recent work of *Page et al (1978)* is a formidable study of the relation between component parts of the fibrocystic disease complex and breast cancer. They found no increased incidence of cancer above the expected in patients with fibroadenoma, in agreement with other observers and as opposed to the findings of Kodlin et al (1977). They studied a total of 1127 subjects and questionnaires were completed for 1058 (94 per cent) during the three-year duration of this careful study. Excluded were 133 patients, for reasons clearly stated by the authors, leaving 925 subjects for final analysis. The biopsies studied had been obtained at least 15 years before the commencement of the study in January 1974: specifically they reviewed all breast biopsies between January 1952 and June 1959, inclusive. They compared the observed with the expected number of cancers in each carefully defined histological category. The 'expected' number was determined using the entire group of biopsied women as the standard population, following the method of Lillienfeld (1976), as well as the incidence rates of breast cancer for Atlanta, Georgia, obtained from the Third National Cancer Survey (1974). This enabled them to work out a standard morbidity ratio (SMR) for each histological category. The SMR was 1.4 for the total study group but this figure is of more significance when broken down into categories. 'Sclerosing adenosis' had an SMR of only 1.1, 'cysts' only 1.2 and the condition they call 'apocrine-like ductal hyperplasia' ('adenosis' of page 25) only 1.3. The SMR increases to 1.5 for apocrine change, 1.8 for 'ductal hyperplasia', 1.8 for 'papillary apocrine change' and 4.2 for 'atypical lobular hyperplasia', with each of the last three categories defined and illustrated. Only the last three figures are statistically significant ($P<0.05$, $P<0.05$ and $P<0.02$ respectively). Statistical significance is analysed as a one-sided significance level testing for whether the SMR is significantly greater than unity. The significance level was calculated assuming the expected number of cases as the mean value of a Poisson distribution.

The findings of Page et al (1978) support the view that hyperplastic mammary epithelium is a marker for an increased likelihood of cancer development. In this careful work, lobular and ductal hyperplasia have been separated in assessing risk factors and the importance of the age group at the time of the initial biopsy stressed, 45 years of age constituting an important dividing line. Three distinct hyperplastic epithelial lesions were found to be associated with an elevated rate of carcinoma development: atypical lobular hyperplasia, 'ductal hyperplasia' and 'papillary apocrine change'. The pattern of elevated risk in women with lobular lesions differs, in both magnitude and relationship to age at biopsy, from that found in ductal hyperplastic lesions. Thus, women with ALH had an overall cancer rate six times greater than the general population in the age group 31 to 45 years at the time of initial biopsy, with a rate one-half that (×3) in women over 45 years of age. This difference just achieves significance ($P<0.05$). By contrast, ductal hyperplasia is not a determinant of increased risk in the age group 31 to 45 years, while in the age group over 45 this lesion is associated with an elevated risk of about two and one-half times (the SMR for the two age groups is 1.06 and 2.65 respectively with a P value of 0.02). Apocrine change with 'papillary tufting' follows a similar pattern with an SMR of 1.03 in the younger age group (no increased risk) and an SMR of 2.71 in the older age group (with a P value of 0.02).

If we omit ALH from consideration, then in none of the histological groups does the increased risk of cancer reach a figure of even ×2 when all age groups are considered. Even in the age group over 45, hyperplastic lesions have an increased cancer risk which does not exceed 2.7. These results show a definite but slight risk from the hyperplastic components of fibrocystic disease only. The figure of 1.4 for the SMR for the whole study group is considerably below the 2.9 figure of Donnelly et al (1975) and the 2.5 figure of Monson et al (1976), and considerable weight must be attached to this figure because of the very critical manner in which the study of Page et al (1978) was conducted.

Remarkably, the group with ductal hyperplasia with marked atypia was not associated with an elevation of risk higher than that in ductal lesions without atypia. This conclusion of Page et al (1978) is at variance with recent studies of Black et al (1972) and of Kodlin et al (1977). Page et al (1978) suggested that the difference might be attributed to the fact that in these previous studies ductal and lobular hyperplasias were grouped together. It appears to the writer that there is an alternative explanation; group 4 of Black and Chabon (1969) and Black et al (1972) appears to me to show more significant cytological atypia than the dysplastic group of Page et al (1978); the writer feels that the type of lesion illustrated by Page et al (1978) in their Figure 4 corresponds to the lesion designated 'epitheliosis' on page 113, which is regarded by the writer as inherently benign. This discrepancy between the findings of Page et al (1978) on the one hand and those of Black et al (1972) on the other may, therefore, be more apparent than real.

Some of the components of fibrocystic disease, when analysed individually, do not increase the subsequent risk of cancer at all. Specifically, this is true of sclerosing adenosis and of cysts (defined as 0.5 mm in diameter or more). That sclerosing adenosis carries no sinister connotation is now generally accepted, the data of Kodlin et al (1977) with a risk factor of ×5 for this condition being at variance with other workers' findings. For 'pure' cystic disease, the SMR of only 1.2 obtained by Page et al (1978) is regarded as not significantly raised above that expected in the general population. It is unfortunately not possible to compare strictly the conclusions of Page et al (1978) about cysts with those of Haagensen, Lane and Lattes (1972): the latter found an increased cancer risk of ×4 with grossly apparent cystic disease, an important increase. The cysts in the study of Page et al (1978) were defined as 'round, usually epithelial-lined structures without obvious relation to the expected site of a duct' and measuring 'at least 0.5 mm in diameter'. Presumably, therefore, some of these cysts were large enough to constitute clinically significant cysts of a size considered to represent 'gross' cystic disease in the sense of Haagensen, Lane and Lattes (1972). There is room for concern that a discrepancy has appeared between the findings of Page et al (1978) and those of Haagensen, Lane and Lattes (1972) even though their results are not strictly comparable. Future work might well be directed towards taking into account the size of the cysts when analysing the results of follow-up.

In considering the recent study of Monson et al (1976) — which extended and brought up-to-date the 1940 study of Shields Warren, showing an increased risk of ×2.5 in patients diagnosed pathologically as having 'chronic mastitis' — Page et al (1978) raised the issue of whether this factor of ×2.5, as opposed to their own of only ×1.4, may not depend to some extent on the selection of women with known increased risk factors, especially a positive family history. For this reason Page et al (1978) were careful to include, in their questionnaire, information on family history of cancer and other factors known or suspected of being related to the risk of breast cancer. Family history was defined as positive if a mother, sister or daughter had had breast cancer. Ninety-one (9.8 per cent) of the 925 subjects in the final analysis had a positive family history. Such a family history was not associated with the presence or absence of any particular lesion and no adjustment for this factor was therefore necessary in the series of Page et al (1978).

Turning finally to the consideration of ALH, this was the histological feature with the highest SMR (4.2) among the categories examined, with an increased risk of ×6 before the age of 45 and of ×3 after the age of 45 years at initial biopsy; this difference depending on the age at biopsy just reached statistical significance ($P<0.05$). Judging by Figure 5 of Page et al (1978), their ALH corresponds to the features recognized by the writer as ALH and described on page 233. It would seem, as indicated in that section, that ALH, as defined, probably represents in most instances an incompletely developed, 'early' form of CLIS. Andersen (1977) established that in CLIS, treated conservatively, there is an increased risk of the order of about ×12. The present writer's interpretation of ALH fits in well with the risk factor of ×4.2 found by Page et al (1978) in this condition.

In conclusion, the studies to date mostly support one another in indicating some increase in cancer risk in patients operated on for fibrocystic disease or cystic mastopathy. Donnelly et al (1975) found an increased risk of ×2.9, although there was a snag in this study which the authors did their best to circumvent. The famous study of Monson et al (1976) indicated an increased risk of ×2.5, a considerable drop from the previous risk factor of ×4.5 in the 1940 Warren paper. Devitt (1976) is almost alone now in maintaining there is no increased risk at all for cystic disease as a whole, but, while his data are open to severe criticism in the way they are interpreted, his argument has certainly been very much strengthened by those who in the past and even now (Renwick, 1976) have greatly exaggerated the potential dangers. The most critical and credible work in this context is that of Page et al (1978); the increased risk is only of the order of ×1.4 for the total study group; it is non-existent in sclerosing adenosis and in pure cystic disease as defined by them (Table 6–1). On the other hand, the increased risk is of the order of ×1.8, ×1.8 and ×4.2 in the three groups with hyperplastic epithelium, viz. ductal hyperplasia, papillary apocrine change and atypical lobular hyperplasia, respectively (Table 6–1).

On this evidence the increased risk for cystic mastopathy as a whole is between 1.5 and 2.5 times the expected, as long as data are not vitiated by the problem of underdiagnosis discussed previously (Table 6–1). *This represents a definite, statistically valid, but very modest risk.* A risk of this order would have to be taken seriously were one dealing with an environmental carcinogen but it cannot be treated with undue anxiety in dealing with individual patients.

Unless the true risk is kept in proportion, its very existence will continue to be denied. Unfortunately Renwick (1976) recently claimed a ×10 risk for clinically diagnosed 'benign dysplasia' and an increased risk of ×5 to ×11 in biopsy-proven disease. This ×11 figure, though correct, applies to a specific age group in the old Warren (1940) paper. The much lower risk indicated by the careful later analysis of Davis, Simons and Davis (1964), though included in his Table 5, is ignored in the conclusion of Renwick's (1976) paper.

On the basis of the best recent work, there is little to recommend that patients with cystic disease should be followed-up indefinitely, except as part of a specific prospective study or as part of a routine screening programme for women above a certain age. All those interested in this problem should consult the work of Davis, Simons and Davis (1964). Their key study is important not only because it is one of the most comprehensive of its kind, but because it analyses the available data critically and approaches the subject with an open mind. Their findings are summarized in their conclusion that 'the risk of carcinoma in women in general is about 63 per 100 000 per year. We do not advise mastectomy in normal women at age 40 to prevent this. Would we if the risk were 125 per 100 000? This is about the case in cystic disease' (Table 6–1).

Future Prospective Studies. A well-designed prospective study would be the only convincing way to elucidate further this complex problem. In order to answer this question a prospective study would have to be carried out by one of the very large centres with abundant facilities. The minimum requirements are a very large series of cases of cystic disease and cystic hyperplasia (preferably several hundred), adequately sampled and studied

Table 6–1   The breast cancer risk factor in cystic disease and other benign breast diseases with some other risk factors for comparison

Disease	Risk factor	Authors
Duct ectasia	× 1.00	
Sclerosing adenosis	× 1.00	
Fibroadenoma	× 1.00	
Cystic disease without hyperplasia	× 1.20	Page et al (1978)
Cystic disease	× 1.40	Page et al (1978)
	× 2.00	Davis, Simons and Davis (1964)
	× 2.50	Monson et al (1976)
('Gross cysts')	× 4.00	Haagensen (1971)
Ductal hyperplasia	× 1.80	Page et al (1978)
Ductal hyperplasia (>45 years)	× 2.65	Page et al (1978)
Papillary apocrine change (>45 years)	× 2.71	Page et al (1978)
'Atypical lobular hyperplasia'	× 4.00	Page et al (1978)
ALH <45 years	× 6.00	Page et al (1978)
ALH >45 years	× 3.00	Page et al (1978)
CLIS	× 12.00[a]	Andersen (1977)
	× 9.00	Rosen et al (1978)
	× 7.20	Haagensen et al (1978)
Contralateral carcinoma	× 4.80	Rosen et al (1978)
Family history	× 1.50 to × 9.00[b]	Petrakis (1977)

[a] The magnitude of risk is regarded as considerably less than this by many workers though the risk factor has not usually been expressed in the form given by Andersen (see section on lobular carcinoma in situ). On the other hand, McDivitt (1978) regarded the magnitude of risk as 'several hundredfold' that of cystic disease.

[b] Depending on whether pre- or postmenopausal and whether uni- or bilateral.

pathologically to exclude already existing malignancy, the collection to be made within a reasonably short period, preferably over not more than five years, with the pathological specimens preserved for retrospective study if, and when, necessary. Accurate statistical information must be available regarding breast cancer morbidity for the general population (preferably checked against mortality figures for breast cancer). Ideally, a suitable control group of patients should be studied in parallel, the control group chosen being one in whom follow-up would be reasonably easy, and also one in whom a priori there was no reason to believe that there was an increased (or decreased) incidence of breast cancer (new knowledge might render this control group of less value, e.g. does reserpine in the treatment of hypertension increase the incidence of breast cancer?). Follow-up for at least 10 and preferably 20 to 30 years is necessary, since the incubation period before invasion of known in situ duct carcinoma can be of the order of five to 10 years and that of CLIS much longer. Thus a 10-year follow-up would be the very bare minimum required, especially as it is almost certainly reasonable to assume that in patients with epitheliosis one, two, or even more decades might have to elapse before any putative increased risk of malignancy declared itself as overt breast cancer.

In fact, whenever malignancy followed only a few years after diagnosis of a benign lesion, it would be highly desirable to re-examine the original material to try and exclude underdiagnosis in the first place. A higher incidence of malignancy than expected would carry greater conviction if the numbers of patients developing cancer were about equally distributed in the successive quinquennia studied. A relatively high percentage of cancers developing in the first five years (say 50 per cent of the total found in a 15-year study-period, with most of these appearing in the first two years) is highly suspect: such evidence vitiates some of the already published studies. Finally, the original pathological study must give some indication of the types and severity of the disease (apart from it being essential to distinguish duct ectasia, fibroadenoma, etc., from all types of cystic mastopathy in the first place). Cysts (apocrine and other), blunt duct adenosis, epitheliosis, sclerosing adenosis, 'infiltrating epitheliosis', with or without special stromal changes, may not have the same connotation in terms of precancerous proclivity. A few small foci of epitheliosis (present in most adequately sampled cases of cystic disease) may have a different significance from that of extensive epitheliosis, and if the epitheliosis is atypical, or accompanied by significant elastosis, this should be indicated. No truly prospective study to date, other than that of Haagensen (1971), has met most of these requirements and they have mostly been singularly poor in analysis of the pathological findings. A properly conducted study would be an immense undertaking but one of infinite value. It may well need 'another Haagensen' to organize a project of this magnitude.

Possible Objections to Prospective Studies. There are certainly many objections that can be raised to the type of study suggested, including the obvious one that it is usually not known whether a small part, most or all of a potentially sinister lesion has been removed by excisional biopsy; but this is one reason why large numbers of cases should be collected. Dossett (1976) stated that 'follow-up studies are unsuitable for the assessment of the malignant potential of individual breast lesions', but this seems too pessimistic a view. Dossett (1976) went on to make a series of assumptions; for instance, he stated that 'proliferative lesions can be divided into *two equal groups* [my italics] one of high grade and

one of low grade. If the not unreasonable assumption be made that 90 per cent of infiltrating tumours will develop in the high grade group . . .'. Dossett (1976) then went on to draw up statistics based on these two assumptions and upon a dubious interpretation of some of the findings of Frantz et al (1951). Basically he concluded that more disturbing lesions behave worse than less disturbing ones, but to go so far as to attach mathematical figures to this method of analysis is very misleading.

6. Specific Histological Features in the Breast

The incidence of specific histological features in the breast in patients with and without breast cancer has been studied by certain workers. *Wellings and Jensen (1973)* found a higher incidence of epithelial abnormalities of all types in the same, or in the contralateral, breast in patients with duct or infiltrating carcinoma compared to patients without mammary cancer. These workers were basically studying a different problem and they gave no details at that time of the types of abnormality found; however, in their more recent extensive work (*Wellings, Jensen and Marcum, 1975; Jensen, Rice and Wellings, 1976*), these authors clearly indicated that there is a larger average number of benign lobular lesions of all types in patients with, compared to those without, breast cancer. Although, for reasons considered on page 106, the number of benign lobular lesions may have been slightly overestimated, their basic contention is thoroughly validated, based as it is on such a detailed and extensive study

The studies of *Izuo et al (1971)* are also pertinent in that these workers found a greater degree of apocrine proliferation in patients with cystic disease who later developed cancer, compared with those who did not. Moreover, the only two patients with an aneuploid DNA distribution pattern in apocrine epithelium were found in the group of patients with cystic disease who later developed carcinoma. While this work suggests fascinating and probably important quantitative and qualitative differences in apocrine epithelium accompanying or preceding the development of carcinoma, it does not imply a precancerous proclivity for cystic disease. The changes observed microscopically are not of a sort which cause a patient to present clinically. Still less do they indicate that cystic disease progresses to carcinoma; rather do they show that patients with carcinoma tend to have greater hyperplastic activity in their apocrine epithelium, but there are many possible explanations for this important finding.

There are two quite fundamental problems which must not be confused. The first, relating to patients who present to a surgeon with cystic disease, has already been considered. The second, equally fundamental problem is the question of whether or not patients with a breast carcinoma have, compared with control groups, an increased incidence of cystic disease or proliferative breast lesions either in the vicinity of the carcinoma, or at some distance in the same or in other breast quadrants. Wellings and Jensen (1973) and Wellings, Jensen and Marcum (1975) found that this is indeed the case as far as proliferative lesions are concerned. *Fisher, Gregorio and Fisher (1975)*

reported on a very careful study of 1000 patients with carcinoma. They found 'proliferative fibrocystic disease' in the quadrant of the dominant mass in 35 per cent of cases and the 'non-proliferative' form in a further 20 per cent. When other quadrants were examined, 'PFC disease' was found in 55 per cent and the 'non-proliferative' in 35 per cent. They concluded that these 'incidences are greater than those cited for the occurrence of fibrocystic disease in "control" breasts of those not harbouring cancer'. Certainly these incidences are very high, but they must be interpreted with some caution in the absence of significant reports of 'control' breasts which have been studied as intensively as in the Fisher, Gregorio and Fisher (1975) study. This study is of particular value in that it carefully defines the terms used and illustrates the different categories of disease. Their further reports will be awaited with eagerness because of the vast scope of the study and the precision with which it is being conducted.

THE ORIGINS OF 'EARLY' DUCTAL CARCINOMA

To the best of my knowledge, there were hardly any published studies of microscopic (? 'early') in situ carcinomas, excluding CLIS, prior to 1969. Study of such lesions, usually incidentally discovered, is obviously of great importance as they may throw light on the site or sites of origin of ductal carcinoma and its mode of origin. They are also important in so far as they have a bearing on the relationship, or otherwise, of in situ carcinoma to epitheliosis. Studies of the latter problem carried out in the past have dealt with infiltrating carcinoma of grossly recognizable form. Such lesions can scarcely be expected to yield reliable information regarding the genesis of the earliest recognizable cancers. *Gallager and Martin (1969a and b)* were one of the first groups of modern workers to apply themselves to the study of the 'early phases' in the development of breast cancer. These workers were essentially correlating mammographic appearances with their histological counterparts, using subserial whole organ sectioning. In the course of this work a host of

other information was unearthed, as a result of which they formulated a number of conclusions with more general applicability.

They described changes in the ductal epithelium similar to those described in the section on 'clinging carcinoma' in Chapter Ten. They found that the 'preneoplastic' or neoplastic changes affected the ducts close to invasive masses most often and most intensively, but that equally advanced changes were often found in more remote parts of the breast. Another important finding was the involvement of mammary lobules, as opposed to ducts, in about 40 per cent of breasts with primary carcinomas. This was an important observation made at a time when there was little stress on the role of the lobule as a site of involvement in ductal type carcinoma. Indeed some of the changes they reported correspond probably to 'cancerization' of lobules as described in Chapter Ten.

Caution is necessary in interpreting some of their observations. The term 'lobular carcinoma in situ' is not used in the conventional, more restricted sense of other authors. It is used in a broader sense to include carcinomas of ductal type as they affect the lobule or, in other words, what Fechner (1971) termed 'cancerization'. This different terminological usage leads to problems in interpreting some of their findings.

Another of their conclusions is that 'the earliest histologically recognizable change in the sequence which eventuates in invasive mammary carcinoma is epithelial hyperplasia'. Few would disagree with this statement as it stands but the crucial question is to decide which forms of hyperplasia are innocuous or nearly so, and which carry a distinctly increased cancer risk. We have already seen that in the types of hyperplasia like sclerosing adenosis and blunt duct adenosis there is no increased cancer risk. Even in the lesion termed 'ductal hyperplasia' by Page et al (1978) and here called 'epitheliosis', the risk factor is only slight. It is therefore not very meaningful to group all hyperplasias together and consider them 'nonobligate preneoplastic lesions'. In the writer's opinion, not only should the different types of hyperplasia be distinguished along the lines of Page et al (1978) and those attempted here, but the epithelial hyperplasias which merge indefinably with the 'early' (e.g. 'clinging') carcinomas should be distinguished from adenosis and epitheliosis. That this distinction is sometimes very difficult is undeniable but it is equally true that it is possible in the vast majority of cases.

Gallager and Martin (1969b), on the basis of their very extensive studies of 60 breasts, were at pains to emphasize that mammary carcinoma is not a focal process but a diffuse disease. One of their major findings was that, of 47 breasts containing invasive carcinomas, 22 showed multiple invasive sites. Rather unexpectedly, in five mastectomy specimens from women without clinical or mammographic evidence to suggest primary carcinoma, in situ carcinoma was present in all five (all these women had had contralateral mastectomies for carcinoma). On this basis they regard it as probable that the rate of bilaterality, at least as a histological lesion, approaches 100 per cent. But the evidence presented on this point is not entirely convincing. Even if this were true as a biological phenomenon, it is not translatable into treatment of an individual patient. The problem of multiple lesions of the breast is a very real and formidable one, and bilaterality is another expression of multicentricity.

Because of the current recognition of non-infiltrating cancer at a much 'earlier' stage than hitherto, the prevalence of multicentricity in these 'minimal' cancers must now be investigated and the significance of these small in situ lesions assessed along the lines indicated by Hutter and Kim (1971) and discussed later.

THE SITE OF ORIGIN OF DUCTAL CARCINOMA

The study of *Wellings, Jensen and Marcum (1975)* is therefore of particular importance and will be considered in detail. Wellings, Jensen and Marcum (1975) carried out a very extensive study of 196 whole human breasts examined by a 'subgross' sampling technique with histological confirmation. Their study originated as a search for precancerous lesions and their rationale was based on their prior experience with rodent models. They had particularly in mind the hyperplastic alveolar nodule (HAN) of the mouse. In the mouse, HAN has several properties that can, with justification, be regarded as having a bearing on the human problem.

The first fundamental conclusion that stems from this superb work is that the vast bulk of breast disease, much of which has been traditionally regarded as of ductal origin, is in fact of lobular and/or terminal duct origin (ductule), a histological complex they conveniently dub 'TDLU' (terminal duct–lobular units). Some of the clinically important duct papillomas are clearly an exception and the present writer would add Paget's disease of the nipple. Nobody who studies the work of Wellings, Jensen and Marcum (1975) can seriously doubt this conclusion. Indeed it is difficult to understand how the traditional view originated and was maintained for the last four decades. The older workers, e.g. Dawson (1933), mostly considered the lobule to be the most frequent site of origin of mammary carcinoma, although Muir (1941) considered intraductal carcinoma to be the usual site of origin. Probably the introduction of the term 'infiltrating duct carcinoma' for the common carcinoma played its part in establishing the traditional view. It is possible also that the study of special types of disease like Paget's disease drew attention to carcinoma of the medium-sized and large ducts and away from the smallest ductal ramifications. Possibly the recognition in 1941 of lobular carcinoma in situ as a distinct entity also played a part, as it was perhaps intellectually easier to conceive of ductal carcinoma and lobular carcinoma as arising in distinct rather than overlapping sites. Whatever the precise reasons, and they are clearly multiple, the notion of ductal carcinoma, with lobular participation excluded, became generally accepted. Once this erroneous belief was firmly entrenched in the literature and in the minds of pathologists it became so sanctified by tradition that it needed the elegant and exhaustive study of Wellings, Jensen and Marcum (1975) to demolish it convincingly.

DISTENSION BY CARCINOMA AND THE CONCEPT OF 'UNFOLDING'

Certainly, at the histological level, it is easy to see why any structure distended by carcinoma cells will appear larger than the original structure on a simple 'inflationary' basis and thus mimic a different part of the parenchyma (Figure 6–1). When to this simple proposition is added the concept of 'unfolding' expounded by Wellings, Jensen and Marcum (1975) the room for error becomes obvious. With 'unfolding', a number of small epithelial units merge to give rise to fewer but larger structures (Figure 6–1). Indeed the vast majority of cysts in the breast form through an

'unfolding' process, though why this occurs with involution remains a mystery.

The origin of most breast carcinomas in the TDLU is best appreciated by the study of 'early' cancers and especially by their examination at a very low scanning magnification. The 'subgross pathology' method of Wellings, Jensen and Marcum (1975) is a simple and ingenious extension of the use of a very low magnification.

ATYPICAL LOBULES AS THE SOURCE OF ORIGIN OF BOTH DUCTAL AND LOBULAR CARCINOMA

Another important finding of Wellings, Jensen and Marcum (1975) was the identification of 'atypical lobules' (AL), which were thought to give rise to both ductal carcinoma in situ and lobular carcinoma in situ by diverging histogenetic pathways. The former, commoner, type was called ALA and the latter ALB. Cancerous breasts and those contralateral to cancer contained many more lesions than did non-cancerous breasts obtained at necropsy. ALA had a lobular morphology and was a terminal structure on the mammary tree; it tended to persist after the menopause whereas normal lobules usually atrophied. If ALA progressed to ductal carcinoma in situ, the unfolded lobule came to resemble a duct and gave the false impression that so-called

Figure 6–1 Sequential alteration in the size and number of lobular units as they become filled with cancer cells. Slight to moderate distension in B is followed by marked distension in C. A normal lobule is shown for comparison in A. In D, unfolding is added to distension so that there are only a few, very much larger cancerized lobular units. These have been mistaken in the past for cancer of the larger ducts because of their large size, lack of obvious lobular grouping, failure to use elastica stains and other reasons. The appearance is apt to mislead the observer into assuming that he is looking at extralobular ducts when he is actually looking at grossly distended and sometimes unfolded lobules. Many structures identified and illustrated in past work as ducts containing carcinoma have in fact been cancerized lobules, the microanatomy of which has been grossly altered.

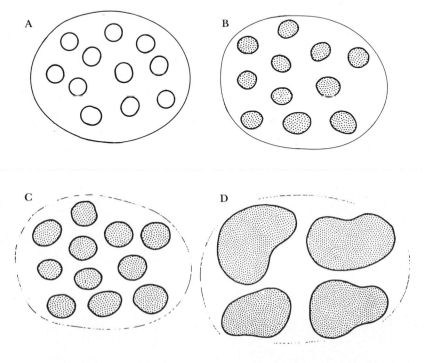

ductal carcinoma had originated as a ductal lesion. Wellings, Jensen and Marcum (1975) also found that ALA showed varying degrees of anaplasia, which formed an arbitrary continuum from normal lobules to ductal carcinoma in situ. This last finding is one of great theoretical and practical importance. It was their search for precancerous lesions which initiated their study in the first place. They adopted a grading system for ALA ranging from grade I (minimal change) to grade V (ductal carcinoma in situ), a grading system based on both histological and cytological criteria. The grades are clearly described and profusely illustrated.

This concept of a continuum from normal lobules to adenosis to in situ carcinoma deserves very close examination, as it is a central tenet of their conclusions. Their grades I and II of ALA correspond to 'adenosis' or 'blunt duct adenosis' as generally understood and as described in Chapter Three. Their grade V ALA represents ductal carcinoma in situ and is illustrated in their Figures 69 to 72 and Figures 77 to 88. There should be no difficulty in accepting this. Grades III and IV, however, are more problematical. Grade IV is illustrated in their Figures 61 to 64: in the opinion of the writer this is probably already in situ carcinoma. 'Clinging carcinoma' is visible in the lower part of Figure 62 and is illustrated at higher magnifications in Figures 63 and 64. Indeed, there is a hint here of peripheral cartwheel formation best seen in the upper part of Figure 62. The same is probably true of their Figure 67, also said to show grade IV atypia, and of Figure 76. This is true also of the lesion illustrated as grade IV atypia in the summarized work of these authors published in 1976 (Jensen, Rice and Wellings, 1976). The writer suspects that most of the grade IV ALA lesions would be called in situ carcinoma by many workers, including him. If this is accepted, *ALA grade III becomes the crucial link essential to sustain the hypothesis of Wellings, Jensen and Marcum (1975)* that ALA is a preneoplastic lesion analogous to HAN in the mouse. Their grade III atypia is not very well illustrated. Figures 58 to 60 illustrate basically an adenosis with some spindle-cell bridging (see their Figure 60) as seen in epitheliosis. It seems to the writer that the distinction between their grade III (Figure 60) and grade IV (Figure 64) is a fundamental qualitative one rather than a mere matter of degree.

In summary, grades I to III appear to be benign lesions (adenosis and some epitheliosis) while most grade IV lesions (as well as grade V) represent in situ carcinoma. The weakness of the argument rests on the fact that the crucial bridging link in the postulated spectrum has not been demonstrated convincingly.

EVIDENCE AGAINST THE CONCEPT OF A CONTINUUM FROM BENIGN HYPERPLASIA TO CARCINOMA

It would have been surprising to find that such a postulated link was easily demonstrable. If it were, we would not have been faced with the prolonged argument over the precancerous proclivities of cystic disease in general and its epithelial hyperplastic component in particular. The very mild increase in cancer risk with adenosis ($\times 1.3$) and the still modest increase with 'ductal hyperplasia' of $\times 1.8$ found by Page et al (1978) are hardly in keeping with the concept of Wellings, Jensen and Marcum (1975). Adenosis and blunt duct adenosis show all types of transitional forms to epitheliosis and to sclerosing adenosis, as indicated in Chapter Three. It is this host of transitional forms which gave rise to the many difficulties and disagreements about the precise, but benign, categories into which individual biopsies should be placed in the study of Page and his co-workers (1978). Nor, if we adopt the concept of a continuous spectrum, would it be as necessary as it is to try and distinguish accurately between epitheliosis and in situ carcinoma, a distinction to which the next chapter is devoted.

Also of interest is the work of Kern and Mikkelsen (1971), who reported on a series of 21 carcinomas less than 10 mm in diameter. This included 16 infiltrating and five non-infiltrating carcinomas. Of relevance here is the finding that 'several of the small carcinomas were also associated with considerable duct hyperplasia in randomly sectioned breast tissue'. Their Figure 7 illustrates, in the opinion of the writer, a definite in situ carcinoma and not merely 'duct papillomatosis'. This lesion was associated with two small carcinomas elsewhere in the breast. In another case, illustrated in their Figure 6, there was 'atypical large duct epithelial hyperplasia' associated with a small intraductal carcinoma elsewhere. But, independently of the issue of where one draws the line between benign and malignant, the value of this work, in the present context, lies in demonstrating that the *'borderline' or premalignant hyperplasias do not merge with or show transitions from foci of epitheliosis or adenosis of any recognized type.* This evidence hardly suggests that 'early' cancers commonly arise in and from foci of adenosis and epitheliosis by imperceptible transitional stages. As with the work of Wellings, Jensen and Marcum (1975), it is best interpreted as indicating that ductal carcinoma has its origin de novo from normal structures passing through a phase of indeterminate or 'borderline' atypical hyperplasia, which is usually distinct from the various types of adenosis and epitheliosis. This point will be discussed more fully later.

It would, of course, be unwise and almost certainly wrong to deny that such benign hyperplasias do occasionally undergo malignant transformation. Any breast lesion may do so, even lesions like sclerosing adenosis and fibroadenoma. What needs to be established is whether they do so more often than would be expected by chance. In the case of sclerosing adenosis and fibroadenoma, the evidence of Haagensen, Lane and Lattes (1972) and Page et al (1978) is that these lesions have no precancerous proclivity. Even in the case of adenosis and epitheliosis, the increased risk is only of the order of $\times 1.3$ and $\times 1.8$ respectively. The view expressed here in no way contradicts the conclusions of Wellings, Jensen and Marcum (1975) that carcinoma is accompanied by an increased incidence of benign epithelial proliferative disorders in other parts of the breast, but this has little bearing on the mode of origin of the actual cancerous focus or foci.

STUDY OF MINUTE DUCTAL CARCINOMAS

With increasing appreciation of the criteria of malignancy, as they apply to the breast, it has become possible in the last 10 to 15 years to recognize accurately minute in situ cancers of ductal type which in a given focus involve only a very few anatomical structures, be they lobules, ductules or ducts. Such cancers are clearly valuable in providing information in a number of ways.

Source of Material. The writer has studied 15 lesions of this type in recent years, the material being derived from 13 patients, two of whom had bilateral lesions (both doctors); four specimens were seen in consultation while 11 were from our own material. In only one case was the malignant lesion itself deemed to be producing symptoms or signs. Six of our 11

lesions were microscopic findings in breasts with other disease processes, either cystic disease or duct ectasia; three were in breasts which were otherwise normal but in which there was some clinical nodularity deemed to warrant biopsy excision. These three lesions were found in two patients, one a doctor with bilateral biopsies who had a very high index of suspicion because of a recent history of maternal breast cancer. Two lesions were picked up on mammography of 'well women'; one also had duct ectasia and hence is listed among the six patients with other breast disease. Interestingly the calcification identified radiologically in these two patients was mainly in benign disease adjacent to the carcinoma. It was situated in sclerosing adenosis in one patient; in the other it was situated in the luminal contents of duct ectasia, and in a duct with ectasia as well as minimal carcinoma affecting the lining. The main focus of carcinoma was not calcified. One patient had nipple discharge probably attributable to malignancy.

Clinical Data and Criteria for Inclusion. The ages of the patients ranged from 26 years to 53 years, with a mean of 38 years; one patient was pregnant at the time of biopsy. No lesion measured more than 3 mm in maximum diameter, an entirely arbitrary cut-off point. The one exception is a patient with duct ectasia and 'clinging carcinoma' in whom the overall lesion measured 4.5 mm; the total tumour volume was so minute that this case was included. At the other extreme one lesion measured only 200 μm, a carcinoma affecting a single ductule adjacent to a ruptured tension cyst. On serial section there was microscopic stromal infiltration over an area no larger than the in situ focus. To varying degree all these lesions were diagnostic problems, as one might expect from the fact that four of the 15 were referred for a second opinion and that all were extremely small. Of our 10 patients, seven had simple or subcutaneous mastectomy (including the doctor with bilateral lesions); three had no further treatment: one cancer, with only two lobules involved, was missed initially and a report of benign disease was issued; in the second patient a report of 'lobular carcinoma' was ambiguous and was interpreted as meaning CLIS (LCIS); in the third patient the nipple discharge was attributed to small benign papillomas while the ductal carcinoma of 'clinging' type was misinterpreted as benign.

The Course of Disease in Untreated Patients.
The course in these three patients is instructive. In the first, with a diagnosis of benign disease only, all was well for about five years, when the patient noticed a small nodule in the biopsy scar. This grew very slowly to a size of about 1 cm. About one year after its appearance it bled slightly when it rubbed on her clothing and it bled on a few further occasions over the next four years. The patient sought no medical advice over this five-year period, an instructive reminder that it is not possible to lay down dogmatic principles in patient management and treatment which have applicability to all social strata and to individuals of all nationalities and temperaments. Eventually she was seen in hospital because of arthritis of her finger joints and the examining physician referred her to a surgeon because of an 'ulcer' of her breast. Biopsy showed a well-differentiated breast carcinoma diffusely infiltrating the dermis, where it had excited a very marked elastotic reaction. Tumour had extended to and breached the basement membrane of the epidermis and had spread into the epidermis focally in pagetoid fashion. The patient received radiotherapy, which has controlled her disease for two years, though at last examination she had a hard, clinically involved lymph node in her supraclavicular fossa.

The second patient, with an initial diagnosis of 'lobular carcinoma' in March 1974, had a biopsy in 1975 which had some dubious changes only, but nothing which any pathologist who saw the slides would call malignant. In January 1978 further biopsy showed involvement of a single lobule by cancerization, including the formation of two unequivocal 'Roman bridges'. Further treatment has not yet been decided upon.

In the third patient, in whom nipple discharge was attributed initially to two microscopic papillomas, these were accompanied by in situ carcinoma which was missed; recurrent discharge four months later led to a diagnosis on biopsy of epitheliosis ('papillomatosis'). The reputed epitheliosis affected a large duct close to the nipple, a fact which should have alerted the pathologist to the possibility of an erroneous diagnosis, as discussed in Chapters Two and Seven. The 'epitheliosis' diagnosed at two biopsies was in fact in situ carcinoma: in the first biopsy it took the form of lobular cancerization with small duct involvement: in the second biopsy a large duct was involved. The patient developed recurrent tumour attached to the surgical scars, presenting at the hospital four and three-quarter years after the first biopsy and nearly four and one-half years after the second biopsy. Unfortunately, she had meanwhile failed to keep several follow-up appointments arranged for her in the second to fourth years post-biopsy, having attended only during the first postoperative year. Infiltrating carcinoma was found at frozen and paraffin section; tumour had infiltrated the dermis. It is unlikely that infiltrating carcinoma, at any rate of significant volume, was present at the time of the previous operations since two careful explorations were undertaken by a very experienced breast surgeon and the tissue biopsied had been very adequately examined pathologically. It is now three years since mastectomy but the final outcome is unknown since the patient emigrated to another country and could not be traced.

Pathology of the Microcancers. These 15 carcinomas showed features of lobular cancerization and usually some evidence of small duct involvement in continuity; hints of a pagetoid spread were sometimes present. Quantitatively, the lobular involvement was generally in excess of the ductal, though the cancer was of the so-called ductal type, as opposed to CLIS, having been deliberately selected in this way. In four lesions it was not possible to identify extralobular ductal involvement with confidence, although the small ducts have traditionally been regarded as the site of origin of these tumours. It is of course possible that evidence of ductal involvement was present in the unsampled tissue and there was no way of identifying the relevant tissue macroscopically. The alternative possibility of an in situ origin for cancerization is considered in Chapter Ten, page 210; this possibility has been given greater credibility since the work of Wellings, Jensen and Marcum (1975).

These microcancers showed mainly 'clinging' and cribriform patterns with occasional solid foci. No comedo cancer was present amongst them, as one might expect in minute carcinomas which posed diagnostic problems. The affected lobules and ducts contrasted sharply with the surrounding normal or benign hyperplastic tissue. Malignant changes affected the epithelial cell layer, while the myoepithelial cell layer was unaltered or flattened, inconspicuous and relatively less prominent or sometimes invisible. The epithelial cells formed only a single layer in parts and were sometimes orientated correctly, but they showed marked hypertrophy, nuclear enlargement with an increased nuclear/cytoplasmic ratio and sometimes conspicuous nucleoli. Frequently epithelial cell layers were multiple, varying between two and six layers or more, after allowing for tangential cuts. Orientation towards the lumen sometimes deviated slightly from the norm but this point was difficult to discern. In the more solid areas, sharper cell margins and the absence of 'streaming' (see Chapter Seven) distinguished the cancers from epitheliosis. The cribriform pattern took the form of early, rigid cartwheel formations, while features like trabecular bars and Roman bridges, even in minute amount, provided absolute evidence of malignancy.

The Absence of a Spatial Relationship Between Microcancer and Epitheliosis

One of the more striking findings was the absence of any evidence of transition from areas of epitheliosis to cancer, except perhaps in a single case. Epitheliosis was either absent, or present in other areas of the same block, or present in different blocks. In fact, though four patients had clinical and pathological cystic disease and a fifth patient had microscopic cysts only, in only two of our 10 patients were there numerous foci of epitheliosis. The 'early' in situ 'ductal' carcinoma appears to arise de novo either by a single step mutation, or by multiple step transformations; this histogenesis is suggested in small ducts, in which it is possible to trace the change from hyperplastic but benign epithelium through indeterminate or 'borderline' epithelium to distinctly malignant epithelium as witnessed by cytological and nuclear characteristics, the presence of pagetoid spread, a trabecular structure and similar unequivocal features of malignancy.

The converse of this is also true. Cases of severe extensive epitheliosis, which may at first sight appear very alarming, especially to the inexperienced pathologist, very rarely show unequivocal transition to definite carcinoma. Indeed, a few 'worrying' cells in a setting of epitheliosis can usually be safely ignored. As more cases of small and even minute in situ carcinoma are identified in the future, we can expect to learn a lot more about the relationship to cystic disease in general and to epitheliosis in particular.

THE NATURAL HISTORY OF INCIDENTALLY DISCOVERED MICROCANCER

More must be learned about the natural behaviour of lesions picked up as incidental findings accompanying other breast disease or picked up at mammography of selected women or of mass populations. Equally difficult is the problem of how to treat the woman whose 'lump' shows no breast pathology other than a minute in situ ductal carcinoma which could not, of itself, have led to the production of a clinical mass. Of our 10 patients discussed here, two were in this category: one, a doctor with bilateral lesions, opted for subcutaneous mastectomies: the other, left untreated because of a misdiagnosis, developed recurrent disease at five years and has persistent disease at 12 years.

THE NATURAL HISTORY OF IN SITU CARCINOMA DETECTED AT MAMMOGRAPHY

Lagios, Margolin and Rose (1977) suggested that occult foci of ductal carcinoma in situ detected by mammography differ substantially from DCIS which presents clinically, and that tylectomy with follow-up examination may represent a legitimate therapeutic option for such patients. If this is true of the type of patient discussed by Lagios, Margolin and Rose (1977), it would be truer presumably of the patients discussed here. It is certainly worth considering this option in all intelligent and well-informed patients who will follow a recommended course of management. It is vitally important in this regard to determine the incidence of multicentricity of ductal in situ lesions picked up by different methods: Lagios, Margolin and Rose (1977) found that six cases of DCIS identified only mammographically and less than 35 mm in size had no significant incidence of multicentricity as opposed to four larger lesions, three of which were palpable clinically. Patchefsky et al (1977) produced some evidence about multicentricity of DCIS which is not entirely in agreement. It is much too early to draw conclusions. The important point is that many centres are now dealing with an increasing amount of 'new pathology'.

This is mainly attributable to two causes: refinements in histological diagnosis and population screening. An entirely new approach to management is needed since so little is known about the behaviour of these 'earlier' and frequently much smaller lesions. As will be discussed below, Hutter and Kim (1971) pointed out one way of approaching this problem.

The Treatment of Cancer Detected by Different Means

Crile (1975) made out a case for partial mastectomy in *selected* cases even in clinically overt cancers. Subsequent clinical carcinomas developed no more frequently on the ipsilateral than on the contralateral side, a surprising finding which suggests that after partial mastectomy the danger of the appearance of a new cancer in the affected breast is less than might have been anticipated on the basis of the multicentricity demonstrated histologically by many workers. The microscopic findings described by the present writer are regarded mainly as of academic importance in relation to the genesis of 'early' cancers. It would be quite wrong to imply that they should necessarily be treated by mastectomy when a reasonable though still highly contentious case has been made for treating selected clinical cancers (Crile, 1975) and a stronger case for treating mammographically detected but non-palpable DCIS by more conservative means (Lagios, Margolin and Rose, 1977).

THE DE NOVO ORIGIN OF DUCTAL CARCINOMA

The concept of the 'atypical lobule' of Wellings, Jensen and Marcum (1975) remains an essentially valid one. But the pathway that leads to blunt duct adenosis, epitheliosis, sclerosing adenosis and so on, is regarded as one of little or no sinister significance. The lobular lesion that can justifiably be regarded as 'preneoplastic', in the sense of Wellings, Jensen and Marcum (1975), parts company with adenosis at an earlier stage than envisaged by those authors. There are qualitative, subtle cytological changes which distinguish the two and these will be considered under the headings of 'clinging carcinoma' and 'cancerization' (Chapter Ten). Thus it is that the 'early' carcinoma rarely has its origin in solid areas of epitheliosis or other types of benign epithelial hyperplasia and

hypertrophy. Rather does it arise by cytological changes in the epithelial cells of the TDLU that do not show the typical features of any type of adenosis. If one wishes to retain the concept of the ALA expounded by Wellings, Jensen and Marcum (1975), it would be better to divide the types of lesion encompassed by it into two more or less discrete entities. The starting point of these two entities is the same but their pathways of differentiation diverge from each other at an early stage, possibly at or even before the grade I ALA described by Wellings et al. This concept of an early divergence at the morphological level is strongly suggested by observations on minute and 'early' cancers, and is also more in keeping with the statistical findings of Page and coworkers (1978) in connection with the relation of the 'fibrocystic disease complex' to breast cancer.

This concept of the usual development of carcinoma from normal or near-normal structures negates the notion of a continuous spectrum of grades of hyperplasia in the lobule terminating in malignancy. This is important both theoretically and from a practical point of view. *The erroneous concept of a continuous spectrum would lead pathologists to search for 'early' malignancy in the more solid forms of benign proliferation.* But, on the contrary, the earliest changes usually take place de novo in epithelium which is not affected by previous solid benign hyperplasia. For these reasons the 'early' forms of carcinoma in situ are usually of the 'clinging' variety (q.v.) with or without early peripheral cartwheel formation. These are the types which are easily missed altogether at low magnification because their presence is not even suspected, and which have to be distinguished from benign hyperplastic lesions when they are studied at higher magnifications. By contrast, the more solid and comedo types of in situ cancer are easier to detect and easier to recognize as malignant lesions, thus posing less of a diagnostic challenge. But these are not the only recognizable 'early' in situ cancers. Nor, with these forms, is there much indication either that they take origin in solid benign hyperplasias. Most 'early' ductal carcinoma in situ has an origin de novo.

THE NEED FOR COMPARABLE NECROPSY STUDIES

Hutter and Kim (1971) discussed the problem of multiple lesions of the breast and selected four case histories to illustrate the extremes of unicentricity and multicentricity. Case 1, with a cancer detected by mammography, had a dominantly intraductal tumour with minimal invasion; the lesion was not only impalpable but was difficult to locate at surgery and could have been missed without the aid of specimen radiography. In their Case 4, whole organ study disclosed 38 additional foci of cancer (32 in situ and 6 infiltrating) in a specimen which was reported as having no residual tumour after 'routine' pathological examination. Cases 2 and 3 were intermediate in terms of multicentricity of the cancers. As Hutter and Kim (1971) emphasize, these cases are in no sense a series but are selected to make several points.

Their findings have an important bearing on the question of the significance of 'early' or minimal lesions. The baseline data on the incidence of multicentricity are constantly changing because of the more general recognition of minimal lesions. The trend is in an upward direction. It is now imperative to investigate the autopsy incidence of these lesions using the same histological criteria, in order to assess the significance of the reported increasing prevalence of multicentric microscopic foci of subclinical, subgross cancers (Hutter and Kim, 1971). If such minimal lesions are found to be as prevalent in autopsy as in surgical specimens, this would indicate either low expressivity or long latency for the development of clinical infiltrating cancers. There is no information on whether promoting factors are necessary for progression to occur to clinical disease. As Hutter and Kim (1971) stress, it is important to determine whether the latent period of the lesion exceeds the life expectancy of the patient. We should not forget the saga of the latent prostatic carcinoma, although the prostatic analogy is probably not a close one, for a number of reasons. For one thing, the minimal breast lesions in question are usually detected a decade or two before the prostatic lesions and this would obviously affect their potential significance. Although it is unlikely that the latent period of these newly recognized in situ breast cancers matches, let alone exceeds, the life expectancy of the patient, it is nevertheless a possibility. Autopsy material should be the best source of data. If the frequency of minimal lesions in autopsy material from non-cancerous patients is the same as in the second breast of patients with cancer in one breast, it would probably mean a long latent period for such lesions, in the absence of special promoting agents. But if, as seems more likely, there is found to be an important difference in incidence between the clinical and autopsy data, there would be a need to detect these lesions by screening procedures and to treat them. The correct method of treatment of this type of lesion is a challenging problem which only future work will determine.

References

Andersen, J. A. (1977) Lobular carcinoma in situ of the breast. An approach to rational treatment. *Cancer*, **39**, 2597–2602.

Black, M. M. and Chabon, A. B. (1969) In situ carcinoma of the breast. In *Pathology Annual* (Ed.) Sommers, S. C. pp. 185–210. New York: Appleton-Century-Crofts.

Black, M. M., Barclay, T. H. C.., Cutler, S. J., Hankey, B. F. and Asire, A. J. (1972) Association of atypical characteristics of benign breast lesions with subsequent risk of breast cancer. *Cancer*, **29**, 338–343.

Bonser, G. M., Dossett, J. A. and Jull, J. W. (1961) *Human and Experimental Breast Cancer*. London: Pitman Medical.

Buhl-Jørgensen, S. E., Fischermann, K., Johansen, H. and Petersen, B. (1968) Cancer risk in intraductal papilloma and papillomatosis. *Surgery, Gynecology and Obstetrics*, **127**, 1307–1312.

Chardot, C., Varroy, A. and Parache, R. M. (1970) Mastose fibro-kystique et cancer. (A propos de 206 mastoses en relation possible avec 12 cancers.) *Bulletin du Cancer*, **57**, 251–268.

Clagett, O. T., Plimpton, N. C. and Root, G. T. (1944) Lesions of the breast. The relationship of benign lesions to carcinoma. *Surgery*, **15**, 413–419.

Crile, G., Jr (1975) Multicentric breast cancer. The incidence of new cancers in the homolateral breast after partial mastectomy. *Cancer*, **35**, 475–477.

Davis, H. H., Simons, M. and Davis, J. B. (1964) Cystic disease of the breast: relationship to carcinoma. *Cancer*, **17**, 957–978.

Dawson, E. K. (1933) Carcinoma in the mammary lobule and its origin. *Edinburgh Medical Journal*, **40**, 57–82.

Devitt, J. E. (1972) Fibrocystic disease of the breast is not premalignant. *Surgery, Gynecology and Obstetrics*, **134**, 803–806.

Devitt, J. E. (1976) Breast cancer and preceding clinical benign breast disorders. A chance association. *Lancet*, **i**, 793–795.

Donnelly, P. K., Baker, K. W., Carney, J. A. and O'Fallon, W. M. (1975) Benign breast lesions and subsequent breast carcinoma in Rochester, Minnesota. *Mayo Clinic Proceedings*, **50**, 650–656.

Dossett, J. A. (1976) Malignant potential of breast lesions. In *Risk Factors in Breast Cancer* (Ed.) Stoll, B. A. Ch. 3, pp. 54–66. London: Heinemann Medical.

Fechner, R. E. (1971) Ductal carcinoma involving the lobule of the breast: a source of confusion with lobular carcinoma in situ. *Cancer*, **28**, 274–281.

Fisher, E. R., Gregorio, R. M. and Fisher, B. (1975) The pathology of invasive breast cancer. *Cancer*, **36**, 1–263.

Foote, F. W. and Stewart, F. W. (1945) Comparative studies of cancerous versus noncancerous breast. II. Role of so-called chronic cystic mastitis in mammary carcinogenesis. Influence of certain hormones on human breast structure. *Annals of Surgery,* **121,** 197–222.

Frantz, V. K., Pickren, J. W., Melcher, G. W. and Auchincloss, H., Jr (1951) Incidence of chronic cystic disease in so-called normal breasts. A study based on 225 postmortem examinations. *Cancer,* **4,** 762–783.

Gallager, H. S. and Martin, J. E. (1969a) The study of mammary carcinoma by mammography and whole organ sectioning. Early observations. *Cancer,* **23,** 855–873.

Gallager, H. S. and Martin, J. E. (1969b) Early phases in the development of breast cancer. *Cancer,* **24,** 1170–1178.

Haagensen, C. D. (1956) *Diseases of the Breast.* First edition. Philadelphia, London, Toronto: W. B. Saunders.

Haagensen, C. D. (1971) *Diseases of the Breast.* Second edition — revised reprint. pp. 169–171, 172–175. Philadelphia, London, Toronto: W. B. Saunders.

Haagensen, C. D., Lane, N. and Lattes, R. (1972) Neoplastic proliferation of the epithelium of the mammary lobules. Adenosis, lobular neoplasia, and small cell carcinoma. *Surgical Clinics of North America,* **52,** 497–524.

Haagensen, C. D., Lane, N., Lattes, R. and Bodian, C. (1978) Lobular neoplasia (so-called lobular carcinoma in situ) of the breast. *Cancer,* **42,** 737–769.

Herrmann, J. B. (1971) Mammary cancer subsequent to aspiration of cysts in the breast. *Annals of Surgery,* **173,** 40–43.

Humphrey, L. J. and Swerdlow, M. A. (1968) Large duct epithelial hyperplasia and carcinoma of the breast. *Archives of Surgery,* **97,** 592–594.

Hutter, R. V. P. and Kim, D. U. (1971) The problem of multiple lesions of the breast. *Cancer,* **28,** 1591–1607.

Izuo, M., Okagaki, T., Richart, R. M. and Lattes, R. (1971) Nuclear DNA content in hyperplastic lesions of cystic disease of the breast with special reference to malignant alteration. *Cancer,* **28,** 620–627.

Jensen, H. M., Rice, J. R. and Wellings, S. R. (1976) Preneoplastic lesions in the human breast. *Science,* **191,** 295–297.

Kern, W. H. and Brooks, R. N. (1969) Atypical epithelial hyperplasia associated with breast cancer and fibrocystic disease. *Cancer,* **24,** 668–675.

Kern, W. H. and Mikkelsen, W. P. (1971) Small carcinomas of the breast. *Cancer,* **28,** 948–955.

Kiaer, W. (1954) *Relation of Fibroadenomatosis ('Chronic Mastitis') to Cancer of the Breast.* Copenhagen: Munksgaard.

Kodlin, D., Winger, E. E., Morgenstern, N. L. and Chen, U. (1977) Chronic mastopathy and breast cancer. A follow-up study. *Cancer,* **39,** 2603–2607.

Lagios, M. D., Margolin, F. R. and Rose, M. R. (1977) Personal communication.

Lillienfeld, A. M. (1976) *Foundations of Epidemiology.* pp. 63–64. New York: Oxford University Press.

MacGillivray, J. B. (1969) The problems of 'chronic mastitis' with epitheliosis. *Journal of Clinical Pathology,* **22,** 340–347.

McDivitt, R. W. (1978) Breast carcinoma. *Human Pathology,* **9,** 3–21.

McDivitt, R. W., Stewart, F. W. and Berg, J. W. (1968) *Tumors of the Breast.* Atlas of Tumor Pathology, Second series, Fascicle 2. Washington, D.C.: Armed Forces Institute of Pathology.

Monson, R. R., Yen, S., MacMahon, B. and Warren, S. (1976) Chronic mastitis and carcinoma of the breast. *Lancet,* **ii,** 224–226.

Muir, R. (1941) The evolution of carcinoma of the mamma. *Journal of Pathology and Bacteriology,* **52,** 155–172.

Page, D. L., Zwaag, R. V., Rogers, L. W., Williams, L. T., Walker, W. E. and Hartmann, W. H. (1978) Relation between component parts of fibrocystic disease complex and breast cancer. *Journal of the National Cancer Institute,* **61,** 1055–1063.

Patchefsky, A. S., Shaber, G. S., Schwartz, G. F., Feig, S. A. and Nerlinger, R. E. (1977) The pathology of breast cancer detected by mass population screening. *Cancer,* **40,** 1659–1670.

Pellettiere, E. V., II (1971) The clinical and pathologic aspects of papillomatous disease of the breast: a follow-up study of 97 patients treated by local excision. *American Journal of Clinical Pathology,* **55,** 740–748.

Petrakis, N. L. (1977) Genetic factors in the etiology of breast cancer. *Cancer* (Supplement), **39,** 2709–2715.

Potter, J. F., Slimbaugh, W. P. and Woodward, S. C. (1968) Can breast carcinoma be anticipated? A follow-up on benign breast biopsies. *Annals of Surgery,* **167,** 829–837.

Renwick, S. B. (1976) The possible relationship between mammary dysplasia and breast cancer. *Australian and New Zealand Journal of Surgery,* **46,** 341–343.

Sandison, A. T. (1962) *An Autopsy Study of the Adult Human Breast.* National Cancer Institute Monograph No. 8. Washington, D.C.: U.S. Department of Health, Education and Welfare.

Steinhoff, N. G. and Black, W. C. (1970) Florid cystic disease preceding mammary cancer. *Annals of Surgery,* **171,** 501–508.

Tellem, M., Prive, L. and Meranze, D. R. (1962) Four-quadrant study of breasts removed for carcinoma. *Cancer,* **15,** 10–17.

Veronesi, U. and Pizzocaro, G. (1968) Breast cancer in women subsequent to cystic disease of the breast. *Surgery, Gynecology and Obstetrics,* **126,** 529–532.

Warren, S. (1940) The relation of 'chronic mastitis' to carcinoma of the breast. *Surgery, Gynecology and Obstetrics,* **71,** 257–273.

Wellings, S. R. and Jensen, H. M. (1973) On the origin and progression of ductal carcinoma in the human breast. *Journal of the National Cancer Institute,* **50,** 1111–1118.

Wellings, S. R., Jensen, H. M. and Marcum, R. G. (1975) An atlas of subgross pathology of the human breast with special reference to possible precancerous lesions. *Journal of the National Cancer Institute,* **55,** 231–273.

Willis, R. A. (1967) *The Pathology of Tumours.* Fourth edition, p. 230. London: Butterworth.

Chapter Seven

Epitheliosis and In Situ Carcinoma

It is obviously essential to comment in detail on the criteria listed in Table 7–1 for distinguishing epitheliosis from in situ carcinoma, for all these criteria, singly or in combination, must be evaluated critically and intelligently. The final histological diagnosis must be based on accurate observations; these observations are then pooled, enabling a pathologist to judge whether a given lesion is benign or malignant. In practice one does not consciously list these criteria in every instance; one relies on one's experience. But 'experience' can be merely the repetition of the same error often enough, which explains why a pathologist who has been badly trained in the first place usually finds it very difficult to relearn his craft. It is therefore most important that all diagnostic criteria employed should be as objective as possible, that the importance of different criteria in different circumstances should be correctly assessed and that a pathologist frequently consults other critical colleagues in order to preserve and increase his diagnostic acumen.

One must be willing, even anxious, to learn from one's errors. This requires a degree of humility, a readiness to listen to the arguments of others, including those of one's juniors, and the inclination to re-examine cases in which a mistaken diagnosis has been made and to analyse the reasons for the original mistake; otherwise there is a grave danger of repeating that same mistake. Perhaps worse than making a preventable error is the easily acquired habit of sitting on the fence and not committing oneself: there is no better way of learning nothing. Of course, very rarely a pathologist will be bound to confess frankly that he is at a loss for an answer, but this is quite different from not making a very determined effort to arrive at an accurate diagnosis. The pathologist who makes a definite diagnosis only when that diagnosis is rather obvious clinically is not of much help to the surgeon; he is not making full use of his training and is not doing justice to either himself or his craft.

In analysing criteria, one must attempt to use a *standardized nomenclature* or, when this is not possible, to define the terms used. This has been dealt with partly in Chapter Three. The reasons for preferring the term 'epitheliosis' to 'papillomatosis' are not by any means academic only, still less are they inspired by

Table 7–1 The differentiation of epitheliosis from 'ductal' carcinoma in situ

Epitheliosis	Carcinoma in situ (ductal type)
1. Solid or fenestrated	*Comedo*, solid, *cribriform* or 'clinging'
2. Necrosis hardly ever	Necrosis frequent
3. Haemorrhage hardly ever	Haemorrhage occasional
4. Foam cells frequent	Foam cells frequent
5. Periductal changes	Periductal changes
Inflammatory infiltrate absent unless other cause	Inflammatory infiltrate sometimes, especially with certain types
Fibroelastosis sometimes, especially with infiltrating variant	Fibroelastosis sometimes
6. *Streaming* frequent but usually subtle	No streaming
Mounds and tufts sometimes	Tufts occasionally
No trabeculae	*Trabeculae*
Spindle-cell bridging only type seen	Both spindle-cell and *trabecular bridging*
	Roman bridge and its variants
Collapsible fenestrated framework	Rigid cribriform framework
7. Spaces ovoid, irregular, sinuous, crescentic or eccentric	Tend to be rounded
Lining cells have blebbed margins (glandular spaces) or convex margins	Lining cells tend to be truncated
8. Syncytial appearance, indistinct cell margins	Cell margins usually more distinct but many exceptions
Ovoid cells or slightly elongated cells	Polygonal, rounded, cuboidal or columnar. Rarely ovoid or elongated
9. Cytoplasm bland and homogeneous, eosinophilic	Cytoplasm very variable between almost colourless and more deeply eosinophilic or amphophilic
	Sometimes faintly granular
10. Nuclei ovoid, delicate membrane, inconspicuous nucleoli, little chromatin beading, slight variation staining, tendency to overlap	Nuclei usually more rounded, hyperchromatic, monotonous (with exceptions, e.g. comedo), evenly spaced, nucleoli often conspicuous
11. Mitoses rare to many	Mitoses rare to very numerous
Atypical mitoses practically never	Atypical mitoses may be present and particularly valuable diagnostically in borderline solid and clinging lesions
12. Pagetoid spread absent	Pagetoid spread may be present, though more conspicuous with CLIS
13. Calcification infrequent	Calcification common
Psammoma bodies rare	Psammoma bodies sometimes
14. Epitheliosis occasionally merges with microscopic papillomas and apocrine foci	Only very rarely seems to merge with apparently benign papillomas, practically never with benign apocrine epithelium

These differential points are mere guides to diagnosis. *They are not meant to be used without the text.* Tabulated criteria, like atlases, have limited usefulness. '*Critical diagnosis requires experience transcending mere tabular guidelines*' (McDivitt, Stewart and Berg, 1968).

Explanatory Notes for Table 7–1

Since this table is regarded as potentially dangerous, some explanatory notes are appended to serve as a link with the text. Even the heading of the right-hand column is potentially misleading. 'Ductal type carcinoma' is not necessarily synonymous with carcinoma in the duct. It has become increasingly clear that much of what has been called 'ductal carcinoma' in the past is situated, in fact, in the lobule (Wellings, Jensen and Marcum, 1975).

1. The term 'fenestrated' epitheliosis is used since 'cribriform' has become synonymous in pathology with the 'punched out' neatly rounded spaces found in malignant tumours of the breast and other appendages and hence has come to signify a malignant tumour. 'Cribriform' literally means a 'sieve-like' appearance, but a sieve actually has rectangular holes and the term which best describes 'cribriform' as currently used in pathology is 'colanderiform' (with round holes like a vegetable strainer or colander). Colloquially, the writer is used to the expression 'holy epitheliosis' but not in the sense that it is sacred, only that it is traversed by spaces.

   The comedo pattern is practically diagnostic of cancer. The *cribriform pattern is diagnostic of cancer if it refers exclusively to the so-called sieve-like but actually colanderiform appearance*, rather than to spaces of any shape within a hyperplastic mass. The 'clinging' pattern is not seen in epitheliosis, but this type of cancer must be distinguished from adenosis: indeed, frequently, the very existence of an abnormal focus is difficult to perceive with 'clinging' carcinoma.

4. Foam cells are slightly commoner in epitheliosis than in carcinoma but the overlap is so great that they are useless as a differentiating criterion.

7. Though the spaces are usually rather neatly rounded in carcinoma, one must never rely heavily on this criterion as exceptions occur and, in occasional cases, irregularly shaped spaces may be found almost exclusively. This can give a deceptively benign impression at low magnification.

   While truncated cells are characteristic of malignancy and are rarely seen in the glandular (fenestrated) part of epitheliosis, luminal blebbing does occur with certain types of carcinoma and is not as rare as would appear from the literature.

8. Indistinct cell margins are of little or no value diagnostically. On the other hand, distinct cell margins can be of value in certain situations.

   A columnar cell is, of course, elongated in the sense that one axis is significantly longer than the other but this is not the meaning of 'elongated' in the sense used here.

10. These differences may be very obvious or extremely subtle. It would be extremely dangerous to attempt to rely on mere tabulated criteria to distinguish benign and malignant lesions. These and the other tabulated criteria have varying value in different circumstances as explained fully in the text. Thus, for instance, in certain clinging carcinomas the nuclei are predominantly ovoid and not strikingly hyperchromatic though there is usually a high N/C ratio, and the nuclei contain prominent nucleoli and may show abnormal mitotic activity.

12. Pagetoid 'spread' is, in a sense, absent by definition in benign conditions including epitheliosis, since it indicates a type of permeation seen only with cancer cells. The question resolves itself, then, into the definition of a pagetoid appearance. The more closely the appearance approximates that seen in Paget's disease of the nipple, the more justified is the use of the term 'pagetoid appearance' and the greater the diagnostic significance. Fortunately, only very rarely do benign conditions simulate this appearance at all closely.

14. This is not meant to imply that benign papillomas become malignant (see Chapter Eight). It indicates that, very rarely, ductal carcinoma may appear to merge with intraductal papilloma. This usually happens only with widespread in situ carcinoma and the possibility that the contiguity of the two lesions is fortuitous is not excluded.

   The writer has never actually seen intraductal carcinoma merge with benign apocrine epithelium and 'practically never' is used here only because the term 'never' is so seldom applicable in pathology.

---

any slavish adherence to narrow-minded nationalism. The true papilloma and the papillary carcinoma are dealt with in the following chapter. Structurally, epitheliosis is not a papillary lesion in the sense that pathologists use this term with reference to, say, papillary carcinoma of the thyroid or to papillary urothelial tumours. It is unfortunate that the term 'papillomatosis' has been so generally accepted in the birthplace of modern surgical pathology, i.e. the USA. This has had regrettable consequences, because many lesions illustrated as 'papillomatosis' and 'atypical papillomatosis' would not be so termed were they in other organs: surely this is, in itself, an indictment of the term. Epitheliosis has to be distinguished from in situ carcinoma in its variant forms and especially from the solid and cribriform varieties. Use of the term 'papillomatosis' for essentially solid lesions has obscured, and not clarified, this important distinction. The term 'cribriform' can be used in a number of alternative senses but, in the strict sense used in the explanatory notes to Table 7–1, a cribriform structure is an important diagnostic criterion.

Another general point to bear in mind is the importance of *cytology and mitotic aberrations*. Pathologists examining breast lesions all too often concentrate exclusively on structure and ignore the cytological and nuclear details. Although structural patterns are generally sufficient to distinguish epitheliosis from malignancy, in a difficult case the fine cellular details can be invaluable. The frequency of mitoses (including prophases) should be estimated; chromosomal breaks, abnormalities of chromosome number, multipolar mitoses, etc., should be diligently looked for in borderline cases and, when present, are ignored at one's peril. Possibly the scant attention paid to cytological appearances as distinct from histological patterns stems largely from a separation of the two disciplines within the same hospital or institute, a situation brought about by historical circumstances. It is paradoxical that in an age of ultrastructural study some pathologists pay too little attention to the use of their ×40 objective lenses and almost ignore their oil immersion lenses. New methods of diagnosis usually supplement, without replacing, older methods.

A further point of general importance is an *awareness of the parts of the breast that can be affected by different diseases.* The schematic representation of this in Chapter Two may seem all too obvious had the writer not accumulated a mass of evidence to the contrary. The major ducts of the nipple region are virtually never affected by epitheliosis, though they may, of course, be the seat of papillomas: one of the many important reasons, incidentally, for not using these terms interchangeably. Solid lesions of the major ducts are thus liable to be underdiagnosed because of failure to appreciate that epitheliosis does not affect these ducts, while carcinoma may and does. A priori, a 'borderline' solid lesion of the ducts of the nipple region is very unlikely to be a benign one. It is unfortunate, therefore, that 'ductal hyperplasia' is illustrated schematically as affecting the area of the lactiferous sinus by Shah, Rosen and Robbins (1973). Shah, Rosen and Robbins (1973) were factually correct in that they were referring to a premalignant hyperplasia in the course of emphasizing the wide field of origin of carcinoma. But the impression left on the reader can unfortunately be misleading.

Clinical data are always important. Sometimes they illuminate pathological processes, as in the distinction between cystic disease and duct ectasia. The pathologist can help the clinician a great deal by drawing attention to the fact that the pathology he has observed does not adequately explain the symptoms and signs recorded. As discussed in Chapter Five, cystic disease is not acceptable as the cause of a nipple discharge, while duct ectasia and ductal papilloma are well-recognized benign causes of such a complaint. Epitheliosis, as opposed to papilloma, does not give rise to discharge from the nipple; this is understandable because of the distal sites involved by epitheliosis and because epitheliosis rarely undergoes infarction or necrosis. If a pathologist encounters a 'borderline' solid lesion which is associated with a history of nipple discharge, he should think and think again before making a diagnosis of epitheliosis. If the diagnosis of epitheliosis is nevertheless correct, then a dual pathology is very likely as an explanation of the discharge. Apart from rarities like adenoma of the nipple ('florid papillomatosis'), duct ectasia and ductal papilloma are virtually the only acceptable benign structural causes of a nipple discharge. The remainder are malignant until proof to the contrary is forthcoming.

EPITHELIOSIS

Necrosis

Necrosis is sufficiently rare in epitheliosis as to cast doubt on the correctness of this diagnosis if it is present. A few degenerate cells with pyknotic nuclei may occasionally be found in epitheliosis on careful scrutiny and, even more rarely, a few loose necrotic cells may be found free in a lumen. But these changes cannot be seen at low magnifications (×2.5 and ×10). They are found, if at all, only after a deliberate search with a ×25 or ×40 objective. In the vast majority of cases of epitheliosis, necrosis is absent or very inconspicuous. Exceptions will occur and I have seen obvious necrosis in two otherwise typical examples of epitheliosis.

Haemorrhage

Frank evidence of haemorrhage, recent or old, is rare in epitheliosis. This is as might be expected, since the lesion very rarely shows obvious necrosis and apparently does not become infarcted. The writer has seen haemorrhage with epitheliosis only once. It was present in one of the two cases with obvious necrosis just mentioned. While haemorrhage, per se, cannot be regarded as a criterion of malignancy, its presence should make an observer suspicious and lead him to examine the specimen with greater care.

Foam Cells

Curiously, foam cells are very frequently found in epitheliosis and are often more prominent a feature than in carcinoma but, since they are found in both conditions, their presence has little differential diagnostic value. The foamy cells are probably macrophages, though this still requires confirmation since alternative explanations have been put forward (Hamperl, 1970; Davies, 1974). The foam cells in epitheliosis rarely contain haemosiderin or other pigments and the source of their lipid content is not clear.

ESSENTIAL FEATURES OF EPITHELIOSIS

The most important features of epitheliosis are the structural configurations, the nature of the luminal spaces, the intercellular relationships, the appearance of the cell cytoplasm and of the nuclei and the presence of divergent differentiation. These are the cardinal criteria in the distinction from carcinoma and empirically they have proved to be very valuable diagnostic features. An

attempt to explain them on theoretical grounds will be made later. In epitheliosis the lumina are partially or completely filled by solid cellular sheets or ones that contain spaces, which are mostly ovoid or irregular in outline (Figures 7–1 to 7–4). Where intraluminal growth is partial, it frequently takes the form of broad polypoid tongues, which protrude eccentrically leaving a crescentic lumen (Figure 7–4).

The Structural Pattern

Epitheliosis has a characteristic *'streaming' growth pattern*, distinct or subtle, meaning that, in some planes of sectioning, the cells and their nuclei have a parallel orientation of their long axes (Figures 7–5 and 7–6). This is a cardinal feature of epitheliosis, invariably present in some areas of the lesion at least in subtle form. It is a feature which serves to

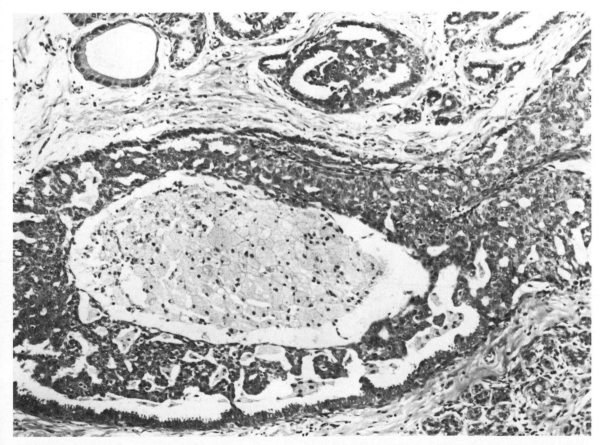

Figure 7–1   Epitheliosis (so-called 'papillomatosis') in a duct. Solid and fenestrated pattern. Lumina have an irregular shape. Foam cells are present centrally. Marked cytoplasmic blebbing is present on one margin of the duct. H and E. ×400.

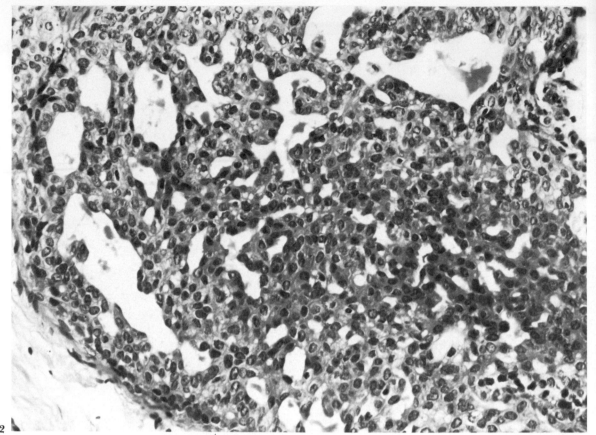

7–2

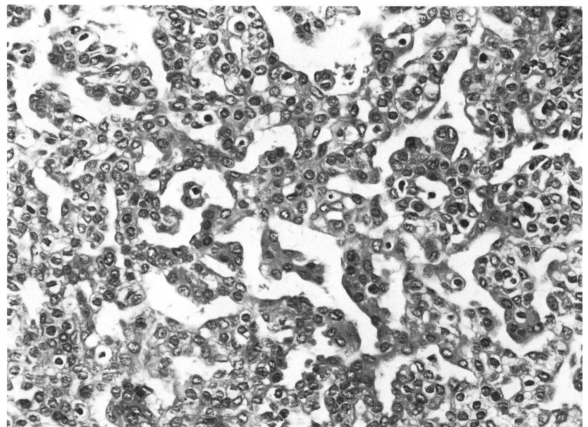

7–3

118

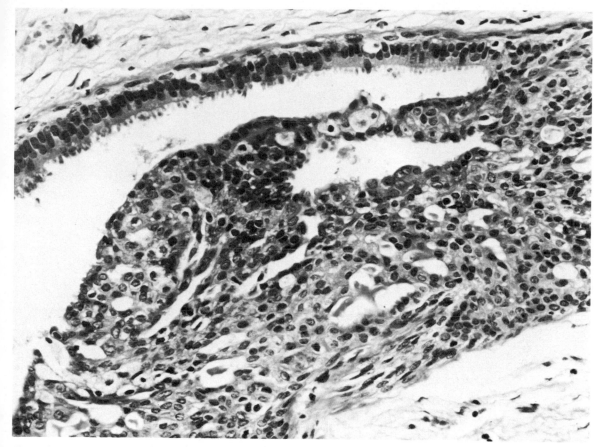

Figure 7–4 Tongue of epitheliosis projecting into lumen eccentrically. It has a collapsible structure. The nuclei have a delicate, bland appearance. There is marked cytoplasmic blebbing of the epithelial cells lining one side of the duct. H and E. ×400.

distinguish it from carcinoma at low magnifications, if only by an unconscious process of pattern recognition.

Cytoplasmic and Nuclear Detail

Cytoplasmic Borders are usually indistinct so that the nuclei appear to lie in a syncytial mass (Figures 7–2 and 7–4). The cytoplasm is weakly to moderately eosinophilic and generally so homogeneously stained, uniform and bland as hardly to impinge upon the observer's consciousness.

Nuclei. It is the nuclear characteristics that strike the observer. Nuclei are not large in absolute terms but the N/C ratio may be high in comparison with normal epithelial cells, partly because of the generally small size of the cells. The character and spacing of the nuclei is very important, for the nuclei vary in shape from ovoid, irregularly ovoid or occasionally nearly bean-shaped to a more spindle form; they are rarely rounded, except where cut transversely. Cells are correspondingly more or less elongated (Figures 7–5 and 7–6). The nuclei sometimes show slight variation in staining intensity (Figures 7–2 and 7–4) but they do not display the pleomorphism of certain varieties of carcinoma. They possess a very delicate nuclear membrane, a delicate internal structure that lacks prominent chromatin markings and, characteristically, they lack prominent or large nucleoli (Figures 7–3, 7–5 and 7–6).

Figure 7–2 (*Opposite, above.*) Typical epitheliosis with 'syncytial' structure traversed by irregularly shaped spaces lined by slightly bulging cells. H and E. ×400.

Figure 7–3 (*Opposite, below.*) Collapsed, as opposed to rigid, trellis characteristic of epitheliosis. Slightly ovoid nuclei have a delicate internal structure and show slight overlap. H and E. ×400.

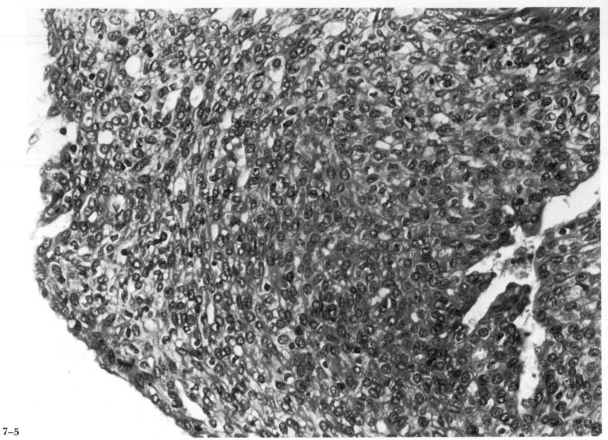

7–5

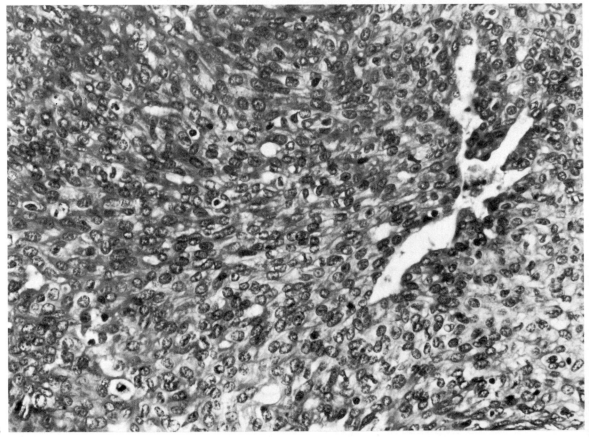

7–6

Nucleoli. Usually in epitheliosis it is difficult to find as many as 10 nucleoli in 50 nuclei. More important than the number is the fact that nucleoli in epitheliosis are mostly small, generally single and very inconspicuous. If, on the other hand, one were to find 10 conspicuous large nucleoli in 50 nuclei, the alternative diagnosis of carcinoma should be seriously considered. In many cribriform carcinomas, nucleolar prominence is not a feature. It is particularly with certain solid and 'clinging' forms of in situ carcinoma that large and prominent nucleoli attain importance. Nucleoli have about the same diagnostic significance as they have in the prostate, perhaps more so, since attention to cytology is of even greater importance in dealing with in situ carcinoma of the breast than it is for the prostate, where the problem is usually the recognition of a small but invasive lesion.

Nuclear Spacing. The nuclei are not evenly spaced in the 'syncytial' mass of epitheliosis, so that they appear slightly crowded in some areas and spaced a little further apart in others (Figures 7–4 and 7–7). Where nuclei are crowded, they often overlap one another very slightly even in a uniformly cut 5 μm section (Figure 7–7). This *irregular nuclear spacing* with slight overlap, the nuclear morphology described, taken in conjunction with the 'streaming' pattern, are the hallmarks of epitheliosis.

Mitotic Activity. The degree of mitotic activity is sometimes of little help but it is a generally underrated feature which can, on occasion, be extremely useful. Mitoses are usually scanty and it is a little surprising, perhaps, how few are usually demonstrable even in a florid epitheliosis. Numerous fields may be searched to no avail, but too much reliance must not be placed on this feature alone since exceptions do occur. For practical purposes, mitoses in epitheliosis are qualitatively normal. On the other hand, in carcinoma in situ, the presence of even a few abnormal forms can be extremely helpful in establishing the diagnosis. Though no rigid

rules apply in pathology, a solid epithelial proliferation containing a mitotic figure in every two or three high-power fields with an occasional field containing three and even more mitoses is not likely to be benign. If mitotic aberrations are found, the diagnostic problem becomes that much easier to resolve. Insufficient attention is paid to mitotic abnormalities and the writer has seen malignancy missed because of such lack of attention. Although practically no criterion can ever be considered in isolation, the quality of the mitotic activity as well as the prominence of nucleoli in a breast lesion deserve greater attention than is usually accorded them.

Tufts and Mounds

When small buds or tufts project into a lumen they assume a distinctive pattern. The tongue-like projections show perpendicular streaming (Figure 7–8), whereas the more rounded mounds, with convex luminal profiles, show varying degrees of onion-skin or concentric lamination. It will be readily understood that these are only adaptations of the basic streaming pattern and many variations on this basic theme may be observed.

Spindle-Cell Bridging

While certain types of luminal bridging are characteristic, indeed diagnostic, of malignancy, luminal bridging of a different kind can be seen in epitheliosis (Figures 7–8 and 7–9). Elongated cells are arranged parallel to the long axis of the bridge, producing in effect a spur which spans the lumen (Figures 7–8 and 7–9). This concept of Spindle-cell Bridging in epitheliosis is essential to an understanding of one of the major features distinguishing it from carcinoma. By contrast, the bridging beams of in situ carcinoma form trabeculae, the cells of which are not necessarily orientated with their long axes in

Figure 7–5 (*Opposite, above.*) Solid epitheliosis with streaming of cells and nuclei. Characteristic nuclei of epitheliosis without chromatin clumping and without prominent nucleoli. H and E. ×400.

Figure 7–6 (*Opposite, below.*) Streaming in epitheliosis with cells and nuclei in parallel array. H and E. ×400.

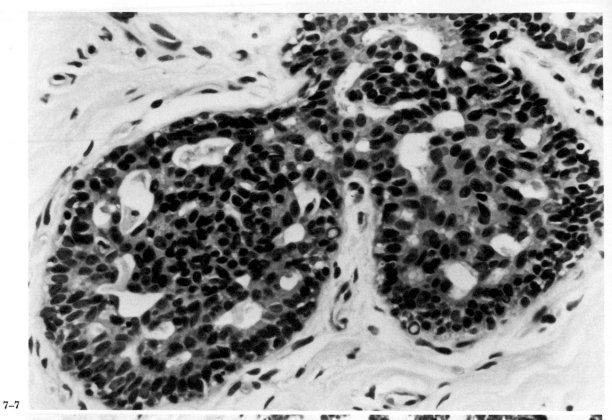

7–7

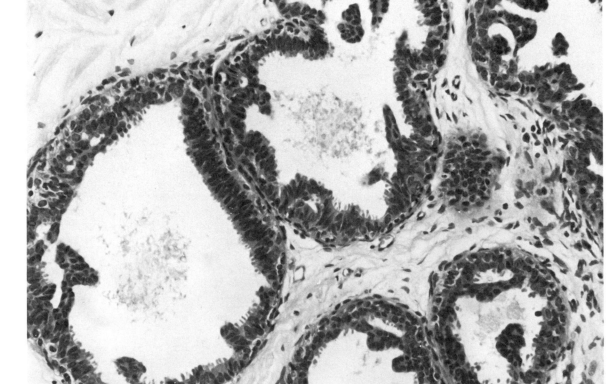

7–8

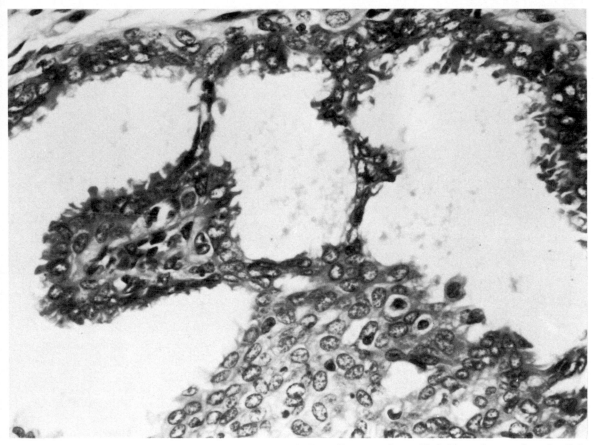

Figure 7–9   In solid area nuclear blandness is striking. In darker cells at margins and in bridges, the cytoplasm is a little more eosinophilic, nuclei overlap and sometimes bulge, cytoplasmic luminal margins show some blebbing. The twisted, 'rough' spindle-cell bridge is characteristic of epitheliosis. H and E. ×400.

the long axis of the beam. The more definite the transverse orientation of cells in such trabeculae, the more definite is the diagnosis of malignancy.

The architectural pattern of epitheliosis can be summarized by the key words Streaming, Spindle-cell Tufting and Bridging, Without Trabecula Formation as here defined.

The Spaces Within a Lesion

The spaces within a lesion of epitheliosis are hardly ever neatly rounded but are usually ovoid, irregular or even serpiginous or crescentic (Figures 7–1 to 7–4 and 7–7). Some of these spaces represent true glandular differentiation, as will be discussed below. Other spaces are not obviously due to glandular differentiation, but the elongated cells which line these spaces have convex luminal margins with a central bulge (Figure 7–2).

Divergent Differentiation

Two cell types are not usually distinguishable with any confidence in areas of solid epitheliosis, so

Figure 7–7   (*Opposite, above.*)   Solid and fenestrated epitheliosis. The nuclei are crowded in many areas. Though they are more deeply staining than average, they lack the pleomorphism of anaplasia and the overall structure conforms to that of epitheliosis. H and E. ×600.

Figure 7–8   (*Opposite, below.*)   Part of a lobule affected by microcystic BDA is shown. There is spindle-cell tufting, spur formation and even bridging of the type seen frequently in epitheliosis. The mounds and peninsulas are of the type seen characteristically in benign disease. No trabeculae or cartwheels. H and E. ×300.

that this criterion is not applicable in the way it is used to distinguish between benign and malignant papillary tumours. At most, in solid epitheliosis there is a hint of variation in the depth of nuclear staining, but it is usually doubtful at light microscopic level whether this represents a two-cell-type differentiation. At ultrastructural level, Ahmed (1978) strongly suggests that it is.

On the other hand, persistence of pre-existing two cell types at the periphery of the containing structure is common enough in epitheliosis, as it is also with in situ carcinoma, especially the less obvious forms. Persistence of such myoepithelial cells at the periphery is, therefore, useless as a differential feature between a benign and a malignant lesion.

Glandular Differentiation. A more obvious differentiation of the lesional tissue, with the formation of *epithelium-lined glandular spaces*, is frequent in the less solid parts of epitheliosis and this can be seen in the centre of a lesion, where the question of 'persistence' does not arise (Figure 7–9). The epithelial cells which line these gland-like spaces show orientation towards a lumen and are characterized by having more copious eosinophilic cytoplasm, which distinguishes them from the surrounding spindled or elongated cells. These epithelial cells display irregular luminal margins or 'fluffy borders', and, at low magnifications, the whole cell appears peg-shaped. The 'fluffy border' is · due to eosinophilic material attached to, or adjacent to, the free cell margins, a phenomenon referred to here as *cytoplasmic blebbing* (Figure 7–9).

Ultrastructural examination has shown that this 'cytoplasmic blebbing', characteristic of, but not restricted exclusively to, benign disease, is caused by 'peninsulas and bays' on the luminal edge as well as by the differentiation of copious and long microvilli (Ozzello, 1971). This establishes that these cells are epithelial in nature since they are endowed with an absorptive type of free surface. There is much more limited evidence that these cells possess secretory activity at the ultrastructural level (Ozzello, 1971). These epithelial cells with blebbing of their free edges are the same cells which have been referred to in the literature as cells with 'apocrine snouts', 'secretory snouts' or more recently as 'apocrine-like cells' (Page et al, 1978). The term 'apocrine snouts' is inappropriate since the resemblance to apocrine

epithelium is superficial at both light microscopic and ultrastructural levels (Harris and Ahmed, 1977). Histochemically also the cells lack the distinctive PAS positive granules which characterize apocrine epithelium. The term 'secretory' is barely appropriate for reasons already stated. But the picturesque designation of 'snouts' is as accurate as 'blebbing' for the appearances actually seen. 'Snouts', 'apical snouts' (Harris and Ahmed, 1977), 'blebbing', 'fluffy borders' are terms which can be used more or less interchangeably for the same phenomenon.

Whatever the precise terms used, there is no doubting the value of this particular type of differentiation in the diagnosis of breast lesions. It is of greater value in the more solid and cribriform hyperplasias than in the distinction of adenosis and 'clinging' carcinoma and other 'early' malignancies (page 199). The convex, peg-shaped snout or fluffy edge is in contrast 'with the sharper, more square-cut or truncated edge usually seen in carcinomas. Widespread and prominent fluffy borders, in conjunction with the correct structural patterns, suggest a benign lesion. Definite truncation of cells, in the correct architectural context, is strong presumptive evidence of malignancy, but the opposite does not always hold because in situ carcinoma may contain foci of distinct microvillous differentiation.

Apocrine Metaplasia

In pure epitheliosis, apocrine metaplasia is uncommon so that, as a negative finding, it is of no value in the distinction from carcinoma. Of course, if present, it very much favours the diagnosis of a benign lesion. The greatest value of apocrine metaplasia is seen in the type of lesion which is transitional between epitheliosis and microscopic papillomas. In such cases the small and ill-defined papillary fronds do not always show two cell types, and their cores are partly occupied by epitheliosis. In this transitional type of lesion, apocrine metaplasia is quite common and is useful as a confirmatory sign that the lesion is benign (Figure 7–10). The nuclei of apocrine epithelium are usually rounded, fairly deeply staining, sometimes variable in size, with rare giant nuclei, and frequently they possess relatively conspicuous nucleoli. These features are not shared by the areas of epitheliosis or by the epithelial cells which cover papillary fronds. In apocrine epithelium such features are not by themselves indicative of malignancy; on the contrary, the presence of apocrine metaplasia points to a benign lesion despite this mild degree of nuclear atypia. The apocrine metaplasia referred to here is the classical obvious form, which is recognizable at a glance and is not seen in carcinoma in situ. It must of course be appreciated that apocrine metaplasia of varying degree may be present with invasive carcinomas as well as with in situ malignant lesions, but the degree of apocrine alteration seen rarely in carcinoma in situ is not likely to cause confusion with benign apocrine metaplasia. Moreover, the degree of cytological atypia seen with apocrine carcinoma is such as to leave little room for doubt about its malignant nature.

Distension

Epitheliosis gives rise to variable degrees of distension of the containing structures, but the very gross degrees of distension sometimes seen with malignancy are less common with epitheliosis. There is, however, so much overlap and so many exceptions that, in practice, this criterion is not often of value. Where distension is so gross as, of itself, to suggest malignancy, there is usually little difficulty in making this diagnosis on other grounds. The questionable 'borderline' in situ lesions often produce little or no distension. Having appreciated that, one must admit that a gross degree of distension may draw attention to a lesion that needs much closer scrutiny. Such gross distension could be regarded as having 'pinpointing' value but it must never be looked upon as more than that.

Calcification

The presence of calcification is important as a positive finding though no deductions can be drawn from its absence. In malignant disease, calcification manifests itself in two main

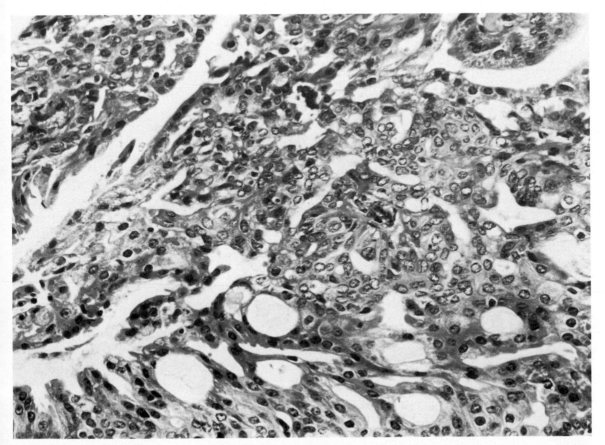

Figure 7–10 Transition between epitheliosis and apocrine differentiation. In the latter areas, the nuclei are rounded, more deeply staining and sometimes have more prominent nucleoli. H and E. ×400.

forms. It is frequently present in granular form in necrotic parts of in situ carcinoma; secondly it may take the form of calcific spherules in in situ or invasive parts of carcinomas. Calcification may be found in ductal and ductular carcinoma and in cancerization of lobules. Calcification is seen also, less frequently, in CLIS. Calcification in carcinoma is discussed in Chapter Eighteen. On the other hand, in epitheliosis there is usually very little or no calcification and, in particular, *there are hardly ever any calcific spherules or psammoma bodies.* This is an important distinguishing point because, in a difficult case with a focus of borderline architecture and cytology, one or two calcific spherules can have almost as much diagnostic significance as the presence of trabecular luminal bridging or of 'punched-out' sieve-like cribriform spaces. For example, in a case of ductal carcinoma with slight but distinct pagetoid spread, a well-defined deeply haematoxyphil calcific spherule was situated amongst the pagetoid cells where they were forming such a thin layer as to be barely detectable. The calcific spherule and the pagetoid spread were each, as it were, confirming the tell-tale significance of the other finding. One must, of course, remember that exceptions which prove the rule will occur. I have seen obvious necrosis with marked calcification in a single instance of otherwise typical epitheliosis, in which no cause for the necrosis could be found. In four out of 60 cases of epitheliosis specifically studied, small flecks of calcium were present in the zones of epitheliosis but in only one of these was the calcification at all conspicuous on haemalum–eosin preparations. *Calcospherites in epitheliosis have apparently not been recorded in the literature* and have correspondingly greater diagnostic significance; the writer has observed them on only two occasions.

Stressing the sparsity of calcification in epitheliosis is not of course meant to imply that calcification does not occur in benign breast disease in general nor that it does not occur in other components of cystic hyperplasia. Sclerosing adenosis, for instance, frequently shows calcification in the distorted glandular spaces, and the calcium deposits are occasionally sufficiently profuse or localized to be confused with the calcification of carcinoma on mammography. In adenosis or 'blunt duct adenosis' small amounts of amorphous and granular calcification are quite common. The luminal contents of cysts are sometimes the seat of calcium deposition and the writer has even seen psammoma bodies in apocrine cysts on several occasions.

Inflammation

Epitheliosis per se is not accompanied by a significant inflammatory response around the lesion. It must, however, be remembered that cystic disease with tension cysts frequently accompanies epitheliosis as part of the cystic hyperplasia complex, and that rupture of tension cysts is a frequent cause of inflammatory infiltration in the breast. If ruptured tension cysts are present in the vicinity, 'spillage' of inflammatory cells into the foci of epitheliosis is frequent and hence allowance must be made for this and similar factors.

Fibrosis and Elastosis

Epitheliosis is usually not associated with either fibrosis or elastosis but exceptions are fairly frequent. Firstly, preceding duct ectasia can lead to periductal fibrosis and even elastosis, and epitheliosis may supervene on these pre-existing changes; this is an uncommon cause of fibroelastosis associated with epitheliosis. More cogently, epitheliosis per se, especially the infiltrating variety, is sometimes associated with fibrosis and elastosis, and this can occur in the absence of other antecedent or concomitant disease, i.e. fibroelastosis can represent a response to epitheliosis. It is particularly important to appreciate that these pathological associations occur and hence that the widely publicized view of Jackson and Orr (1957) that periductal fibrosis and elastosis are always precancerous stromal changes must be rejected. Nevertheless, severe and prominent fibroelastosis with epitheliosis is a relatively uncommon finding and cases showing marked fibroelastosis deserve further study. Fibroelastosis around foci of epithelial proliferation has about the same significance as an inflammatory infiltrate. It cannot be regarded as an indicator of malignancy but it should be regarded as a finding which focuses attention on areas in need of closer scrutiny. It is on a detailed study of structural patterns and cytology that a definitive diagnosis must be based.

Accompaniments of Epitheliosis

As part of a general hyperplasia, epitheliosis is quite commonly accompanied by microscopic papillomas, which are either separate from, or contiguous with, areas of epitheliosis. The presence of such well-formed, two-layered papillomas suggests that the adjacent epithelial hyperplasia is also probably benign, but this can be regarded only as very circumstantial evidence from the company kept by the focus in question. It is not definitive evidence since in situ carcinoma may on occasion coexist side-by-side with a papilloma or an area of epitheliosis, if only by chance. The same arguments apply to accompanying sclerosing adenosis and other benign hyperplasias. The foregoing arguments about the 'company kept' as circumstantial evidence of a benign lesion applies only, and that in a very limited way, to the differentiation of epitheliosis and in situ ductal carcinoma. It does not apply to the diagnosis of CLIS. Since this is almost always an incidental finding when some other lesion is resected, cystic disease often with some degree of benign hyperplasia is a usual accompaniment of CLIS.

SPECULATIONS ON THE NATURE OF EPITHELIOSIS

It is tempting to speculate about the reasons for the 'streaming' pattern of epitheliosis and its many variations, its cytological, nuclear and other characteristics, the relative paucity of calcification, and its other positive and negative characteristics. The last 15 years have seen an intensive search for evidence of myoepithelial cell differentiation in every type of breast carcinoma, a search which has yielded evidence of a dubious nature, evidence which has sometimes stretched credibility to breaking point and which has later been mostly rejected. No attempt has, to my knowledge, been made to study epitheliosis with the same possibility in mind; this is curious because, a priori, there are perhaps better grounds for suspecting myoid differentiation in epitheliosis than in most carcinomas. *A plausible hypothesis is that we might be dealing here with a very rudimentary and imperfect attempt at myoid differentiation.* Such a hypothesis would explain the shape of the cells and their nuclei, together with their orientation one to another. The streaming pattern, the spindle-cell tufting and the spindle-cell bridging would all be explicable on this basis. These cells show no very concrete evidence of epithelial differentiation in many cases of solid 'epitheliosis'. The most definite epithelial

differentiation in 'epitheliosis' is manifested by the gland-like structures lined by cells showing polarity and possessing microvilli on their luminal borders.

Epitheliosis represents a benign proliferative process showing some divergent differentiation into clearly recognizable epithelial cells, on the one hand, and a larger mass of indeterminate or perhaps transitional cells, on the other, the latter possibly showing greater similarities to myoid cells than to epithelial cells. The paucity of calcification in epitheliosis, and in particular the rarity of calcospherites, are consistent with this view. Sclerosing adenosis and benign papillomas can be regarded as proliferative processes with an advanced form of differentiation into two cell types, while epitheliosis could be viewed as a hyperplasia with a much lesser degree of differentiation and tending to be mainly myoid though at a very rudimentary level. Histochemical evidence which might lend support to this view was provided by the demonstration of intense alkaline phosphatase activity in areas of solid epitheliosis (Ahmed, 1974) but a lot more evidence is obviously necessary before this can be regarded as anything more than a tentative hypothesis.

The alternative possibility, which on current evidence seems more likely, is that we are dealing here with a mass of indeterminate cells of the type identified by Ozzello (1971) even in the normal breast. On this hypothesis, the hyperplastic tissue could be regarded as of indeterminate type and uncommitted to an epithelial or myoepithelial line of differentiation. The spindle-cell streaming and bridging are certainly consistent with the growth pattern which such uncommitted tissue would be likely to assume. It would clearly be rash to postulate myoid differentiation only on the grounds previously mentioned here, though the demonstration of alkaline phosphatase activity makes this an attractive hypothesis. It is, nevertheless, salutary to remind oneself of the potential fallacy of relying on only one piece of evidence. Thus, the demonstration of ATPase in 'scirrhous' carcinoma had been regarded as definitive evidence of myoepithelial differentiation in such tumours until recent work demonstrated that this concept is invalid (see Chapter Twelve).

Ultrastructural studies of fibrocystic disease and cystic hyperplasia have concentrated mainly on the changes of sclerosing adenosis and the alterations found in apocrine epithelium (Wellings and Roberts, 1963; Ozzello, 1971). Even in the comprehensive and detailed account of Ozzello (1971) on the ultrastructural pathology of the human breast, the section on 'mammary dysplasia' deals largely with sclerosing adenosis and cystic disease. In the description of ductal and lobular hyperplasia, however, Ozzello (1971) does state that in some instances myoepithelial cells, though still recognizable as such because of the presence and orientation of filament bundles with dense zones, do seem to lose most of their other distinguishing characteristics. As a result of this, they attain the features of 'indeterminate cells' and may be very difficult to separate from the epithelial cells. The distinct possibility of the existence of an 'indeterminate cell' even in the normal breast is an important one, as stressed by Ozzello (1971). These cells are difficult to categorize either because of lack of distinguishing features or because they exhibit characteristics of both cell types. Indeterminate cells could represent the progenitors of both epithelial and myoepithelial cells or might represent a transitional form between the two cells.

Since indeterminate cells have been identified by Ozzello (1971) in dysplastic breasts, there is a need to study specifically the lesion of epitheliosis in an effort to determine its precise cellular composition. This would be no mean task but should prove most rewarding.

As will be seen, *the main structural and cytological traits of carcinoma, as opposed to epitheliosis, can be firmly attributed to exclusive or almost exclusive epithelial differentiation*, with the exception of certain rare specific entities like adenoid cystic carcinoma and related tumours. These rare exceptions are not germane to the argument as it relates to the vast majority of cancers of the breast.

IN SITU CARCINOMA

General Patterns

In situ carcinoma has a number of distinctive patterns which may be present singly or in combination. The *comedo, solid* and *papillary* patterns are self-explanatory. Papillary carcinoma in its pure form is relatively rare (Fisher, Gregorio and Fisher, 1975): its distinction from papilloma will be considered in Chapter Eight. The *cribriform* pattern is used here to include the so-called adenocystic and tubular patterns of some authors (e.g. Fisher, Gregorio and Fisher, 1975). The very rare true adenoid cystic carcinoma is considered on page 335. The *'clinging'* pattern is one which is not generally recognized and deserves much wider recognition. It is a descriptive term we have adopted for in situ cancers in which there are only one, two or just a few layers of cells lining the structure of origin — hence 'clinging' in the sense that malignant cells are present peripherally while the lumen is empty or virtually empty. A clinging carcinoma often merges into other carcinomatous patterns but when it is the dominant pattern it is very easily missed. Cytological features assume great importance in the correct identification of this type. Clinging carcinoma arises in at least two ways: firstly, as a variation of comedocarcinoma in which the necrotic debris has been largely removed, leaving a largely empty lumen. In other instances, there is no evidence of necrosis and the epithelial linings of ducts, ductules and/or lobules consist of a single layer of malignant epithelial cells with some degree of orientation towards the lumina. Whether these malignant cells have originated in situ, or have resulted from a 'creeping replacement' as a single cell layer is not clear, for both processes may play a role in the development of this type of lesion. In cancerization of lobules, the pattern may be of comedo, cribriform or solid type but a clinging pattern is also common. Clinging carcinoma is considered in Chapter Ten.

All the patterns of in situ carcinoma share certain features which distinguish them from benign hyperplasias, but the criteria that are valuable in differentiation do vary somewhat with the different patterns. The comedo and some of the clinging patterns can usually be differentiated from epitheliosis on the basis of obvious necrosis, cytological pleomorphism and other cellular characters. The solid and cribriform varieties are usually easily recognized provided that the changes are typical and widespread. But some of these varieties and most of the clinging types are very difficult to identify, especially if the tumour foci are small.

Necrosis

Necrosis is frequent in many forms of ductal carcinoma, conspicuous in some cases, slight in others, and as a positive finding it is of great diagnostic value. In contrast, necrosis in epitheliosis is distinctly rare, with the exception of the type of necrosis described on page 116. In a borderline case, necrosis is important enough to warrant a thorough search for its presence. Necrosis is often more conspicuous in the larger epithelial structures so that there may be little or no necrosis at the periphery of cancerized lobules, while necrosis is present in cancer involving the intra- or extralobular ductules and is even more prominent in the larger ducts. Apart from obvious necrosis it is important, in a difficult case, to take note of ragged crevices in a solid mass; these crevices may contain a rare single necrotic cell, or a small cluster of necrotic cells, or simply portions of necrotic cells. Such ragged crevices sometimes represent the only tell-tale evidence of necrosis.

Haemorrhage

Haemorrhage is valuable as a potential indicator of malignancy. Though haemorrhage is more frequent with carcinoma than with epitheliosis, it is not a very frequent feature even in carcinoma, so that it is useful only as a positive finding. The writer has seen haemorrhage once in an otherwise typical instance of epitheliosis.

Foam Cells

Foam cells may be found in carcinoma, usually in association with either haemorrhage or necrosis, but they are rather less common and usually less conspicuous than in epitheliosis. This very fact has given rise to problems of interpretation about the source of

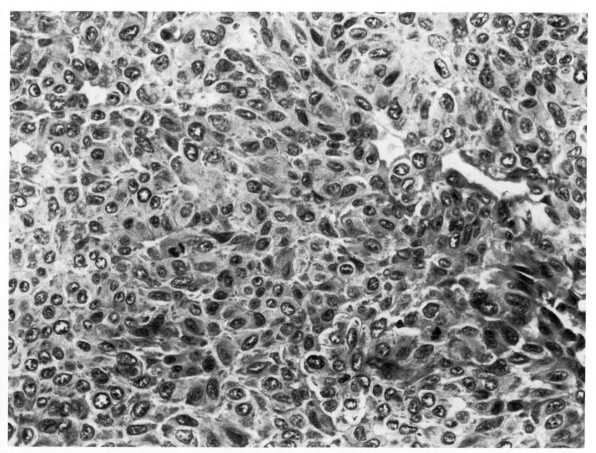

Figure 7–11   Solid variant of in situ carcinoma. The distinction from epitheliosis is frequently a good deal more subtle than seen here. Sharper cell margins, the appearance of the nuclear chromatin, more conspicuous nucleoli, the degree and nature of the mitotic activity, the pleomorphism *within one cell type*, the hint of cytoplasmic granularity are among the important distinguishing points. H and E. ×400.

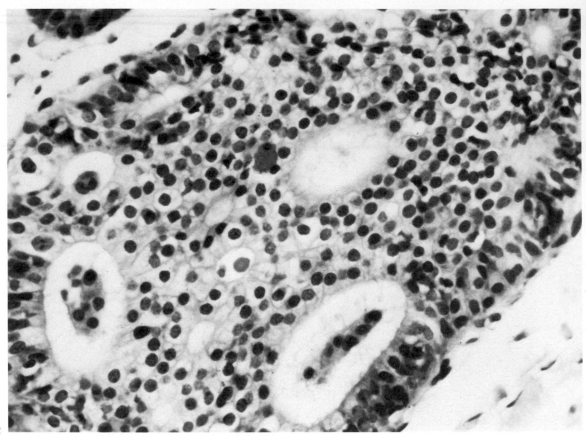

7–12

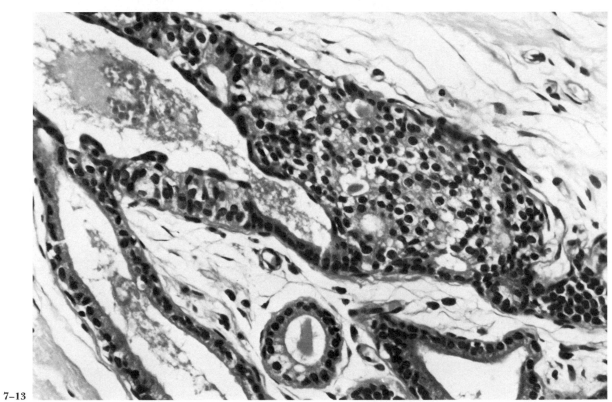

7–13

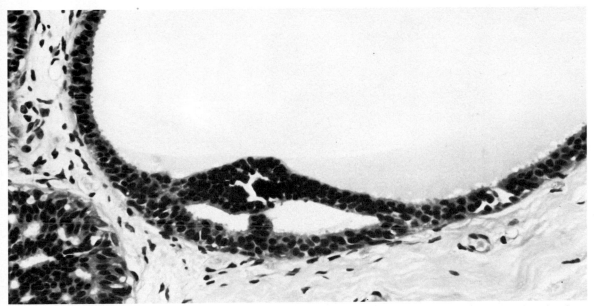

Figure 7–14 Clinging carcinoma lining a cystic structure: this is a type of carcinoma which is frequently missed, as happened in this case. The trabecular bridge with a trabecular support is diagnostic of carcinoma. Calcification is present where the bridge and its supporting pillar meet. H and E. ×400.

the foam cells in epitheliosis. They have very limited usefulness in differential diagnosis.

THE STRUCTURAL PATTERN: TRABECULAR BARS AND ROMAN BRIDGES

The main distinction between in situ carcinoma and epitheliosis lies in the differing structural patterns and cytology, and important positive as well as negative points have to be looked for. Solid in situ carcinoma is truly patternless and shows *no 'streaming'* (Figures 7–11 to 7–13). Rarely, streaming can be closely mimicked by a squash artefact but one must beware of artefacts with any tissue diagnosis. Streaming is not an essential characteristic of carcinoma, while it is a characteristic of epitheliosis.

On the positive side, differentiation in carcinoma is towards the formation of *trabecular bars*, a trabecula being defined as a row of cells with their long axes arranged more or less perpendicular to the long axis of the row. The cell nuclei are orientated similarly and it is the orientation of the nuclei that the pathologist ordinarily notices in the recognition of trabeculae (Figures 7–14 to 7–17). These malignant epithelial trabeculae are responsible for the *cartwheel formations, radial spokes* and *curvaceous serpentine structures* reminiscent of the contours of a piece of antique furniture (Figures 7–18 to 7–23). *Bridges with robust and rigid supporting pillars* and fine filigree patterns are among the structures formed (Figures 7–14, 7–20 and 7–21). The *Roman bridge* is the hallmark of in situ carcinoma of cribriform type (Figure 7–24). Most of these cartwheel and 'early' cribriform patterns are aesthetically pleasing while the heaps, mounds, sheets and tongues of epitheliosis are 'ugly' patterns which lack the sharp lines and boldly etched contours of malignancy. Robustness with delicacy of

---

Figure 7–12 (*Opposite, above.*) Lobular cancerization, solid and cribriform. Rounded nuclei are mostly evenly spaced in a clear cytoplasm. The sharply delineated cell margins should lead one to suspect that this is malignant. This is carcinoma in situ in a lobule but it is *not* CLIS. H and E. ×600.

Figure 7–13 (*Opposite, below.*) 'Clinging' and solid carcinoma in a small duct just outside the limits of the lobule. Hyperchromatic, rounded nuclei are centrally placed in pallid cells. Fairly sharp cell margins. There is a distinct hint of pagetoid spread where the tumour is less bulky. H and E. ×400.

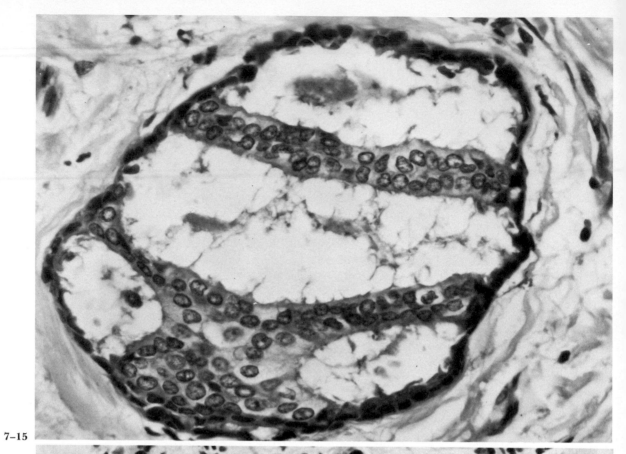

7-15

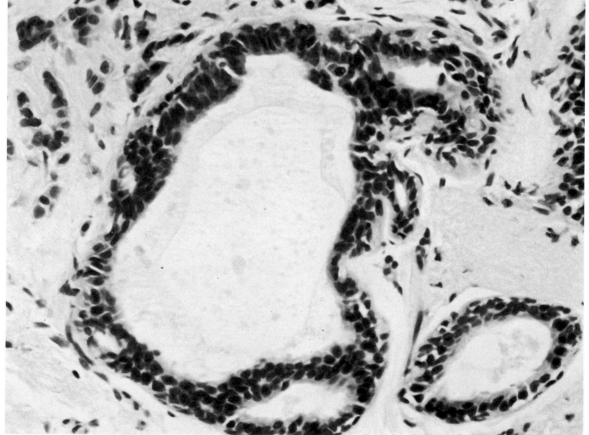

7-16

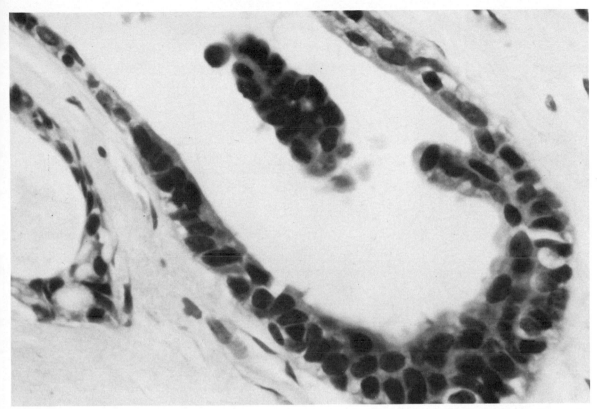

Figure 7–17 The essentials for a diagnosis of carcinoma in situ are shown here. The heaping up of a single cell type, the large hyperchromatic nuclei, are very suspicious, as is the abrupt change between normal and abnormal epithelium at one point: note the change at this point of both nuclear and cytoplasmic staining. The solitary projecting spur is highly suggestive of malignancy because of its rigidity and cellular composition. Particularly crucial is the nucleus at its tip, orientated at right angles to the axis of the spur. H and E. ×450.

structure is a characteristic of cribriform carcinoma (Figures 7–19, 7–21 and 7–24). Fundamentally, all these structures can be traced back to the formation of trabeculae. Luminal bridging is a well-known feature of carcinoma, but it is the type of bridging which is of diagnostic importance. Spindle-cell bridging, as seen in epitheliosis, is also found with carcinoma and can, at times, even be prominent in a given area. Probably spindle-cell bridging is the more 'obvious' form of growth, irrespective of whether a lesion is benign or malignant. The same is true of spindle-cell tufts, mounds and other non-bridging structures. Spindle-cell bridging is, therefore, also found with carcinoma while trabecular bridging is present *only* with carcinoma. Trabeculae represent positive differentiation in a malignant tissue which is

committed to the epithelial path. Spindle-cell growth may represent the natural growth pattern of 'uncommitted' or 'indeterminate' tissue, as well as the definitive growth pattern of myoid tissue. Luminal bridging in epitheliosis, if present, is always of spindle-cell type, whereas luminal bridging in carcinoma has cells which may or may not be orientated in the axis of the bridge and it is those that are *not* which constitute clear evidence of malignancy. When cuboidal cells form a bridge or spur, the question of orientation does not arise.

The Spaces Within a Lesion

The 'spaces' of carcinoma tend to be of the neatly rounded, 'punched out' variety reminiscent of

---

Figure 7–15 (*Opposite, above.*) Trabecular bars of carcinoma. This field is virtually diagnostic of cancer. H and E. ×600.

Figure 7–16 (*Opposite, below.*) Heaping up of epithelial cells with inconspicuous myoepithelial cells. The neoplastic cells have relatively large, deeply hyperchromatic and monotonous nuclei. The long bridge with a trabecular arrangement is highly suspect. Trabeculae of infiltrating carcinoma are also present in the adjacent stroma. H and E. ×450.

133

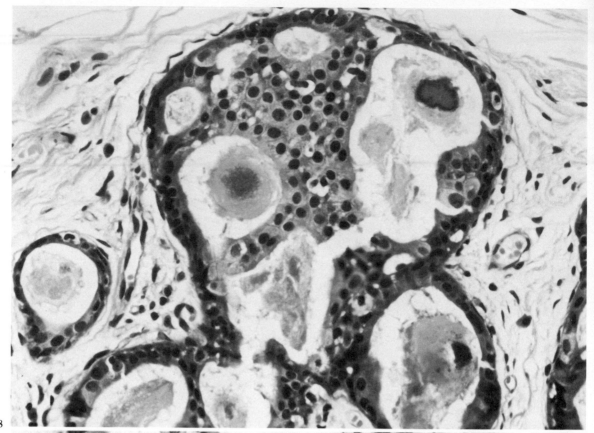

7–18

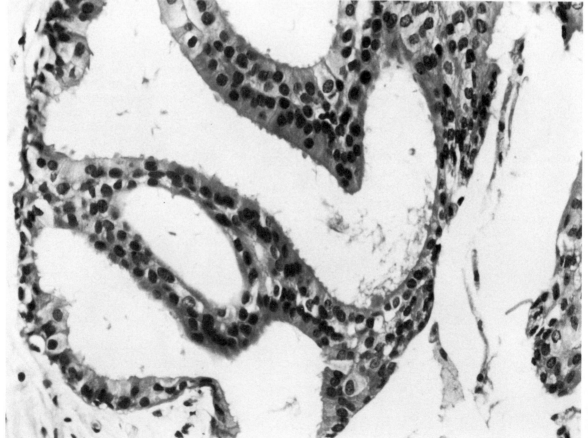

7–19

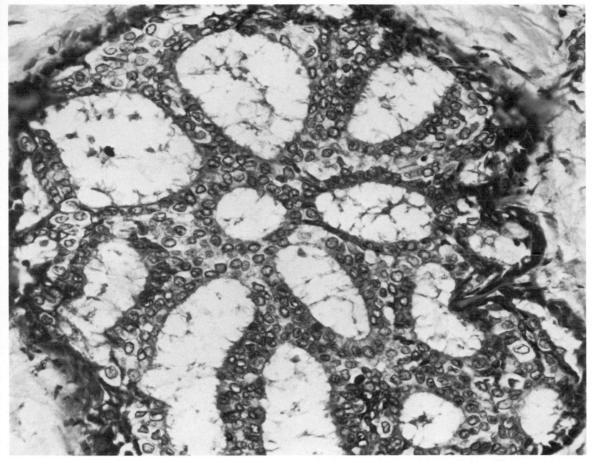

Figure 7–20   The rigidity of this cribriform structure is among the features which enable it to be identified as carcinoma. Note the 'radial spokes of a wheel' appearance. The nuclei lack many of the characteristics usually seen in malignant cells. H and E. ×400.

those of adenoid basal cell carcinoma of the skin, variably sized and rather uniformly spaced (Figures 7–11, 7–25 and 7–26) or, alternatively, they represent true glandular lumina with orientation of the cells around them. In either case *a sieve-like (or strainer like) appearance* is produced. The spaces are usually more or less rounded, while those of epitheliosis are ovoid or irregular, and frequently eccentric and crescentic. Carcinoma tends to 'fill in' from the periphery, only rarely leaving large eccentric spaces as seen in epitheliosis. But ovoid and irregular spaces are occasionally seen in carcinoma and the

shape of the spaces must not be allowed to override other considerations.

CYTOPLASMIC AND NUCLEAR DETAIL

Cytoplasmic Borders. Carcinoma does not usually have the 'syncytial' character of epitheliosis. Cytoplasmic borders vary considerably, from the barely definable to the distinct and easily seen. While indistinct cell margins do not, by any means, rule out carcinoma, sharp cell edges are very suggestive of malignancy in a borderline lesion

---

Figure 7–18   (*Opposite, above.*)   Lobular cancerization with specialized lobular connective tissue still apparent. Convex margin indicates the limit of the lobule. Clinging and incipient cribriform pattern. Note rounded deeply stained nuclei and sharp luminal cell margins. Inspissated material and calcific bodies are present in the lumina. This is 'ductal type' carcinoma but situated in the lobule not in the extralobular ducts. H and E. ×450.

Figure 7–19   (*Opposite, below.*)   Carcinomatous bridges, delicate but firm and rigid, with curvaceous and serpentine outlines. The two or three cell *layers* in some bridges must be distinguished from the two cell *types* seen with divergent differentiation in certain benign breast diseases. H and E. ×400.

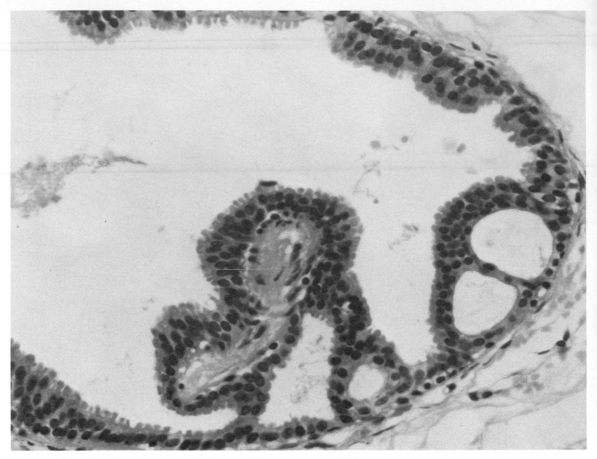

Figure 7–21 Part of a lobule containing well-shaped and moulded structures representing early cartwheel and Roman-bridge formation. Note the robust nature of the delicate formations. This is a type of well-differentiated in situ carcinoma which is very easily missed. H and E. ×525.

(Figures 7–11 and 7–12). Conversely, one should hesitate before making a diagnosis of epitheliosis in the presence of very distinct cell margins in solid areas.

Cell Shape and Staining Characteristics are very variable in carcinoma. Fusiform cells as the dominant type are distinctly unusual in carcinoma; they are the usual form in solid epitheliosis. In some ductal carcinomas there is marked *pallor of the cytoplasm* or, rarely, almost absent staining, sufficient to attract attention at low magnification (Figures 7–12 and 7–24). In other tumours the cytoplasm is moderately to intensely *eosinophilic or am-*

phophilic, with an opacity more striking than that seen in epitheliosis (Figures 7–11 and 7–18). The cytoplasm is usually homogeneous as in epitheliosis; however, *slight granularity,* even focal, should arouse one's suspicions; while distinct cytoplasmic granularity is a conspicuous feature of relatively few carcinomas, it is sufficiently characteristic to have diagnostic value (Figures 7–11 and 7–18).

Nuclei vary from case to case but much less so in different blocks from the same case. Absolute nuclear size is often rather similar to that found in epitheliosis. There are important differences of *shape, spacing, and staining*

Figure 7–22 (*Opposite, above.*) Carcinomatous bulges, sprouts and bridges. Note nuclear staining qualities and structure. All the luminal projections seen here are suspect. One part of the long bar bridging the lumen just enables it to qualify as a trabecular bar diagnostic of malignancy. H and E. ×645.

Figure 7–23 (*Opposite, below.*) 'Early' cribriform carcinoma. The neoplastic bars are joined to form cartwheels and curvaceous structures, leaving lumina bordered mainly by cells with truncated margins. There is a calcified mass with 'shatter effect' in the centre. H and E. ×420.

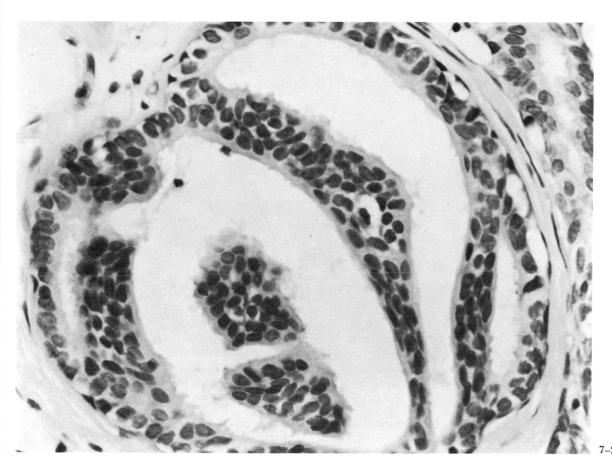

7-22

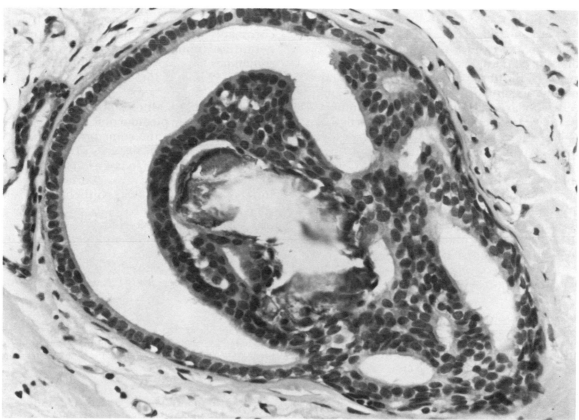

7-23

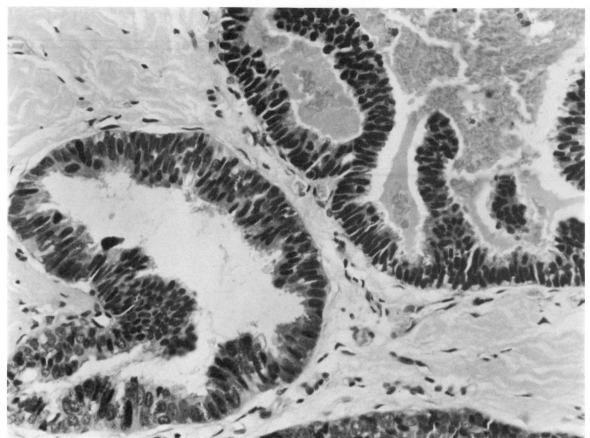

7-30

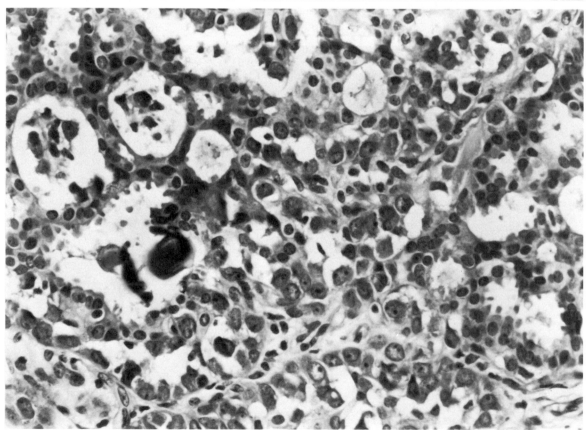

7-31

142

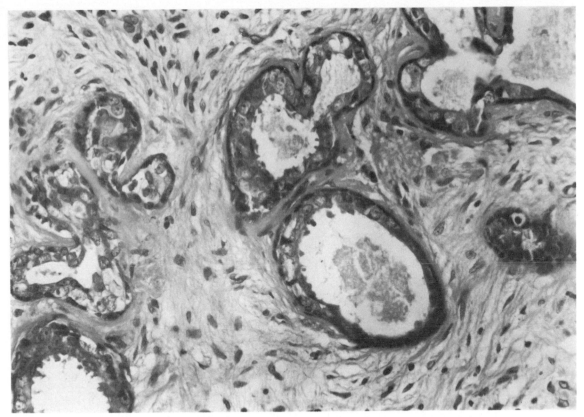

Figure 7–32 Clinging cancerization affecting parts of two lobules. The neoplastic epithelial cells have prominent nucleoli while persistent myoepithelial cells outline most of the epithelial units. A little cell debris is present in some lumina. H and E. ×400.

Mitotic Aberrations. Even more significant is the *quality of the mitoses,* for atypical mitoses are of diagnostic value (Figures 7–27 and 7–29). In comedocarcinomas they are often present but they are not usually critical in establishing the diagnosis, as this can usually be made on other grounds; but in solid lesions especially, atypical mitoses are a critical finding. The writer has searched in vain for atypical mitoses in many cases of severe and florid epitheliosis and it needs stressing that it is extremely difficult to find even a single convincingly abnormal mitosis. For this reason, the presence of even three or four distinctly abnormal mitoses in a borderline lesion is a finding of diagnostic significance. In clinging carcinoma also, the presence of abnormal mitoses can be the clinching feature in making the correct diagnosis.

Absence of Divergent Differentiation

In carcinoma there is no differentiation into two cell types as frequently found in epitheliosis, and glandular spaces lined by peg-shaped epithelial cells with fluffy borders are usually absent. It is nevertheless true that *pre-existing myoepithelial cells at the periphery may persist,* and they may even appear to be more prominent than normal (Figures 7–32 and 7–33); such persistence, and even prominence, in no way excludes carcinoma.

Figure 7–30 (*Opposite, above.*) Recurrent in situ carcinoma eight years after a local excision with an erroneous pathological diagnosis of benign disease. From the same patient as the three preceding illustrations. Carcinomatous stalactites have nuclei orientated transversely to the long axis of the bars. H and E. ×400.

Figure 7–31 (*Opposite, below.*) Cribriform and lacy in situ carcinoma. Apical snouts and shattered psammoma bodies are present. Prominent nucleoli are present in many malignant cells, especially in the less well differentiated parts. H and E. ×450.

143

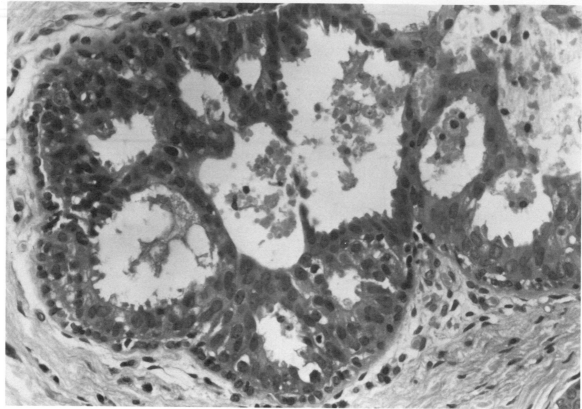

Figure 7–33   Carcinoma in situ in a lobule. Residual myoepithelial cells are present at the periphery: their presence in no way excludes in situ cancer. In the absence of the necrosis here present, the structural and cytological traits shown in this field would be suggestive rather than diagnostic of malignancy. Adjacent fields, however, showed unequivocal carcinoma, in situ and infiltrating. H and E. ×400.

That myoepithelial cell persistence at the periphery of the containing structure, as opposed to differentiation in the centre of an epithelial mass, does not exclude malignancy in the in situ context was regarded by the writer as a well-known finding, and is certainly known to many surgical pathologists with whom the writer communicates or corresponds. It came, therefore, as something of a surprise to find this observation contradicted in a recent disputation between Rosier (1976) on the one hand and Jensen, Rice and Wellings (1976) on the other. Rosier (1976), like the writer (see page 106), believes that the lesion described and illustrated by Jensen, Rice and Wellings (1976) is carcinoma and not merely 'atypia'; in their reply to Rosier's letter, Jensen, Rice and Wellings (1976) state that 'when myoepithelial cells persist, we call the lesion severely atypical'. The writer, like Rosier (1976), rejects this view entirely. This is not a matter of semantics but a question of fundamental principle. Myoepithelial cell persistence is sometimes easily detectable at the light microscope level; when it is dubiously present or apparently absent, it can still frequently be demonstrated at the ultrastructural level, as was so elegantly demonstrated by Ozzello (1971).

On the other hand, the writer is in complete agreement with Jensen, Rice and Wellings (1976) about the site of origin of ductal carcinoma from the TDLU (Chapter Six). Rosier (1976) says 'whether or not so-called intraductal carcinoma originates from breast lobules appears to be irrelevant'. The fundamental conclusion of Jensen, Rice and Wellings (1976) in this respect is both true and important. While the 'truth' on this point is uncomfortable and has undermined the cosy traditional belief that 'ductal carcinoma' and 'lobular carcinoma' arise in quite different sites, it is nevertheless an important truth which Jensen, Rice and Wellings (1976) have taken great pains to establish beyond reasonable doubt.

It is a pity that two such vital problems, one entirely practical, the second largely but by no means entirely academic, have been juxtaposed in this manner and that this has been done under the singularly uninformative title of 'Breast Lobules'! The writer agrees entirely with Rosier (1976) on the practical diagnostic issue and entirely with Jensen, Rice and Wellings (1976) on the histogenetic issue.

Cellular Orientation

This is absent in many forms of in situ carcinoma, e.g. in the comedo and solid forms. There are two growth patterns, however, in which good glandular orientation is present: in many forms of clinging carcinoma, especially when involving lobules in lobular cancerization, there is distinct and easily recognizable orientation; secondly, true tubular spaces are found in some cribriform duct carcinomas, with the epithelial cells lining them taller than the surrounding cells and containing ovoid nuclei orientated around the luminal space. In the latter the observer may get the erroneous impression of a two-cell-type differentiation, but in effect there is only a single cell type showing varying degrees of differentiation. These orientated carcinoma cells differ from the glandular lining cells of epitheliosis by being for the main part truncated and clean-cut and lacking fluffy luminal edges. The nuclear/cytoplasmic ratio is increased, chromatin markings are heavy and nucleoli may be conspicuous.

Truncation versus Blebbing

While truncation suggests malignancy, a few, some or even many areas in a carcinoma may show fluffy edges due to peninsular and microvillous differentiation (Figure 7–31), a feature which is most extensive and conspicuous in some of the cribriform varieties, which are only distinguishable from epitheliosis on the basis of architectural traits such as trabecular bars, cartwheel formation and similar patterns.

None of these criteria is all-or-none and, in different cases, one has to rely on different groups of criteria. Certainly some features are of greater diagnostic significance than others. It cannot be emphasized too strongly that attention must be paid to overall structure and cytology rather than to isolated fields and cells. It is only very rarely that the diagnosis of malignancy is based on a few high-power fields and this generally applies only to minute lesions. Similarly, no single criterion is infallible taken on its own though a few, such as the formation of trabeculae, cartwheels, etc., are virtually diagnostic. For example, distinctly ovoid nuclei may be found in some areas and are even the dominant shape in some varieties of carcinoma, especially with the clinging types of carcinoma as they affect both lobules and ducts; they are also seen in the tubular areas of some more solid forms of in situ carcinoma. Ovoid nuclei are often not as hyperchromatic as the rounded ones. Thus, two major typical features, viz. roundness of nucleus and deep haematoxyphilia, can be absent in some carcinomas. In cases of this type the chromatin markings, nucleoli, and features like truncation and other cytological parameters assume paramount importance.

Calcification

Calcification, as a positive finding, is important in distinguishing in situ carcinoma from epitheliosis, as already emphasized (page 125) and discussed in Chapter Eighteen (Figures 7–14, 7–23 and 7–31).

Pagetoid Spread

Pagetoid spread is sometimes seen in carcinoma — especially, but not exclusively, in the lobular variety — and it can provide very useful confirmatory evidence of malignancy in a dubious or borderline case (Figure 7–13). Pagetoid spread is virtually diagnostic of malignancy, for there are hardly any non-malignant lesions which mimic it or could be mistaken for it. The concept of pagetoid spread and its value in distinguishing carcinoma from epitheliosis is discussed in Chapter Ten.

Chronic Inflammatory Cells

A cuff of chronic inflammatory cells may surround in situ carcinoma, especially the comedo, some of the clinging and a few of the solid variants (Figures 7–34 and 7–35). This may represent a reaction to dead or living tumour cells, and may possibly, more rarely,

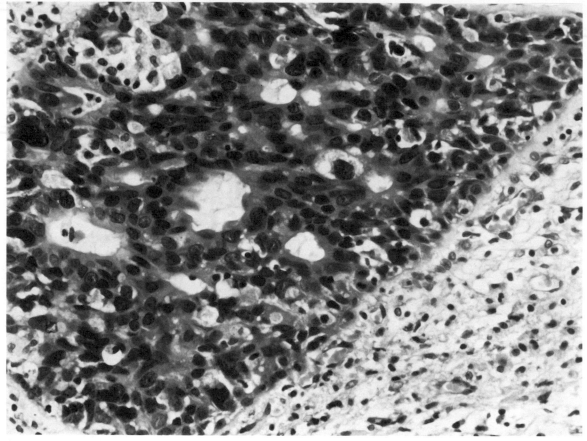

Figure 7–34   A microscopic focus of ductular carcinoma in situ found 'incidentally' adjacent to a ruptured tension cyst. Note nuclear characteristics of carcinoma cells. H and E. ×400.

represent a host defence reaction to tumour, as is strongly suspected for certain forms of infiltrating carcinoma.

Fibrosis and Elastosis

Similarly, some in situ carcinomas are associated with fibrosis, either as a consequence of inflammation or as a more direct desmoplastic response to cancer. Elastosis may surround duct cancer; it is even more frequently seen in infiltrating carcinoma (Azzopardi and Laurini, 1974), and its presence in localized aggregates, accompanying duct cancer, should always arouse one's suspicion that invasion may have occurred. But since fibroelastosis may also accompany epitheliosis and its variant 'infiltrating epitheliosis', it does not by itself indicate that a lesion is malignant. Areas of fibroelastosis are nonetheless useful in pinpointing foci that require further careful scrutiny.

THE ROLE OF ULTRASTRUCTURAL STUDIES IN THE DIFFERENTIATION OF BENIGN AND MALIGNANT BREAST DISEASE

Attempts have been made over the last 15 years to detect ultrastructural differences which would help refine the diagnostic criteria used to distinguish benign and malignant breast disease. In this effort, attention has been directed mainly to three ultrastructural parameters (Ozzello, 1971):

1. The Presence of Intracytoplasmic Lumina (ICL). These are further discussed in the section on CLIS (lobular neoplasia). Luminal spaces within the cytoplasm of epithelial cells, with microvilli lining the space, have been described frequently in breast carcinomas (Wellings and Roberts, 1963; Sykes et al, 1968; Carter, Yardley and Shelley, 1969; Goldenberg, Goldenberg and Sommers, 1969). While

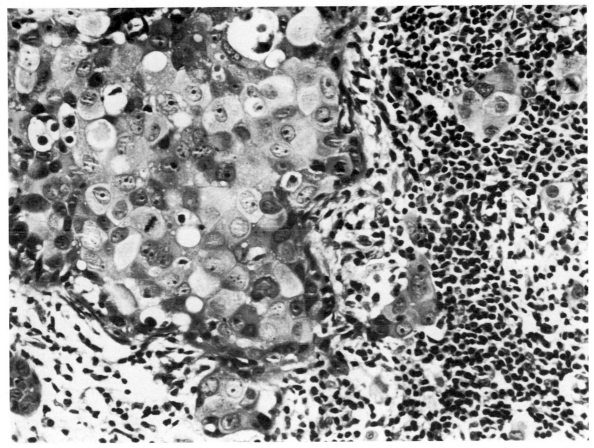

Figure 7–35   Deeper level of the focus depicted in Figure 7–34. Microinvasive cancer is present in addition. Nucleolar prominence is especially striking. Mitoses are visible in both in situ and invasive parts. H and E. ×400.

Busch and Merker (1968) came to the conclusion that there are no ultrastructural qualitative signs that could be considered diagnostic of malignancy, Goldenberg, Goldenberg and Sommers (1969) suggested that ICL may be a qualitative criterion which distinguishes malignant from benign lesions. It is true that, generally speaking, ICL are commoner with cancer, but they can also be found in non-neoplastic epithelium, for instance in sclerosing adenosis (Ozzello, 1971). ICL do not, therefore, constitute a reliable or clear-cut indicator of malignancy. ICL are, incidentally, not always strictly intracellular; in many cases they represent intracytoplasmic extensions of the intercellular spaces (Wellings and Roberts, 1963). That the latter view is correct in most cases was demonstrated on serial sections by Ozzello (1971). But a few are genuinely intracytoplasmic. In any case, if they appear as intracellular lumina in a given plane of section, they have come to be called ICL by most authors. This is a valuable and meaningful term inasmuch as these ICL are so frequent a feature of breast carcinomas (Battifora, 1975). They are particularly frequent in the lobular variety (Gad and Azzopardi, 1975). Tschubel and Helpap (1976) confirmed the greater frequency of ICL in carcinoma compared with benign diseases. But, in the present context, they cannot be regarded as evidence of the malignant nature of an epithelial lesion of the breast.

It is possible, nevertheless, that further work may indicate greater diagnostic value for ICL in the context of certain specific lesions. Certainly sclerosing adenosis must first be excluded by conventional methods. The distinction between florid epitheliosis and in situ carcinoma can be a very difficult one and it is in this setting that the presence of ICL might be a valuable indicator of the diagnosis. In epitheliosis, solid or fenestrated, ICL are uncommon (personal observations); in CLIS they are very common and further work is indicated to determine whether they are of any value in distinguishing epitheliosis from in situ ductal carcinoma.

2. The Presence of Abundant Tonofibrils. Sykes et al (1968) considered that not only ICL but also abundant 'tonofibrils' were pathognomonic of cancer. It is true that in benign hyperplasias, while cytoplasmic filaments in epithelial cells may be more numerous, their individual size and distribution are similar to those of normal epithelial cells in the breast. On the other hand, in cancers, including the in situ variety, cytoplasmic filaments are not only increased in number but vary also in their form. Some form straight bundles of fine filaments comparable to those found in benign epithelium; some of these converge on desmosomes. But other filaments in malignant cells are much thicker and arranged in prominent groups or wavy bundles. These coarser filaments resemble the filaments of keratinizing cells (Ozzello, 1971) and have been considered to represent tonofibrils by some authors (e.g. Sykes et al, 1968). While this variation in the character of the cytoplasmic fibrils appears to be more conspicuous in malignancy, Ozzello (1971) did not regard it as a definite indicator of malignancy but rather as providing supporting evidence.

Some general comments are in order here about these possible indicators of malignancy. In the nature of things more work has been done on the malignant than on the benign lesions so that the finding of so-called pathognomonic indicators of malignancy must be tempered with caution, lest optimism and enthusiasm in the quest for the ultimate goal defeat realism and a more objective truth. Secondly, and again understandably, most of the observations have been made on lesions which are patently benign or obviously malignant rather than on dubious or 'borderline' lesions, though there are a few notable exceptions (e.g. Goldenberg, Goldenberg and Sommers, 1969). Thus, although reasonably defined differences may be identifiable in the 'typical' benign and malignant lesions, it is by no means clear as yet whether these differences are of any diagnostic value in the truly 'borderline' case.

3. The Absence of Basal Laminae. There is a feature which Ozzello (1971) regards as potentially more important than either 1 or 2

in the diagnosis of malignancy. This is the usual absence of basal laminae around clusters of invasive malignant cells. Basal laminae are intact in non-neoplastic breast tissues and in benign tumours of the breast. They are mostly absent in infiltrating carcinomas and may be focally missing in in situ carcinomas, both ductal and lobular. The latter observation is one of the more fundamental ones made by Ozzello (1971). Alterations of the basal laminae, and indeed of the epithelial–stromal junctions in general, are almost as important in benign and malignant breast disease as the epithelial changes themselves. Herein lies one of the most valuable contributions of this study. Ozzello (1971) suggested that *absence of basal laminae probably indicates that a given epithelial lesion is malignant though it does not differentiate between in situ and invasive cancers.* On the other hand, the persistence of a basal lamina cannot be of any diagnostic value. Ozzello's (1971) suggestion is based on very sound evidence and a very critical approach to and careful appraisal of all the work in this field. He was cautious in his suggestion and maintained that his findings were still in need of further confirmation.

The reader is referred to Ozzello (1971) for a comprehensive account of the ultrastructure of the human breast in health and disease. He provides a wealth of observations, the significance of which is critically assessed from every angle. The value and limitations of the findings are analysed most lucidly and a very valuable attempt is made to bring together the many discordant views in the literature. Ozzello (1971) points the way to unexplored and challenging aspects in this field and his work is obligatory reading for all those wishing to have a deeper understanding of things established, things probable or likely, as well as aspects which remain unsolved.

References

Ahmed, A. (1974) The myoepithelium in cystic hyperplastic mastopathy. *Journal of Pathology,* **113,** 209–215.

Ahmed, A (1978) *Atlas of the Ultrastructure of Human Breast Diseases.* pp. 31–33. Edinburgh, London and New York: Churchill Livingstone.

Azzopardi, J. G. and Laurini, R. N. (1974) Elastosis in breast cancer. *Cancer,* **33,** 174–183.

Battifora, H. (1975) Intracytoplasmic lumina in breast carcinoma. A helpful histopathologic feature. *Archives of Pathology,* **99,** 614–617.

Busch, W. and Merker, H. J. (1968) Elektronenmikroskopische Untersuchungen an menschlichen Mammacarcinomen. *Virchows Archiv A: Pathologische Anatomie,* **344,** 356–371.

Carter, D., Yardley, J. H. and Shelley, W. M. (1969) Lobular carcinoma of the breast: an ultrastructural comparison with certain duct carcinomas and benign lesions. *Johns Hopkins Medical Journal,* **125,** 25–43.

Davies, J. D. (1974) Human colostrum cells: their relation to periductal mononuclear inflammation. *Journal of Pathology,* **112,** 153–160.

Fisher, E. R., Gregorio, R. M. and Fisher, B. (1975) The pathology of invasive breast cancer. *Cancer,* **36,** 1–263.

Gad, A. and Azzopardi, J. G. (1975) Lobular carcinoma of the breast: a special variant of mucin-secreting carcinoma. *Journal of Clinical Pathology,* **28,** 711–716.

Goldenberg, V. E., Goldenberg, N. S. and Sommers, S. C. (1969) Comparative ultrastructure of atypical ductal hyperplasia, intraductal carcinoma, and infiltrating ductal carcinoma of the breast. *Cancer,* **24,** 1152–1169.

Hamperl, H. (1970) The myothelia (myoepithelial cells). In *Current Topics in Pathology,* Vol. 53. Berlin: Springer-Verlag.

Harris, M. and Ahmed, A. (1977) The ultrastructure of tubular carcinoma of the breast. *Journal of Pathology,* **123,** 79–83.

Jackson, J. G. and Orr, J. W. (1957) The ducts of carcinomatous breasts, with particular reference to connective-tissue changes. *Journal of Pathology and Bacteriology,* **74,** 265–273.

Jensen, H. M., Rice, J. R. and Wellings, S. R. (1976) Preneoplastic lesions in the human breast. *Science,* **191,** 295–297.

McDivitt, R. W., Stewart, F. W. and Berg, J. W. (1968) *Tumors of the Breast.* Atlas of Tumor Pathology, Second series, Fascicle 2. Washington, D.C.: Armed Forces Institute of Pathology.

Ozzello, L. (1971) Ultrastructure of the human mammary gland. In *Pathology Annual* (Ed.) Sommers, S. C. Vol. 6, pp. 1–59. London: Butterworth.

Page, D. L., Zwaag, R. V., Rogers, L. W., Williams, L. T., Walker, W. E. and Hartmann, W. H. (1978) Relation between component parts of fibrocystic disease complex and breast cancer. *Journal of the National Cancer Institute,* **61,** 1055–1063.

Rosier, R. P. (1976) Breast lobules. *Science,* **193,** 918–919.

Shah, J. P., Rosen, P. P. and Robbins, G. F. (1973) Pitfalls of local excision in the treatment of carcinoma of the breast. *Surgery, Gynecology and Obstetrics,* **136,** 721–725.

Sykes, J. A., Recher, L., Jernstrom, P. H. and Whitescarver, J (1968) Morphological investigation of human breast cancer. *Journal of the National Cancer Institute,* **40,** 195–223.

Tschubel, K. and Helpap, B. (1976) Intracytoplasmatische Einschlüsse in Abklatschpräparaten von der Mamma und ihre diagnostische Verwertbarkeit. *Virchows Archiv A: Pathological Anatomy and Histology,* **371,** 265–271.

Wellings, S. R. and Roberts, P. (1963) Electron microscopy of sclerosing adenosis and infiltrating duct carcinoma of the human mammary gland. *Journal of the National Cancer Institute,* **30,** 269–987

Wellings, S. R., Jensen, H. M. and Marcum, R. G. (1975) An atlas of subgross pathology of the human breast with special reference to possible precancerous lesions. *Journal of the National Cancer Institute,* **55,** 231–273.

the disadvantages of 'papillomatosis'. It encompasses solid and fenestrated lesions. 'Epitheliosis' is, literally as well as in practice, a shorthand expression to describe epithelial hyperplasia of solid and glandular (fenestrated) forms. As such, it is convenient, brief and expressive and suffers from no apparent disadvantages. If a better alternative can be found, so be it: the writer cannot think of one, nor does there appear to be the necessity to coin one.

MICROSCOPIC PAPILLOMAS

Microscopic Apocrine Papillomas

By general consent, the very common, often numerous, and minute — even at the microscopic level — apocrine papillomas seen so frequently as part of cystic disease are not usually referred to as papillomas. Structurally, despite their small size, they do qualify to be called papillomas, but for practical purposes it is sensible to follow the established convention; otherwise, in the majority of cases of cystic disease one would have to specify each time that apocrine papillomatosis was present.

Microscopic Non-apocrine Papillomas

If the practice of describing epitheliosis as papillomatosis is discontinued, then *properly defined papillomas of the non-apocrine variety* are not as frequent as they would appear to be from most of the current literature. Nevertheless, it is true that if cases of cystic hyperplasia are extensively sampled, one or more microscopic papillomas are not infrequent as part of the complex hyperplastic process. But generally they form only a minor component of the total hyperplasia, they do not give rise to problems in diagnosis and there is no reason to believe that their significance is different from that of the epitheliosis they accompany.

MACROSCOPIC PAPILLOMA

More important to clinician and pathologist are the papillomas of all sizes, usually solitary, but occasionally multiple, in the ductal system: I am referring here to papillomas which are sufficiently large to be seen macroscopically. Rarely, these isolated papillomas may be found even in cysts, i.e. in structures derived from lobules. The solitary papilloma will be discussed first. Multiple papillomas will be considered separately at the end, for reasons which will become evident.

SOLITARY MACROSCOPIC PAPILLOMA

The solitary papilloma is frequently symptomatic, producing a nipple discharge which is blood-stained in about one-half of the cases. Solitary ductal papilloma is the most frequent structural cause of a nipple discharge, serous or blood-stained. Of course ductal carcinoma may also produce a nipple discharge and must always be considered in the diagnosis. The surgeon's problem is localizing the tumour to the correct segment of the breast and performing the right operation in a patient who is frequently young. As he dissects the specimen from the nipple outwards he must mark the base of the nipple with a stitch so that the pathologist can localize the area correctly. The problem of the pathologist is to localize the lesion and, secondly, to make a correct diagnosis. The localization of the lesion by the pathologist is easy only if the surgeon has marked the specimen correctly. He then opens the relevant duct and continues with a fine pair of scissors until he exposes the soft friable tumour. This is usually an elongated lesion perhaps only 2 or 3 mm in diameter and measuring in length usually no more than 1 or 2 cm. In other cases he may find a more rounded lesion where the duct has become blocked off. It is essential that the pathologist should recognize the tumour macroscopically. If the surgeon merely 'hacks out' a piece of breast tissue and does not mark the base of the nipple in the appropriate way the task of the pathologist becomes near impossible. He then has to slice randomly through the resected tissue and it is only luck that might enable him to find this small soft lesion, if indeed it has been removed by the surgeon. It is worth noting that, while symptomatic large-duct papillomas are not common after the age of 60 years, they do occur in the sixties and even in the seventies and the writer has seen them, in consultation, in women aged 80 and 84 years. Asymptomatic incidental papillomas can be found in old women, of course, when breast tissue is resected for some other disease. At the other end of the scale, solitary ductal papilloma is found very rarely even in patients in their teens. Even a male child of seven months with an intraductal papilloma is recorded (Simpson and Barson, 1969).

The Relationship of Papilloma to Carcinoma

Before embarking on a consideration of the differentiation of benign papilloma from papillary carcinoma, one must consider whether the differentiation is justifiable. It is the opinion of most recent workers that it is theoretically justifiable and, in the great majority of cases, practically feasible to make the distinction. If there were a continuous spectrum from a solitary papilloma to a papillary carcinoma, the distinction would hardly be valid. If a papillary carcinoma could be shown to arise not infrequently from a pre-existing papilloma or, more importantly perhaps, if a papilloma, when locally excised, was followed by recurrent malignant tumour with greater than chance frequency, the differentiation between benign and malignant lesions, although valid, would not be as important as it would be if the two tumours were quite distinct.

The literature on this subject reveals very widely divergent views. The controversy is akin to that concerning the precancerous proclivities of cystic disease of the breast. If anything, the stand taken by different workers differs more sharply in relation to the papillary neoplasms.

If one takes the five major series of Hart (1927), Haagensen, Stout and Phillips (1951), Lewison and Lyons (1953), Hendrick (1957) and Kraus and Neubecker (1962), comprising 427 patients, only two developed breast cancer during the follow-up study (0.4 per cent). The follow-up periods varied between only one and as much as 25 years. If one considers only the three series with a minimum five-year follow-up period, there were still only two cancers among 300 patients, an incidence of 0.7 per cent. Ideally a minimum 10-year follow-up is needed but this ideal is met in only one large series referred to later. These cancer incidences are very low indeed and Carter (1977) analyses possible causes of this low incidence. He points out that between 30 and 80 per cent of patients with ductal papillomas in some of these series were treated by mastectomy and were thus not eligible for the development of carcinoma on the ipsilateral side. If these cases are subtracted from the

series of Hart (1927), Lewison and Lyons (1953) and Haagensen, Stout and Phillips (1951), there were no cancers at all developing in 121 patients. But Carter's (1977) argument is that there would almost certainly have been some selection in treating the larger or more atypical lesions more aggressively and the smaller or more typical ones more conservatively. This might give the impression that the ductal papilloma has less malignant potential than it actually possesses. Carter's (1977) point is valid but one must not overstate the case; his criticism could apply only to the development of ipsilateral carcinoma and not, of course, to contralateral carcinoma. Since contralateral carcinoma occurs at least as frequently as ipsilateral in these patients, mastectomy, as opposed to local excision, could at the very most halve the incidence of subsequent development of breast cancer. The gross discrepancy between the 0.7 per cent cancer incidence cited above and the 14 per cent incidence in some other series cannot be explained entirely, or even mainly, on this basis.

At the other end of the scale from the series considered above are those of Buhl-Jørgensen et al (1968) and of Kilgore, Fleming and Ramos (1953). In the former series, seven of 53 patients (13.2 per cent) and, in the latter, eight of 57 patients (14 per cent) developed cancer, for a total of 15 cases in 110 patients. The conclusions of Buhl-Jørgensen et al (1968) have already been questioned in Chapter Six and the criticisms of this paper will not be reiterated. The paper of Kilgore, Fleming and Ramos (1953) is in a very different category. It was written at a time when the criteria for distinguishing between benign and malignant lesions were not as sharply defined as they are now. This brings one to consider the important question of whether the discrepancies in the findings of different authors can be attributed to the use of different diagnostic criteria at different epochs or even at the same time in different centres. The writer believes that there is very good evidence that this is probably the most important single factor. The work of Kilgore, Fleming and Ramos (1953) is very well illustrated and their Cases 4 and 5 will be recognized *now* as malignant tumours (e.g. their Figure 11 is a good illustration of 'clinging' carcinoma with some trabecular bar formation). The more usual error in the older literature, in cases with this sequence, was underdiagnosis of the original cancerous

Table 8–1   The differential diagnosis of benign papilloma and papillary carcinoma

Papilloma	Papillary carcinoma
May be intricately arborescent: sometimes complex glandular pattern	Cribriform and trabecular patterns commonly present in addition
Well-developed stroma in fronds	Stroma scanty, delicate or absent in parts but can be well developed sometimes
Two cell *types* in *parts* at least: outer type sometimes myoid	One cell type only: number of cell layers very variable, can be two *layers* but not types
Pleomorphism of divergent differentiation frequent	Usually more monotonous or shows pleomorphism of anaplasia
Nuclei normochromatic N/C ratio not high Mitoses usually scantier	Nuclei hyperchromatic N/C ratio often high Mitoses usually more numerous
Apocrine metaplasia frequent	Apocrine metaplasia absent
Infiltration surroundings usually spurious due to haemorrhage and fibrous distortion or takes form of 'infiltrating epitheliosis' with spindle-cell formations	Infiltration, if present, takes carcinomatous form
Sometimes has benign accompaniments	Usually lacks benign accompaniments while other forms of ductal carcinoma may be present

NOTE: It remains true that 'Critical diagnosis . . . transcends mere tabular guidelines'. McDivitt, Stewart and Berg, 1968).

papillomas studied in detail by Carter (1977) ranged in size from 0.3 to 3.5 cm. The largest seen by the writer measured 3.2 cm. Exceptions occur as, for instance, with a papilloma arising in a tension cyst; the papilloma, by obstructing the outlet of the cyst, can cause enlargement of the cyst, as in a personally studied case which measured 4 cm. Even in such cases it is almost invariably the cyst rather than the tumour itself which reaches this size; in my own case the actual tumour measured 1.5 cm. That more genuine exceptions do occur is illustrated by a 4.5 cm tumour mentioned by Smith and Taylor (1969); this was one of a highly selected group of ductal papillomas with chondroid and osseous metaplasia of the stroma; this metaplastic change might itself have been partly responsible for the relatively bulky size of this particular tumour.

The papilloma has an arborescent architecture with a well-developed connective tissue component which supports the blood vessels and occupies the centres of the branches (Figures 8–1 to 8–3). Some collagen is almost invariably present between the smallest blood vessels in the fronds and the basement membrane of the epithelial covering. This feature is more easily appreciated in the villous component of a tumour. There is a variant of papilloma frequently referred to as '*papillary cystadenoma*' or '*multiradicular papilloma*' (Figures 8–4 and 8–5). The term 'cyst' is not meant to indicate that the tumour

Figure 8–1   (*Opposite, above.*)   Papilloma of nipple duct with partial extrusion of tumour from orifice on nipple. This should not be confused with 'adenoma of the nipple', which is a distinct entity. H and E. ×30.

Figure 8–2   (*Opposite, below.*)   Two-cell-type differentiation in a papilloma. The distinction between the two cell types seen here is very obvious but in practice it is often subtle. Weigert elastic and HVG. ×300.

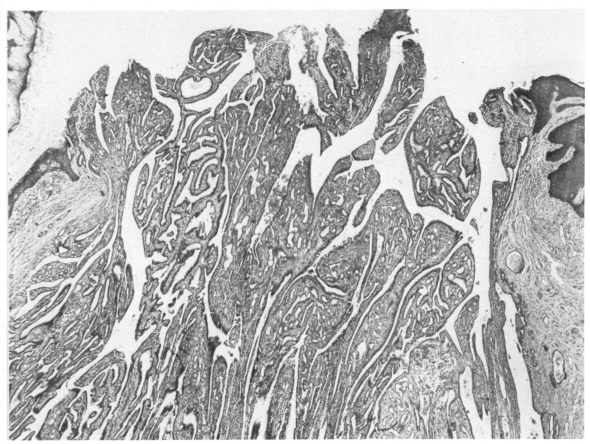

8–1

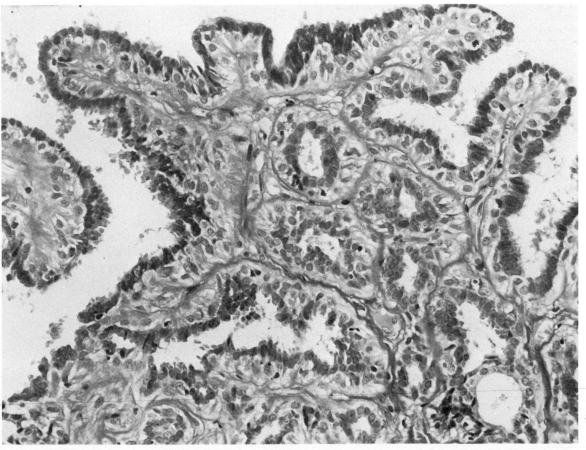

8–2

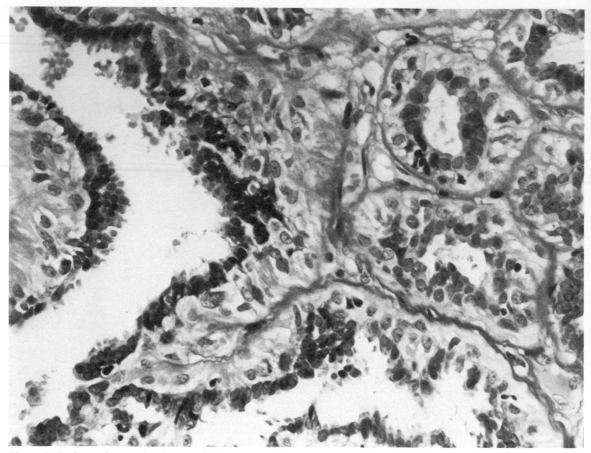

Figure 8–3 Same tissue as in Figure 8–2. There are variations in the distinctness of two-cell-type differentiation even in the same field. Weigert elastic and HVG. ×525.

originates in a cyst but that the grossly distended, blocked, rounded duct has a cystic configuration in a descriptive sense. The term 'adenoma' has been introduced into this name to indicate that, apart from papillary fronds, the tumour contains glandular adenomatous spaces in its interior. The precise histogenesis of the adenomatous component is debatable. This so-called papillary cystadenoma can be even more difficult to differentiate from papillary carcinoma than the less complex papilloma. The adenomatous structures may be very closely apposed one to another but they do not merge (Figure 8–6); fine vessels and usually a small amount of connective

tissue separate them. The 'glands' do not share party walls; if there is a strong indication that they do, the alternative diagnosis must be seriously considered.

PAPILLARY CARCINOMA

The papillary carcinoma, by contrast, has in general a less bulky, finer stroma, often consisting of little more than thin-walled vessels and scanty collagen fibres (Figures 8–7 and 8–8). In some areas, it may, however, contain abundant and even sometimes hyaline stroma in the cores of the fronds (Figure 8–9).

Figure 8–4 (*Opposite, above.*) Multiradicular papilloma or papillary 'cystadenoma', a more complex neoplasm than the simple arborescent papilloma. The protuberances, associated with fibrosis, at the margin of the containing duct can be misinterpreted as malignant infiltration. H and E. ×40.

Figure 8–5 (*Opposite, below.*) Same tissue as in Figure 8–4. An adenomatous structure with apocrine metaplasia predominates here. H and E. ×150.

158

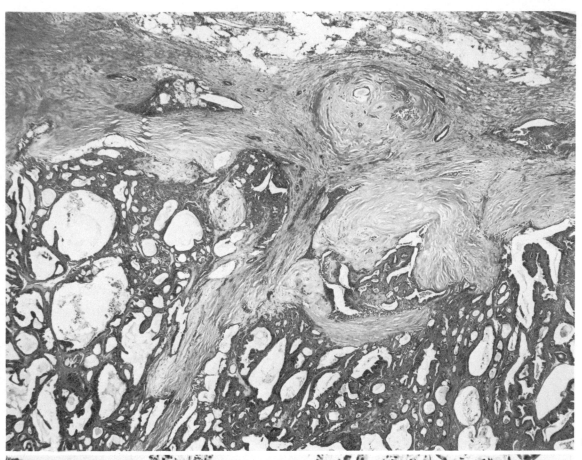

8–4

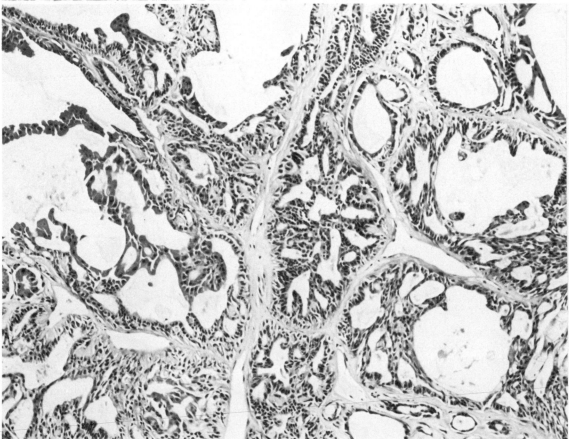

8–5

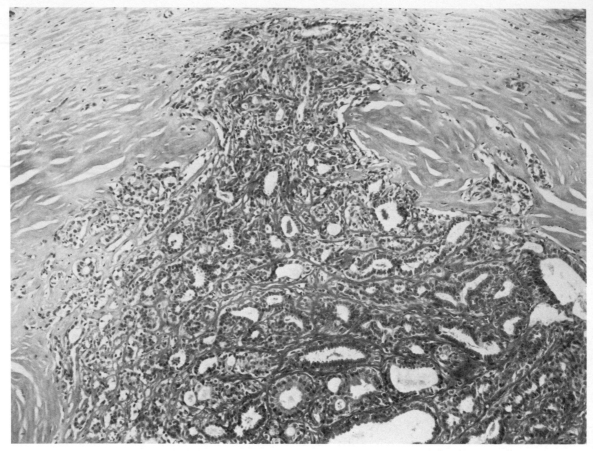

Figure 8–6   A ductal 'cystadenoma' with a mushroom-shaped extension into the fibrous wall. H and E. ×120.

When considering the stroma in differential diagnosis, it is vital to take into account the overall picture rather than isolated fields. Isolated fields can be deceptive rather than helpful (Figures 8–7 to 8–9). Glandular spaces separated by blood vessels only without any collagen fibre should be regarded with suspicion. This is even more true of the sharing of party walls. In papillary carcinoma, buds of neoplastic cells may project individually from the duct wall or appear free in the lumen in a given plane of section. There is frequently little or no stroma in these buds and clusters, partly because of tangential cutting and partly because of a genuine dearth or total absence of stroma. When stroma is absent from such structures, they appear as neoplastic columns or 'stalactites' projecting into the lumen (Figure 7–30). When such structures are numerous the term 'papillary' hardly remains applicable and the appearances merge with the bridges and cartwheels of cribriform carcinoma. This is the other end of the spectrum from the well-fronded papillary carcinoma and the diagnosis is correspondingly easier. The presence of other patterns in a papillary carcinoma serves as a reminder that there is no sharp dividing line between the different types of ductal carcinoma. The divisions into distinct types are useful but largely man-made.

PLEOMORPHISM IN PAPILLARY TUMOURS

Two Cell Types and the Pleomorphism of Divergent Differentiation. It is well known that the benign papilloma is frequently more

---

Figure 8–7   (*Opposite, above.*)   Arborescent neoplasm easily mistaken for a benign tumour by the inexperienced. Note monotonous appearance of the nuclei. H and E. ×150.

Figure 8–8   (*Opposite, below.*)   Higher magnification of part of field seen in Figure 8–7. Despite nuclear monotony, perhaps partly because of it, this is papillary carcinoma. Compare chromatin with that of tumour cells in Figures 8–2 and 8–3. H and E. ×400.

160

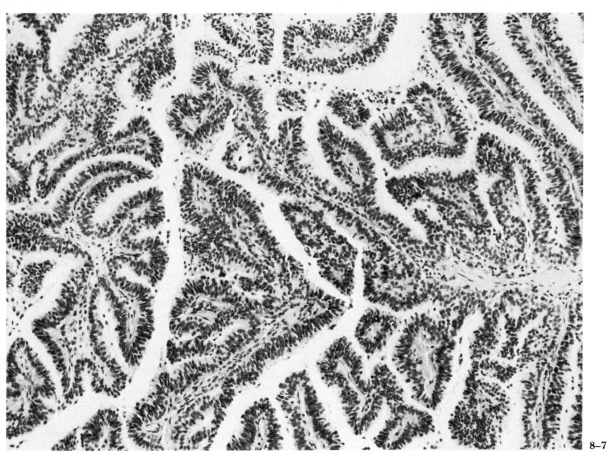

8–7

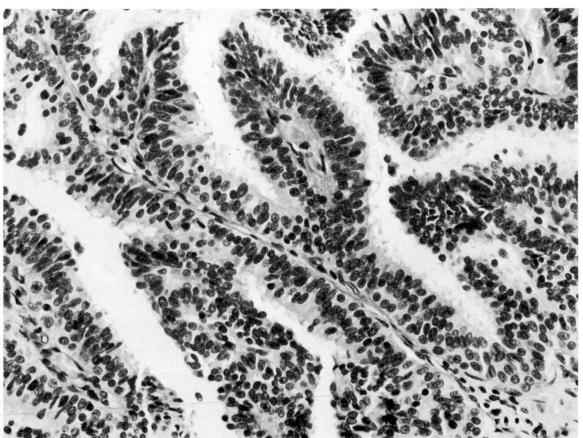

8–8

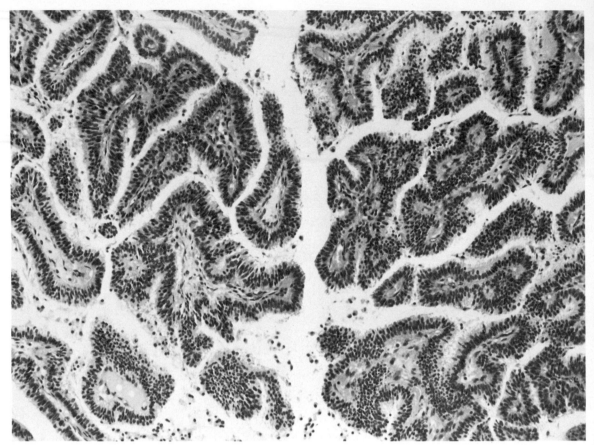

Figure 8–9   Same tumour as illustrated in Figures 8–7 and 8–8. Because of bulky connective tissue cores in some papillae, this type of tumour can be confused with a benign papilloma: this was so misdiagnosed. H and E. ×150.

pleomorphic in appearance than its malignant counterpart (Figures 8–2, 8–5 and 8–6). This is not as paradoxical as might appear at first sight. The pleomorphism of the papilloma is the pleomorphism of divergent differentiation. It is caused partly by the divergent differentiation into two cell types, which is so characteristic a feature of benign breast tumours and hyperplasias (Figures 8–2 and 8–3). It is a constant feature of at least some parts of a papilloma. The prominence and prevalence of this feature is, however, extremely variable, so that it can be very conspicuous or, at the other extreme, require a careful and sometimes extensive search. As a positive finding, it has great diagnostic significance. Two cell types are usually not detectable with any certainty in apocrine areas, at any rate at the light structural level.

The Distinction Between Two Cell Layers and Two Cell Types. Two-cell-type differentiation is, for practical purposes, not a feature of papillary carcinoma. Two qualifying pro-

visoes must be made: firstly, two cell types may be present in the lining of the duct wall as opposed to the centrally situated luminal mass; this is due to a *persistence* of the normal pre-existing outer cell type but the latter is not an integral part of the neoplasm. Secondly, 'two cell *layers*' is not synonymous with 'two cell *types*'. The papillae, 'glands' and other formations of papillary carcinoma are frequently lined by two cell layers, in the same way as they may be lined by one or three or more cell layers. In addition to genuine stratification, pseudostratification may be present also; difficulties in interpretation are very substantial. It is the presence of two distinctive epithelial cell types and not merely the number of epithelial cell layers which distinguishes papilloma from papillary carcinoma.

In view of this importance of two-cell-type differentiation in making the diagnosis of a benign papillary neoplasm, it is unfortunate that Murad, Swaid and Pritchett (1977) state that myoepithelial cell differentiation is also present in papillary carcinomas. With the provisoes made here, this statement must be rejected as misleading. They appear to make this claim on the same grounds they used for regarding scirrhous cancer as a myoepithelial cancer, but the evidence for these claims is rejected for reasons given in Chapter Twelve.

The Pleomorphism of Anaplasia. Papillary carcinoma is sometimes pleomorphic but, when it is, it is the pleomorphism of anaplasia as opposed to the pleomorphism of divergent differentiation. In these circumstances there will be little difficulty in distinguishing it from a papilloma.

A Deceptively Monotonous Appearance. Just as frequently, or perhaps more often, papillary carcinoma has a rather monotonous, uniform appearance which structurally, if not cytologically, can be very deceptive (Figures 8–7 and 8–9). This is reminiscent of the deceptive monotony of many cribriform and even some solid in situ carcinomas.

APOCRINE METAPLASIA IN PAPILLARY TUMOURS

Apocrine metaplasia is frequently seen in the papilloma and virtually never seen in the papillary carcinoma (Figure 8–5). I am referring here to distinct apocrine metaplasia of the type seen in cystic disease. Defined in this way, it is dubious whether it is ever seen in papillary carcinoma; at any rate the writer is unaware that it has ever been described in the literature. Of course, in the rare apocrine carcinoma, the in situ carcinoma component may show apocrine features. But, firstly, apocrine carcinoma in situ is mostly non-papillary and, even if papillary foci are present, the overall pattern is not that of a papillary carcinoma. Secondly, the neoplastic apocrine epithelium differs cytologically from apocrine epithelium of the type seen in cystic disease. The finding of apocrine foci is sufficiently useful as a confirmatory sign that a papillary tumour is benign that, in a difficult situation, it is worth studying multiple levels to search for it.

CYTOLOGY OF PAPILLARY TUMOURS

Nuclear and other cytological details are of paramount importance in the differentiation. In the papilloma, nuclei are orthochromatic, ovoid, with a delicate nuclear membrane and a lack of heavy chromatin stippling (Figures 8–2

and 8–3). Mitoses are usually scanty but too much significance should not be attached to a few normal mitoses. It is important to note that in apocrine foci the nuclei may be larger, more rounded and hyperchromatic. This has no sinister connotation in this setting, just as it has none in apocrine cystic disease and in apocrine foci within sclerosing adenosis. The cytoplasm is usually distinctly eosinophilic in the epithelial cells and very pallid in the outer myoepithelial cells (Figures 8–2 and 8–3). The luminal edges almost always show snouts or apical blebbing. This is conspicuous in most papillomas but in some, although present, it is less well developed. In papillary carcinoma, on the other hand, the neoplastic cells are columnar to cuboidal with nuclei which are correspondingly ovoid to rounded. Whatever the nuclear shape, the N/C ratio tends to be high and the nuclei hyperchromatic (Figure 8–8). The cytoplasm varies between moderately eosinophilic and rather clear, with the emphasis sometimes on the latter. The deeply staining nuclei tend to stand out in stark relief compared with the blander nuclei of the papilloma. Mitoses vary between few and numerous; in general they are found with considerably greater ease than in the benign papilloma. As already indicated, there is an overlap in the number of mitoses and too much reliance should not be placed on this criterion. Truncated luminal cell margins are commonly present in part or most of the tumour and this is a useful indicator of malignancy. Although truncation is an important pointer to malignancy, an irregular luminal edge with blebbing or snouts does not always indicate a benign lesion. The same applies in the consideration of non-papillary in situ ductal lesions, e.g. the cribriform and 'clinging' varieties. Parts of a well-differentiated papillary carcinoma may have fluffy ill-defined luminal margins. This parameter of differentiation must, like many others, be interpreted on the overall structure rather than on the basis of isolated microscopic fields. Even then, while widespread truncation points to malignancy, if fluffy luminal margins are present in a tumour, the possibility of malignancy remains and has to be rejected or sustained on other grounds.

SPURIOUS INFILTRATION IN PAPILLOMA

The Difficulty Caused by the Spurious Appearance of Infiltration at the Base of a Benign Papilloma (Figures 8–4 and 8–6) is so important that it is considered under the heading of 'overdiagnosis' in the next chapter. Suffice it to say here that malignant infiltration of the duct wall from a papillary neoplasm which looks benign overall does not occur or, if it does, it is so very rare that it has not yet been described.

ACCOMPANIMENTS OF PAPILLARY TUMOURS

Papilloma is sometimes accompanied by other benign disease in the surrounding tissue, mostly cystic disease and cystic hyperplasia. With papillary carcinoma, such changes are less frequent but may, of course, be found, if only by chance. Such benign accompaniments provide, at best, only corroborative evidence and little reliance should be placed on them. If, on the other hand, the papillary tumour is accompanied by other types of ductal carcinoma the diagnosis is correspondingly easier. But, in the final analysis, the nature of the papillary tumour must be judged on its own structural and cytological traits.

MAIN SOURCES OF ERROR

This subject is so fraught with difficulties that it is worth considering the main sources of error.

Overdiagnosis of a Papilloma can be caused by:

1. Haemorrhage, fibrosis and distortion at the base of the tumour, trapping epithelial elements in the duct wall so as to simulate invasion.
2. The erroneous expectation that apocrine epithelium will be found invariably.
3. The expectation that the two cell types will be obvious or at least easily found. This may be so and these cases are easily recognizable and, because they are photographable, are reproduced in books, giving the impression that identification of the two cell types is relatively easy. This is by no means always the case. The most difficult papillomas to identify as benign are the tumours with little or no apocrine metaplasia and those in which two-cell-type differentiation is fairly subtle and not ubiquitous.
4. Too much reliance on frozen sections in deciding whether a papillary tumour is benign or malignant. This problem has been discussed in Chapter One.

Underdiagnosis of a Papillary Carcinoma can be caused by:

1. Failure to appreciate that the connective tissue in the fronds is not always scanty or delicate; in a few fronds at least the stroma can be bulky.
2. Confusion between two cell layers and two cell types, a distinction which has not always been emphasized.
3. The absence of truncated luminal margins; truncated luminal margins suggest malignancy, but their absence and the presence instead of snouts or at least of irregular margins does not exclude malignancy.
4. The monotonous low-power appearance, which may be deceptively 'benign-looking' to the untutored eye.

Clinicopathological Correlation. The importance of clinicopathological correlation is illustrated by a problematical papillary lesion studied a few years ago. A drill biopsy was carried out and subsequently an open biopsy performed in the same year and a pathological diagnosis of benign papilloma made on both occasions. The pathologists concerned had not been alerted by the monotonous uniformity of the cytology and the subtle but distinct increase of the N/C ratio: a rather pallid H and E preparation with inadequate haematoxylin staining had masked the hyperchromasia present. The skin incision failed to heal for two years but, almost incredibly, no approach was made to have the microscopic sections reviewed. After two years a further biopsy was diagnosed as papillary carcinoma and a review of all the previous material showed that the previous biopsies had been essentially similar. Modified radical mastectomy unfortunately revealed infiltrating carcinoma with nodal metastases. Two pathological errors were compounded by an unfortunate lack of clinical liaison. This is a good, though sad, illustration of the necessity for proper clinicopathological correlation at all times.

MULTIPLE PAPILLOMAS OF BREAST DUCTS

Solitary papilloma of a breast duct is a benign lesion and there is no evidence that it becomes transformed into cancer with a greater frequency than might be expected by chance.

By contrast are the rare cases with multiple, macroscopically visible, papillomas affecting the breast ducts. This clinical and pathological condition requires separate identification for a number of reasons. Only one of these cases will be seen to each 10 or 12 solitary papillomas. Because they are rare, Haagensen and colleagues (1971) appear to be the only group of workers who have reported on these lesions. They managed to collect 39 cases of this type. They are lesions which have a great capacity for recurrence and a great liability to be associated with malignancy at the same site; 15 of their 39 cases (38 per cent) were so associated. Of 24 patients who did not have carcinoma, 13 were followed for 10 years or more after local excision; only four were apparently cured by one operation while nine had local recurrence; three had only one recurrence but the other six had between two and five local recurrences. The main differences between solitary papilloma and multiple papillomas can be summarized in accordance with Haagensen (1971) as in Table 8–2.

Haagensen (1971) used conservative surgery even in this unusual group of patients but adopted several safeguards. Very great care must be taken to excise all the diseased tissues, using a fastidious operative technique. Usually a whole sector of breast tissue has to be resected. If this conservative surgery is adopted, the patients must be carefully followed every three months for the rest of their life. If for any reason this type of planned care is not feasible, simple mastectomy obviously needs very serious consideration.

There is need for careful documentation of further cases of this type from other centres in order to make comparison with Haagensen's experience (1971).

Table 8–2   The main differences between single and multiple papillomas

Clinical feature	Solitary papilloma	Multiple papillomas
Mean age of patient	48 years	40 years
Nipple discharge	80.0%	35.0%
Subareolar location	95.0%	25.0%
Bilaterality	1.5%	25.0%

CONCLUSION

Basically, in discussing the precancerous potential and other features of papillomas of the breast, one must distinguish *three distinct types of pathology*. Failure to do this has contributed to the immense confusion and some completely conflicting views in the literature on this subject. The confusion and disputes are chiefly attributable to (1) erroneous pathological diagnoses, especially in the older work, a problem already discussed, (2) a residue of intrinsic pathological difficulties and statistical problems and (3) a failure to distinguish between three distinct forms of pathology:

(i) The solitary papilloma of a major duct, which presents with nipple discharge and/or a palpable lump which is almost always situated in the subareolar region. This lesion is benign and there is no good evidence that it is associated with malignancy with a greater than chance frequency.

(ii) The *rare* type of patient with multiple macroscopic papillomas of the ducts, as described by Haagensen (1971), requires segregation. These lesions are associated with or develop into carcinoma with greatly increased frequency.

(iii) Microscopic papillomas recognized by the pathologist only, and not identifiable by the surgeon or on macroscopic study of the pathological specimen, constitute the third distinct type of papillary breast disease. These papillomas are part of the cystic disease and cystic hyperplasia complex. Their significance is the same as that of other forms of benign epithelial hyperplasia of the breast. The whole question of the precancerous proclivity of cystic disease is considered in Chapter Six.

References

Buhl-Jørgensen, S. E., Fischermann, K., Johansen, H. and Petersen. B. (1968) Cancer risk in intraductal papilloma and papillomatosis. *Surgery, Gynecology and Obstetrics,* **127,** 1307–1312.

Carter, D. (1977) Intraductal papillary tumors of the breast. A study of 78 cases. *Cancer,* **39,** 1689–1692.

Forrest, H. (1966) Intraduct papilloma of the breast. *British Journal of Surgery,* **53,** 1028–1032.

Gatchell, F. G., Dockerty, M. B. and Clagett, O. T. (1958) Intracystic carcinoma of the breast. *Surgery, Gynecology and Obstetrics,* **106,** 347–352.

Haagensen, C. D. (1971) *Diseases of the Breast.* Second edition — revised reprint. pp. 262–266, 290. Philadelphia, London, Toronto: W. B. Saunders.

Haagensen, C. D., Lane, N. and Lattes, R. (1972) Neoplastic proliferation of the epithelium of the mammary lobules. Adenosis, lobular neoplasia, and small cell carcinoma. *Surgical Clinics of North America,* **52,** 497–524.

Haagensen, C. D., Stout, A. P. and Phillips, J. S. (1951) The papillary neoplasms of the breast. 1. Benign intraductal papilloma. *Annals of Surgery,* **133,** 18–36.

Hart, D. (1927) Intracystic papillomatous tumours of the breast. *Archives of Surgery,* **14,** 793–835.

Hendrick, J W. (1957) Intraductal papilloma of the breast. *Surgery, Gynecology and Obstetrics,* **105,** 215–223.

Kilgore, A. R., Fleming, R. and Ramos, N. (1953) The incidence of cancer with nipple discharge and the risk of cancer in the presence of papillary disease of the breast. *Surgery, Gynecology and Obstetrics,* **96,** 649–660.

Kraus, F. T. and Neubecker, R. D. (1962) The differential diagnosis of papillary tumors of the breast. *Cancer,* **15,** 444–455.

Lewison, E. F. and Lyons, J. G., Jr (1953) Relationship between benign breast disease and cancer. *Archives of Surgery,* **66,** 94–114.

MacGillivray, J. B. (1969) The problem of 'chronic mastitis' with epitheliosis. *Journal of Clinical Pathology,* **22,** 340–347.

Moore, S. W., Pearce, J. and Ring, E. (1961) Intraductal papilloma of breast. *Surgery, Gynecology and Obstetrics,* **112,** 153–158.

Murad, T. M., Swaid, S. and Pritchett, P. (1977) Malignant and benign papillary lesions of the breast. *Human Pathology,* **8,** 379–390.

Page, D. L., Zwaag, R. V., Rogers, L. W., Williams, L. T., Walker, W. E. and Hartmann, W. H. (1978) Relation between component parts of fibrocystic disease complex and breast cancer. *Journal of the National Cancer Institute,* **61,** 1055–1063.

Pellettiere, E. V., II (1971) The clinical and pathologic aspects of papillomatous disease of the breast: a follow-up study of 97 patients treated by local excision. *American Journal of Clinical Pathology,* **55,** 740–748.

Simpson, J. S. and Barson, A. J. (1969) Breast tumours in infants and children. *Canadian Medical Association Journal,* **101,** 100–102.

Smith, B. G. and Taylor, H. B. (1969) The occurrence of bone and cartilage in mammary tumors. *American Journal of Clinical Pathology,* **51,** 610–618.

Chapter Nine

Overdiagnosis of Malignancy

SEVERE EPITHELIOSIS

It is in cases of extensive and severe epitheliosis that the pathologist may be tempted to issue an equivocal report. This temptation must be avoided as frequently as is feasible. Leaving aside here the question of whether patients with cystic hyperplasia have or have not got an increased liability to develop cancer at a later date, the pathologist's function, when dealing with an individual patient, is to decide whether the case is one of epitheliosis or carcinoma. Of course very rarely, for various reasons, he may have to admit that, after consultation with others, he is unable to state definitely whether a case is benign or malignant. But, in the vast majority of cases, the distinction can be made and the clinician should be told as unequivocally as possible whether the pathologist considers that the lesion is benign or malignant. Terms like 'atypical epitheliosis' and 'atypical hyperplasia' should be avoided as far as possible, as should 'atypical papillomatosis'. Such terms sometimes frighten surgeons into performing unnecessary mastectomies.

It is in instances of severe and extensive epitheliosis especially that the pathologist may lean towards a diagnosis of malignancy. He is more likely to do this if he has been led to believe that this condition is markedly 'precancerous' and that transitional forms between it and carcinoma are quite common. In these cases there is quite likely to be very minor evidence of cellular necrosis of the type described in Chapter Seven. The epitheliosis may be associated with dense fibrous sclerosis, and sometimes even with elastosis, and these stromal changes may add to the doubt about the true nature of the lesion. It cannot be stressed too strongly that *if the general architecture and cytology correspond to that described in Chapter Seven, these additional changes should not make a difference to the diagnosis of the lesion as benign.* There is certainly justification for coding or indicating separately cases of this type for purely laboratory and research purposes, but, from the surgeon's point of view, they should be reported as benign. Equivocal reports will be less frequent as the pathologist's acquaintance with sclerosing adenosis in its variant forms grows and as the type of lesion discussed later under the heading of 'infiltrating epitheliosis' becomes more widely recognized.

SCLEROSING ADENOSIS

Adenosis accompanied by stromal proliferation and fibrosis to an extent that tubular structures are distorted is called sclerosing or fibrosing adenosis. It is generally stated that the proliferation affects lobules, i.e. that it is a type of lobular hyperplasia. Some authors, notably Bonser, Dossett and Jull (1961), maintain that there is no real increase in the number of epithelial units in this disorder and that the observed increase in cellularity is entirely stromal. These authors regard the whole process as a purely regressive one and they therefore coined the name 'lobular sclerosis' for the condition. Their view that sclerosing adenosis does not have a component of epithelial hyperplasia must be rejected in view of the infiltrative propensities of this lesion, as discussed below.

The view that sclerosing adenosis represents a hyperplasia in pre-existing lobules is certainly true of most cases. In some cases of sclerosing adenosis variants, studied by the writer by step sectioning and the use of elastic tissue stains, it is clear that the epithelial proliferation can also take the form of outgrowths from small and medium-sized ducts. Tanaka and Oota (1970), using a stereomicroscopic technique, also reached the conclusion that budding occurs from the duct walls with the formation of a series of intertwined tubules, running more or less parallel with the axis of the duct. Budding also occurs at less acute angles with the ducts, resulting in the formation of reasonably localized glandular foci. As a result there are both diffuse glandular units and rather discrete glandular arrangements; the latter can be interpreted as an abnormal development of lobule-like structures. Thus, while sclerosing adenosis, especially in its more classical forms, originates in lobules, some ductal participation is not excluded. Scleros-

ing adenosis is correctly recognized as showing both epithelial efflorescence and stromal overgrowth to varying degrees and these, combined with the different modes of origin and structural patterns, give rise to an immense variety of overlapping appearances. When it is realized that additional processes like epithelial hypertrophy and epitheliosis can be superimposed on sclerosing adenosis, the complexity of the appearances will be appreciated.

When a palpable focus of sclerosing adenosis is excised, often from the breast of a relatively young woman, the microscopic diagnosis can be difficult. It is important, as always, that the specimen be carefully examined macroscopically, preferably with a magnifier and good incident light. Sclerosing adenosis tends to have a multinodular rather well-circumscribed outline, compared with the carcinomas with which it can be confused microscopically. Though usually firm, it is generally not as hard on palpation as a cancer. But there are exceptions to this and, like the typical 'scirrhous', it may even show yellow streaks of elastosis. When sections are examined with a hand lens or a very low power of the microscope, *the nodular and whorled configuration* can usually be clearly discerned (Figure 9–1); high-power examination from the start is likely to be very deceptive (Figure 9–2). The nodules tend to be more cellular centrally, while at the periphery there is frequently increasing stromal proliferation and fibrosis separating the tubules (Figure 9–1); the reverse is true of a scirrhous carcinoma. Highly cellular areas in sclerosing adenosis differ from those in carcinoma by the absence of the pleomorphism of anaplasia, necrosis, etc., while the more sclerosing areas differ in that the epithelial elements are disposed *in elongated and compressed tubules and strands as opposed to the trabeculae and angulated or irregular glands of carcinoma* (Figure 9–2). The tubules of sclerosing adenosis are lined by two cell types though this may require some subtlety of detection; carcinomatous tubules are made up of a single cell type. In some areas the outer cell type of the tubules of sclerosing adenosis may show differentiation to myoid

Figure 9–1   (*Opposite, above.*)   Classical type of sclerosing adenosis with nodular whorling of the hyperplastic tissue. H and E. ×40.

Figure 9–2   (*Opposite, below.*)   Higher magnification of part of field shown in Figure 9–1 showing compactly arranged whorls of glandular tissue. This should no longer be mistaken for carcinoma, granted that the sections are technically adequate and the principles laid down in Chapter One are strictly adhered to. H and E. ×150.

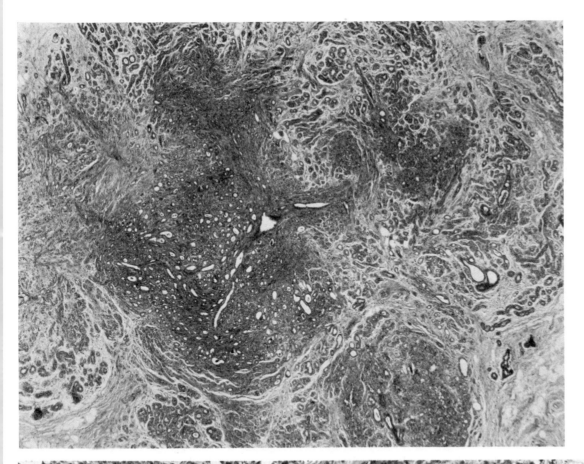

9–1

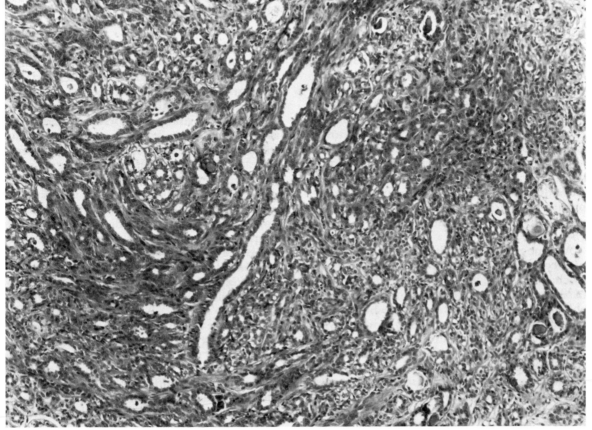

9–2

169

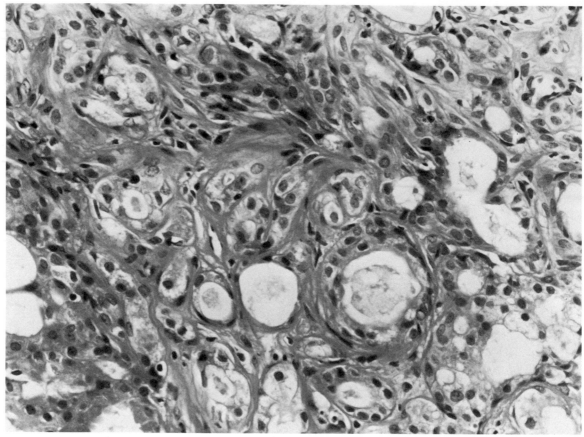

Figure 9–5 Partial apocrine metaplasia in a setting of sclerosing adenosis. This can be differentiated from cancer if it is remembered that minimal atypia of this kind is common with apocrine metaplasia and that apocrine metaplasia can assume partial, less obvious, forms. Also focal changes should be assessed in the context of the entire picture. H and E. ×400.

Apocrine Metaplasia

Apocrine change in sclerosing adenosis is uncommon, and, partly because of its infrequency, when present it can be open to misinterpretation. Occurring in 'closed' or strangled tubules, the larger eosinophilic cells may mimic malignant cells, especially since the outer cell layer is often virtually invisible in such areas (Figures 9–4 and 9–5). One may thus be faced with foci consisting of larger cells, of one cell type, with nuclei which are hyperchromatic and slightly pleomorphic. Apocrine epithelium may show these features even in ordinary apocrine cysts. The reasons for this are not clear, but it is a feature which metaplastic benign apocrine epithelium shares with other metaplastic mitochondrion-rich cells, i.e. oncocytes or oxyphil granular cells in other organs. Areas of slightly pleomorphic epithelium with rounded, deeply staining nuclei, which are recognizably apocrine in type, should not, therefore, be regarded with too much concern: their presence in foci of sclerosing adenosis is

unusual and will attract attention, but the basic diagnosis and ultimate prognosis are not altered. These areas of slightly pleomorphic epithelium are apt to be particularly confusing when, as is often the case, apocrine metaplasia is only *partial*, because in these circumstances cytoplasmic eosinophilia is less pronounced and the fact that there is a tendency to apocrine differentiation may not be appreciated (Figure 9–5). The danger of overdiagnosis is increased if the nuclei of these cells have conspicuous nucleoli, but as long as the epithelium in question is recognized as metaplastic apocrine epithelium in a setting of sclerosing adenosis, the lesion must be regarded as benign unless there is independent evidence of malignancy.

Neural and Vascular Infiltration

Only just over a decade ago, perineural infiltration by epithelium was synonymous with malignancy. Admittedly as early as 1960, Ackerman stated at the International Meeting

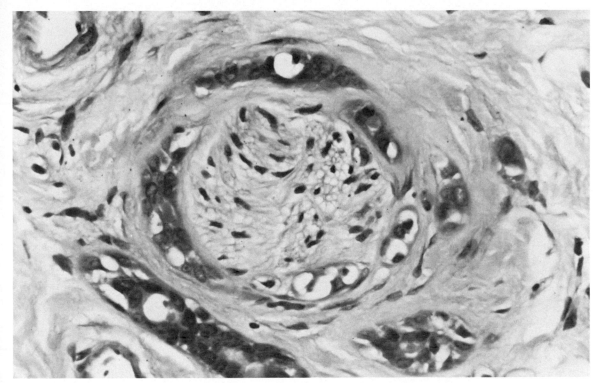

Figure 9–6 Perineural infiltration in sclerosing adenosis. H and E. ×600.

of the I.A.P. held in London, England, that he had observed perineural infiltration in benign breast disease. Taylor and Norris (1967) deserve the credit for first documenting fully the occurrence of perineural infiltration in sclerosing adenosis; they found it in 20 of 1000 cases (Figure 9–6). It is remarkable in retrospect that it took such a long time for this phenomenon to be recognized. Pathologists were not attuned to the idea that benign hyperplastic processes could infiltrate, having been brought up to believe that only malignant tumours infiltrated. The shackling of the thought processes imposed by such teaching was considerable and extended into all spheres of pathology. Davies (1973) found an even higher incidence of 4 per cent of perineural and neural infiltration in sclerosing adenosis. The infiltrating tubules are cytologically benign and have an easily demonstrable two-cell-type structure. The perineural infiltrate is indeed indistinguishable from typical benign mammary epithelium except for its location. This infiltration of perineural spaces and of nerves in sclerosing adenosis is benign and must not be misinterpreted as carcinoma. Gould, Rogers and Sommers (1975) referred to the same phenomenon as epithelial–nerve intermingling in benign breast lesions.

By courtesy of Professor G. Bussolati of

Turin, Italy, the writer has studied a case of sclerosing adenosis with quite remarkable neural involvement. Of three contiguous nerve trunks, one was virtually completely occupied by a collection of benign mammary ductules, which lay within the nerve substance completely ensheathed by perineurium: this localized collection simulated a breast lobule. A second nerve was half occupied by a benign lobule-like structure; in this case, the lobule-like structure was in continuity with similar epithelium in the stroma outside the nerve. The lobule-like structure had apparently transgressed the perineurium and extended wholesale into the nerve substance. The third nerve trunk was normal. Unfortunately it was not possible to trace the events in serial studies.

Perineural infiltration in sclerosing adenosis militates strongly against the view that this process is basically a 'lobular sclerosis' with stromal but no epithelial proliferation (Bonser, Dossett and Jull, 1961); in fact it renders this hypothesis quite untenable. This finding also makes the view that sclerosing adenosis represents lobular hyperplasia followed by sclerosis appear to be an oversimplification. Sclerosing adenosis in its proliferative phase is a more infiltrative process than has been assumed hitherto. It can form grossly enlarged lobules or lobule-like structures,

173

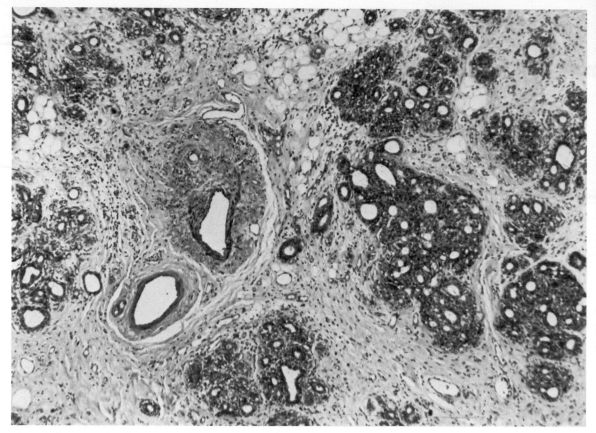

Figure 9–7 Arterial intimal penetration by benign mammary tissue in 'nodular adenosis', a variant of sclerosing adenosis. See Figure 9–8. H and E. ×80.

which, aggregated together, may give rise to a palpable breast lump; it can also infiltrate rather more diffusely into periductal tissues and breast stroma generally and sometimes invades neurovascular bundles. With this view in mind, it is not surprising to find that sclerosing adenosis can even infiltrate the *walls of blood vessels* (Eusebi and Azzopardi, 1976). Figures 9–7 to 9–10 show infiltration into the intima of an artery by two-layered tubules. Figures 9–11 to 9–14 show infiltration of vein walls by similar structures. Invasion of nerve sheath and of vein wall by a benign infiltrative process is less surprising than the unique penetration of an arterial wall illustrated in Figures 9–7 to 9–10. In a systematic study we found venous wall infiltration in four out of 44 consecutive cases of sclerosing adenosis, an incidence of 9 per cent, which is higher than

our 2 per cent incidence of perineural infiltration (Eusebi and Azzopardi, 1976). Taking into account the limited extent of sampling, the true incidence of venous infiltration in sclerosing adenosis is almost certainly higher. *Neurovascular infiltration of this type is benign* and does not alter the prognosis.

INFILTRATING EPITHELIOSIS

This is the name chosen to describe a lesion which is not uncommon but which has not received adequate recognition in the literature until recently. As far as can be ascertained, this is the lesion which McDivitt,

---

Figure 9–8 (*Opposite, above.*) Same tissue as in Figure 9–7. Two benign glandular structures (arrowed) are present internal to the internal elastic lamina within a thickened intima. H and E. ×80.

Figure 9–9 (*Opposite, below.*) Higher magnification of part of field shown in Figures 9–7 and 9–8. H and E. ×550.

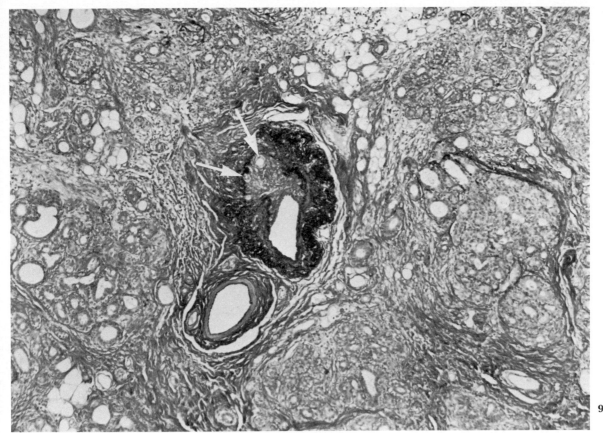

9–8

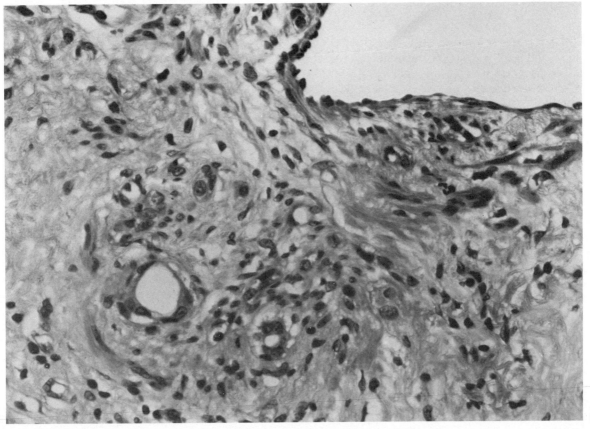

9–9

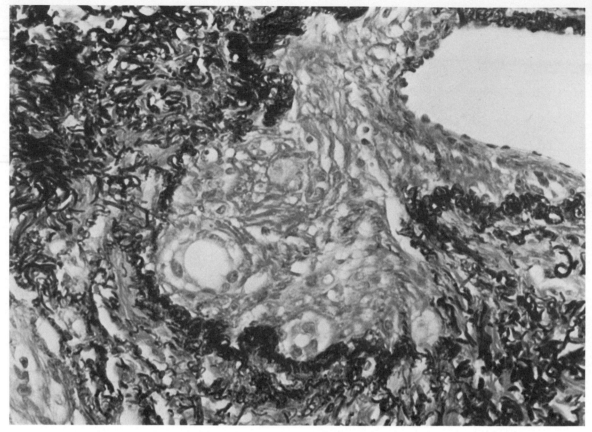

Figure 9–10 Same tissue as in Figure 9–9. The benign glandular epithelium is situated within the arterial intima. Weigert elastic and HVG. ×550.

Stewart and Berg (1968) termed 'sclerosing adenosis with pseudo-infiltration'. It seems reasonably certain that most of the lesions called 'sclerosing papillary proliferations' by Fenoglio and Lattes (1974) represent the same entity. This is apparently the first detailed description of this condition. For reasons which will be discussed, the name chosen for this lesion by Fenoglio and Lattes (1974) is unsatisfactory.

MICROSCOPIC APPEARANCE

Basically, the histological picture is one of epitheliosis, with or without accompanying cystic disease (Figures 9–15 to 9–17).

Epitheliosis affects the ductal system and often the lobules also. The proliferative process is usually severe so that occupied structures are to some extent distended and, frequently, the hyperplastic process is also extensive. On the other hand, the lesion sometimes involves only a few high-power fields or scattered minute foci may be present.

By contrast with classical epitheliosis, the epithelial structures affected do not all have the regular, well-defined, sharply delineated, blunt edges with a well-preserved basement membrane (Figures 9–15 to 9–18). Instead, the edges of the foci of epitheliosis are sometimes jagged and irregular with triangular or pointed 'juts' abutting on the stroma. The basement membrane, as delineated by

Figure 9–11 (*Opposite, above.*) Benign glands present in the intima of a vein wall in sclerosing adenosis. This is difficult to detect in routine preparations. See Figure 9–12. H and E. ×750.

Figure 9–12 (*Opposite, below.*) Benign infiltration of venous wall in sclerosing adenosis. The glandular tissue forms a crescent internal to the elastic coat of the vessel wall. The vascular lumen is eccentric and narrowed. At some levels it is reduced to a narrow slit. Weigert elastic and HVG. ×750.

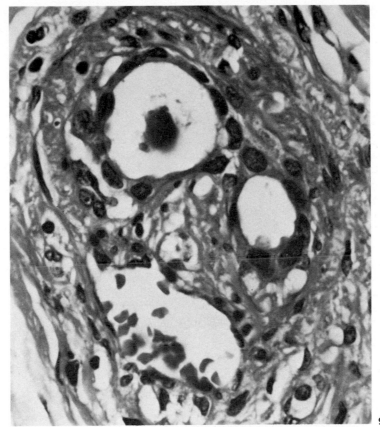

9–11

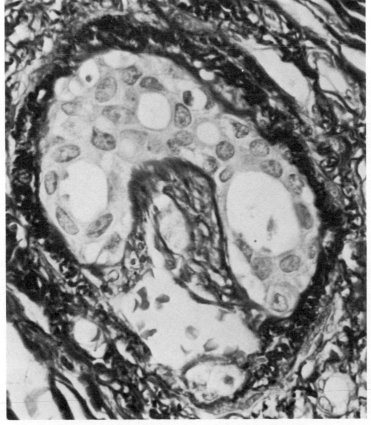

9–12

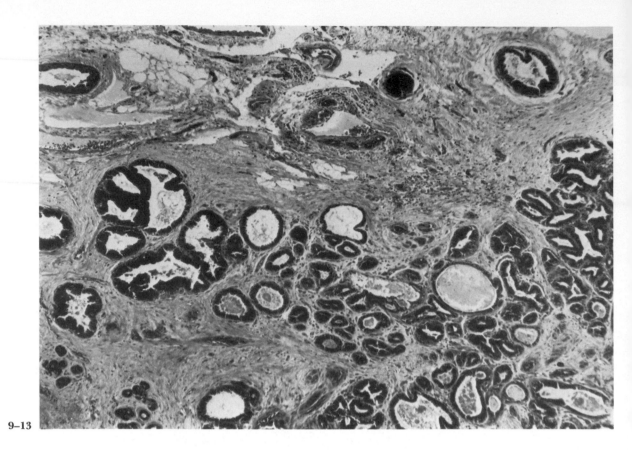

9–13

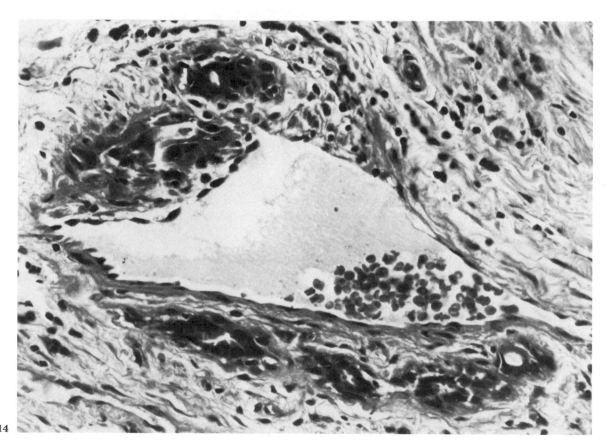

9–14

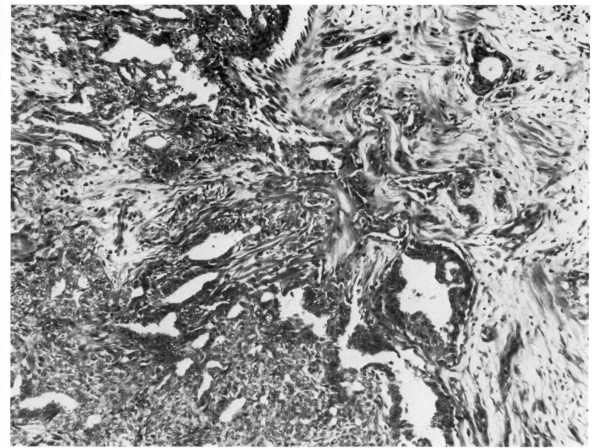

Figure 9–15 'Infiltrating epitheliosis'. The solid portions are identical with ordinary epitheliosis. The margins of the sheets are, however, irregular and jagged rather than smooth and blunt so that the hyperplastic tissue appears to flow into the adjacent stroma. H and E. ×150.

PAS and other stains, is sometimes intact, sometimes thin and indistinct, or it may appear to be frankly defective in some parts. Assessment of the integrity or otherwise of the basement membrane is frequently obscured by the fibrosis and elastosis which is often present immediately adjacent to the epithelial foci. Investigation of the basal lamina by electron microscopy has not, to my knowledge, been carried out in this condition. In view of the findings of Ozzello (1971) that a defect in the basal lamina at ultrastructural level indicates malignancy, the apparent lack of a basement membrane found by the writer

in parts of the lesions of 'infiltrating epitheliosis' needs confirmation. It is possible that the basal lamina is intact at ultrastructural level and that the proliferating cells of epitheliosis do not establish direct contact with the connective tissue without the interposition of basal lamina.

The proliferating epithelium appears to 'flow out' into the adjacent stroma and it is in these regions especially that the basement membrane sometimes appears defective. The proliferating tissue that streams into the stroma may or may not appear to be in continuity with the main mass, in any given

Figure 9–13 (*Opposite, above.*)   A non-organoid type of adenosis and microcystic adenosis with infiltration of the wall of a vein at top centre at some distance from the main hyperplastic tissue. See Figure 9–14. H and E. ×75.

Figure 9–14 (*Opposite, below.*)   Higher magnification of part of field shown in Figure 9–13. The venous intima is partly occupied by benign two-layered breast epithelium forming a corona of glands. At one point the infiltrating epithelium together with a little fibrin forms a small mound immediately below hypertrophic and slightly elevated endothelial cells. Diastase–PAS. ×550.

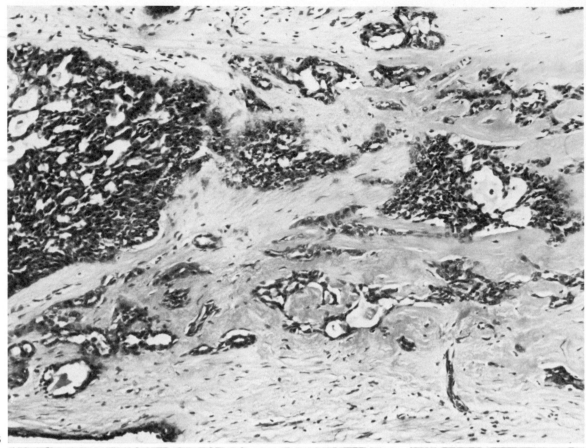

9–16

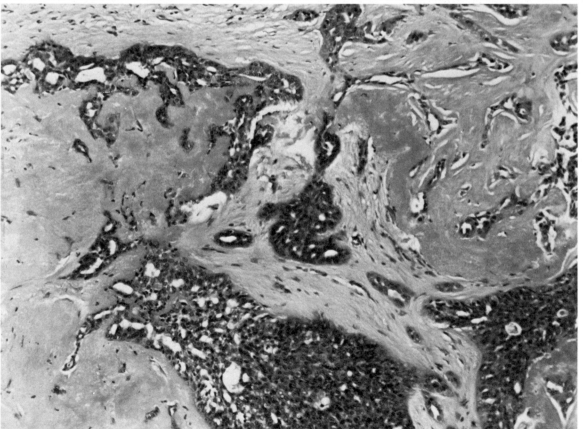

9–17

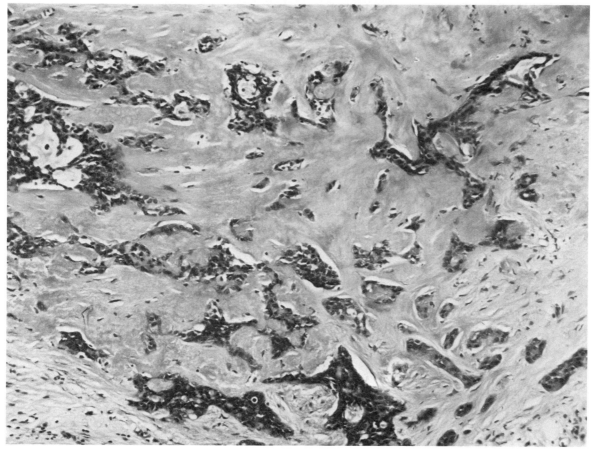

Figure 9–18 Marked fibrous sclerosis and some elastosis associated with infiltrating epitheliosis. Trabeculae of cancer are absent and the spindled cells are elongated in the axis of the cell bundles. H and E. ×150.

plane of section. It infiltrates the surrounding tissue as tubules, elongated strands, clumps and as single isolated cells (Figures 9–15 to 9–20). The tubules are elongated but a few are angulated and these may mimic malignant tubules, sometimes very closely. Careful examination will reveal that in some tubules two distinct cell types can usually be distinguished. The strands of cells consist of plump cells with large ovoid vesicular nuclei containing prominent nucleoli or spindled cells with darker nuclei. The cytoplasm of these cells varies from faintly eosinophilic and nondescript to an opaque deeply eosinophilic cytoplasm, strongly suggestive of myoid

differentiation. The constituent cells are elongated in the long axes of the cords (Figures 9–16 and 9–18). The strands may be cut longitudinally, obliquely or transversely and, in the latter cases, appear as clumps of ovoid or even rounded cells. Where there are clusters of rounded eosinophilic cells, small nerves may be mimicked if the cytoplasm is mistaken for myelin sheaths. The cell groups that mimic small nerves are the ones that show myoid differentiation. The isolated single cells have the same characteristics as the cells in the strands (Figure 9–20). Myoid cells can be identified by their eosinophilia but some of the cells that show little or no differentiation

Figure 9–16 *(Opposite, above.)*   Infiltrating epitheliosis centred on a duct which runs in the long axis of the illustration. The amorphous, 'hyaline' sparsely cellular zones contain abundant elastic tissue. This is a benign lesion frequently mistaken for cancer, a diagnosis seriously entertained by the contributing pathologists. H and E. ×150.

Figure 9–17 *(Opposite, below.)*   Solid and slightly fenestrated epitheliosis merging with infiltrating epitheliosis. There are large pools of elastic tissue which appear as denser, more homogeneous and less cellular zones than the fibrous tissue. H and E. ×150.

181

term is that this lesion is not one which pathologists will easily recognize as sclerosing adenosis and it must be emphasized that the pattern is very different from that of classical sclerosing adenosis. Many pathologists who see this condition fail to recognize it as sclerosing adenosis and they have frequently been a little reluctant to agree that it is closely related. The qualification 'with pseudo-infiltration' was descriptively apt in 1968, before it was recognized that genuine infiltration of structures like nerves occurred with benign breast disease. Since both neural and venous infiltration have been seen by the writer in the lesion described here, the qualification 'infiltrating' is appropriate now. The term *'infiltrating epitheliosis'*, which has been in use at Hammersmith Hospital since 1970, adequately describes the appearances and has the merit of being distinctive. The only disadvantage of this name, and it is a significant one, is that the qualifying 'infiltrating' might suggest malignancy to a clinician.

This name must be accompanied in a report by a rider to the effect that the lesion is benign, until surgeons have been taught to appreciate that infiltration is not uncommon in sclerosing adenosis and that the term 'infiltrating' applied to breast disease does not indicate malignancy when it qualifies a lesion like epitheliosis.

GROSSLY DETECTABLE LESIONS

Many of these lesions are recognized only microscopically but, when a lesion is extensive, it can form a grossly detectable firm to hard nodule with yellow streaks, which, like sclerosing adenosis, can mimic infiltrating carcinoma on gross examination. With a large lesion, the resemblance to a carcinoma can be even closer than with sclerosing adenosis. One must depend on microscopy for differentiation.

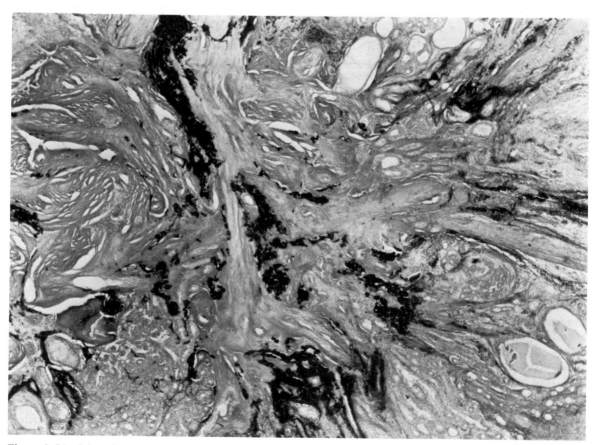

Figure 9–21 Scleroelastotic scar, mammographically and macroscopically simulating carcinoma, of the type reported by Eusebi, Grassigli and Grosso (1976). Weigert elastic and HVG. ×45.

FREQUENCY OF LESIONS AND PROBLEMS IN
DIAGNOSIS

It is of considerable interest that the
histology of this lesion was not described in
detail until 1974, although McDivitt, Stewart
and Berg (1968) had illustrated what was
almost certainly the same condition. Over a
period of a few years the writer collected more
than 30 lesions of this type from nearly 1000
breast specimens (local excisions and mastectomy specimens but excluding excisions of
fibroadenoma). This includes some very small
lesions of this type but, from the way the
material was collected, many lesions must have
been missed since only one-third of the total
material was systematically screened by the
writer and, for the rest, he relied on referral of
specimens which were considered difficult to
interpret or which contained unusual
findings. The incidence of approximately one
lesion in 30 surgical breast specimens
(excluding fibroadenoma) is thus a minimum
figure; infiltrating epitheliosis is therefore a
fairly common lesion. Judging by consultations from other hospitals, the larger lesions of
infiltrating epitheliosis cause considerable
difficulty in diagnosis and this has obviously
been the experience also of Fenoglio and
Lattes (1974). Infiltrating epitheliosis is
probably responsible for a high proportion of
diagnoses like 'atypical hyperplasia' and
'atypical epitheliosis' or of equivocal reports,
and even erroneous diagnoses of infiltrating
carcinoma. Three or four of our more florid
examples caused considerable anxiety a few
years ago and pathologists in other centres
have experienced the same difficulties.
Colleagues have expressed surprise that they
were unable to find a detailed description of
this lesion in the literature before 1974.

*Does this lesion ever become malignant? Perhaps
more important, is the lesion ever malignant ab
initio?* To the second question, the work of
Fenoglio and Lattes (1974) strongly suggests
that the correct answer is no. A curious finding
in their series was that two out of five patients
undergoing mastectomy also had synchronous or subsequently developing lobular
carcinoma in situ. A further two patients,
among those who underwent local excision
only, also had CLIS. This apparently high
incidence of lobular neoplasia may well have
been pure coincidence, but it leaves open the
possibility that infiltrating epitheliosis is
associated with other lesions of a more sinister
nature more often than would be expected by
chance. Nevertheless, the only definite
conclusion that can be drawn at present is that
this lesion is inherently benign.

McDivitt, Stewart and Berg (1968) clearly
reached the same conclusion since they used
the expression 'pseudo-infiltration' and classified the lesion under benign conditions.
These authors did, however, go on to suggest
that, very rarely, a carcinoma could originate
in such a lesion. In our own material, this
lesion is also apparently benign in its
behaviour but the follow-up periods are too
short for definite conclusions. In a solitary
case only was there a possibility that a
well-differentiated carcinoma had evolved
(Figure 9–22); in the centre of an area of
infiltrating epitheliosis associated with elastosis there was what appeared macroscopically
and microscopically to be a miniature
scirrhous carcinoma, 2.5 mm in diameter. The
angulated tubules in this area were all single
layered, as far as could be ascertained, but in
the absence of trabeculae or other pathognomonic evidence of malignancy, the
evidence for malignant transformation is
equivocal and remains unconvincing. It
cannot yet be regarded as proven that a
carcinoma can evolve from a lesion of
infiltrating epitheliosis. Further study is
clearly required.

RELATIONSHIP TO OTHER BENIGN HYPERPLASIAS

Infiltrating epitheliosis is related to
epitheliosis on the one hand and to sclerosing
adenosis on the other. It differs from
sclerosing adenosis in showing little or no
lobular or even nodular formations, in having
a less organized arrangement, in being
regularly associated with epitheliosis, and in
being only partly arranged in two layered
tubules. It could perhaps be looked on as a
rather diffuse form of poorly organized
sclerosing adenosis, but even this view is an
oversimplification as it disregards the strong
links it has with epitheliosis. Intermediate
forms between sclerosing adenosis and
infiltrating epitheliosis do occur but they are
not common. More common is the coexistence
of both types of lesion in different parts of the
same breast. There is no doubt that, if this
lesion is to be identified correctly, it must have
a distinct label. It is a common benign lesion,
and an important one, because it is so easily
confused with carcinoma. 'Infiltrating epitheliosis' best describes its essential characteristics.

RELATED OR IDENTICAL LESIONS DESCRIBED RECENTLY

There are three more recent papers with a bearing on this complex pathological lesion. The first is by Hamperl (1975), who described 18 cases with 'radial scars and obliterative mastopathy'. Hamperl regarded these lesions as similar to those described by Fenoglio and Lattes (1974). He also disapproved of the designation 'papillary' to describe the epithelial proliferation which was usually, but not invariably, present in his cases. Hamperl (1975) regarded the central scar as the primary lesion, on which there was sometimes superimposed an epithelial hyperplasia which radiated from a fibroelastotic centre. Eusebi, Grassigli and Grosso (1976) described similar lesions under the heading of 'scleroelastotic lesions of the breast simulating infiltrating carcinoma'. The latter workers stressed especially the mammographic and macroscopic resemblance to a miniature infiltrating carcinoma: even fine stippled calcification could be present. Like Hamperl (1975), they regarded these lesions as originating in obliterated ducts, with a secondary epithelial hyperplasia which sometimes took origin within the damaged ducts and penetrated the duct walls to extend into the surrounding stroma.

The lesions described by Hamperl (1975) and by Eusebi, Grassigli and Grosso (1976) appear to be identical. By courtesy of Dr V. Eusebi, the writer has been able to study all four of their cases. We are in agreement on the factual data. What is not clear is whether the Hamperl–Eusebi lesions represent one end of a spectrum, the other end of which was described by Fenoglio and Lattes (1974); my own cases correspond more closely to most of those described by Fenoglio and Lattes (1974).

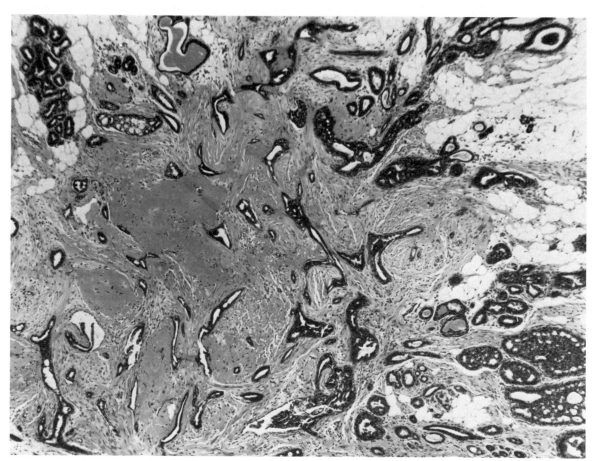

Figure 9–22   Infiltrating epitheliosis with gross elastosis. Yellow flecks were visible grossly in a minute puckered focus which was thought to be malignant on macroscopic examination. The angulated glands were difficult to distinguish from a miniature carcinoma in this case. The patient is well more than six years after a local excision for cystic disease. H and E. ×60.

The alternative possibility is that these lesions represent two pathogenetically distinct entities; one with infiltrating epitheliosis as the primary lesion with secondary stromal alterations, the other with a primary scleroelastotic scar based on obliterative duct disease. The former type is more likely to be overdiagnosed microscopically as carcinoma, the latter is more likely to be overdiagnosed on mammographic examination. Both types can simulate cancer on macroscopic examination. Even if the possibility that these two types represent separate entities were to prove correct, it would appear that the end stages can be indistinguishable. Further study is essential in view of the risk of overdiagnosis, both radiographic and pathological, as stressed by Eusebi, Grassigli and Grosso (1976).

Tremblay, Buell and Seemayer (1977) more recently described 17 cases of 'elastosis in benign sclerosing ductal proliferation of the female breast'. The lesions they described and illustrated correspond very closely to and are probably identical with those studied by the writer. These authors stressed that the gross appearance, as well as the microscopic, can mimic infiltrating carcinoma. These workers, unlike Hamperl (1975) and Eusebi, Grassigli and Grosso (1976), regarded the epithelial hyperplasia as the primary lesion, though they stress desmoplasia, which is greatest centrally, and the constant finding of elastosis. They also found nodular masses of elastic tissue which probably represent completely obliterated ducts. Rather wisely, in the writer's opinion, they refrained from being too specific about the pathogenesis of these lesions. There is much we still need to know about them.

PAPILLARY CYSTADENOMA WITH PSEUDO-INFILTRATION

The differentiation of benign and malignant papillary tumours has been discussed in Chapter Eight. Pathologists tend to be divided into those who believe that papillary carcinoma of the breast practically always arises de novo and those who believe that a significant proportion of papillomas and papillary 'cystadenomas' undergo malignant alteration and become invasive. There is one particular complication of cystadenoma which can easily lead to the tumour being erroneously interpreted as malignant. Benign papillary

tumours frequently bleed into the lumen because of damage to fronds by infarction or other trauma. Hence a nipple discharge may be blood-stained. Histological evidence of previous haemorrhage may be found in such circumstances. Haemorrhage occurring at the site of attachment of the tumour to the duct wall can lead to a very disturbing appearance. The haemorrhage can result in fibrosis and, as this contracts, it can draw out and distort parts of the periphery of the tumour (Figures 8–4 to 8–6). This leads to projecting nubbins of tissue or even angulated tubules isolated in fibrous tissue in the duct wall, not always in obvious continuity with the main tumour mass, an appearance which is easily interpreted as incipient invasion. Haemosiderin deposits, siderophages and the cholesterol clefts which are often present give a strong hint as to the true sequence of events. A few foci of chronic inflammatory cells are frequently also present but these do not aid in the diagnosis. If the apparently isolated tubules are carefully scrutinized, they will be seen to possess the two cell layers that are present in the rest of the tumour. In these circumstances one can make a confident diagnosis of a benign lesion. This potentially deceptive appearance represents 'pseudo-infiltration' of the duct wall brought about by cicatricial fibrosis secondary to haemorrhage. *In practice, if a papillary tumour in the ductal lumen is judged to be benign, a nubbin of apparent infiltration of the wall can safely be disregarded,* and is usually the result of the process described. This cautionary note should hardly be necessary but this mistake is still sometimes made even by experienced pathologists. It is this type of evidence which has contributed to the view that solitary papilloma of the breast is prone to malignant change.

FIBROSIS AND ELASTOSIS

'Subepithelial Collagenosis' and Elastosis. Because elastosis is very common with carcinoma of the breast there is a danger that, in certain circumstances, its presence can bias the observer towards a diagnosis of malignancy. Askanazy (1931) proposed that fibrosis and elastosis of duct walls associated with stagnant secretion might represent a premalignant state. Although, in retrospect, Askanazy (1931) was describing a stage of duct ectasia,

his views were strenuously supported by Jackson and Orr (1957) and again by Orr in 1958. These workers believed that '*subepithelial collagenosis*' was a precancerous state that was followed by the development of cancer and they attached similar significance to *elastosis*. The implication of this work was that elastosis was a sinister finding irrespective of any epithelial change. Their interpretation influenced workers in the field of tissue interactions in experimental carcinogenesis and the present writer was also nearly misled by this interpretation.

The significance of elastosis is discussed in Chapter Fifteen. Suffice it to say here that *elastosis in the breast cannot be equated with malignancy*. Its presence certainly calls for a search for the provoking stimulus. There are both benign and malignant causes of elastosis in the breast and the significance of the elastosis has to be interpreted in the context of the overall picture.

Epitheliosis is sometimes accompanied by fibrosis and elastosis and the combination of severe epitheliosis and a marked stromal reaction can appear formidable and worrisome. There is no evidence to suggest that the behaviour is any different from that of epitheliosis of similar quality without the stromal changes.

Sclerosing Adenosis is one of the commoner benign diseases to be associated with elastosis. Elastosis may be absent or negligible, or it may be a prominent feature that is sometimes recognizable even macroscopically. The presence of elastosis makes no difference to the behaviour of the lesion.

Infiltrating Epitheliosis is usually accompanied by a fibroelastotic stromal reaction. It is a benign disease which is relatively frequently overdiagnosed as malignant. The accompanying elastotic reaction might add to the tendency to overdiagnose the condition, especially in view of the sinister connotation that has been placed on elastosis by some workers. A few years ago we suspected that rare florid examples of infiltrating epitheliosis might represent 'early' carcinoma, influenced by the infiltrative nature of the lesion and especially by the presence of marked degrees of elastosis. To prevent potential errors, one must be acquainted with the features of infiltrating epitheliosis, recognize that stromal infiltration in the breast is not a feature

restricted to malignant disease and understand current views on the significance of elastosis as expounded in Chapter Fifteen.

When marked fibrosis and elastosis are present with one of the three benign conditions mentioned, *circumstances may combine to simulate malignancy*. The marked stromal change may lead to a clinical suspicion of malignancy and, at operation especially, the firmness may add to this suspicion. The lesion may cut with a hardness which mimics carcinoma and, if yellow streaks and flecks are present on the cut face, the imitation can be very close. The macroscopic appearances combined with unusual histological features can lead to the pathologist entertaining very seriously a diagnosis of malignancy (Tremblay, Buell and Seemayer, 1977).

CALCIFICATION

The significance of calcification in the differentiation of epitheliosis and in situ carcinoma has already been discussed. There is no doubt that calcification can be a very important pointer to malignancy, but this is true only when it is present in the right setting. Like any other criterion, it can be abused and, because certain types of mammographic microcalcification are so useful as a pointer to probable malignancy, there is *a distinct danger that pathological calcification of certain types might be equated with malignancy*. The position is analogous to the finding of elastosis; it requires a search for an explanation and it may pinpoint areas requiring detailed study but it certainly does not mean that a lesion is automatically malignant.

Sclerosing adenosis is an example of a benign lesion in which microspherules of calcified material are frequent in the distorted tubular proliferation (Figure 9–23). The behaviour of sclerosing adenosis alters not a jot in the presence of such microcalcification and yet calcification in sclerosing adenosis can mimic so-called 'malignant calcification' very closely indeed radiographically (MacErlean and Nathan, 1972).

When the presence of calcification is being utilized as a differential point in favour of malignancy, it is essential to *localize precisely the site of the calcification*. Calcification in duct ectasia or in a fibroadenoma is not relevant here. It is important to remember that

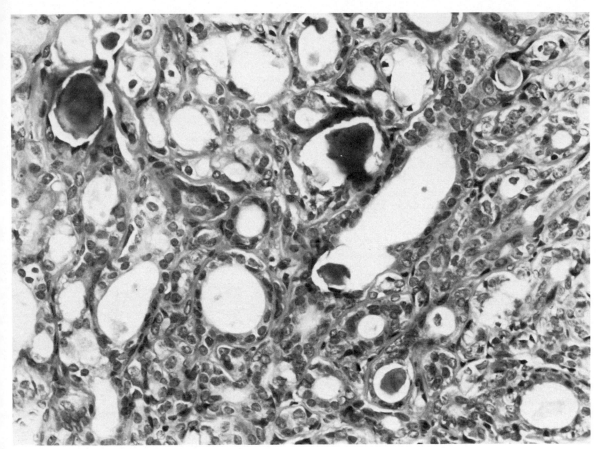

Figure 9–23   Calcospherites in sclerosing adenosis. H and E. ×400.

calcification in a papillary tumour is not necessarily an indication that it is malignant. In the cystic hyperplasia complex, calcification is found in sclerosing adenosis, in cysts, in blunt duct adenosis and in microscopic papillomas. Less frequently calcifications in cystic disease may be visible on the mammogram and a suspicion of malignancy may have already been entertained on that score. In practice, more complex situations arise, as when calcification is present in a ductal carcinoma as well as in immediately adjacent benign disease. Calcification, as a positive finding, has its greatest value in the differentiation of duct carcinoma and cancerized lobules from epitheliosis. Epitheliosis rarely exhibits a significant degree of calcification although there are a few exceptions; it is important to remember that *the psammomatous type of calcification is especially rare in epitheliosis.*

Unfortunately there is very little information in the mammographic literature on the question of radiologically visible calcification in epitheliosis. The mammoth work of Koehl et al (1970) lists duct papilloma and duct hyperplasia together as causes of radiographically visible calcification in 28 of 1034 specimens with benign disease. If their term 'duct hyperplasia' equates with the British term 'epitheliosis', it would have been extremely useful to know whether there were only a very few such cases with calcification; if this were so, radiologically visible calcification in areas of epitheliosis would be quite exceptional, but if the number of such cases were, say, 10 or 15 it would make radiologically visible calcification of marginally less value in the differentiation of carcinoma from epitheliosis than is currently believed. This is worth bearing in mind in future correlative mammographic–pathological studies. On present information the writer regards radiographically visible calcification in epitheliosis as rare. In the presence of such calcification, the pathologist has a duty to exclude the presence of in situ carcinoma.

For present purposes it is important to

emphasize that microscopic calcification is found in a variety of benign breast diseases. In some instances of diseases like sclerosing adenosis it can be profuse and, when localized, it can mimic radiographically the microcalcifications of malignancy. The same is true of the calcification in breast scars of the type described by Eusebi, Grassigli and Grosso (1976). Calcification per se, even psammomatous calcification, does not indicate malignancy (Figure 9–23). Microcalcifications of a certain type *suggest* it radiographically but it is only microscopic examination which will determine the precise significance in a given case. Its greatest value to the pathologist is in the distinction between 'borderline' carcinoma and epitheliosis. Calcification is discussed in detail in Chapter Eighteen.

PSEUDO-LOBULAR CARCINOMA

Mimicry Due to Artefacts

The colloquial term 'pseudo-lobular carcinoma' does not represent a pathological entity but merely the conditions or circumstances which may lead to a close mimicry of CLIS. The commonest cause is lobular distortion caused by poor fixation or a traumatic or other artefact. Squeeze artefact, autolysis with shedding of cells and similar circumstances may produce a solid appearance in the lobular units that can be misconstrued as malignant disease. With autolysis, it will be recognized that the desquamated normal epithelial cells and not neoplastic cells are plugging the lumina. Traumatic artefacts should be recognized from the distortion caused to the whole lobular outlines and the fact that the lobules are usually small, while careful cytological examination will show ovoid rather than rounded nuclei, with an overlapping which is related to distortion, rather than the even spacing usually seen in CLIS. It is a good working rule that 'doubtful CLIS' should be regarded as benign. This is particularly true if processing is less than perfect.

Mimicry Due to Genuine Changes

There is another situation, unrelated to poor fixation or artefact, in which CLIS may be overdiagnosed. With simple lobular involution, the epithelium usually disappears at the same time as the basement membranes are undergoing thickening. Occasionally,

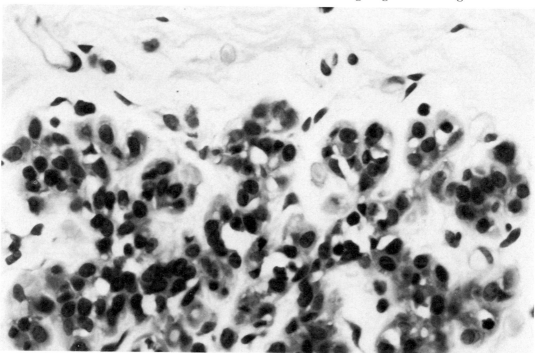

Figure 9–24 'Pseudo-CLIS'. Apparent filling of lumina caused in part by marked artefactual contraction. The basement membrane is thickened rather than thinned. A diagnosis of CLIS should not be made in the presence of a thickened basement membrane. H and E. ×600.

however, the epithelium persists while the basement membrane is undergoing thickening (Figure 9–24). This early thickening can be mistaken for the eosinophilic cytoplasm of the epithelial cells and, if there is a virtual absence of lumina, the whole appearance can mimic CLIS (Figure 9–24). The simplest way to distinguish this with certainty is with a basement membrane stain; the basement membranes are thickened in the situation under consideration while in CLIS they are attenuated to a degree which depends on the extent of distention. Again, for practical purposes, 'doubtful CLIS' should be regarded as benign. This statement does not really clash with the view on 'atypical lobular hyperplasia' expressed in Chapter Ten. Before diagnosing atypical lobular hyperplasia, all artefacts must be excluded, fixation should be excellent and there should be no basement membrane thickening. Unless these criteria are satisfied, the diagnosis of 'atypical lobular hyperplasia' is best avoided.

References

Askanazy, M. (1931) Die Beziehungen der gutartigen Erkrankungen der Brustdrüse zum Mamma Karzinom. *Beiträge zur pathologischen Anatomie und zur allgemeinen Pathologie*, **87**, 396–424.

Bonser, G. M., Dossett, J. A. and Jull, J. W. (1961) *Human and Experimental Breast Cancer*. London: Pitman Medical.

Davies, J. D. (1973) Neural invasion in benign mammary dysplasia. *Journal of Pathology*, **109**, 225–231.

Eusebi, V. and Azzopardi, J. G. (1976) Vascular infiltration in benign breast disease. *Journal of Pathology*, **118**, 9–16.

Eusebi, V., Grassigli, A. and Grosso, F. (1976) Lesioni focali scleroelastotiche mammarie simulanti il carcinoma infiltrante. *Pathologica*, **68**, 507–518.

Fenoglio, C. and Lattes, R. (1974) Sclerosing papillary proliferations in the female breast. A benign lesion often mistaken for carcinoma. *Cancer*, **33**, 691–700.

Gould, V. E., Rogers, D. R. and Sommers, S. C. (1975) Epithelial-nerve intermingling in benign breast lesions. *Archives of Pathology*, **99**, 596–598.

Hamperl, H. (1975) Strahlige Narben und obliterierende Mastopathie. *Virchows Archiv A: Pathological Anatomy and Histology*, **369**, 55–68.

Hutter, R. V. P. and Kim, D. U. (1971) The problems of multiple lesions of the breast. *Cancer*, **28**, 1591–1607.

Jackson, J. G. and Orr, J. W. (1957) The ducts of carcinomatous breasts, with particular reference to connective-tissue changes. *Journal of Pathology and Bacteriology*, **74**, 265–273.

Koehl, R. H., Snyder, R. E., Hutter, R. V. P. and Foote, F. W., Jr (1970) The incidence and significance of calcifications within operative breast specimens. *American Journal of Clinical Pathology*, **53**, 3–14.

MacErlean, D. P. and Nathan, B. E. (1972) Calcification in sclerosing adenosis simulating malignant breast calcification. *British Journal of Radiology*, **45**, 944–945.

McDivitt, R. W., Stewart, F. W. and Berg, J. W. (1968) *Tumors of the Breast*. Atlas of Tumor Pathology, Second series, Fascicle 2. Washington, D.C.: Armed Forces Institute of Pathology.

Orr, J. W. (1958) The significance of connective tissue changes within the ducts in relation to mammary carcinoma. In *International Symposium on Mammary Cancer* (Ed.) Severi, L. p. 209. Perugia, Italy: Division of Cancer Research.

Ozzello, L. (1971) Ultrastructure of the human mammary gland. In *Pathology Annual* (Ed.) Sommers, S. C. Vol. 6, pp. 1–59. London: Butterworth.

Tanaka, Y. and Oota, K. (1970) A stereomicroscopic study of the mastopathic human breast. I. Three-dimensional structures of abnormal duct evolution and their histologic entity. *Virchows Archiv A: Pathology*, **349**, 195–214.

Taylor, H. B. and Norris, H. J. (1967) Epithelial invasion of nerves in benign diseases of the breast. *Cancer*, **20**, 2245–2249.

Tremblay, G., Buell, R. H. and Seemayer, T. A. (1977) Elastosis in benign sclerosing ductal proliferation of the female breast. *American Journal of Surgical Pathology*, **1**, 155–159.

Chapter Ten

Underdiagnosis of Malignancy

The carcinomas that are most likely to be underdiagnosed are those which of recent years have come to be called '*minimal breast cancer*' (Gallager and Martin, 1971). This includes all forms of non-invasive cancer and cancers which are infiltrating but smaller than 5 mm in diameter, an arbitrary but convenient cut-off point (Hutter, 1971). In addition, *certain cancers are prone to be underdiagnosed because of their morphology.* Thus papillary carcinoma belongs in this group because it can be confused with benign papilloma, and tubular carcinoma because it can be mistaken for sclerosing adenosis by those who are unfamiliar with it.

In general, infiltrating carcinomas of the NOS variety (Fisher, Gregorio and Fisher, 1975) which are larger than 5 mm in diameter will not be misdiagnosed by competent and reasonably experienced pathologists. Small infiltrating carcinomas can, however, be missed when the pathologist is examining the gross specimen and he may fail to sample them. This is much less likely to happen if there is good liaison between surgeon, radiologist and pathologist, if the resected specimen is properly examined and blocks are selected from the correct parts and if, in certain cases at least, specimen x-rays are utilized to localize abnormalities. Case 4 of Hutter and Kim (1971) is a reminder that as many as six additional infiltrating carcinomas can be found in a specimen which is reported as having no residual tumour after 'routine' examination. As these authors stated, what constitutes an adequate routine examination is a subject in itself: a lot depends on the training, competence and conscientiousness of the individual pathologist.

In this chapter ductal carcinoma in situ will be considered first, followed by cancerization of lobules — a close relative of ductal carcinoma. The concept of pagetoid spread will be considered next and then lobular carcinoma in situ will be discussed. This is often called LISC or LCIS for short in the literature, but the term CLIS, coined by Hamperl (1972) and short for carcinoma lobulare in situ, will be used here as a more euphonious term. Finally the recognition of tubular carcinoma will be dealt with.

DUCTAL CARCINOMA IN SITU

Ductal carcinomas, and their differentiation from benign hyperplasias, have already been

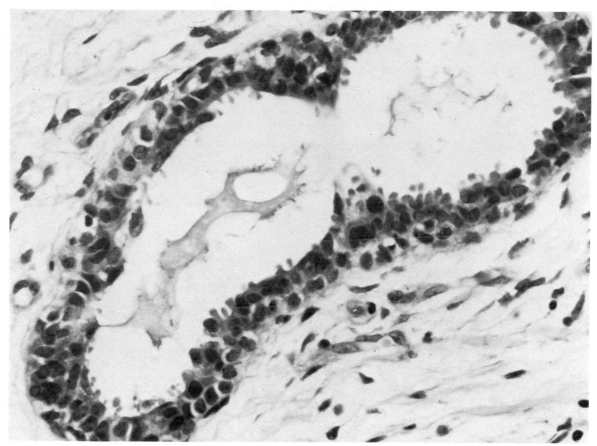

Figure 10–1 'Clinging carcinoma'. Loss of polarity and anaplasia of the lining epithelial cells is present but the bulk of the neoplastic tissue is much less than usually seen in comedo cancer and there is no obvious luminal necrotic debris. H and E. ×600.

considered. The basic patterns are the *comedo,* the *solid,* the *cribriform* and the *papillary* varieties, occurring either singly or in various combinations. Cancers with comedo patterns are perhaps the least likely to be underdiagnosed. The solid and cribriform patterns give rise to greater diagnostic problems but their recognition has already been discussed in detail in Chapter Seven, while papillary carcinoma has been dealt with in Chapter Eight.

An excellent paper on the recognition of difficult in situ cancers is that of McDivitt, Holleb and Foote (1968). The present writer's diagnostic criteria match very closely those outlined by these workers. Their Figures 1 to 4 illustrate definite in situ cancers and yet these authors feel obliged to state 'we have the impression . . . that many pathologists still are reluctant to interpret such lesions as malignant'. The writer is in complete agreement and has had the same experience. Their

Figures 5 and 6 illustrate a less common pattern of cancer, also identifiable on objective criteria. Their Figures 7 and 8 represent a still less common variant, which is easily underdiagnosed and will be referred to again later. All these subtypes are malignant tumours capable of infiltrating and metastasizing. This paper by McDivitt, Holleb and Foote (1968) deserves very careful study.

'CLINGING CARCINOMA'

There is a fifth type of in situ ductal cancer which has not received specific mention in the literature. This is a type which we, at our institute, have for some years termed 'clinging carcinoma'. This is merely a descriptive term to indicate that the neoplastic cells are limited to the periphery of the containing structures,

cancer, as already mentioned. Yet, if this focus had lacked the neoplastic buds projecting into the lumen, and had little or no necrotic detritus, it would still constitute an in situ cancer of the type referred to here as 'clinging'. At low magnification the malignant focus can in these circumstances be easily missed altogether, but, provided that the abnormal focus is detected, the pleomorphism and anaplasia of the lining cells should be clearly discernible as testimony to its malignancy.

There is another, more common, form of clinging carcinoma in which the lesion shows no evidence of having originated as a comedo cancer and this is indeed the most difficult type to recognize (Figures 10–3 to 10–6). The involved structures are lined by a single or a few layers of neoplastic epithelial cells (excluding the non-neoplastic myoepithelial cell layer), showing orientation towards the lumen, whilst there is no obvious necrosis. The malignant cells appear to have originated in situ or perhaps to have spread as a single well-orientated layer of cells by a process of 'creeping replacement'. While the former genesis seems the more likely, it is possible that the latter also plays a part. 'Creeping replacement', as a mode of spread, is accepted in lobular cancerization of solid, comedo and other types. Hence it may also be involved in this orderly form of clinging carcinoma, though it is a little less easy to visualize than in the case of the patternless solid and comedo forms.

RECOGNITION

Importance of Recognition. The recognition of clinging carcinoma is of dual importance. Firstly it is important for diagnostic reasons. Secondly it has a bearing on the genesis of 'early' carcinoma in situ and on the vexed question of its relationship to benign hyperplasia of the epitheliosis type (see Chapter Six).

Difficulty of Recognition. In the case of clinging carcinoma the distinction is mainly not from epitheliosis, as it is in the solid and cribriform varieties of in situ carcinoma. *The diagnostic problems are two-fold.* At low magnification, the lesion can be missed entirely since *the alteration is cytological rather than anatomical.* To try and avoid this pitfall, a high degree of awareness is necessary as well as the more frequent use of a high-power objective whenever the observer's suspicion is aroused. Once the lesion is localized, the cytology is in some cases clearly indicative of malignancy, but *in many cases, even when the lesion is identified, its malignant nature is often difficult to recognize.* It may be recalled that two decades ago there was a great deal of disagreement among pathologists as to the characteristics of in situ carcinoma of the uterine cervix but this problem has since been very largely resolved. Similarly, a careful study of the cytology of the breast lesions in question, and comparison with known cases of adenosis and other benign lesions, will reveal distinct though frequently subtle differences. Attention must be paid to nuclear enlargement, the N/C ratio, chromatin structure, nucleolar prominence, mitotic activity and the presence of abnormal mitoses: these features will be considered in greater detail. A search at deeper levels, without trimming of the tissue block, is frequently necessary to provide the clinching evidence. A few necrotic epithelial cells in the lumen, a tripolar mitosis, a few giant nuclei or pagetoid spread may provide the clinching evidence of malignancy in an otherwise highly suspect focus.

Clinging carcinoma is particularly easy to miss within the lobule. Several lobules are usually involved, with or without duct involvement in any given plane. This therefore comes into the general category of cancerization of the lobules. When cancerization is of the solid, comedo or cribriform varieties, it is both easier to detect the alteration and to recognize it as malignant. But in the 'clinging' variety there is no solidification, no characteristic growth

---

Figure 10–5 (*Opposite, above.*) Between one and three layers of abnormal epithelial cells line this part of a terminal lobular unit. Truncated cell margins, rounded nuclei and pallid cytoplasm are noteworthy features. Haematoxyphilic mucin in the lumen first drew attention to this focus. This field is not convincing of malignancy taken in isolation but is regarded as probably malignant in the context of carcinoma in situ in neighbouring fields. H and E. ×600.

Figure 10–6 (*Opposite, below.*) One of the most difficult varieties of clinging carcinoma to identify. Hyperplasia affects the epithelial layer at the expense of the myoepithelial. The epithelial layers are increased in number and they have densely staining nuclei. Diagnosis is based largely on cytological criteria. H and E. ×375.

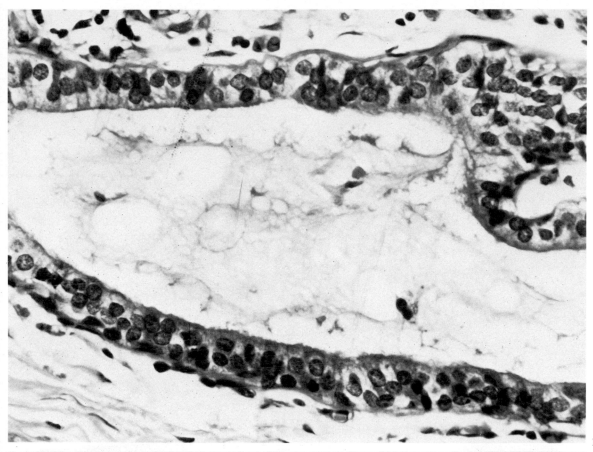

10–5

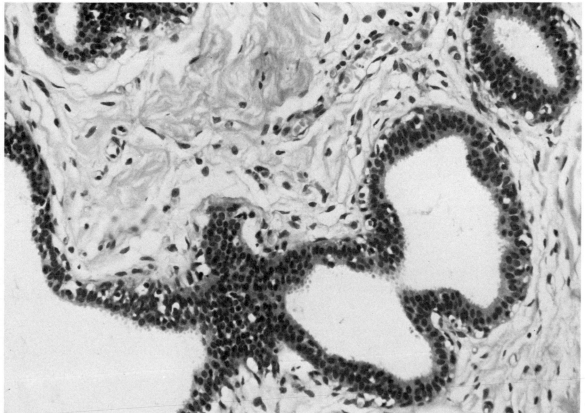

10–6

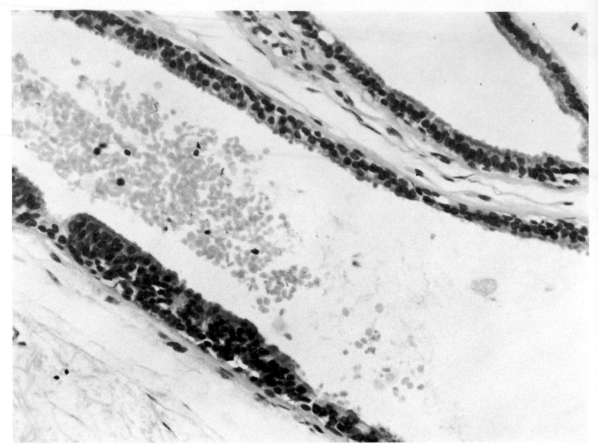

Figure 10–7   Mural or clinging carcinoma in a small duct. On one side of the duct there is an abrupt change to a neoplastic stratified epithelium at two points. On the other side there is an imperceptible gradation. Both types of change are seen with 'early' carcinoma. H and E. ×400.

pattern, no necrosis and frequently there is no marked alteration in the size of the lobular epithelial units (Figure 10–3). In order to become fully acquainted with the typical diagnostic features, it is essential to study a few cases of ductal carcinoma with obvious cancerization of lobules. Many of the lobules which at low magnification appear to be normal or, at any rate, hyperplastic but benign will show definite cytological evidence of malignancy at higher magnifications (Figure 10–3).

SITE OF LESIONS

The 'earliest' change usually affects apparently normal lobules and/or small ducts (e.g. ductules). The changes are, therefore, not to be sought mostly in solid areas of epitheliosis or even in areas of florid adenosis in its many forms.

The individual lobular epithelial units are usually larger than normal but the degree of enlargement is very variable and frequently quite minor. Indeed sometimes there is no enlargement of the lobular units whatever and the changes are entirely cytological without any microanatomical alteration.

CYTOLOGICAL CHANGES

The main changes, and those on which the diagnosis is based, *affect epithelial cells as opposed to myoepithelial cells.* The change in the epithelial cells from normal to neoplastic may be very gradual with a barely perceptible transition over a strip of about 20 or 30 cells between normal and neoplastic tissue (Figure 10–7). In other areas there is sometimes a more abrupt change in morphology at one, two or rarely even more points in the epithelial lining, giving the impression of a 'step' mutational change (Figure 10–7).

Changes in Cytoplasmic Staining. The epithelial cells are increased in volume, due in part usually to an increase in the volume of the cytoplasm. There is in most cases a change in the staining properties of the cytoplasm. This takes the form either of *amphophilia* or of *pallor.* The slightest degree of retention of the haematoxylin during the decolorization process is responsible for the amphophilia (Figures 10–2 and 10–3). This amphophilia may affect the cytoplasm diffusely but there is often focal accentuation towards the luminal margin, accounting for a dense appearance in this region. The cytoplasm frequently appears slightly cloudy or reticulated or even very finely vacuolated (Figures 10–2, 10–3 and 10–5). This is in contrast to the bland cytoplasmic staining in adenosis and other benign hyperplasias. A more distinct granularity of the cytoplasm is less frequent but even more suspect when present. The *reticulated character of the cytoplasm* is a feature to which considerable importance is attached.

In other cases, instead of slight amphophilia and increased staining density, the cytoplasm stains palely and sometimes the pallor alone will draw one's attention to such an atypical focus (Figure 10–5). This cytoplasmic pallor is an important characteristic which deserves emphasis since it appears to have received little attention in the literature. It is of course a well-known feature of some forms of CLIS, but very pallid, almost clear cytoplasm can also be seen with certain forms of in situ carcinoma of ductal type. The round or ovoid hyperchromatic nuclei stand out in stark relief against a nearly colourless cytoplasmic background. When only a single layer of such cells is present, their identity as neoplastic cells is almost impossible to establish without other corroborative evidence. But frequently a search, at the same or deeper levels, will reveal two or multiple layers of epithelial cells of this type and the significance of this finding will be considered later. The important point to make here is that cytoplasmic pallor is a danger signal which should alert one to make a closer study of a particular focus. The writer has found this a useful sign in unearthing the cribriform type of carcinoma in particular.

The Luminal Margins tend towards truncation; this is always a highly suspect manifestation and one which must be accorded due weight (Figures 10–2, 10–3 and 10–5). Marked convexity and blebbing of the luminal margin is characteristic of benignity and is typically seen in adenosis. But the equating of blebbing with benignity has possibly been overemphasized. Blebbing can be found in some very 'early' neoplastic lesions and even in more obvious in situ cancers of well-differentiated type (Figures 10–6 and 10–8). This luminal blebbing has been regarded as a partial apocrine change (Page et al, 1978) and the blebs are frequently referred to as 'apocrine snouts'. It is premature to decide whether this interpretation is correct, but, whether it is or not, its presence does not automatically exclude malignancy.

The Nuclei are both absolutely and relatively large (Figures 10–3 and 10–4) but this is very difficult or even impossible to appreciate at low magnifications. It is also difficult to appreciate when there is no residual normal tissue for comparison in the same lobule or at least in adjacent lobules (Figure 10–3). The nuclei are often ovoid (Figures 10-4, 10–7 and 10–10), rounded forms being more characteristic of the cribriform and solid cancers and, of course, more typical of malignancy. *The nuclei are either hyperchromatic* (Figures 10–4, 10–6, 10–7 and 10–10) *or they have prominent nucleoli* (Figure 10–2). They characteristically possess a *prominent* filamentous, granular or punctate *chromatin* net. These nuclear characteristics of size, staining quality, nucleolar prominence and chromatin structure are more or less essential to the diagnosis of malignancy when one is assessing a single layer of epithelial cells which are correctly orientated.

The *position* of the nucleus is variable. Nuclei may be present at different levels in adjacent cells, as with benign hyperplastic tissue, but sometimes they assume a basal polarity (Figure 10–8); why this should be the case is unknown. At the other end of the scale, the enlarged nuclei bulge at the luminal edge, producing an Arias–Stella-like appearance (Figure 10–10); this is uncommon. When this nuclear bulging becomes exaggerated there is a hobnail appearance, but this is distinctly rare.

Mitoses in small numbers are of course common enough in epitheliosis, but in the degree of hyperplasia known as adenosis they are usually sparse and a significant number should make one pause and consider the

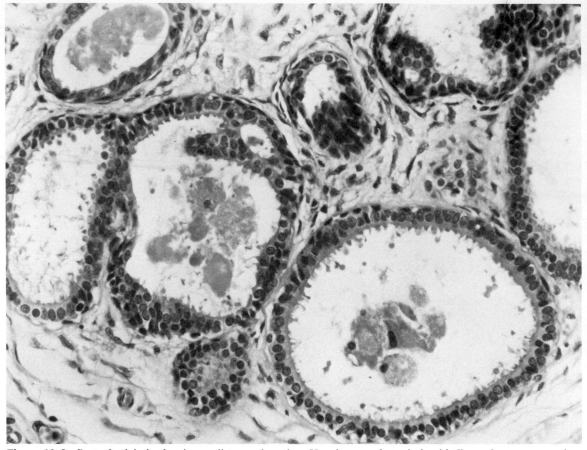

Figure 10–8 Part of a lobule showing malignant alteration. Heaping up of atypical epithelium of one type, nuclear hyperchromasia and the luminal detritus are all suspicious. Trabecular bars and incipient cartwheels confirm a diagnosis which should already have been suspected. H and E. ×400.

alternative diagnosis. Even a very few atypical mitoses can assume great importance in reaching a correct diagnosis.

The Epithelial Bud or Embryo Roman Bridge

There may, in addition, be epithelial bud formation (Figures 10–8 and 10–9) towards the lumen, or cartwheels, but such changes are indicative of a merger with other, better-recognized patterns and the diagnosis becomes correspondingly easier. When using the epithelial bud or bulge as a criterion of cancer, it must be sharply differentiated from the 'stalactite tufts' of epitheliosis. An

extension of the stalactite tuft is spindle-cell bridging. On the other hand, the epithelial bud, when elevated, becomes the Roman bridge and this is diagnostic of cancer.

Heaping up of the Epithelial Layer

The presence of more than one epithelial cell layer lining the lobular–ductal system of the breast is significant (Figures 10–5, 10–6, 10–7 and 10–10). Obviously this does not apply to epitheliosis which has specific identifying features. It refers to a lining, two or more cells in thickness, with distinctly epithelial features and excluding mere

Figure 10–9 (*Opposite, above.*) Clinging carcinoma in a lobule. A few tell-tale trabecular bars are present. The dense eosinophilic material in one lumen drew attention to the focus. H and E. ×375.

Figure 10–10 (*Opposite, below.*) Clinging carcinoma in a duct. Multiple epithelial layers with atypia show transition to less atypical epithelium. Most of the nuclei are ovoid but hyperchromatic. In one area the nuclei bulge at the luminal margin. Comedo necrosis is gross and obvious in this case. H and E. ×375.

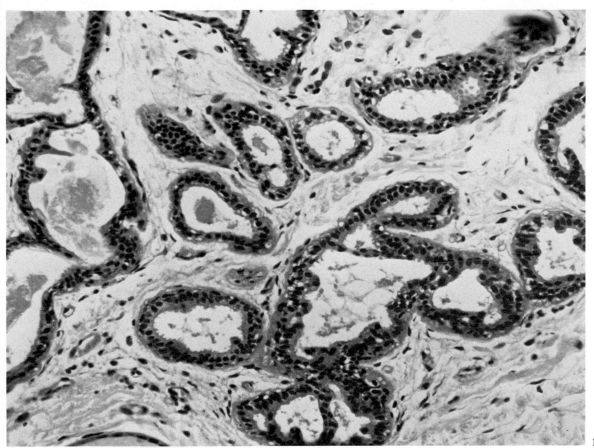

10–9

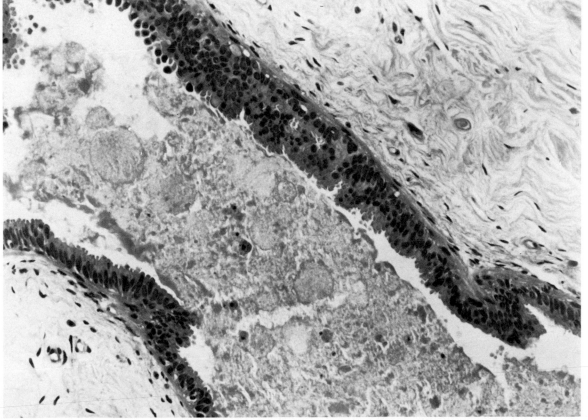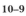

10–10

tangential artefacts. Such an epithelial hyperplasia is always worthy of critical examination. With four such layers, the alteration is usually detectable at low magnification, but with only two or three it is very difficult to appreciate and can be missed almost as easily as a single layer of altered cells. Once the abnormal focus is detected, a clinging carcinoma with two or more layers of abnormal epithelium is generally more easily recognized as malignant than one with only a single layer, but the problems are still very formidable.

Loss of Polarity. There is often some degree of loss of the normal orientation, so adjacent nuclei, when ovoid, tend to point in slightly different directions (Figures 10–1 and 10–4). Loss of polarity becomes a criterion to be added to the cytological alterations previously considered.

Luminal Contents

The contents of the lumina can reveal valuable information concerning the nature of the surrounding epithelium. Any deviations from the normal, usually eosinophilic, uniformly staining, rather glassy, homogeneous, usually thin-looking secretion of the lobular–ductal system must be examined. Comedo necrosis (Figure 10–10) is only the extreme manifestation of a luminal alteration which is much more commonly seen in a very minor, but important, form (Figures 10–8 and 10–9). Inspissated densely staining material, variations in staining intensity and texture of the material in a given lumen (Figures 10–8 and 10–9), granular and fragmented products sometimes with stippled or other types of calcification, and the presence of even small amounts of nuclear debris (Figure 10–8), parts of cell cytoplasm or a remote hint of the ghosts of dead cell outlines in the eosinophilic content all need careful evaluation (Figure 10–2). It is arguable whether a proportion of this material is a secretory product or whether it mostly represents the residue of cell necrosis, but of its diagnostic value there can be no doubt.

THE RELATIONSHIP BETWEEN EPITHELIAL AND MYOEPITHELIAL CHANGES

There is an additional point which helps to distinguish most 'clinging' lobular malignancy

from adenosis: in the malignant condition *the atypical changes affect only the luminal or inner cell layer*, i.e. only one cell type is affected by the changes described. The outer cell layer may be invisible in parts, it may be scarcely identifiable or it may be easily discernible, but, if the latter, it is usually not hypertrophic. By contrast, in adenosis, both cell types usually undergo simultaneous changes, so that there is an organoid hypertrophy of all elements. In many cases of adenosis the hypertrophy of the outer cell type is less marked than that of the inner, but the outer cell type is nevertheless easily recognizable. In the uncommon situation in which the outer cell type is inconspicuous, e.g. in some microcystic adenosis with luminal distension, even the epithelial layer tends to be low with obviously benign characteristics so there is little or no diagnostic problem. *It is in the presence of a tall columnar epithelium that the changes in the myoepithelial layer are of greatest significance.* In adenosis, the outer cell layer is easily identified and frequently hypertrophic. In clinging carcinoma, by contrast, it is often barely discernible and usually not hypertrophic, with some exceptions to be mentioned below. To appreciate these differences between benign and malignant disease, one must compare lobular cancerization with several good examples of adenosis.

One should not, however, assume from the foregoing that the outer cell layer is never prominent in clinging carcinoma. Certainly *with in situ cancer, the outer cell layer* may not only be visible (Figure 10–2) but it *can actually be hypertrophic in a minority of cases* (Figure 7–33). Whether this change is induced by the neoplastic epithelial cells themselves, or is attributable more directly to the cancerigenic agent, or is sometimes induced by surrounding infiltrating carcinoma (for it is in these circumstances that the writer has observed it most often), or whether it is caused by all of these factors or by some other is not known. What matters in the present context is that the outer cell layer is *usually* inconspicuous in in situ carcinoma, and that this contrasts with the usual appearances in adenosis, in which the outer cell layer is easily detectable and frequently conspicuous.

CONCLUSION

It must be appreciated that the diagnosis of clinging carcinoma is often a difficult one. No single criterion can be relied upon. All cytological parameters must be carefully assessed as must the number of epithelial cell layers, the relationship of epithelial to myoepithelial cell change and the character of any luminal content. In the final analysis it is the cytological changes in the epithelial layer which are the crucial factor in making a decision. For this reason it is essential that biopsy tissue be studied at a higher scanning magnification than is frequently used, a point which will be enlarged upon after cancerization is dealt with in the ensuing section.

CANCERIZATION OF LOBULES

'Cancerization of lobules' is a term meant to indicate that the lobular units are occupied by cancer cells which are morphologically indistinguishable from cancer cells as seen in ducts (Fechner, 1971). The morphological appearances are generally distinct from those seen in CLIS. Malignant cells are thought to arise in the small ducts and ductules and spread secondarily into the lobules. It is presumably for this reason that the term 'cancerization' was coined, as it *indicates both a histological appearance and a mode of spread of the cancer.* The acceptance of this view coincided with the acceptance, until very recently, of a ductal origin for the vast majority of breast cancers, hence the term 'infiltrating ductal carcinoma'. It is only lobular carcinoma as a histologically defined entity, i.e. CLIS, that has long been regarded as a tumour which arises in the lobule. While Fechner's (1971) concept of the site of origin of the carcinoma needs slight modification in view of recent work, the coining of the term 'cancerization' of lobules constituted an important step forward, both in stressing the frequency of lobular involvement by carcinoma and in distinguishing it from CLIS.

Four problems relating to cancerization need discussion: its frequency and its recognition, its histogenesis and, lastly, its relationship to CLIS.

Frequency

The frequency of lobular cancerization is easier to estimate in cases of pure in situ carcinoma and carcinoma with only minimal invasion. With the usual invasive carcinoma,

the precise localization of the in situ lesion may be largely obscured. Because of the size of the structures concerned and special factors like the elastic content of the duct wall, it can be reasonably assumed that residual evidence of in situ carcinoma in the ducts would be easier to detect than residual evidence of lobular involvement. Studies of predominantly or exclusively in situ lesions demonstrate without question that cancerization of lobules is a frequent and often extensive lesion, whereas a review of the literature shows that it has often been mistaken for ductal carcinoma with a few noteworthy exceptions. Bonser, Dossett and Jull (1961) found an incidence of about 20 per cent of carcinomas restricted to structures of lobular derivation. These figures apply only to those infiltrating cancers in which it was considered possible to determine the sites of origin. It is worth reflecting on why certain workers recognized the frequency of lobular cancerization while others did not. Dawson (1933, 1948) and Parks (1959) appreciated the frequent occurrence of carcinoma within the lobules. Cheatle and Cutler (1931) found that small duct cancer was very frequently accompanied by cancer within the lobule, and Bonser, Dossett and Jull (1961) also stressed the frequency of lobular cancerization. These workers shared the emphasis they placed on thorough study of the normal structure and on the usefulness of elastic tissue stains in the study of breast disease.

Cancerization of lobules is commonly mistaken for carcinoma in ducts. One of the major reasons for such misinterpretation is the expansion of the containing structure by tumour. Foote and Stewart (1946) recognized that small ducts are frequently expanded by contained carcinoma so as to mimic larger ducts. Similarly, cancerized units of a lobule often become grossly distended, up to five or even ten times the normal diameter, and thus come to resemble cancerized ducts. However, when examined with a scanning lens, the grouping of the distended units into focal aggregates will be appreciated because cancerized lobules still retain the architectural grouping and the relationship to ducts that is seen in the normal breast. When it is realized that cysts may also be the seat of cancerization and that many cysts have lost most traces of their original lobular configuration, the potential for confusion between cancerized cysts and carcinoma in ducts will be appreciated.

The foregoing is not intended to detract

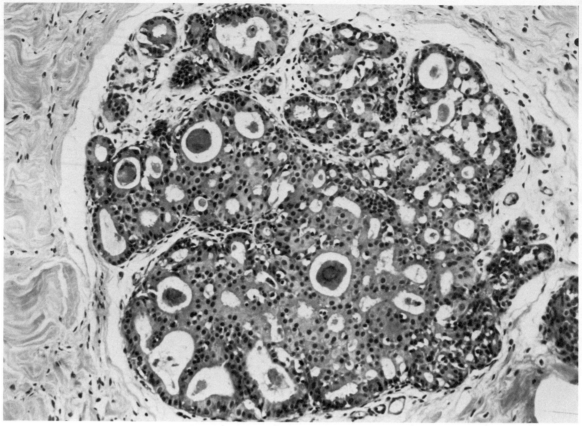

Figure 10–11 Lobular cancerization: so-called ductal carcinoma in situ. The outline is that of a lobule with a little residual specialized connective tissue. The slight separation from the interlobular connective tissue marks the boundary of the altered lobule. Mainly cribriform pattern with sharp luminal margins. Inspissated secretion and some calcification in lumina. H and E. ×180.

altogether from the role played by the medium- and even larger-sized ducts in the initiation of infiltrating cancer of the breast. Duct carcinoma of the galactophores, which open onto the nipple surface, in patients with Paget's disease is an obvious example of carcinoma of large ducts. Comedo cancer of the large ducts has such a striking macroscopic appearance on slicing that it gained this distinctive name, which now has a histological connotation in addition to the original one indicating that worms of necrotic tumour could be expressed from ducts distended by carcinoma. But this tells us nothing about the sites of origin of the common breast cancers.

Wellings and Jensen (1973) tried to answer this question by a three-dimensional study of 60 breasts using a method which attempted to define the sites of the smallest malignant lesions. Nine breasts with in situ carcinoma were discovered, one of these with as many as 91 distinct malignant foci. Each of the in situ malignant lesions studied was in the TDLU (terminal duct–lobular unit) complex, this complex being affected in continuity. *This perceptive work emphasized smallest duct and lobular involvement in the incipient stages of carcinogenesis* (Figures 10–11 to 10–15). These workers also drew the conclusion that lobular cancerization was frequently misinterpreted

Figure 10–12 (*Opposite, above.*) Lobular cancerization. Clinging and incipient cribriform patterns. Specialized lobular connective tissue is very conspicuous here. This is 'ductal type' carcinoma but situated in the lobule not in the extralobular ducts. H and E. ×150.

Figure 10–13 (*Opposite, below.*) Cancerized lobule, frequently mistaken for carcinoma situated in the ducts until the work of Wellings, Jensen and Marcum (1975). Clinging, bridging and cribriform carcinoma. Same case as shown in Figure 7–19. H and E. ×60.

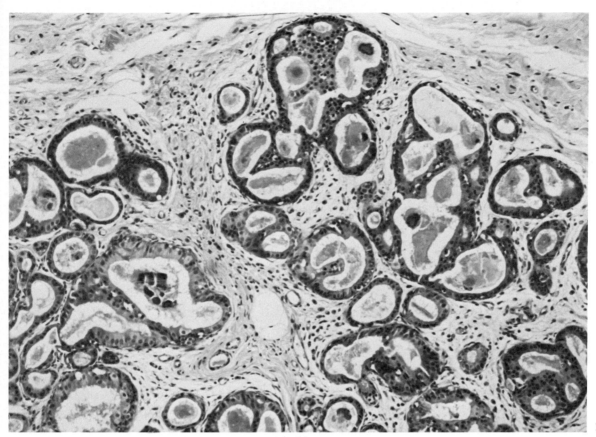

10-12

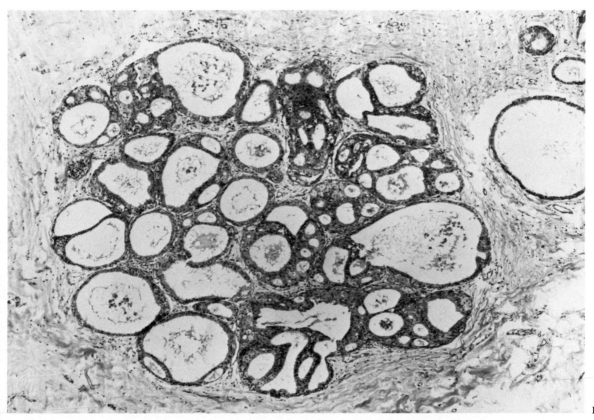

10-13

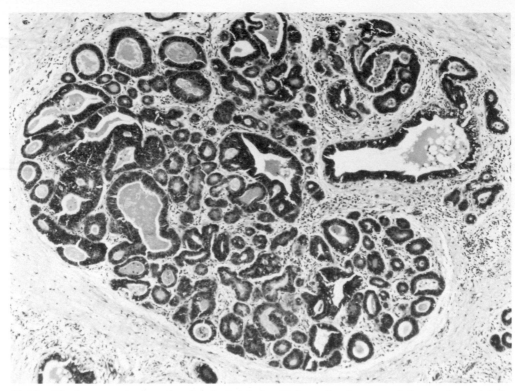

Figure 10–14 Clinging cancerization of entire single lobule with lesser involvement of elongated extralobular duct at right, probably the ductule leading to this lobule. H and E. ×90.

as ductal because of the gross distension of the lobular units (Figure 6–1). Wellings and Jensen (1973) showed diagrammatically how smaller units, when distended, can 'unfold' into fewer larger ones, thus mimicking ducts even more closely (Figure 6–1). Their three-dimensional findings complement two-dimensional findings using elastic tissue stains. Hence all past work needs to be re-examined in the light of these important observations. Wellings, Jensen and Marcum (1975) elaborated on their previous findings and showed beyond question that *the TDLU complex constitutes the site of origin of most breast cancers.*

Recognition

With the emphasis on diagnosis of breast cancer at earlier stages of the disease, the microscopic identification of cancerization of lobules is vital. Cancerization can be missed as easily as CLIS but, because cancerization has the same significance as ductal carcinoma, failure to recognize it is, in practice, more serious than failure to recognize CLIS. The statement that cancerization of lobules is easily missed is based on a prospective study by the writer of material which had previously been reported on by other pathologists, as well as by retrospective surveys. Cancerization is particularly easily missed when the foci are small or widely scattered. The in situ malignancy is sometimes merely an incidental finding when breast tissue is excised for another reason. In other cases, lobular cancerization is found in the neighbourhood of or remote from foci of invasive carcinoma of ductal type. In cancerization it is rare to see transition from epitheliosis to malignancy; on the contrary, the malignancy generally appears to arise de

Figure 10–15 (*Opposite, above.*) Two adjacent cancerized lobules. In one the pattern is mainly solid with focal cribriform and clinging carcinoma. The other lobule shows only partial involvement by clinging carcinoma. H and E. ×200.

Figure 10–16 (*Opposite, below.*) Dominantly clinging type of lobular cancerization. Two lobules and part of a third are shown. Contrast the dominant dark-cell type with the clear-cell type in one corner. H and E. ×90.

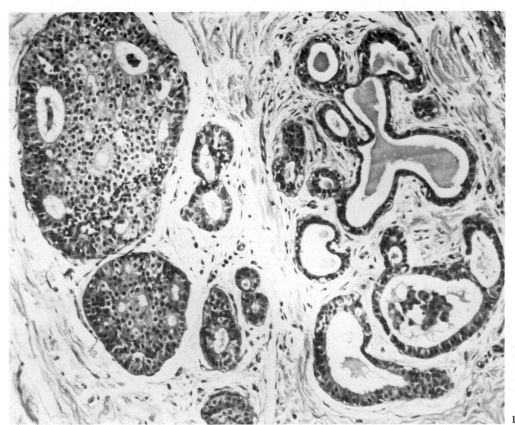

10–15

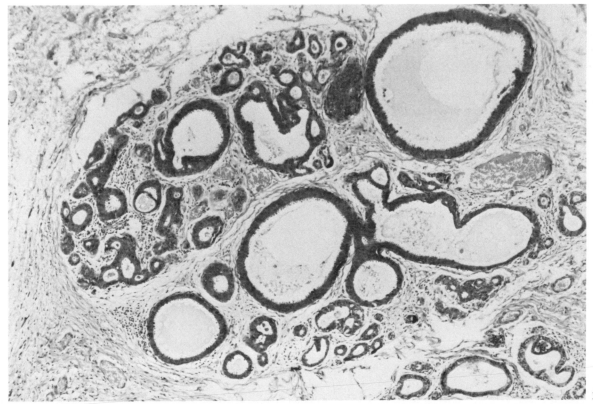

10–16

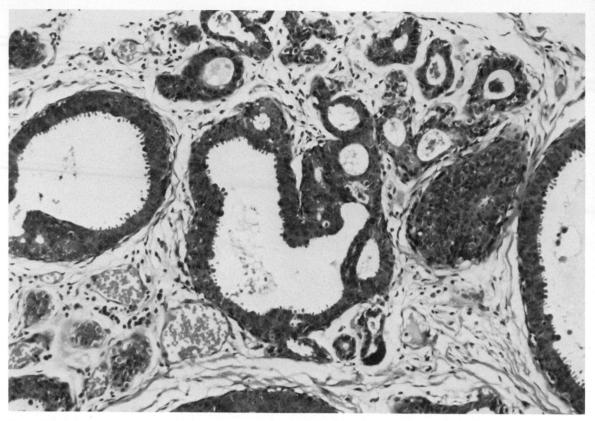

Figure 10–17 Higher magnification of part of field shown in Figure 10–16. Clinging carcinoma with a little bridging. The periphery of the lobule shows less involvement than the centre: this contrasts with CLIS. Note that cytoplasmic blebbing does not exclude cancer. H and E. ×225.

novo (Chapter Six). It involves one or, more usually, a number of adjacent lobules and, in most cases, ductules and sometimes the smaller ducts are also affected.

Recognition requires very careful scanning of all the tissue sampled. Any deviation from the normal and from the various types of adenosis must be examined at a high magnification. Lobules which show alteration of only part of their architecture are suspect (Figures 10–15 and 10–16); apparent loss of two cell layers in the lobule is likewise suspect, as are deviations from the normal staining quality of the epithelium (Figures 10–11, 10–14 and 10–16), already considered in the section on clinging carcinoma. Absence of cytoplasmic luminal blebbing may be significant (Figures 10–11 and 10–15), especially when localized to certain lobules while adjacent lobules display this feature. Blebbing can be inconspicuous or even absent in benign adenosis. When it is absent in adenosis, luminal cell margins generally still have a tendency to be slightly convex rather than very sharply cut. But even this is not invariable and, if all other features point to benignity, truncation is not by itself an indicator of

malignancy. It is true to say that, in a 'borderline' situation, truncation is a pointer to possible malignancy and that, other things being equal, blebbing, especially if marked, favours a benign condition. The criterion of the presence or absence of blebbing in the differential diagnosis of benign and malignant disease has to be interpreted with great caution since there are many exceptions in both directions. In the presence of marked blebbing, a diagnosis of malignancy is permissible only if there are definite cytological traits (Figures 10–16 and 10–17) or structural features of malignancy like trabecular bars.

Nuclear monotony (Figures 10–11 and 10–15) or hyperchromasia (Figures 10–14 and 10–16) are suspect, as is any hint of luminal trabecular bridging (Figures 10–12 and 10–13) or cribriform pattern (Figures 10–11 to 10–13). Changes like an increase in the N/C ratio (Figures 10–14 and 10–17) are likely to be noticed only when attention has already been drawn to certain lobules because of subtle structural alterations, and this is also true of conspicuous nucleoli.

When, in addition, small duct involvement

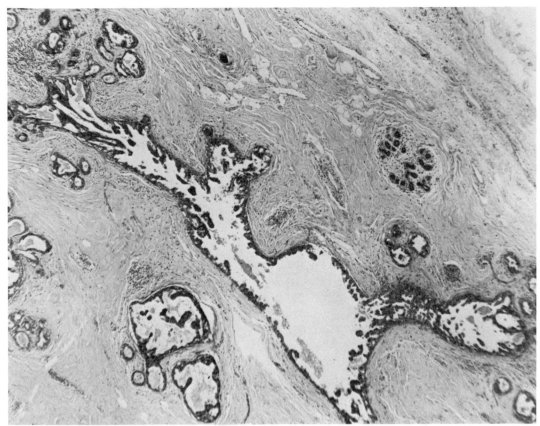

Figure 10–18 Ductal carcinoma with cancerization of lobules. Changes of pre-existing duct ectasia were also present. H and E. ×45.

is also present the diagnosis is correspondingly easier (Figures 10–14 and 10–18). The contrast between neoplastic epithelium and normal epithelium is more easily observed in the ducts than in the lobule, where little or no normal epithelium may have remained.

Haematoxyphilic mucin may sometimes draw attention to lobules requiring closer scrutiny. By itself, haematoxyphilic mucin is of course not an indication of malignancy; it may be present, for example, in some cases of epitheliosis. But its presence in the lumina of lobules which are not displaying epitheliosis, while surrounding lobules contain eosinophilic mucin, is an indication to examine the former more closely.

It is the composite picture that matters, for there is practically no single criterion which is totally reliable. All deviations from the normal lobule must be recognized and their significance understood if lobular cancerization is to be identified correctly.

Histogenesis

'Cancerization of lobules', as defined here, means the spread of tumour from ducts or ductules into lobules. When the term was coined, the possibility of a reverse mode of spread was not even entertained, reflecting the prevailing view that 'duct carcinoma' as a pathological entity arose in ducts and not in lobules. When, therefore, lobules were found affected by the same type of neoplasm, it was usually assumed that the lobules were only secondarily affected and that the primary lesion was extralobular. Nevertheless, Fechner (1971), ahead of his time, considered the possibility that 'cancerization' came about by malignant change simultaneously in both sites as part of a wider field change.

The discovery in the last few years (Wellings, Jensen and Marcum, 1975) that most breast cancers arise in the TDLU complex necessitates a fresh look at this subject. The study of very small in situ cancers shows that they involve the ductules (both extra- and intralobular parts) and the terminal ramifications in the lobule in continuity. It probably remains true that in cancerization the spread of tumour is generally from the ductule to the acini (Figures 10–16 to 10–19), i.e. from the centre of the lobule to the periphery, but the possibility that carcinoma

209

GENERAL COMMENTS ON THE DETECTION AND
IDENTIFICATION OF CLINGING CARCINOMA AND
CANCERIZATION

In the last few years there has been an intense interest in lobular carcinoma in situ (LCIS or CLIS) not only from a diagnostic, prognostic and therapeutic viewpoint but also from an ultrastructural and histochemical angle. This interest has been accentuated by the finding of a positive correlation between lobular carcinoma and the presence of oestrogen receptor sites and the consequent hormone dependency of most of these tumours. Yet it remains a fact that there is justifiable and wide disagreement among different workers about the management of every new patient in whom CLIS is diagnosed. Some workers insist that CLIS should not be called a carcinoma, with all that this usually implies (Haagensen, Lane and Lattes, 1972). In view of this, the underdiagnosis of CLIS is not quite as serious as the underdiagnosis of ductal carcinoma. In the writer's view there should be far greater concern at the underdiagnosis of lobular cancerization in its variant forms and in the virtual neglect of clinging carcinoma. These are forms of cancer which are relatively common, very frequently missed and of great importance to the patient.

In the recognition of clinging carcinoma there are some general points that should be made which apply also, to some extent, to other forms of in situ carcinoma. There is a tendency to scan breast tissue under the microscope at too low a magnification. Of course a very low power scanning of the tissue is essential in order to get a bird's eye view and to identify single or multiple foci of gross pathology, be they cysts, infiltrating carcinoma or any other type of pathology. But it is not possible to exclude in situ carcinoma on this basis. Obviously the more extensive and easily recognizable types of in situ carcinoma will be identifiable at very low magnifications, but this is certainly not true of clinging carcinoma and even of some very 'early' cribriform and other patterns. Most types of lobular cancerization can also be missed quite easily at low magnifications even by the most experienced pathologists. This is especially true when cancerization or clinging carcinoma affects only one or a very few adjacent lobules or other structures. An identical difficulty is experienced if, although multiple lobules or ducts are involved, these structures are scattered rather than being clustered in sizable foci.

The increased identification in the last decade of 'early' and small lesions has led to an increased incidence of multicentricity of carcinoma being reported than hitherto. In addition, among the cases with multicentric cancer, increased numbers of cancerous foci in a single breast have been recognized. Thus Hutter and Kim (1971) identified 38 additional foci of cancer (32 in situ and 6 infiltrating) in a specimen which had been reported as having no residual tumour after 'routine' pathological examination. This remarkable finding can be attributed both to whole organ study in this highly selected case and to the identification of in situ lesions which were not universally recognized as malignant as recently as 10 years ago.

It is essential that breast sections be scanned at a magnification of at least ×40 to 50 and, in certain cases, ×80 or thereabouts. Obviously a generalization of this type has to be qualified and tempered by common sense. Such detailed examination is not necessary for an enucleated fibroadenoma and, perhaps, in a case of duct ectasia with complete lobular atrophy and no signs of anything untoward in the epithelial lining, the pathologist might be exempt from the rigidity of this ruling. The minor structural and important cytological changes of clinging and some other forms of in situ carcinoma will frequently be missed if this rule is not adhered to in the study of most biopsy specimens.

Using this magnification, deviations and aberrations not readily identifiable as benign disease will be spotted. These abnormalities must then be examined at a very high power and assessed along the lines already indicated. Certain forms of in situ cancer can be identified only in this way. Of course, this method is more time consuming than that frequently employed but it does ensure that one does not miss a cancer at a stage when it is eminently curable. As a spin-off, there is the additional advantage of the recognition of ill-understood lesions which can be utilized for prospective research studies.

The importance of recognizing clinging and other types of in situ cancer is self-evident as far as the individual patient is concerned. But this recognition is important in other ways also. It will lead to a better understanding of the sites of origin of breast carcinoma, the frequency and significance of multicentricity, the incidence of the various patterns of involvement and so on. More cases of 'early' carcinoma of the type discussed in Chapter Six will be identified and this will allow study of the precise genesis of these lesions. We will be able to determine how many arise de novo as opposed to an origin in foci of epitheliosis. The over-emphasis in the past on a relationship between cystic disease and cystic hyperplasia, on the one hand, and carcinoma, on the other, led pathologists to look for 'early' cancer in foci of solid and fenestrated epitheliosis and other forms of florid benign hyperplasia. But, with rare exceptions, these lesions are and remain benign. In other words, carcinoma has too often in the past been sought in the wrong sites and on false premises. One needs to scan the tissue at a reasonably high magnification because the 'early' changes of carcinoma cannot otherwise be identified. With tumours of this type, the writer has retrospectively attempted to identify the lesions with the more customary lowest scanning magnifications. Instead of discovering means of recognizing them at these very low magnifications, he has mostly been impressed by the impossibility of the exercise.

ATYPICAL HYPERPLASIA

An interesting study of 'atypical lesions' of the breast is that of Ashikari et al (1974). In a group of 296 patients, nearly 10 per cent developed cancer at four years. They calculated that the risk of breast cancer in patients with these lesions was almost 18 times greater than expected. Their descriptions and illustrations appear to show that their concept of 'borderline' malignancy is close to, but not identical with, my own. In studies of this nature it is very important to be sure that cases of clinging carcinoma and of cancerization are not included among the merely 'atypical lesions'. The writer suspects that some of the lesions of the type illustrated in Figures 8 to 12 of Ashikari et al (1974) would be classified by him as cancerization. The problem of where to draw the dividing line is obviously an extremely difficult one (Gallager, 1972), but no less important because of that.

Wellings, Jensen and Marcum (1975) regarded the hyperplastic changes as a continuous spectrum from grade I to grade V. Were this correct, the finding of a dividing line would be as theoretically undesirable as it would be practically impossible. But, for reasons discussed in Chapter Six, the writer regards this view as erroneous. The distinction between benign and malignant ductal hyperplasia is possible in the vast majority of cases along the lines indicated by McDivitt, Holleb and Foote (1968). It is for this reason that the distinction has been considered in detail in Chapter Seven.

Atypical 'Ductal' Hyperplasia

There is a type of lesion, affecting lobules mainly, the significance of which is unknown. This lesion does not appear to have been described specifically in the literature and, pending further study, is regarded as an 'atypical hyperplasia' of ductal type (ADH). For reasons already discussed, the term 'atypical hyperplasia' is used with reluctance but in the present state of knowledge there is not much option. Since it affects the lobule, it should logically be termed 'atypical lobular hyperplasia', but this would be most confusing since this designation is already used for the type of lobular hyperplasia which is probably related to CLIS (page 233).

This ADH differs from the recognized forms of adenosis, as a study of Figure 10–22 will indicate. It does not, on the other hand, possess the requisite characteristics that would identify it as carcinoma. In ADH there is hyperplasia of epithelial cells without significant change in the myoepithelial cells. The hyperplasia results in a very markedly pseudostratified epithelium with crowding of the nuclei. The nuclei are ovoid to elongated, slightly hyperchromatic, usually without conspicuous nucleoli. The cells maintain good orientation towards the lumen. Mitoses are generally sparse. The luminal cell margins tend to be truncated. In addition there is sometimes an appearance which suggests 'gland-within-gland' formation, with the inherent implication that this might indicate some trabecular bar formation. But this evidence is merely suggestive and there is a lack of convincing evidence of malignancy.

Two questions need investigation. Are atypical hyperplasias of this type more frequent in cancerous compared with non-cancerous breasts? More important perhaps, is this type of hyperplasia a preneoplastic or even, in certain cases, already a neoplastic lesion? These are important questions and we many levels, in a dubious focus in the breast and, if found, it should be regarded as strong evidence in favour of malignancy. The writer has only once seen a benign hyperplasia which had an appearance in parts which could be mistaken for pagetoid spread. This is still under study in an endeavour to establish criteria that will distinguish it objectively from pagetoid spread. A unique instance of this sort in no way detracts from the value of the phenomenon in the diagnosis of malignancy.

LOBULAR CARCINOMA IN SITU ('LOBULAR NEOPLASIA')

Infiltrating lobular carcinoma accounts for between 6 and 10 per cent of all infiltrating breast carcinomas, though it is still classified under the generic title of 'scirrhous' carcinoma in some laboratories. It is agreed that this type of tumour arises on the basis of an in situ phase, but the frequency with which a diagnosis of CLIS is followed by ipsilateral or contralateral infiltrating carcinoma after *local* resection of a lesion is a matter of considerable dispute (Hutter and Foote, 1969; Hamperl, 1971; Wheeler et al, 1974).

It is a pity that a subject of such intrinsic difficulty should be confused by the recent coinage of terms like 'small-cell dysplasia' of solid and cribriform varieties (Toker, 1974). Figures 3 to 8 of Toker (1974) illustrate CLIS, while Figures 10 and 11, said to show 'Type II and Type III dysplasia' of cribriform type, illustrate cribriform duct carcinoma, which is a distinct entity. By lumping these two conditions together, the otherwise important conclusion about the apparently bad prognostic significance of CLIS has been completely vitiated. This confusion serves to underline the need for accurate diagnosis in the first place. Andersen (1977) has made similar criticisms of this work.

Lobular carcinoma in situ has, until recently, always been an *incidental finding* when an operation is performed for some other condition, usually cystic mastopathy. Some cases may possibly be suspected on mammographic examination. The diagnosis of CLIS depends on *a high degree of alertness* when a pathologist is scanning sections. Pathologists must be well acquainted with the condition from a thorough study of some

good examples. *Very good fixation* is even more essential for the diagnosis of CLIS than it is for some other in situ malignancies. It cannot be stressed too strongly that many of the problems of diagnosis and differentiation from other conditions are greatly minimized by excellent fixation, processing and staining. The emphasis placed on this by Wheeler and Enterline (1976) is wholly justified. The author agrees with these authors that the type of fixative used is of less importance than the time that must be allowed for thorough tissue penetration. Too many diagnoses of CLIS are based on inadequately fixed material.

HISTOLOGICAL APPEARANCES

Typical CLIS shows more or less total involvement of one or more lobules (Figure 10–24). If lobular involvement is not total, the uninvolved part is limited to the centre of the lobule (i.e. intralobular part of the ductule). The acini or 'lobular units' ('terminal ductules' of many authors) are completely plugged without any sign of residual lumen (Figures 10–24 to 10–26). The cells are small to medium-sized (about 8 to 10 μm in diameter, occasionally up to 12 μm), usually but not always uniform in size in a given case, rather rounded, with only moderately eosinophilic (Figure 10–26) to pallid cytoplasm (Figures 10–24 and 10–25). The nuclei are relatively large for the cell size, uniform, distinctly rounded, moderately deeply staining with uniform staining especially within the same lobule, central in the cell and uniformly spaced, so as to give an uncrowded appearance (Figures 10–25 and 10–26). Nucleoli are usually distinguishable but small (Figure 10–26). Mitoses are generally very sparse to rare. The cells usually give the impression of being lightly cohesive so that, even though the lumina are completely filled, the cells frequently do not appear tightly packed (Figures 10–24 and 10–26). This is in contradistinction to epitheliosis, which is tightly cohesive, and also, to a certain extent, to cancerization of lobules. The lobular units are distended to varying degrees between different lobules and in different cases. At first their shape is not greatly altered, but, with greater distension, the units become globular and, as they expand, they abut on one another but without becoming confluent. When this degree of involvement is present, the

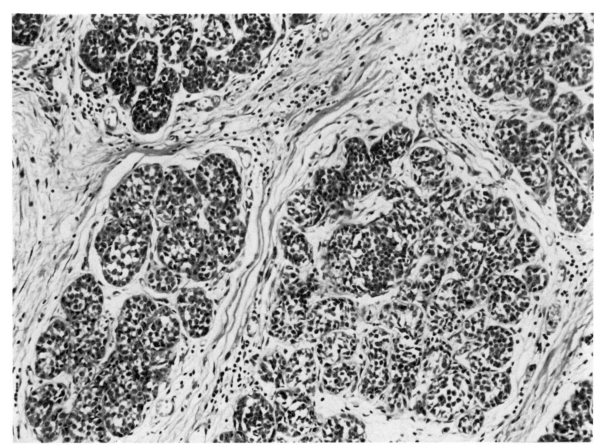

Figure 10–24   CLIS with moderate distension of all acini (terminal ductules) in the lobules. H and E. ×180.

specialized connective tissue of the lobule is barely recognizable.

Pagetoid Spread

An important feature of CLIS is pagetoid spread, which is diagnostic of malignancy in general and a very frequent finding with CLIS in particular (Figure 10–27). The ductule or a duct of larger size contains malignant cells insinuated between a preserved but attenuated luminal epithelium and the basement membrane of the duct; the myoepithelial layer may or may not persist. These neoplastic cells are indistinguishable from those filling the lobule. They are virtually always in continuity with CLIS, often the neoplastic cells appearing to trail away in the duct as the distance from the 'feeding' lobule increases: that is to say, maximum involvement is in the lobule and there is progressively less in intralobular ductule, extralobular ductule, small duct and larger duct (Figure 10–28). This strongly suggests that the

tumour cells have spread between pre-existing normal structures and represent invaders from elsewhere — hence the term 'pagetoid spread'. The writer has seen four cases in which pagetoid spread extended into a lactiferous sinus but he has never seen it reach the nipple surface. In a difficult or 'borderline' case, serial sections to demonstrate the presence of pagetoid spread can be invaluable in confirming a diagnosis of CLIS.

The Importance of Epithelial Alterations in the Extralobular Ducts

These changes were stressed by Fechner (1972a). Changes in the extralobular ducts were present in 34 of 45 breasts with lobular carcinoma. Wheeler and Enterline (1976) also regarded involvement of extralobular ducts as very frequent and cited incidences varying between 75 and 100 per cent. Fechner (1972a) described *mural, solid, cribriform* and *papillary* patterns.

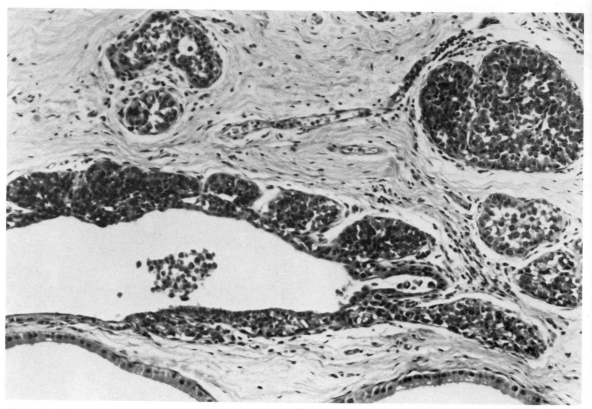

Figure 10–28   CLIS with involvement of an adjacent duct. Note the clover-leaf pattern of ductal involvement. H and E. ×90.

sections and processing of the remainder of the tissue revealed typical CLIS.

The Solid Pattern. Fechner (1972a) found the solid pattern (Figure 10–29) to be present even more frequently than the mural lesion; it probably represents, in some cases, intraluminal extension of mural lesions and, as such, might represent a later or more florid phase of the same lesion. Sometimes the ductal involvement may be solid from the start, without a preliminary pagetoid or mural phase (see Figure 5 of Fechner). This solid pattern of ductal involvement in CLIS should be distinguished from the solid type of ductal carcinoma, not always an easy task. The usually clear cytoplasm and frog-spawn appearance of the nuclei (Figure 10–25) are important indicators, as is the mucin content (Gad and Azzopardi, 1975).

The Cribriform and the Papillary Patterns are regarded by Fechner (1972a) as probable variations of the solid pattern. The cribriform type shows an open lace-like arrangement or lattice pattern. It is not known what occupies the rounded 'punched-out' spaces in vivo. The cribriform pattern in isolation would be difficult to distinguish from that of cribriform duct carcinoma, but Fechner (1972a) was helped in his interpretation by the fact that in no case were the cribriform or papillary lesions present alone. This cribriform type of duct involvement accompanying CLIS may be related to the lesion described by McDivitt, Holleb and Foote (1968) and illustrated in their Figures 7 and 8. The writer has no personal knowledge of the papillary pattern described by Fechner (1972a). These less common patterns clearly deserve further study.

It is ironic in many ways that at about the same time as Fechner (1972a) was stressing the frequency and importance, as well as the variable patterns, of extralobular *ductal* involvement in *lobular* carcinoma in situ, Wellings and Jensen (1973) and Wellings, Jensen and Marcum (1975) were stressing that the terminal duct *lobular* unit complex was the site of origin of the bulk of *duct* cancers.

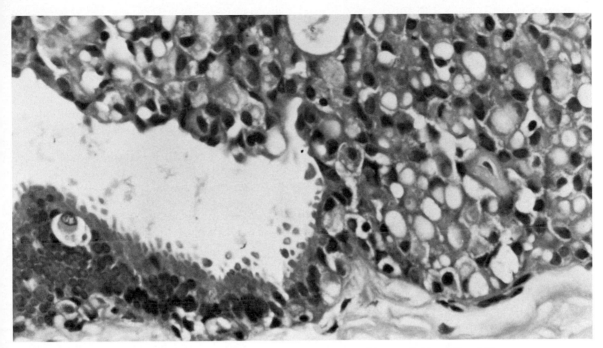

Figure 10–29   Solid focus of CLIS in a duct with a mere hint of pagetoid spread. H and E. ×600.

AGE INCIDENCE

Lobular carcinoma in situ is generally considered to be a neoplasm of premenopausal women. Indeed it has been recorded in a girl of 15 years of age (Bosincu and Eusebi, 1972). An unexpected finding in Fechner's (1972a) study was the number of elderly patients with lobular carcinoma, for an observer of Haagensen's experience (1971) had not seen CLIS in a postmenopausal woman. Fechner (1972a) found infiltrating lobular carcinoma in eight women aged between 70 and 83 years and three of these eight patients had concomitant CLIS. Furthermore, two additional patients had contralateral CLIS. The data from this group of elderly women verifies the observation of Newman (1966) that CLIS and infiltrating lobular carcinoma can be found in the elderly and it demonstrates that the potential for bilaterality of CLIS, well recognized in younger women, extends also into the eighth and ninth decades. The writer has twice seen CLIS accompanying infiltrating lobular carcinoma in patients in the ninth decade.

RELATIONSHIP TO CANCERIZATION

CLIS differs from cancerization of lobules in a number of respects. Cancerization implies a spread into the terminal lobular units from carcinoma of the intralobular ductule, i.e. a spread which is thought to occur in the reverse direction to that which takes place with CLIS. Indeed, in cancerization the cytology and, to a large extent, the architecture are identical with those seen in ductal carcinoma. Cancerization may have comedo, solid, cribriform or clinging patterns. In the latter, lumina are present and the epithelial units are not completely filled, tumour cells tend to be columnar, sometimes with orientation of their ovoid nuclei, and their luminal edges tend to be truncated. In the solid forms of cancerization there is more cellular cohesiveness than in CLIS and a search almost always reveals other patterns as well, with some cribriform areas or areas of necrosis. In typical cases the distinction is easy but it must be admitted that rarely, especially with small foci, indeterminate forms occur in which it is possible to state confidently that in situ carcinoma is present but in which it is not possible to say whether it is CLIS, cancerization, an indeterminate type or even a transitional form which links the two (Figures 10–20 and 10–21).

WHAT LINE OF DIFFERENTIATION DOES CLIS TAKE?

This occasional difficulty in distinguishing between CLIS and cancerization leads to a consideration of what CLIS represents. The commoner duct carcinomas and lobular cancerization show differentiation towards epithelial cells with variably successful attempts at secretion of mucin and at production of absorptive surfaces. The view that 'scirrhous' duct carcinomas are myoepithelial cancers (Murad and Scarpelli, 1967; Murad, 1971b) cannot be sustained. Ahmed (1974) showed that ATPase is localized to the plasma membrane of breast cancer cells, showing definite evidence of epithelial differentiation, and he suggested that ATPase activity may represent a rather non-specific property of carcinoma cells. Further evidence against the view that infiltrating duct carcinoma is a myoepithelial cell cancer is given on page 275.

Hamperl (1972) suggested a myoepithelial origin for CLIS. This is inherently less unlikely than a myoepithelial origin for infiltrating duct carcinoma. In CLIS any residual normal cells seen at the light microscopic level are mostly epithelial, consistent with the view that the tumour *might* arise in the outer cell layer. Ultrastructurally, though, a preserved myoepithelial layer has been demonstrated at the periphery of lobules involved with CLIS (Murad, 1971a; Ozzello, 1971) and this can be seen occasionally at light structural level (Figure 12–9). Even with CLIS and infiltrating lobular carcinoma, a lot more evidence would be necessary before the concept of myoepithelial differentiation could be seriously considered, let alone sustained.

Though lobular carcinoma is distinctive at light microscopic level, ultrastructural studies have failed to distinguish it convincingly from ductal carcinoma (Fechner, 1971 and 1972b; Ozzello, 1971). Carter, Yardley and Shelley (1969) found large numbers of cytoplasmic fibrils in lobular carcinoma; these were similar to those seen in myoepithelial cells, and Carter, Yardley and Shelley (1969) regarded the appearances as distinctive enough to separate lobular from ductal carcinoma. Wellings and Roberts (1963), however, had described the same appearances in infiltrating duct carcinoma. This dispute has not yet been satisfactorily resolved.

Murad (1971a) put the case for CLIS, which he called 'ductular carcinoma', being regarded as an epithelial rather than a myoepithelial cancer. He identified morphological similarities between the carcinoma cells and 'ductular epithelial cells in rats during pregnancy and involution'. In the in

situ stage, Murad (1971a) identified persistent myoepithelial cells by the positive ATPase reaction localized to their plasma membranes, while the neoplastic cells showed a negative reaction.

There is nothing to suggest myoid differentiation in either the in situ or the infiltrative phase of lobular carcinoma. Two examples studied personally at the ultrastructural level showed intracytoplasmic lumina with microvilli and no suggestion of myofilaments. We have demonstrated that CLIS and its infiltrating analogue are *special variants of a mucin-secreting carcinoma* (Gad and Azzopardi, 1975). Tumour cells contain alcianophilic haloes and often a central core of neutral mucosubstance (Figures 10–30 and 10–31). This 'target' or 'bull's-eye' appearance is most clearly demonstrated with an Alcian blue/PAS combination. It must be appreciated that excellent fixation is vital for the proper recognition of these intracellular mucinous vacuoles. We have noted loss of most of the staining of the delicate haloes when part of the tissue removed for frozen section was not fixed for a bare 20 minutes. Alcian blue staining is superior to mucicarmine in this regard.

Intracytoplasmic lumina have indeed come to be recognized as a characteristic though not pathognomonic feature of lobular carcinoma (Battifora, 1975), to the extent that they can be useful in predicting the site of an occult primary carcinoma from the appearances in metastatic disease. Such lumina with 'thick edges' (Battifora, 1975) can be recognized in haemalum–eosin sections (Figures 10–29 and 10–30) and sometimes the lumen contains a central or eccentric eosinophilic dot which corresponds to the neutral mucosaccharide, identifiable histochemically. The cytoplasmic lumina described by Spriggs and Jerrome (1975) in pleural effusions from breast cancer patients appear to represent the same phenomenon.

It is interesting to note how these histochemical, light microscopic, cytological and ultrastructural studies have led to almost identical conclusions from different approaches. Gad and Azzopardi (1975) suggested that the rare signet-ring cell carcinoma of the breast might sometimes represent the extreme end of the spectrum of an infiltrating lobular carcinoma.

CLIS *may* arise from the basal or outer layer or alternatively from the 'indeterminate cells'

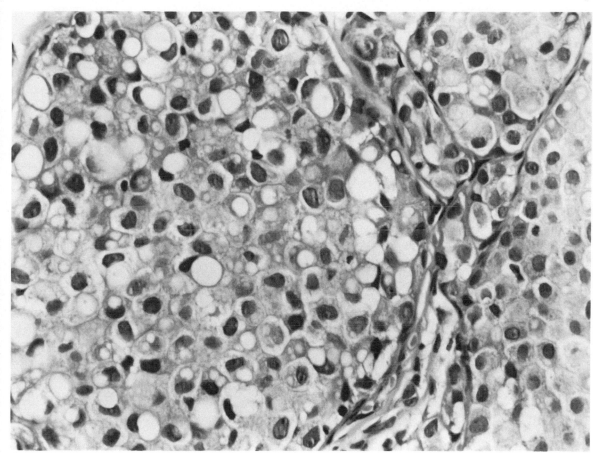

Figure 10–30   Grossly enlarged lobular units affected by CLIS. Intracytoplasmic lumina are numerous and vary from small and barely visible to large lumina indenting the nucleus. H and E. ×600.

of Ozzello (1971) but, in any case, there is no evidence that it shows myoepithelial differentiation. Contrary to a very widespread belief, glandular tumours are mostly classified according to how they differentiate rather than their microscopic site or cells of origin (and the two are not necessarily synonymous) which is frequently unknown and purely speculative. *There is little evidence to date for regarding CLIS as a myoepithelial cell cancer and it is doubtful whether any will be forthcoming.*

Commendable accounts of lobular carcinoma in situ are those of Newman (1966), Warner (1969), Giordano and Klopp (1973), Kahn and Webber (1974), Wheeler et al (1974), Andersen (1974) and Dall'Olmo et al (1975).

FREQUENCY

Retrospective studies, many of them extending back to the years when sampling of

biopsy specimens was minimal by present standards, indicated an incidence of CLIS of between 0.3 and 0.8 per cent of all biopsies. Other studies found an incidence of CLIS in biopsies from patients with otherwise benign breast disease of 1.5 per cent (Lambird and Shelley, 1969; Andersen, 1974). Haagensen et al (1972) stated that the incidence in their laboratory was much less than 1.5 per cent. Wheeler and Enterline (1976) found an incidence of 0.8 per cent of CLIS and a further 0.4 per cent of ALH (ALH implies similar qualitative changes to CLIS but 'not reaching a level sufficient to qualify as LCIS'): thus, their combined incidence of CLIS and ALH is 1.2 per cent. One of the highest figures — 2.6 per cent — is given by Giordano and Klopp (1973). Differences in the incidence of CLIS in biopsy specimens are probably nowadays not attributable for the main part to differences in diagnostic criteria, as these have become reasonably standardized. The number of blocks taken is a crucial factor in

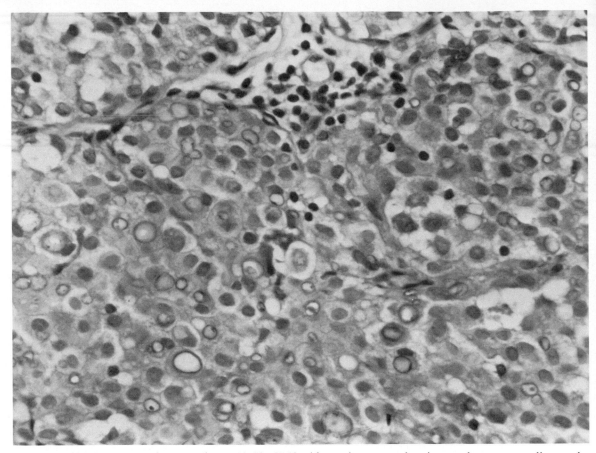

Figure 10–31   From same tissue as Figure 10–30. CLIS with mucinous cytoplasmic vacuoles corresponding to the intracytoplasmic lumina. In addition to the delicate but sharp-edged haloes, an eccentric mucinous globule is sometimes situated in the lumen and encompassed by the halo. Alcian blue and diastase–PAS. ×600.

determining this figure, as demonstrated by Giordano and Klopp (1973). Another factor is the thoroughness with which material is scanned and scrutinized. Haagensen et al (1978) found an incidence of no less than 3.8 per cent, the highest figure on record. This is based on the re-study of 5560 cases of 'benign' breast disease. There are racial differences, lobular carcinoma being less common in Negroes (Ashikari et al, 1973) and it is possible that geographical and other unknown factors also play a part.

It appears from the best evidence that an incidence of CLIS in breast biopsy specimens of anything less than 0.8 per cent is almost certainly too low and that the true figure with even average sampling in most countries in which the problem has been adequately studied lies somewhere between 1 and 1.5 per cent. Allowance must be made for the possibility of some regional variation, as suggested by Giordano and Klopp (1973), and

for the extent of sampling and care with which the material is studied as suggested by the *recent* work of Haagensen et al (1978). There is ample scope for the determination of comparative frequencies in different races and countries.

RECENT STUDIES OF LOBULAR CARCINOMA

An excellent account of lobular carcinoma of the breast is that of Wheeler and Enterline (1976). They gave a historical outline of the problems as they developed. They insisted on the necessity of lobular distension for a diagnosis of CLIS. When lobular changes of similar or identical type are found but the change does not reach 'a level sufficient to qualify' as CLIS, these workers termed the lesion 'atypical lobular hyperplasia', a term employed also by the present writer. This is the 'atypical terminal duct hyperplasia' of

McDivitt, Stewart and Berg (1968). Wheeler and Enterline (1976) made a diagnosis of ALH, rather than of CLIS, when (1) some normal epithelial or myoepithelial cells remain (presumably at light structural level — my qualification), (2) a lumen persists, and (3) there is lack of distension of the terminal ductules (acini). Although future experience may well show that the distinction between CLIS and ALH is unnecessary, they considered it preferable to keep the terms strictly separate, for the present at least.

Wheeler and Enterline (1976) discussed the variations in the qualitative and quantitative criteria employed by different workers to make the diagnosis of CLIS. Hutter, Foote and Farrow (1970) agreed arbitrarily not to accept a mere two or three lobules with changes of CLIS as quantitatively sufficient to make the diagnosis. One can appreciate their reasons for doing this since their treatment of patients with CLIS at that time was less conservative than that of many other surgeons dealing with this disease. Nevertheless, as Wheeler and Enterline (1976) pointed out, it is not easy to justify this policy on theoretical grounds and it is a unique policy in the morphological diagnosis of cancer. Wheeler and Enterline (1976) made a diagnosis of CLIS even in the presence of only one involved lobule, as long as the qualitative criteria were fully satisfied. Apart from the theoretical justification for this, they also pointed out that, at that time, the little evidence available suggested that there was no relationship between the number of involved lobules and the prognosis. This relationship will be discussed again later, in the light of the more recent work of Toker and Goldberg (1977) and Carter and Smith (1977).

There is an abundance of other useful information on CLIS in all its aspects in this work of Wheeler and Enterline (1976). Their critique of other workers' data and conclusions is as valuable as their own.

One of the most elegant studies of lobular carcinoma of the breast is that of Eusebi et al (1977). These workers obtained positive results in the intracytoplasmic lumina (ICL) with ruthenium red staining, a well-known marker for the glycocalyx (Figure 10–32). This indicated a probable continuity between the ICL and the extracellular space, a suggestion in conformity with the ultrastructural studies of Ozzello (1971) in serial sections of the ICL. Eusebi et al (1977) suggested that the alcianophilic haloes described by Gad and Azzopardi (1975) in fact represent the glycocalyx, and the writer agrees with this. The glycocalyx is a recognized specialized cell product and reflects the epithelial nature of these cells. In addition these workers found 'villous polarity' in as many as 20 per cent and 60 per cent of two of three cases examined ultrastructurally; this took the form of a covering of one pole of the cell by numerous long thin microvilli and represents further evidence of cell surface specialization.

Casein and Other Milk Protein Synthesis

Eusebi and co-workers (1977) studied milk protein and especially casein production in lobular carcinoma, using the immunofluorescent and immunoperoxidase methods. They demonstrated abundant casein in all 26 cases examined: five CLIS and 21 infiltrating lobular carcinomas (Figure 10–33). A positive reaction for casein was present in between 40 and 90 per cent of tumour cells. Particularly striking is the cytoplasmic localization and the abundance of the material demonstrated, though they do caution that the method used for detection is a very highly sensitive one. The cytoplasmic localization contrasts with the dominantly intraductal and intercellular localization in infiltrating duct carcinoma found by Pich, Bussolati and Di Carlo (1977).

Eusebi et al (1977) drew attention also to the presence of α-lactalbumin and lactoferritin in lobular carcinomas, indicative of a more general milk protein synthesis by these tumours. They speculated about a relationship between this synthesis and the virtually constant presence of oestrogen receptors in this type of tumour, though the relationship is not likely to be causal.

It would seem, therefore, that lobular carcinoma has not only distinctive histological, histochemical and histogenetic features but also exhibits a more or less constant and intensive synthesis of milk proteins. As the methods for milk protein detection become more refined and their specificity can be relied upon, the differences between the types of carcinoma in relation to this synthesis of milk proteins will probably become sharper and their significance clearer.

Oestrogen Receptors

Observations by Rosen and co-workers (1975) on the presence of oestrogen receptors

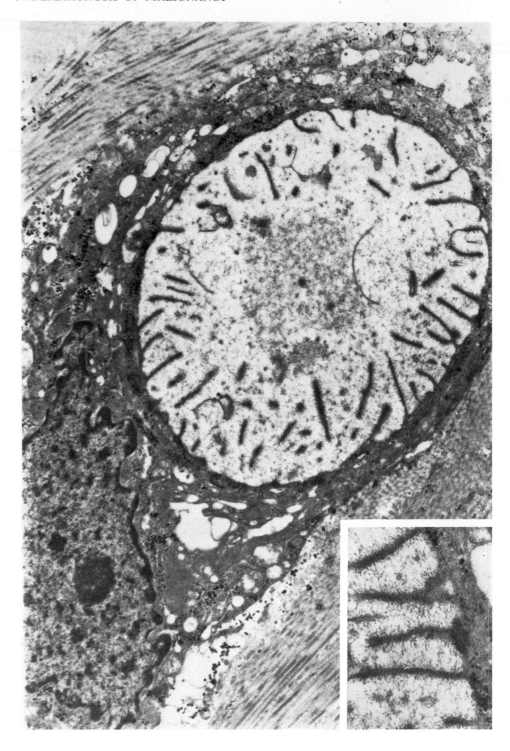

Figure 10–32   Infiltrating lobular carcinoma. 'Intracytoplasmic' vacuole showing numerous thin microvilli. The inset shows electron-dense 'fuzzy' deposits around the villi. Exposed to ruthenium red during postfixation with osmium tetroxide. E.M. ×15000. Inset ×43000. (From Eusebi et al (1977) with kind permission of the authors and the editor of *Histopathology*.)

in different types of breast cancer showed that a large majority of infiltrating lobular carcinomas (12 out of 13) were positive for oestrogen receptors, as opposed to only 55 per cent of infiltrating duct tumours. These findings were confirmed by Pich, Bussolati and Di Carlo (1977). Eusebi et al (1977) analysed 10 cases of lobular carcinoma for oestrogen receptor activity and obtained positive results in all cases. Values obtained ranged between 5 and 104 fmoles/mg cytosol protein with a mean value of 34 fmoles, findings which confirmed and extended the observations of Rosen et al (1975) and of Pich, Bussolati and Di Carlo (1977). Eusebi et al (1977) discussed the significance of the almost constant presence of oestrogen receptors in lobular carcinoma, which contrasts with the great variability of the results obtained with infiltrating duct carcinoma and other tumour types.

The histochemical findings of Murad (1971a and b) are of considerable interest in relation to this almost constant endocrine pattern in respect of its oestrogen receptor content. In 'scirrhous' and in medullary carcinoma, acid phosphatase activity was found restricted to lysosomes: by contrast, in lobular carcinoma, acid phosphatase was found both in the cytoplasm and the nucleus. In the cytoplasm, acid phosphatase activity was found diffusely in the cytoplasmic ground substance as well as in any rare lysosomes present. In the nucleus, acid phosphatase was localized to areas of heterochromatin and, in the nucleolus, it was localized on the nucleonema. This distribution of acid phos-

phatase activity was regarded by Murad (1971a and b) as characteristic of infiltrating lobular carcinoma and he adopted it as a means of specific identification of this tumour type. The presence of nuclear acid phosphatase could be related to the site of phosphorylation of sex hormones. In experimentally produced breast cancer, tritiated oestradiol uptake has been demonstrated in the nuclei of cancer cells (Sander and Attramadal, 1968) and, in human breast carcinoma, tritiated oestradiol uptake has similarly been shown to occur in the tumour tissue (Ellis et al, 1969). Murad (1971b) postulated that lobular carcinoma arises from hormonally sensitive epithelial cells, and that the finding of nuclear acid phosphatase in tumour cells may suggest that the carcinoma cells maintain their hormonal response. Murad admitted that this hypothesis was speculative and that further study was needed. The writer is unaware of other work which corroborates these important histochemical findings of Murad (1971b). Certainly it would be premature to adopt his proposed new classification of breast cancer, especially since one of its essential findings has been disputed as a basis for classification by Ahmed (1974) and by Buell, Tremblay and Rowden (1976).

MULTICENTRICITY AND BILATERALITY AND ITS BEARING ON TREATMENT

All authors are agreed on the frequency of multicentricity and of bilaterality of lobular carcinoma. Benfield, Jacobson and Warner

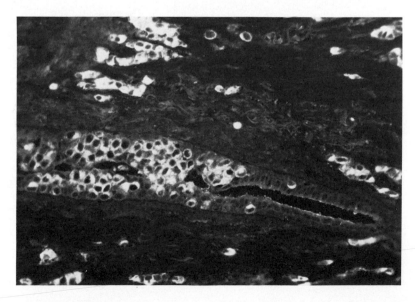

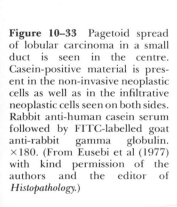

Figure 10–33 Pagetoid spread of lobular carcinoma in a small duct is seen in the centre. Casein-positive material is present in the non-invasive neoplastic cells as well as in the infiltrative neoplastic cells seen on both sides. Rabbit anti-human casein serum followed by FITC-labelled goat anti-rabbit gamma globulin. ×180. (From Eusebi et al (1977) with kind permission of the authors and the editor of *Histopathology*.)

(1965) pointed out that the mastectomy specimens, after local resection of tissue containing CLIS, contained residual tumour in 39 of a total of 44 cases they found reported in the literature at that time. Warner (1969) concluded that the *frequency of multicentricity*, determined in a similar way, was *in the region of 70 per cent*. This type of data is the main reason for the recommendation of simple mastectomy by most authors prior to 1975. Because of the frequency of bilaterality, most workers recommended either contralateral biopsy or very careful follow-up, clinical and mammographic, of the contralateral breast. Benfield, Fingerhut and Warner (1969) went so far as to recommend bilateral mastectomy as a primary procedure.

BEHAVIOUR OF CLIS AND PATIENT MANAGEMENT

Andersen (1974) tabulated the available data, from three large series, on the risk of the development of ipsilateral and contralateral invasive carcinoma in patients with CLIS who underwent only local resection. This risk was of the order of 23 per cent on the same side and about 10 per cent on the opposite side. There is a lot of very valuable information tabulated by Andersen (1974) on the behaviour of this quixotic disease. McDivitt et al (1967) found that the cumulative risk of infiltration was 35 per cent and 25 per cent after twenty years, on the same and opposite sides respectively. Though the aggressive potential of CLIS is not in question, the frequency with which it displays such aggressiveness in unselected material is decidedly contentious, as is the best mode of treatment. The number of patients developing infiltrating carcinoma after conservative surgery is not as high as might be expected from the available knowledge of the multicentricity of the disease, a paradox not yet satisfactorily explained. Even though Hutter and Foote (1969) and Haagensen, Lane and Lattes (1972) had similar experiences with the behaviour of this neoplasm, Haagensen, Lane and Lattes (1972) adopted a much more expectant and conservative attitude.

The position was further complicated by the findings of Wheeler et al (1974): they concluded that the risk of subsequent development of infiltrating carcinoma in the breast with biopsy-proven CLIS is substantially less than had been indicated by previous authors. Only a single patient (4 per cent) developed ipsilateral invasive carcinoma in a complete follow-up study, averaging 17.5 years: of 32 women with a contralateral breast at risk, only three (9.7 per cent) developed infiltrating carcinoma. Wheeler et al (1974) believe that there is no statistically valid evidence that the cumulative risk of developing invasive carcinoma in the ipsilateral breast, following biopsy-proven CLIS, is any greater than in the contralateral breast. This has very important therapeutic implications. Wheeler et al (1974) pointed out probable fallacies in the contradictory evidence presented by other workers, and Andersen (1977) also detailed problems concerning the material from the Memorial Hospital for Cancer in New York, in terms of the manner in which it was collected. This *may* have marginally biassed their prognostic data. It is fair to state, however, that the evidence of Andersen (1974) is only in partial agreement with that of Wheeler et al (1974). Nevertheless, even Andersen (1974) considered alternatives to mastectomy in the treatment of this condition. The same dilemma has faced many workers in this field, as exemplified by the provocative title of Dall'Olmo et al (1975): 'Lobular carcinoma of the breast in situ: are we too radical in its treatment?'.

Wheeler and Enterline (1976) studied in depth the extremely complex problems of prognosis, after a very careful analysis of all the data. While there is no doubt that these workers can be classified as 'mammary conservationists', they argued their case very convincingly. Even those like Andersen (1977), who found a greater risk from CLIS than Wheeler and Enterline (1976), argued in favour of a more conservative approach than that adopted only a few years ago. Wheeler and Enterline (1976) stated that 'The Connecticut State Department of Health . . . has shown that a 44-year-old woman has . . . a 2.6 per cent risk' of developing invasive breast cancer over a 15-year period. 'If a 44-year-old woman with fibrocystic disease has 2 to 4 times the risk of developing carcinoma as compared with the general population, then her risk will be about 5 to 10 per cent over a 15-year period'. 'If one takes into account that women who are discovered to have LCIS [CLIS] are almost uniformly operated upon for fibrocystic disease, then the extra risk from LCIS may be so limited as to afford both patient and surgeon a valid reason to avoid an unwanted mastectomy.'

There are obviously many dangers in this

type of reasoning but the arguments of Wheeler and Enterline (1976) must be seriously considered by all those treating patients with this disease. The writer thinks that they slightly overstate the risks from cystic disease (see Chapter Six) and slightly understate the risks from CLIS (see Andersen, 1977). No less an authority than McDivitt (1978) has stated that 'one should not simply state that both fibrocystic disease and lobular carcinoma in situ increase infiltrating carcinoma risk, since the magnitude of risk associated with these lesions differs at least by *several hundred-fold*' (my italics). The writer does not accept this last italicized figure but inserts it here to indicate the magnitude of the disagreement among leading experts in the field.

Andersen (1977) has reassessed the position from the world literature and his own experience. Out of 172 cases with only biopsy-treated CLIS, 26 (15.1 per cent) developed ipsilateral invasive carcinoma with a mean follow-up of about ten years, while 19 (9.3 per cent) developed contralateral invasive carcinoma. These new figures, compared with Andersen's 1974 data, were arrived at by making certain corrections on the basis of the potential flaws revealed by Wheeler et al (1974) and by Andersen (1977) himself. The corresponding figures in Andersen's (1977) own material are 20.4 per cent and 9.1 per cent respectively with a mean follow-up of 15.9 years. Of his 44 patients treated by biopsy alone, 11 (25 per cent) developed invasive disease after indefinite follow-up. This is *calculated to be about 12 times the frequency expected in comparable Danish women* without a previous history of CLIS (Table 6–1, Chapter Six). Andersen (1977) concluded that women with CLIS are 'high risk' patients with a considerable danger of developing invasive cancer. Despite the high risk involved he favours close and lifelong follow-up, arguing his case cogently. Four clinical examinations and one mammogram each year are recommended. No doubt this policy can be advised in some parts of the world and with intelligent women who are informed of the problem. In individual cases, lack of facilities, the personality of the patient, the dangers of cancerphobia or other factors may lead the surgeon to follow a different course. On present evidence the decision will often be a difficult one and must ultimately depend to a large extent on the views of the patient herself. Ackerman and Katzenstein (1977), quoting

the evidence of Wheeler et al (1974), Andersen (1977) and a personal communication from Haagensen, suggested a conservative approach to treatment. They rightly stressed that pathologists should be conservative in making the diagnosis of CLIS. It is not clear that these authors are right to conclude that CLIS should not be considered 'minimal' cancer and it is unfortunate that they go on to state that 'it may be only a marker for cystic disease'. Andersen (1977) does not hold this view for, by indicating an increased breast cancer risk of about ×12, he is suggesting that the level of risk is at least three to four times and possibly six times greater than it is in cystic disease. Put a different way, the increased risk with CLIS is of about twice the order seen in women with a contralateral infiltrating carcinoma. Ackerman and Katzenstein (1977) dismissed the significance of CLIS a little too sweepingly and this seems to be almost as bad as to err in the other direction and overestimate its potential dangers.

Toker and Goldberg (1977), in their dissertation on 'The Small Cell Lesion of Mammary Ducts and Lobules', decided to consider only the solid proliferations as distinct from the cribriform. This was a wise decision, since the earlier work of Toker (1974) in this regard was somewhat confusing for reasons already discussed. Toker and Goldberg (1977) also dropped the previous division into grades of dysplasia, coming to the conclusion that there is 'no present basis for the division of the lesions into the categories of dysplasia and in situ carcinoma'. Toker and Goldberg (1977) found a 20-year cumulative risk of 28 per cent of developing a first invasive breast cancer in either breast among 178 women (this figure is based on 25 events in 178 women). However, it should be noted that no fewer than 11 invasive tumours were contralateral growths which were resected *simultaneously* with the biopsy that detected the in situ lesion in the ipsilateral breast. For those 165 patients who were free of any simultaneous contralateral tumour, either invasive or non-invasive, at the time of biopsy, the 20-year cumulative risk was 23 per cent (a figure based on 14 events in 165 patients). The 23 per cent figure is more meaningful and more in agreement with the recent data of other workers. Toker and Goldberg (1977) also calculated the risks of invasive cancer in the two breasts independently, in women without prior contralateral mastectomy or bilateral biopsy. The 20-year cumulative risk for the ipsilateral breast was 19 per cent and for the contralateral breast 14 per cent. In agreement with most recent authors, they found that the risks of invasive cancer were not statistically different in the two breasts. This has an important bearing on the correct treatment of patients with CLIS.

Relationship of 'Maximum Lesion Size' to Subsequent Behaviour

Toker and Goldberg (1977) applied themselves in particular to a measurement of the maximum lesion size in an attempt to determine the relationship of this to other parameters, clinical and pathological, and especially to the prognosis. The 15-year cumulative risk of developing invasive cancer in either breast was the same with small and moderate-sized lesions (under 5.0×10^3 μm^2 and 5.0 to 9.9×10^3 μm^2 respectively). A somewhat elevated risk for the 43 women with large lesions (greater than or equal to 10.0×10^3 μm^2) was not statistically significant. This study suggested that the lesion size may not be related to the risk of subsequent invasive cancer, although these authors did conclude that the risk *may* be slightly greater in the ipsilateral breast in women with large lesions.

Relationship of Bilaterality of Disease to Subsequent Behaviour

It is of considerable interest that of eight patients with bilateral CLIS in the series of Toker and Goldberg (1977) not subjected to mastectomy at the time of diagnosis, no fewer than three developed subsequent invasive cancer. This represents a 12-year cumulative rate of developing invasive breast cancer of 36 per cent in this special subgroup.

Carter and Smith (1977) studied 49 patients with CLIS. Of these 49, 39 patients had bilateral breast biopsies: 25 were found to have CLIS in one breast only, while 14 had bilateral lesions, an incidence of bilaterality of 36 per cent. Of the 25 patients with unilateral disease only, all underwent mastectomy: 13 had residual in situ disease but none showed invasion. Of the 14 patients with bilateral CLIS, 13 underwent bilateral mastectomy: 12 had residual disease, in situ only in nine but invasive in three; this represents an incidence of 21 per cent of invasion in the group of 14

patients with *bilateral* biopsy-proven CLIS. In view of these findings, Carter and Smith (1977) suggested that the presence of bilateral disease may be a rough estimate of the extent and severity of the disease and they also suggested that the extent of the changes *may* correlate with the risk of invasive cancer. While the findings of Carter and Smith (1977) are by no means strictly comparable with those of Toker and Goldberg (1977), the findings of both groups *suggest that bilateral in situ disease is potentially more sinister in its implication.*

Relationship of Quantity and Quality of CLIS to Subsequent Behaviour

Carter and Smith's (1977) broader suggestion that the extent of the changes may have prognostic significance is only partly supported by the data of Toker and Goldberg (1977) on the significance of the 'maximum lesion size' in evaluation of the prognosis in an individual patient. Fisher and Fisher (1977) commented on their failure to find any association between invasive lobular carcinoma and the occurrence of multicentric disease in other quadrants. It should be emphasized, however, that their starting point was quite different from that of Carter and Smith (1977) and of Toker and Goldberg (1977).

One of the most definitive works in this regard is that of Rosen et al (1978), who, in a very careful analysis, concluded that *the number of lobules found to be affected by CLIS had no significant predictive value* in terms of the risk of subsequent development of invasive carcinoma. The degree of lobular distension, sometimes accorded importance, as well as the presence or absence of ductal involvement by tumour, also had no predictive value.

These workers investigated 10 clinical and pathological features of, or associated with, CLIS to establish possible predictive value in terms of subsequent invasive cancer. Disappointingly, none of the 10 features, individually or in combination, proved to have a convincing association with a substantial higher or lower risk of subsequent carcinoma. Even 'small' cell and 'large' cell type in CLIS offered no help, though in a small group of 12 cases with mixed small and large cells no fewer than eight (67 per cent) developed subsequent carcinoma. However, because this observation was based on so few cases, Rosen et al (1978) were inclined to discount it until confirmation is obtained in a larger series.

The other features which were each separately associated with a *trend* to greater risk of subsequent carcinoma that was less than significant statistically were: nulliparity, *clinically* detected cysts, six or more lobules with CLIS, and marked lymphocytic infiltration in CLIS.

The Risk of Missing Invasive Cancer with a Biopsy Diagnosis of CLIS

The incidence of three cases of invasive cancer at mastectomy in the whole series of 49 women with only CLIS at biopsy, studied by Carter and Smith (1977), indicates that about 6 per cent of patients who apparently have CLIS only at the time of biopsy have an infiltrating carcinoma at the time, a somewhat worrying finding if one opts for a conservative approach in treatment. That this is not an isolated finding of one group of workers is borne out by the similar incidence of 5 per cent in the series studied by Shah, Rosen and Robbins (1973): two patients out of 40, with a diagnosis of CLIS on biopsy excision, were found to have infiltrating carcinoma at mastectomy. These findings have a bearing on the wider problems of local excision in the treatment of carcinoma of the breast, a controversial issue well discussed by Shah, Rosen and Robbins (1973). The risk of missing synchronous invasive cancer when a patient with biopsy-proven CLIS is treated expectantly is clearly small but nevertheless significant.

Recent Views on Management

Fisher and Fisher (1977) gave an excellent account of the surgical management with a review of the widely divergent views of different workers. Based on the principles they outlined, they made out a strong case for segmental resection as opposed to total mastectomy, and a less clearcut case for low axillary dissection. Prophylactic mastectomy of the contralateral breast, as recommended by some workers (Benfield, Fingerhut and Warner, 1969, 1972) has no place in their therapeutic approach. Fisher and Fisher (1977) stressed the importance of obtaining mammograms of both breasts prior to operation to provide a baseline for comparison with subsequent examinations. With their approach to treatment, interval mammography of both the contralateral and ipsilateral breasts is mandatory.

Rosen et al (1978) contributed a masterly study of the problem based on a detailed analysis of 99 patients with an average follow-up of 24 years. Because the frequency of subsequent breast carcinoma is nine times greater than expected, these workers considered it prudent in most cases to recommend ipsilateral mastectomy with low axillary dissection, as well as concurrent biopsy of the opposite breast.

For a different view of the problem the reader is referred to Haagensen, Lane and Lattes (1972). The views of these experienced workers have to be taken very seriously. It is impossible to summarize accurately their approach to the doctor's dilemma. It involves not only accurate description, a critical analysis, statistical evaluation and so on, but a great deal of incisive logic and a considerable element of psychology. Particularly relevant is their contention that when invasive carcinoma does evolve from 'lobular neoplasia' it is usually a favourable type. 'Lobular neoplasia' is the name they chose for what others call CLIS because they believe that it is wrong to regard it as a true carcinoma. Indeed they state that the name 'lobular carcinoma in situ' is 'a most unfortunate choice for the disease entity'. Many of their arguments are convincing and perhaps their only fault is that they slightly overstate the case for conservative management. But their interesting and forceful views must be read in their entirety.

Haagensen et al (1978), finding a frequency of subsequent breast carcinoma seven times greater than expected, again strongly advocated conservative management as long as certain stringent procedures and safeguards were adopted. These workers state that: 'when a patient with lobular neoplasia consults us, we present our data regarding the disease fully and sympathetically to her. All of our patients have chosen follow-up rather than bilateral mastectomy.'

Conclusion on Management

Rosen et al (1978) concluded that: 'A decade has already been spent in the dispute between follow-up and mastectomy. Neither of these choices is ideal and each has important risks and deficiencies. The decision . . . in any one case must be arrived at after providing ample opportunity to consider the known facts about the disease, the physician's recommendation, and the patient's desires and response to her condition'. That succinctly states the present position.

The papers by Haagensen et al (1978) and Rosen et al (1978) state the opposing points of view admirably. Both should be consulted in full.

The Most Appropriate Name

One cannot leave this subject without discussing which term is most appropriate to designate the condition currently called CLIS. The writer is in agreement with the increasing number of workers who are dissatisfied with the designation 'carcinoma' for this condition. Even for those who do not follow too conservative a policy in treating patients, the term 'carcinoma' is too emotive and alarming to patient and to surgeon. Certainly there is no room at all for the use of the word 'carcinoma' unless the pathologist is assured that the surgeon is fully acquainted with its significance *in the context of CLIS*. The necessity for stating this might not be as apparent in North America as it is outside that continent. The reason is not that our surgeons are less knowledgeable, merely that pathologists have failed, for various reasons, to communicate the knowledge which has accrued over the last two decades or so.

Toker (1974) suggested small-cell 'dysplasia' but decided to withdraw this designation later (Toker and Goldberg, 1977). Probably he was right to do so, for a variety of reasons. Wheeler and Enterline (1976) tentatively suggested adopting this term. But for one thing, the term 'dysplasia' is already used for breast disease of quite a different type (Chapter Three), although the present writer thoroughly disapproves of its current usage in relation to breast disease. But it will take a very long time to change current practice and, for this reason alone, use of the term 'dysplasia' for what is now called CLIS would introduce inordinate confusion.

The dissatisfaction with the term 'carcinoma' in this context remains and is to a great extent justified. The writer has seen a mastectomy performed on a 75-year-old woman because of a diagnosis of CLIS made by an experienced and competent pathologist. Surely this cannot be right in view of what is known about the natural behaviour of the condition.

It seems to the writer that *the name 'lobular neoplasia'*, adopted by Haagensen (1971) with his formidable intuition, *satisfies our need for a different name.* It does not dismiss CLIS almost contemptuously as a 'marker for cystic disease' while, at the same time, it does not elevate it to the frightening stature of a 'carcinoma'. It is short, accurate and reasonably distinctive, and is a name which is not likely to cause confusion with other pathological processes. It has the additional merit that a surgeon who is unfamiliar with the disease entity will feel constrained to consult his pathologist when meeting this term in a report.

The 30 Per Cent Deficit

One fascinating aspect of 'lobular neoplasia' merits consideration. We know that following discovery of CLIS on biopsy, about 60 per cent of subsequently studied mastectomy specimens yield residual CLIS (Shah, Rosen and Robbins, 1973; Dall'Olmo et al, 1975). And yet, apparently, only 25 to 30 per cent of patients will develop ipsilateral infiltrating carcinoma if followed-up indefinitely after biopsy only (Andersen, 1977). There seems to be an unbridgeable gap of at least 30 per cent. The only exception to the finding of this gap is in the calculations of McDivitt et al (1967) in their classical paper which called attention to the problem of CLIS in a very real way and stimulated so much of the subsequent research. But the statistical calculations of these workers have been challenged by a number of groups of other workers on what appear to be legitimate grounds (Wheeler et al, 1974; Wheeler and Enterline, 1976; Andersen, 1977). Assuming that the latter workers are correct, there is an unexplained 'deficit' of 30 per cent or more.

Postmenopausal Disappearance? One possibility is that CLIS persists as such into old age without giving rise to problems in the lifetime of the patient. It is now known that, contrary to previous belief, CLIS can persist into the later decades of life and be found with or without infiltrating carcinoma (Wheeler and Enterline, 1976; and personal observations). In the vast majority of cases, however, CLIS is discovered in the premenopausal period. The scarcity of CLIS in the later decades may reflect postmenopausal lobular disappearance. But abnormal lobules, e.g. apocrine cysts, tend to persist into old age. We are dealing with the possibility of a post-menopausal disappearance of CLIS. If this disappearance does indeed take place, the 30 per cent 'deficit' would be explained away. We would then require to know the mechanism of this disappearance. In view of what is already known about the ERP content in lobular carcinomas, there are some obvious challenging possibilities to be faced. There must be scope here for collaborative work with the hormone chemists.

'ATYPICAL LOBULAR HYPERPLASIA'

This heading is chosen with great reluctance because, for reasons explained in Chapter Nine, names like 'atypical hyperplasia' should be avoided as far as possible. The writer believes that this is possible in the vast majority of cases with ductal disease, but that there is a residuum of lobular disease in which uncertainty exists. These cases are currently referred to under this heading so that, for the present at least, it is a term that must be used.

Some cases under this heading are probably examples of lobular cancerization in which the evidence for malignancy is inconclusive or only borderline. But, for the most part, they are examples of CLIS which do not fulfil all the requisite criteria. The lobule or lobules may show only partial involvement, lumina may persist, distension may be minimal, nuclei may appear partly ovoid or may show slight overlap. Some of these features may be caused by minor defects of processing, including less-than-perfect fixation, but, if these causes are excluded, the remainder mostly represent cases of very focal, partial or 'early' CLIS, a belief based on the fact that, in cases of obvious CLIS, lobules of this type with only minor involvement can also be found.

Wellings, Jensen and Marcum (1975) also found a spectrum of atypia in the lobules leading up to CLIS (their grade V atypia). Their Figures 98 to 100, illustrating grades I to III atypia, correspond to the types of lesion discussed here. Their concept of a continuous spectrum between the mild degrees of hyperplasia and atypia and full-blown CLIS corresponds to that of the writer. Their data were, however, insufficient to draw any conclusion about the possible precancerous potential of these lesions.

Page et al (1978) reached very important conclusions about the significance of atypical lobular hyperplasia. They concluded, on very good evidence, that atypical lobular hyperplasia has a greater predictive value for subsequent development of carcinoma than other epithelial lesions of the type seen in the fibrocystic disease complex. The increased risk is of the order of about ×4 (Table 6–1, Chapter Six). The superbly documented work of these authors must be read in its entirety because of the number, importance and validity of their conclusions.

There is evidence from the work of Wellings, Jensen and Marcum (1975) and from personal observations that most instances of ALH represent incomplete forms of CLIS. Andersen (1977) found an increased risk of ×12 in CLIS. The finding by Page et al (1978) of an increased risk of ×4 in atypical lobular hyperplasia fits neatly into the concept of ALH as an incomplete form of the disorder.

For academic purposes, ALH should be regarded as probably malignant. *For practical and therapeutic purposes* the answer is not so simple. From a practical point of view, Hutter, Foote and Farrow (1970) decided not to treat patients in whom only two or three lobules were affected by changes which qualitatively qualified as CLIS. A prospective study of 43 patients was started. The behaviour of even florid CLIS is disputed (Wheeler et al, 1974) and in these circumstances a conservative approach to therapy for the type of case under consideration is logical. If CLIS were known to lead to invasive carcinoma (on the same or opposite side) in, let us say, 70 per cent of cases within ten years; it is likely that most cases of so-called 'atypical lobular hyperplasia' would be given their more proper designation of 'incomplete' CLIS. But with the known facts about the behaviour of fully established CLIS, a term like 'atypical lobular hyperplasia' will unfortunately have to be retained until further knowledge renders it obsolete.

TUBULAR CARCINOMA OF THE BREAST

Tubular carcinoma also goes by the names of 'well-differentiated' or 'orderly' carcinoma. 'Tubular carcinoma' is probably marginally preferable as it is descriptively accurate and a little less vague than the alternatives. Definitive accounts of this entity were given by

Taylor and Norris (1970) and by Carstens et al (1972).

Clinical Findings

The clinical findings do not differ very significantly, according to most workers, from those in women with other types of mammary carcinoma. However, Carstens (1978), in a study of 42 tumours, found that 34 tumours measured between 1 and 2 cm, four were smaller than 1 cm and only four out of the total of 42 were larger than 2 cm.

Incidence

The incidence of tubular carcinoma has yet to be determined. It has generally been regarded as a rare entity but very recently Carstens (1978) reported an incidence of 10.3

per cent among all invasive mammary carcinomas seen over a one-year period. Carstens (1978) recognized three histological types of tubular carcinoma and made some interesting observations about this neoplasm. Further data are awaited from other centres for comparison with these findings.

Tubular carcinoma of the male breast was discussed by Taxy (1975).

Diagnosis

The diagnosis of tubular carcinoma is a microscopic one and the main differential diagnosis is from sclerosing adenosis. There is an infiltrative proliferation of small, tubular, duct-like structures haphazardly arranged in an abundant, generally loose and cellular stroma (Figures 10–34 and 10-35). The neoplastic tubules are lined by a single layer of uniform cuboidal cells with spherical, more

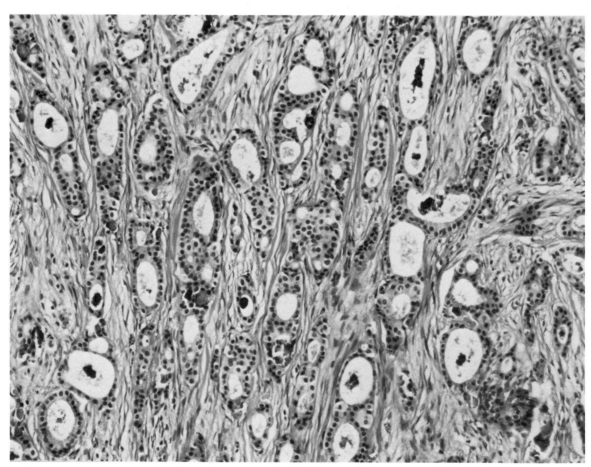

Figure 10–34 Tubular carcinoma with microcalcification. The stroma is mostly of the loose variety, and the glandular lumina widely patent, not compressed as in sclerosing adenosis. H and E. ×200.

or less centrally placed nuclei. Even at the ultrastructural level, myoepithelial cells are rarely observed (Erlandson and Carstens, 1972). The nuclear–cytoplasmic ratio is usually rather high but subtlety and considerable experience are required to detect this. There is a striking absence of cytological atypia and mitoses are extremely sparse. The cytology is 'bland'. The luminal edge of the cells is not usually clean-cut or truncated: on the contrary, it frequently shows blebbing or apical snout differentiation.

The ultrastructural features of tubular carcinoma have been particularly studied by Erlandson and Carstens (1972), Gould, Miller and Jao (1975), Jao, Recant and Swerdlow (1976), Fisher (1976) and Tobon and Salazar (1977). A striking feature is the pattern of peninsulas and bays at the luminal margin of the epithelial cells, usually covered by numerous long microvilli coated with a finely particulate glycocalyx. These luminal protrusions covered by microvilli represent the apical snouts or blebs seen at the light microscope level.

A feature stressed by Tobon and Salazar (1977) is the finding of vast numbers of fine filaments, arranged in bundles, almost completely filling the cytoplasm of most neoplastic epithelial cells. These filaments bore no definite resemblance to tonofilaments or to myofilaments. Their presence in epithelial cells is a timely reminder against an all-too-ready acceptance of filaments as an indicator of myoepithelial differentiation.

The various authors do not agree on some of the ultrastructural data. Thus intracytoplasmic lumina were sometimes found by Tobon and Salazar (1977) (one of three cases), Erlandson and Carstens (1972) and Jao, Recant and Swerdlow (1976) but they were not found by Gould, Miller and Jao (1975) and Fisher (1976). Differences even in the reports

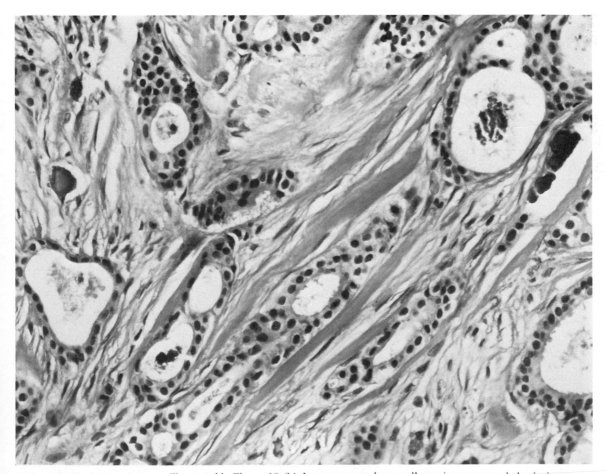

Figure 10–35 Same tumour as illustrated in Figure 10–34. In some areas dense collagen is present and elastic tissue may also be found. The nature of the stroma cannot be relied upon in differentiating tubular carcinoma from sclerosing adenosis. H and E. ×400.

of the same authors illustrate the caution needed in interpreting some of the minute details.

A much more substantial difference is the question of the presence or absence of myoepithelial cells in tubular carcinoma. They are absent according to Gould, Miller and Jao (1975) and Jao, Recant and Swerdlow (1976) and rare according to Erlandson and Carstens (1972). This is what the writer would expect on theoretical grounds, on accurate light-microscopic study of several cases and on ultrastructural study of one case of tubular carcinoma. However, Tobon and Salazar (1977) claimed that it is not unusual to see myopithelial cells either singly or even in complete rows at the periphery of neoplastic tubules: their Figure 2 is certainly convincing on this point. One should, however, bear in mind the possibility that these myoepithelial cells could represent residual non-neoplastic cells in an in situ component of the tumour. Pending further clarification, it would be wise to regard the tubular carcinoma as being composed exclusively or, at any rate, almost exclusively of epithelial cells in its infiltrative part, since the absence of a two-type epithelium is such an important point in the differentiation from sclerosing adenosis.

Differential Diagnosis

The differential diagnosis of tubular carcinoma is from sclerosing adenosis in its variant forms and the main distinguishing points are the following:

1. In tubular carcinoma the neoplastic tubules are haphazardly distributed, lacking any pattern (Figure 10–34). In sclerosing adenosis parts of the lesion usually show a lobular or at least a nodular configuration, the former denoting a lobular origin, the latter denoting a tendency to an organoid arrangement. Any such organization is completely lacking in tubular carcinoma.
2. Single-cell epithelial tubular linings in tubular carcinoma (Figure 10–34) contrast with the bicellular lining pattern common to all types of adenosis, including sclerosing adenosis. In sclerosing adenosis, the bicellular lining may be conspicuous or quite subtle but it is definitely present in some parts.
3. The small but 'open' lumina of tubular carcinoma (Figure 10–34) usually contrast

with the distorted, narrowed, collapsed or 'closed' lumina of sclerosing adenosis. In tubular carcinoma, the tubules 'fail to fade out into sclerotic stroma' (McDivitt, Stewart and Berg, 1968).
4. Trabecular bars, as defined in Chapter Seven, can be found partitioning an occasional tubular lumen (Figures 10–34 and 10–35): these are not present in sclerosing adenosis.
5. The finding of intraductal carcinoma within the lesion in two-thirds of the cases of tubular carcinoma constitutes corroborative but not absolute evidence of the nature of the infiltrative lesion.
6. The loose, abundant, cellular stroma (Figure 10–34) has been regarded by some workers as a useful diagnostic criterion. Other workers mention hyalinization of the stroma (Figure 10–35) and claim to have identified amyloid in these carcinomas. In the writer's opinion, this is elastic tissue and not amyloid (page 391). Though it is true that the stroma of tubular carcinomas is usually loose and cellular, it can also contain abundant elastic tissue. The writer is not wholly convinced that a truly valid distinction between tubular carcinoma and sclerosing adenosis can be made on the quality of the stroma.

The first four points listed are the most crucial, with corroborative evidence sometimes provided by the fifth. That the diagnosis of a tubular carcinoma can present formidable problems is emphasized by the fact that eight of the 35 lesions studied by Taylor and Norris (1970) were initially interpreted as sclerosing adenosis.

Nodal Metastasis

Patients with tubular carcinoma have a relatively good prognosis. Axillary node metastases were present in 9 per cent, 25 per cent and 30 per cent respectively in the series of Carstens et al (1972), Kouchoukos, Ackerman and Butcher (1968) and Taylor and Norris (1970). Of the 10 patients in the Taylor and Norris (1970) series with axillary node metastasis, only two women had more than two lymph nodes involved and, in all patients, involved lymph nodes were confined to the lower axillary region. An exception to this last statement is seen in Case 1 of Carstens et al (1972).

Association with Other Forms of Breast Cancer and Prognosis

Carstens et al (1972) stressed the frequency with which other types of breast carcinoma are found in association with tubular carcinoma of the breast: the prognosis for such patients is then largely dependent upon the associated carcinoma. Although the prognosis with tubular carcinoma is very good, except when it is accompanied by a more aggressive tumour, and although nodal metastases are usually very limited, when they occur, Taylor and Norris (1970) warned against assuming a lack of potential for the tumour to disseminate. One of their patients died of metastatic mammary carcinoma, as did four patients studied by Kouchoukos, Ackerman and Butcher (1967). Taylor and Norris (1970) concluded that this type of tumour is ideally suited for treatment by modified radical mastectomy as described by Auchincloss (1963) and by Patey and Dyson (1948).

Caesar's Due

The writer is not qualified to dictate the type of operation to be performed with particular kinds of tumour. Pathologists can only advise surgeons about the facts and data in the literature as they apply generally, and about any special circumstances that appertain to a particular tumour being reported on. It is a foolish surgeon who does not take full account of pathology, which constitutes the scientific backbone of surgery as it does of medicine. A continuous dialogue between surgeon, pathologist and colleagues in other disciplines is essential to the practice of any type of good medicine. But, when all that is said, the writer feels strongly that in the last resort the clinician must decide on the precise treatment of an individual patient. One might as well render unto Caesar the things that are Caesar's since he will take them anyway!

References

Ackerman, L. V. and Katzenstein, A. L. (1977) The concept of minimal breast cancer and the pathologist's role in the diagnosis of 'early carcinoma'. *Cancer* (Supplement), **39**, 2755–2763.

Ahmed, A. (1974) The myoepithelium in human breast carcinoma. *Journal of Pathology*, **113**, 129–135.

Andersen, J. A. (1974) Lobular carcinoma in situ. A long-term follow-up in 52 cases. *Acta Pathologica et Microbiologica Scandinavica*, Section A, **82**, 519–533.

Andersen, J. A. (1977) Lobular carcinoma in situ of the breast. An approach to rational treatment. *Cancer*, **39**, 2597–2602.

Ashikari, R., Huvos, A. G., Urban, J. A. and Robbins, G. F. (1973) Infiltrating lobular carcinoma of the breast. *Cancer*, **31**, 110–116.

Ashikari, R., Huvos, A. G., Snyder, R. E., Lucas, J. C., Hutter, R. V. P., McDivitt, R. W. and Schottenfeld, D. (1974) A clinicopathologic study of atypical lesions of the breast. *Cancer*, **33**, 310–317.

Auchincloss, H. (1963) Significance of location and number of axillary metastases in carcinoma of the breast. A justification for a conservative operation. *Annals of Surgery*, **158**, 37–46.

Battifora, H. (1975) Intracytoplasmic lumina in breast carcinoma. A helpful histopathologic feature. *Archives of Pathology*, **99**, 614–617.

Benfield, J. R., Fingerhut, A. G. and Warner, N. E. (1969) Lobular carcinoma of the breast—1969. A therapeutic proposal. *Archives of Surgery*, **99**, 129–131.

Benfield, J. R., Fingerhut, A. G. and Warner, N. E. (1972) A multidiscipline view of lobular breast carcinoma. *American Surgeon*, **38**, 115–116.

Benfield, J. R., Jacobson, M. and Warner, N. E. (1965) In situ lobular carcinoma of the breast. *Archives of Surgery*, **91**, 130–135.

Bonser, G. M., Dossett, J. A. and Jull, J. W. (1961) *Human and Experimental Breast Cancer*. London: Pitman Medical.

Bosincu, L. and Eusebi, V. (1972) Carcinoma della mammella insorto in fibroadenoma. *Tumori*, **58**, 195–202.

Buell, R. H., Tremblay, G. and Rowden, G. (1976) Distribution of adenosine triphosphatase in infiltrating ductal carcinoma and non-neoplastic breast. *Cancer*, **38**, 875–887.

Carstens, P. H. B. (1978) Tubular carcinoma of the breast. A study of frequency. *American Journal of Clinical Pathology*, **70**, 204–210.

Carstens, P. H. B., Huvos, A. G., Foote, F. W. Jr and Ashikari, R. (1972) Tubular carcinoma of the breast: a clinicopathologic study of 35 cases. *American Journal of Clinical Pathology*, **58**, 231–238.

Carter, D. and Smith, R. R. L. (1977) Carcinoma in situ of the breast. *Cancer*, **40**, 1189–1193.

Carter, D., Yardley, J. H. and Shelley, W. M. (1969) Lobular carcinoma of the breast: an ultrastructural comparison with certain duct carcinomas and benign lesions. *Johns Hopkins Medical Journal*, **125**, 25–43.

Cheatle, Sir, G. L. and Cutler, M. (1931) *Tumours of the Breast — Their Pathology, Symptoms, Diagnosis and Treatment*. London: Edward Arnold.

Dall'Olmo, C. A., Ponka, J. L., Horn, R. C. Jr and Riu, R. (1975) Lobular carcinoma of the breast in situ. Are we too radical in its treatment? *Archives of Surgery*, **110**, 537–542.

Dawson, E. K. (1933) Carcinoma in the mammary lobule and its origin. *Edinburgh Medical Journal*, **40**, 57–82.

Dawson, E. K. (1948) Genesis and spread of mammary cancer. *Annals of the Royal College of Surgeons of England*, **2**, 241–247.

Ellis, F. G., Bern, T. C., Deshpande, N., Belzer, F. O. and Bulbrook, R. D. (1969) The uptake of tritiated steroids by human breast carcinoma. *Surgery, Gynecology and Obstetrics*, **128**, 975–984.

Erlandson, R. A. and Carstens, P. H. B. (1972) Ultrastructure of tubular carcinoma of the breast. *Cancer*, **29**, 987–995.

Eusebi, V., Pich, A., Macchiorlatti, E. and Bussolati, G.

(1977) Morphofunctional differentiation in lobular carcinoma of the breast. *Histopathology*, **1**, 301–314.

Fechner, R. E. (1971) Ductal carcinoma involving the lobule of the breast. A source of confusion with lobular carcinoma in situ. *Cancer*, **28**, 274–281.

Fechner, R. E. (1972a) Epithelial alterations in the extralobular ducts of breasts with lobular carcinoma. *Archives of Pathology*, **93**, 164–171.

Fechner, R. E. (1972b) Infiltrating lobular carcinoma without lobular carcinoma in situ. *Cancer*, **29**, 1539–1545.

Fisher, E. R. (1976) Ultrastructure of the human breast and its disorders. *American Journal of Clinical Pathology*, **66**, 291–375.

Fisher, E. R. and Fisher, B. (1977) Lobular carcinoma of the breast: an overview. *Annals of Surgery*, **185**, 377–385.

Fisher, E. R., Gregorio, R. M. and Fisher, B. (1975) The pathology of invasive breast cancer. *Cancer*, **36**, 1–263.

Foote, F. W. and Stewart, F. W. (1946) A histologic classification of carcinoma of the breast. *Surgery*, **19**, 74–99.

Gad, A. and Azzopardi, J. G. (1975) Lobular carcinoma of the breast: a special variant of mucin-secreting carcinoma. *Journal of Clinical Pathology*, **28**, 711–716.

Gallager, H. S. (1972) The pathologist and modern breast cancer management. In *Pathology Annual* (Ed.) Sommers, S. C. Vol. 7, p. 237. New York: Appleton-Century-Crofts.

Gallager, H. S. and Martin, J. E. (1971) An orientation to the concept of minimal breast cancer. *Cancer*, **28**, 1505–1507.

Giordano, J. M. and Klopp, C. T. (1973) Lobular carcinoma in situ: incidence and treatment. *Cancer*, **31**, 105–109.

Gould, V. E., Miller, J. and Jao, W. (1975) Ultrastructure of medullary, intraductal, tubular and adenocystic breast carcinomas. Comparative patterns of myoepithelial differentiation and basal lamina deposition. *American Journal of Pathology*, **78**, 401–407.

Haagensen, C. D. (1971) *Diseases of the Breast.* Second edition — revised reprint. pp. 503–519. Philadelphia, London, Toronto: W. B. Saunders.

Haagensen, C. D., Lane, N. and Lattes, R. (1972) Neoplastic proliferation of the epithelium of the mammary lobules. Adenosis, lobular neoplasia, and small cell carcinoma. *Surgical Clinics of North America*, **52**, 497–524.

Haagensen, C. D., Lane, N., Lattes, R. and Bodian, C. (1978) Lobular neoplasia (so-called lobular carcinoma in situ) of the breast. *Cancer*, **42**, 737–769.

Hamperl, H. (1971) Das lobuläre Carcinoma in situ der Mamma. *Deutsche Medizinische Wochenschrift*, **96**, 1585–1588.

Hamperl, H. (1972) Zur Kenntnis des sog. Carcinoma lobuläre in situ der Mamma. Beiträge zur pathologischen Histologie der Mamma V. *Zeitschrift für Krebsforschung*, **77**, 231–246.

Hutter, R. V. P. (1971) The pathologist's role in minimal breast cancer. *Cancer*, **28**, 1527–1536.

Hutter, R. V. P. and Foote, F. W., Jr (1969) Lobular carcinoma in situ. Long term follow-up. *Cancer*, **24**, 1081–1085.

Hutter, R. V. P. and Kim, D. U. (1971) The problem of multiple lesions of the breast. *Cancer*, **28**, 1591–1607.

Hutter, R. V. P., Foote, F. W. and Farrow, J. H. (1970) In situ lobular carcinoma of the female breast,

1939–1968. In *Breast Cancer: Early and Late.* pp. 219, 220. Chicago: Year Book Medical Publishers.

Jao, W., Recant, W. and Swerdlow, M. A. (1976) Comparative ultrastructure of tubular carcinoma and sclerosing adenosis of the breast. *Cancer*, **38**, 180–186.

Kahn, L. B. and Webber, B. (1974) Lobular carcinoma of the breast: a review. *South African Journal of Surgery*, **12**, 51–55.

Kouchoukos, N. T., Ackerman, L. V. and Butcher, H. R., Jr (1967) Prediction of axillary nodal metastases from the morphology of primary mammary carcinomas. *Cancer*, **20**, 948–960.

Lambird, P. A. and Shelley, W. M. (1969) The spatial distribution of lobular in situ mammary carcinoma. *Journal of the American Medical Association*, **210**, 689–693.

McDivitt, R. W. (1978) Breast carcinoma. *Human Pathology*, **9**, 3–21.

McDivitt, R. W., Holleb, A. I. and Foote, F. W., Jr (1968) Prior breast disease in patients treated for papillary carcinoma. *Archives of Pathology*, **85**, 117–124.

McDivitt, R. W., Stewart, F. W. and Berg, J. W. (1968) *Tumors of the Breast.* Atlas of Tumor Pathology, Second series, Fascicle 2. Washington, D.C.: Armed Forces Institute of Pathology.

McDivitt, R. W., Hutter, R. V. P., Foote, F. W., Jr and Stewart, F. W. (1967) In situ lobular carcinoma. *Journal of the American Medical Association*, **201**, 96–100.

Murad, T. M. (1971a) Ultrastructure of ductular carcinoma of the breast (in situ and infiltrating lobular carcinoma). *Cancer*, **27**, 18–28.

Murad, T. M. (1971b) A proposed histochemical and electron microscopic classification of human breast cancer according to cell of origin. *Cancer*, **27**, 288–299.

Murad, T. M. and Scarpelli, D. G. (1967) The ultrastructure of medullary and scirrhous mammary duct carcinoma. *American Journal of Pathology*, **50**, 335–360.

Newman, W. (1966) Lobular carcinoma of the female breast. Report of 73 cases. *Annals of Surgery*, **164**, 305–314.

Ozzello, L. (1971) Ultrastructure of the human mammary gland. In *Pathology Annual* (Ed.) Sommers, S. C., Vol. 6, pp. 1–59. London: Butterworth.

Page, D. L., Zwaag, R. V., Rogers, L. W., Williams, L. T., Walker, W. E. and Hartmann, W. H. (1978) Relation between component parts of fibrocystic disease complex and breast cancer. *Journal of the National Cancer Institute*, **61**, 1055–1063.

Parks, A. G. (1959) The micro-anatomy of the breast. *Annals of the Royal College of Surgeons of England*, **25**, 235–251.

Patey, D. H. and Dyson, W. H. (1948) The prognosis of carcinoma of the breast in relation to the type of operation performed. *British Journal of Cancer*, **2**, 7–13.

Pich, A., Bussolati, G. and Di Carlo, F. (1977) Production of casein and presence of oestrogen receptors in human breast cancers. *Journal of the National Cancer Institute*, **58**, 1483–1484.

Rosen, P. P., Lieberman, P. H., Braun, D. W., Jr, Kosloff, C. and Adair, F. (1978) Lobular carcinoma in situ of the breast. Detailed analysis of 99 patients with average follow-up of 24 years. *American Journal of Surgical Pathology*, **2**, 225–251.

Rosen, P. P., Mendez-Botet, C. J., Nisselbaum, J. S.,

Urban, J. A., Miké, V., Fracchia, A. and Schwartz, M. K. (1975) Pathological review of breast lesions analyzed for estrogen receptor protein. *Cancer Research*, **35**, 3187–3194.

Sander, S. and Attramadal, A. (1968) The in vivo uptake of oestradiol-17β by hormone responsive and un-responsive breast tumors of the rat. *Acta Pathologica et Microbiologica Scandinavica*, **74**, 169–178.

Shah, J. P., Rosen, P. P. and Robbins, G. F. (1973) Pitfalls of local excision in the treatment of carcinoma of the breast. *Surgery, Gynecology and Obstetrics*, **136**, 721–725.

Spriggs, A. I. and Jerrome, D. W. (1975) Intracellular mucous inclusions. A feature of malignant cells in effusions in the serous cavities, particularly due to carcinoma of the breast. *Journal of Clinical Pathology*, **28**, 929–936.

Taylor, H. B. and Norris, H. J. (1970) Well-differentiated carcinoma of the breast. *Cancer*, **25**, 687–692.

Taxy, J. B. (1975) Tubular carcinoma of the male breast. Report of a case. *Cancer*, **36**, 462–465.

Tobon, H. and Salazar, H. (1977) Tubular carcinoma of the breast. Clinical, histological and ultrastructural observations. *Archives of Pathology and Laboratory Medicine*, **101**, 310–316.

Toker, C. (1961) Some observations on Paget's disease of the nipple. *Cancer*, **14**, 653–672.

Toker, C. (1974) Small cell dysplasia and in situ carcinoma of the mammary ducts and lobules. *Journal of Pathology*, **114**, 47–52.

Toker, C. and Goldberg, J. D. (1977) The small cell lesion of mammary ducts and lobules. In *Pathology Annual* (Ed.) Sommers, S. C. and Rosen, P. P. Vol. 12, pp. 217–249. New York: Appleton-Century-Crofts.

Warner, N. E. (1969) Lobular carcinoma of the breast. *Cancer*, **23**, 840–846.

Wellings, S. R. and Jensen, H. M. (1973) On the origin and progression of ductal carcinoma in the human breast. *Journal of the National Cancer Institute*, **50**, 1111–1118.

Wellings, S. R. and Roberts, P. (1963) Electron microscopy of sclerosing adenosis and infiltrating duct carcinoma of the human mammary gland. *Journal of the National Cancer Institute*, **30**, 269–287.

Wellings, S. R., Jensen, H. M. and Marcum, R. G. (1975) An atlas of subgross pathology of the human breast with special reference to possible precancerous lesions. *Journal of the National Cancer Institute*, **55**, 231–273.

Wheeler, J. E. and Enterline, H. T. (1976) Lobular carcinoma of the breast in situ and infiltrating. In *Pathology Annual* (Ed.) Sommers, S. C. Vol. 11, pp. 161–188. New York: Appleton-Century-Crofts.

Wheeler, J. E., Enterline, H. T., Roseman, J. M., Tomasulo, J. P., McIlvaine, C. H., Fitts, W. T., Jr and Kirshenbaum, J. (1974) Lobular carcinoma in situ of the breast: Long-term follow-up. *Cancer*, **34**, 554–563.

Chapter Eleven

Classification of Primary Breast Carcinoma

No classification is perfect nor is it likely that it will ever be. Any classification should be reasonably simple, easy to understand, reproducible in the hands of different workers and as comprehensive as is compatible with simplicity. All classifications depend on our knowledge of the pathology and histogenesis of the tumours being classified and, since this knowledge is far from perfect or complete, no classification can be other than a reasonable working compromise.

Topographical Histogenetic Basis. In general, the writer has found that the virtues and disadvantages of different classifications are outlined clearly and succinctly by van Bogaert and Maldague (1978). These workers opted for a topographical histogenetic classification which placed emphasis on histogenetic knowledge, however incomplete, and on the topography of the structures primarily involved.

Main Primary Divisions. The first important division should thus be into lobular and ductal carcinomas, with further subdivision into in situ and invasive forms (Table 11–1). This conforms with the views of van Bogaert and Maldague (1978), but a slightly different view of the meaning of lobular and ductal carcinoma has had to be adopted since the distinction is not entirely a topographical one, as will be explained later.

Table 11–1 Classification of primary breast carcinoma

I. **Lobular Carcinoma**

    A. *In situ (LCIS or CLIS)*

    B. *Invasive (ILC)*

        (1) Classical ILC including Histiocytoid Carcinoma and ILC with Focal Signet-ring Cell Differentiation

        (2) Variants of ILC: 'Alveolar', Tubular and ? Solid Variant of Fechner; some Signet-ring Cell Carcinomas

Table 11–1—*continued*

II. **Ductal Carcinoma**
  A. *In situ (DCIS)*
      (including Intracystic Carcinoma)
      (including Paget's Disease of the Nipple if Unaccompanied by Invasive Cancer)

  B. *Invasive (IDC)*
      (1) Not Otherwise Specified (NOS)
          (a) Stellate or Irregular (the 'Crab')
          (b) Multinodular, Knobby or Circumscribed but of no special histological type

  SPECIAL TYPES OF IDC (Categories 2 to 14):

  CIRCUMSCRIBED TUMOURS OF SPECIFIC HISTOLOGICAL TYPES
      (2) Medullary Carcinoma with Lymphoid Infiltration, Atypical Medullary Carcinoma
      (3) Pure Mucoid or Colloid Carcinoma

  IDC IN WHICH THE EXTENT AND TYPE OF THE IN SITU COMPONENT QUALIFIES THE NAME OF THE TUMOUR
      (4) Infiltrating Comedocarcinoma
      (5) Infiltrating Cribriform Carcinoma

  ---

      (6) Tubular Carcinoma
      (7) Squamous, Spindle-cell and Sarcomatoid Metaplasia in Carcinoma, excluding Sarcomatoid
          Metaplasia of the Type listed under (8) (Category 7 includes the Commoner Form of Pseudo-
          carcinosarcoma)
      (8) Tumours Analogous to Similar Malignant Tumours in Other Organs
          (a) Carcinoma with Cartilaginous and/or Osseous Metaplasia (Malignant 'Mixed' Tumour
              of Salivary Gland Type)
          (b) Malignant Adenomyothelioma
          (c) Leiomyosarcoma of Myothelial Origin and certain other very rare 'Sarcomas' and so-
              called 'Carcinosarcomas' (Category 8 includes the Rarer Forms of Pseudocarcino-
              sarcoma)
      (9) Adenoid Cystic Carcinoma
      (10) Apocrine Carcinoma
      (11) Lipid-rich or Lipid-secreting Carcinoma
      (12) Glycogen-rich Carcinoma
      (13) Juvenile Carcinoma
      (14) Carcinomas with Noteworthy Clinical Manifestations or Their Pathological Equivalents
          (a) Paget's Disease of the Nipple (Clinical or microscopic, accompanying invasive carcinoma)
          (b) Inflammatory Carcinoma or Dermal Lymphatic Carcinomatosis (The two overlap but
              do not always coincide)
      (15) Mixtures of any Two or More of the Types of IDC listed above

III. **Invasive Carcinoma of Uncertain Type: Ductal or Lobular**

IV. **Definite Mixtures of IDC and ILC in the Same Tumour Mass**

V. **Carcinoma of Type I or II which differs in that it is borne by a Distinct or Pre-existing Tumour,
    viz: Carcinoma in Fibroadenoma or Cystosarcoma Phyllodes**

VI. **True Carcinosarcoma**

VII. **Unclassified Carcinomas, Malignant Tumours in which Carcinomatous Nature is In Doubt
    and Lesions which could represent Pseudo tumours or Carcinomas (in each case give
    reasons for doubt)**

GENERAL COMMENTS ON THE CLASSIFICATION

NECESSITY FOR SEVEN MAJOR DIVISIONS THOUGH TWO ONLY ACCOUNT FOR MOST TUMOURS

Although seven major divisions may seem excessive, Sections V and VI in Table 11–1 are either very rare or extremely rare. Thus there are *only five major divisions of any frequency. Sections I and II will account for most tumours.* The reasons for having Sections III and IV are to prevent tumours from being artificially forced into Sections I and II merely because there is no appropriate place for them. Fisher, Gregorio and Fisher (1975) also tried to overcome this problem by recognizing the frequency of mixtures of different types of carcinoma. There is obviously a need for Section VII, the category of unclassified tumours, perhaps one of the most important categories in any classification.

THE MEANING OF 'DUCTAL TYPE CARCINOMA'

The division into lobular and ductal type carcinomas (I and II in Table 11–1) needs no justification and should command universal support. It must, however, be understood that lobular and ductal *types* of carcinoma refer to histologically and cytologically identifiable entities and not necessarily to sites of origin, since the classical work of Wellings, Jensen and Marcum (1975) and as stressed also by Toker and Goldberg (1977). Thus it is no longer correct to speak of tumours of 'ductal epithelial *origin*' and of 'lobular epithelial *origin*' as if the sites of origin of the two were completely distinct. Ductal carcinomas sometimes have their origin within the lobule, hence the insistence of Wellings, Jensen and Marcum (1975) on the recognition of the TDLU (terminal duct–lobular unit) as a single unit from the point of view of the site of origin of most ductal carcinomas. Most small 'early' ductal carcinomas arise in the TDLU complex and the failure to recognize this in past years is due to many causes, as explained in Chapter Ten.

The vast bulk of, possibly all, lobular carcinomas arise in the lobules, as has been explained in Chapter Ten, although a few authors maintain that lobular carcinoma can have an origin in extralobular ducts. On the other hand, ductal type carcinomas can arise in any part of the ductal–lobular structures from the largest ducts opening at the nipple to the intralobular epithelial units (acini or terminal ductules, depending on the nomenclature used). Most ductal carcinomas arise in the smaller ramifications of the system and involve especially the ductule (extra- and intralobular) and the more central parts of the lobule, usually sparing the extreme periphery of the lobule initially. Thus, while there are probably usually minor differences in the site of origin of ductal and lobular carcinomas, there is a very large overlap, so that the major pathological distinction in most cases depends more on structural configurations and cytological features than on the precise localization of the earliest changes.

It is essential that this is clearly understood from the start, since some types of carcinoma which arise in structures of lobular derivation, e.g. the rare intracystic carcinomas, are universally classified under ductal carcinomas. This is perfectly justifiable but only on the basis of the explanation given here.

THE DIVISION INTO IN SITU AND INVASIVE TYPES

The subdivision of lobular and ductal type carcinomas into in situ and invasive varieties (A and B in Table 11–1) will also command universal support. Indeed it could be argued that the primary division of all carcinomas should be into in situ carcinoma and invasive carcinoma, with subdivision into lobular and ductal types. The opposite course has been followed here in order to try and adhere to the topographical histogenetic classification of van Bogaert and Maldague (1978).

I. A. LOBULAR CARCINOMA IN SITU (LCIS OR CLIS)

This has already been dealt with in Chapter Ten. Its place in the classification is not at issue. The problem of nomenclature is.

I. B. INVASIVE LOBULAR CARCINOMA

A tumour should be classified as invasive lobular carcinoma (ILC) quite independently of the presence or absence, and the nature, of any in situ component. In practice 70 to 80 per cent of ILC will show foci of CLIS as well, if sampling is adequate and the criteria for the recognition of ILC are correct (Wheeler and Enterline, 1976). But ILC can occur in the absence of detectable CLIS (Fechner, 1972; Wheeler and Enterline, 1976), presumably either because of a sampling failure or because there is very little or no residual CLIS left to be found. Alternatively, both CLIS and ductal carcinoma in situ (DCIS) can be present accompanying ILC and, least commonly, DCIS can accompany ILC when no CLIS is detectable, but this is distinctly rare. The classification of a given tumour as ILC, independently of the presence and nature of an in situ component, is very easily justified since the invasive tumour is clearly the more important for a variety of reasons.

I. B. (1) CLASSICAL INVASIVE LOBULAR CARCINOMA

ILC of the classical form presents few serious problems of classification. Although '*histio-cytoid carcinoma*' is in my opinion an ILC, there is a place for its separate identification under this general heading. Firstly, it is apt to be confused with lesions like xanthoma, histiocytosis and, when metastatic to the eyelid, with xanthelasma (Hood, Font and Zimmerman, 1973); it has even been confused with somewhat less justification with granular-cell 'myoblastoma'. I have seen histiocytoid carcinoma metastatic to the skin which mimicked mastocytosis, a resemblance which, it is worth recalling, was pointed out in the original work on lobular carcinoma (Foote and Stewart, 1941). Secondly, 'histiocytoid carcinoma' has unfortunately been confused in the literature with 'lipid-rich carcinoma' and the two terms have sometimes been used synonymously. This terminological muddle can be grossly misleading and the reasons for it will be explained in the relevant sections. For these two reasons, 'histiocytoid carcinoma' should probably be identified separately under the heading of ILC.

I. B. (2) VARIANTS OF INVASIVE LOBULAR CARCINOMA

The recently recognized variants of ILC, including the *solid* variant of Fechner (1975) and the *tubulolobular* variant of Fisher et al (1977b), will be considered in the section on ILC, as will a variant of ILC which we have called '*alveolar*' (Martinez and Azzopardi, 1979). These variants, if such they be, require separate recognition on a number of grounds. Firstly, they are quite unlike the classical forms of the tumour as the designations 'solid' and 'tubulolobular' will immediately indicate. Indeed Fisher et al (1977b) found it extremely difficult to allot this tumour type to the pigeon-hole of ILC as distinct from tubular carcinoma. With the solid variant there are also problems, since Cubilla and Woodruff (1977) raised the possibility that some of these carcinomas may be related to the carcinoid tumours of the breast described by them. Provisionally these solid and tubular forms can be classified as variants of ILC on the basis of the criteria provided by Fechner (1975) and by Fisher et al (1977b) respectively, while recognizing that their nosological position is not by any means certain. The second reason for identifying these variants separately is the suggestion by both groups of workers that the variants they described may have a better prognosis than the classical form of ILC, at least in the short term (Fechner, 1975; Fisher et al, 1977b).

Signet-Ring Cell Carcinoma. Signet-ring cell differentiation in breast carcinoma requires consideration here, since focal signet-ring cell differentiation is fairly common in ILC (Gad and Azzopardi, 1975). Carcinomas with the overall structure of ILC and focal signet-ring cell differentiation only should be classified with ILC of the classical variety. When signet-ring cell differentiation is dominant in a carcinoma or with the very rare pure signet-ring cell carcinoma, problems in classification begin to arise. Gad and Azzopardi (1975) suggested that some cases may represent variants of ILC, a suggestion which is supported by further observations (Martinez and Azzopardi, 1979). The writer believes that some signet-ring cell carcinomas should be so classified. This is not, however, meant to indicate that signet-ring cell carcinoma cannot arise as a variant of invasive ductal carcinoma, so this question will be raised again under Section III (invasive carcinoma of uncertain type).

Should Dominant CLIS with 'Minimal' Infiltration be Segregated?

Before leaving the topic of ILC, it should be mentioned that a case could be made for a separate category of *dominant CLIS with less than 10 per cent of stromal infiltration,* analogous to the category of dominant intraductal carcinoma with 'less than 10 per cent' of stromal infiltration of Silverberg and Chitale (1973). It is not known whether such a category would be useful for prognostic and other purposes but it may be, judging from some observations made in the literature. It will need a working party, possibly internationally based, to determine the desirability and feasibility of such a category. Should it be desirable, it will have to be determined whether 'less than 10 per cent' or 'less than 5 per cent' is the best cut-off point or whether some term as with 'focal' or 'minimal' infiltration is more desirable and how this can best be defined so as to be reproducible in different centres. No such separate category has been included in the classification though the writer uses it in practice and suspects that it might prove useful.

II. A. DUCTAL CARCINOMA IN SITU

Ductal carcinoma in situ (DCIS) is largely self-explanatory. For reasons previously stated, it includes carcinoma of ductal type which has originated in the lobules or which has spread into the lobules secondarily. The term DCIS should be applied to all the patterns recognized, viz. *comedo, solid, cribriform, clinging* and *papillary* and to *any combination* of these patterns. No particular purpose is served by distinguishing comedocarcinoma separately, although a case could be made for it for reasons which will be apparent by referring to the category on 'infiltrating comedocarcinoma' (below).

Intracystic Carcinoma. DCIS includes the rare intracystic carcinoma of the type described by Gatchell, Dockerty and Clagett (1958). This carcinoma arises in a macroscopically identifiable cyst and, as such, has its origin in a structure of lobular derivation, and yet it is a carcinoma of 'ductal type': there are no reports of lobular carcinoma arising in apocrine or other cysts of the breast. Intracystic carcinoma should be classified as DCIS (Intracystic).

Paget's Disease Without Invasion. If Paget's disease is unaccompanied by any invasive cancer, it should be classified as DCIS (Paget's).

II. B. INVASIVE DUCTAL CARCINOMA

A tumour should be classified as invasive ductal carcinoma (IDC) quite independently of the presence or absence, and the nature, of any in situ component. In practice DCIS will be found in a large majority of cases provided that sampling is adequate; with most tumour types, the incidence of DCIS will increase appreciably with increased sampling. In some cases IDC will be accompanied by both DCIS and LCIS, reflecting a dual in situ neoplastic response of the mammary epithelium. In other tumours IDC is found accompanied by LCIS in the absence of detectable DCIS. In the latter cases, there is presumably no direct relationship between the LCIS and the IDC. Sometimes no in situ component of any type can be detected accompanying IDC. This is true of some 20 per cent of cases of IDC even with the very extensive sampling carried out in highly specialized laboratories. The absence of an in situ component with IDC is especially common with medullary carcinoma with lymphoid infiltration and with mucoid carcinoma. In about 90 per cent of typical medullary carcinomas, as strictly defined by Ridolfi et al (1977), there is no in situ component. Indeed originally Ridolfi et al (1977) excluded any tumour with an in situ component from their 'typical medullary' group, but they changed their minds on this point in the course of their study and concluded that there was no reason to exclude a tumour from this category, if all other criteria were satisfied, merely because of the presence of an in situ component. The writer agrees that occasionally a tumour which qualifies fully as a typical medullary carcinoma with lymphoid infiltration can be shown to contain DCIS in ducts and/or lobules. The classification of a given tumour as IDC, independently of the presence and nature of an in situ component, is perfectly justifiable since the behaviour and other important aspects are clearly *mainly* dependent on the invasive neoplasm. One should say 'mainly', rather than 'only', because the presence of CLIS accompanying IDC *may* modify the method of management of the contralateral breast.

II. B. (1) INVASIVE DUCTAL CARCINOMA, NOT OTHERWISE SPECIFIED

The large majority of IDC comes into the category of *invasive ductal carcinoma of no special type*, also called carcinoma, not otherwise specified or *carcinoma NOS* (Fisher, Gregorio and Fisher, 1975). There are two subdivisions of this based on the macroscopic configuration of the tumour in the gross specimen or, better, the configuration of the tumour as seen in stained histological sections examined with the naked eye or with a hand lens. These can be identified as (a) *stellate carcinoma* and (b) *circumscribed or multinodular carcinoma*. Both of these terms, and especially the second, need further definition. These tumour types are best considered in a historical context.

Stellate Carcinoma

The *stellate carcinoma* (irregular carcinoma, infiltrating duct carcinoma with productive fibrosis) is also sometimes known for historical reasons as scirrhous carcinoma and has also been called 'carcinoma with diffuse fibrosis' by the Pathology Working Group, Breast Cancer Task Force (Friedell et al, 1973). This is the classical 'crab', the cancer with tentacles radiating outwards into surrounding tissues. Lane et al (1961) at the Columbia–Presbyterian Medical Center, New York, were one of the earliest groups of workers to consider classifying breast carcinomas of no distinctive microscopic type into two categories, 'irregular carcinomas' and 'well-delimited carcinomas'. The irregular carcinomas are those with a serrated, grossly irregular, often stellate periphery. They were called 'infiltrating duct carcinoma with productive fibrosis' by McDivitt, Stewart and Berg (1968) and 'stellate carcinoma' by Gallager and Martin (1969). These are the carcinomas which exhibit what a distinguished group of authorities called 'prosaic, yet authentic striate, yellowish, chalky streaks . . .'. These yellowish streaks and flecks are caused by elastosis of the ductal and vascular walls and they have more of a poetic than a prosaic aura to them in view of the chequered interpretation of both their composition and their significance during the last five decades and more (see Chapter Fifteen). The terms 'scirrhous carcinoma' and 'carcinoma with diffuse fibrosis' are considered less desirable since, as a number of authors have pointed out recently, these names could apply also to invasive lobular carcinomas and hence are best avoided. Of course, when the name 'scirrhous carcinoma of the breast' was first used, lobular carcinoma had not yet been described and the problem did not exist. 'Stellate carcinoma' is probably the best name for this tumour type and it appears to have been popularized by Gallager and Martin (1969).

Circumscribed or Multinodular Carcinoma

Circumscribed or multinodular carcinoma is characterized by a well-delimited, rounded, lobulated or multinodular contour and has what pathologists have come to call a 'pushing' margin and what is possibly a largely expansile type of growth. This is the tumour type which Gallager and Martin (1969) called, somewhat picturesquely, 'knobby carcinoma' and the present writer tends to think of it in these terms. 'Multinodular carcinoma' was the name chosen by Friedell et al (1973) and this is considered to be one of the best synonyms in common use to describe this tumour. Friedell et al (1973) listed carcinoma NOS as a synonym, but it is best to use carcinoma NOS as a more comprehensive term to include the commoner stellate as well as the less common multinodular carcinoma: this is in accordance with the practice of Haagensen (1971) and of Fisher, Gregorio and Fisher (1975). Friedell et al (1973) also listed medullary carcinoma as a synonym, presumably because of the inclusion of medullary carcinoma by Lane et al (1961) in their 'well-delimited' carcinoma group, and possibly because of a looser usage of medullary carcinoma in the older literature when the term meant only a soft carcinoma, hence the old term 'encephaloid carcinoma of the breast'. It is crucial that 'medullary carcinoma with lymphoid infiltration' be given its rightful place as an independent entity along the lines clearly enunciated by Ridolfi et al (1977). The important clinicopathological differences between irregular and well-delimited carcinoma (Lane et al, 1961) should be re-examined after 'medullary carcinoma with lymphoid infiltration' and any other specific entities have been hived off: the markedly better prognosis of Lane's (1961) well-delimited carcinomas will probably be slightly diluted in this process. But, independently of the question of prognosis, multinodular carcinoma still deserves recognition not only in a descriptive sense, but also because of the imaginative work of Gallager and Martin (1969) suggesting that its mode of origin, progression and possibly its growth rate differs from that of stellate carcinoma.

The 'circumscribed infiltrating duct carcinoma associated with peripheral plasma cell infiltration' distinguished by McDivitt, Stewart and Berg (1968) constitutes a subtype of the multinodular carcinoma.

II. B. (2) MEDULLARY CARCINOMA WITH LYMPHOID INFILTRATION

The circumscribed carcinomas of a distinctive histological type require segregation as separate entities. One of these is medullary carcinoma with lymphoid infiltration. The criteria for its identification should be very strict and are fully discussed on page 286. 'Atypical medullary carcinoma', as defined by Ridolfi et al (1977), is probably worthy of separate recognition but this is still debatable. The alternative course consists of including it with the NOS carcinoma of multinodular type, but separate recognition as suggested by Fisher, Gregorio and Fisher (1975) is probably marginally to be preferred. Admittedly, as Ridolfi et al (1977) concluded, atypical medullary carcinoma is almost certainly composed of a heterogeneous group of tumours since the reasons for the designation 'atypical' vary from tumour to tumour. The argument is a very finely balanced one.

II. B. (3) MUCOID CARCINOMA

Another circumscribed carcinoma of distinctive histological type is mucoid carcinoma: synonyms include colloid carcinoma, mucinous carcinoma, gelatinous carcinoma and mucin-producing carcinoma. A tumour should be labelled mucoid or colloid carcinoma only if adequate sampling shows it to be *completely pure in composition*. Any mixture with, or transition to or from, carcinoma NOS alters the prognosis and possibly the treatment that will be adopted. *If a carcinoma consists of a mixture of mucoid carcinoma and carcinoma NOS, problems in classification arise.* If the mucoid component is only focal or relatively minor, the tumour should be classified as carcinoma NOS. If the mucoid component is substantial (? 25 per cent or more of the tumour), it is best classified under category 15 of mixtures of two or more types of invasive ductal carcinoma, under the heading of impure mucoid carcinoma or what some workers term 'mixed colloid carcinoma'. It must be pointed out that there is no accepted convention as to what proportion of a given tumour should be of colloid type in order that it qualifies for this category rather than for carcinoma NOS. This is the type of problem which arises with all tumour classifications and notably in the breast, the tumours of which are in general a good deal more difficult to classify than in many other organs.

II. B. (4) INFILTRATING COMEDOCARCINOMA

'Infiltrating comedocarcinoma' constitutes nearly 5 per cent of all infiltrating breast carcinomas treated by mastectomy (McDivitt, Stewart and Berg, 1968). It is a designation which takes into account the extent, and the nature, of the intraductal component, which is the dominant feature of the carcinoma, even though invasive carcinoma is also present. There are clinicopathological differences between this tumour type and carcinoma NOS which make its separate recognition desirable. There is a lower incidence of nodal metastases and a considerably higher survival rate with this type of carcinoma than with carcinomas NOS.

It was mentioned in discussing ductal carcinoma in situ that there is no particular merit in distinguishing comedocarcinoma as a type separate from the other varieties of in situ ductal carcinoma. Since McDivitt, Stewart and Berg (1968) consider 'non-infiltrating solid or comedocarcinoma' under a single heading, it would seem logical to follow the same procedure with the corresponding infiltrating types. Thus 'infiltrating solid or comedocarcinoma' could equally well constitute the full title of this tumour type. Presumably McDivitt, Stewart and Berg (1968) omitted the name 'solid' to avoid confusion. The term 'comedocarcinoma' is not open to any misinterpretation, which is precisely why it has stood the test of time. The term 'solid' is easily understood when applied to an intraductal carcinoma but is open to all sorts of misinterpretation in the context of an infiltrating tumour. Thus, in order to avoid confusion, the full name would have to be 'infiltrating carcinoma accompanying dominantly in situ solid or comedocarcinoma', which is clearly far too cumbersome. Nevertheless it must be understood that there is *no difference of substance between the solid and the comedo varieties of ductal carcinoma in situ* and that the two merge imperceptibly. The same is true when they are accompanied by invasive carcinoma, though, for logistic reasons, the name has to be abbreviated to 'infiltrating comedocarcinoma' in accordance with McDivitt, Stewart and Berg (1968).

II. B. (5) INFILTRATING 'PAPILLARY' (CRIBRIFORM) CARCINOMA

'*Infiltrating papillary carcinoma*' is slightly less easy to justify as a separate heading than the last tumour type discussed, not because it is less common, which it is, but because in attempting to define it one becomes entangled in very substantial difficulties of terminology. It is the name chosen by McDivitt, Stewart and Berg (1968). As with the preceding tumour type, the name takes account of the extent and nature of the intraductal component. This tumour is associated with a substantially better prognosis than carcinoma NOS and clearly requires some separate identification. In the writer's view, since this carcinoma is not papillary in its invasive phase and is more correctly termed cribriform in its in situ component, there is little justification for using this name. This is another example of the incorrect use of the term 'papillary', detailed in previous chapters. If the word 'cribriform' is substituted for 'papillary', the problem is largely resolved. This tumour should be labelled '*infiltrating cribriform carcinoma*' as long as it is understood that the cribriform architecture applies to the intraductal component, analogous to infiltrating comedocarcinoma, in which only the intraductal component has a comedo pattern. If this name is not entirely clear, the alternative is 'invasive carcinoma accompanying cribriform duct carcinoma', although the shorter version is obviously more desirable. In the context of this nomenclatural argument, it is pertinent to recall that the Committee on Tumour Nomenclature of the International Union Against Cancer (1965) recommended the use of the term 'cribriform carcinoma' for the lesion termed 'non-infiltrating papillary carcinoma' by McDivitt, Stewart and Berg (1968).

It might be pointed out here that at the time of writing (November 1978) the W.H.O. are considering a heading of 'intraductal carcinoma with invasion' for all invasive ductal carcinomas in which the in situ component constitutes at least 50 per cent of the epithelial tumour mass. This category would presumably include both infiltrating comedocarcinoma and infiltrating cribriform carcinoma. For the present, it is considered by the writer that the two groups are better kept separate along the lines indicated by McDivitt, Stewart and Berg (1968), if only because of the significantly different median survival of treatment failures in the two groups: 2.7 and 5 years for infiltrating comedo and cribriform carcinomas respectively (McDivitt, Stewart and Berg, 1968). This might indicate a slower growth rate of the cribriform carcinomas and a slower progression to death in those which prove fatal.

Tumour categories 6 to 15 should not generate too much controversy and, with the exception of category 12, are included in virtually all the classifications currently in use.

II. B. (6) TUBULAR CARCINOMA

Tubular carcinoma is a distinctive histopathological entity and few would argue against its specific recognition. It has been discussed in Chapter Ten.

Categories 7 to 10 could all be regarded as *metaplastic carcinomas*, though adenoid cystic carcinoma is not usually so considered.

II. B. (7) SQUAMOUS, SPINDLE-CELL AND SARCOMATOID CARCINOMA EXCLUDING THAT LISTED UNDER (8)

If one excludes apocrine carcinomas, the commonest type of metaplasia is squamous and spindle-cell differentiation and these metaplastic forms are frequently combined in the same tumour. Squamous, spindle-cell and pseudosarcomatous differentiation are discussed in Chapter Twelve. Carcinoma of the breast with sarcomatoid metaplasia is not synonymous with carcinosarcoma, as listed by Friedell et al (1973). *Pseudosarcomatous carcinoma of the breast is commoner than*, and must be sharply distinguished from, the extremely rare *true carcinosarcoma*, which is discussed in Chapter Fourteen.

Carcinomas of the breast with extensive giant-cell metaplasia are not common. Some belong in the category of carcinoma NOS, multinodular type, while a very few find their home in the medullary carcinoma with lymphoid infiltration niche. Particularly interesting but difficult are tumours with epulis-like or osteoclast-like giant cells. Very rarely these are seen in medullary carcinoma of the breast as in a case of McDivitt, Stewart and Berg (1968). In other cases, the osteoclast-like cells have been regarded as reactive stromal cells rather than neoplastic cells (Factor et al, 1977). The so-called adeno-osteoclastoma illustrated by Willis (1967) in his Figure 58 is in my collection: I regard it as quite unclassifiable as have other pathologists to whom I have shown this remarkable tumour. Carcinomas with osteoclast-like giant cells are discussed later in Chapter Twelve. Unless they are identifiably part of the rare carcinomas with cartilaginous and osseous metaplasia, I think they should be left as unclassified tumours and placed in Section VII.

II. B. (8) TUMOURS ANALOGOUS TO SIMILAR MALIGNANT TUMOURS IN OTHER ORGANS

Category 8 consists of tumours analogous to similar malignant tumours of the salivary glands and skin apart from those identified separately under categories 9 and 10. These are considered together in Chapter Thirteen. The most important tumours in category 8 are the carcinomas with cartilaginous and/or osseous metaplasia. Also included here is the malignant adenomyothelioma (Hamperl, 1970). Leiomyosarcoma of myoepithelial origin and certain other sarcomas and so-called carcinosarcomas probably also belong in this category.

II. B. (9) ADENOID CYSTIC CARCINOMA

Adenoid cystic carcinoma of the breast is an extremely rare but distinct entity. It must, under no circumstances, be confused with 'adenocystic patterns' in cribriform in situ carcinomas. It is discussed in Chapter Thirteen.

II. B. (10) APOCRINE CARCINOMA

Category 10 consists of apocrine carcinomas. The term 'apocrine carcinoma' is preferred to 'oncocytic carcinoma' for reasons discussed in Chapter Thirteen.

II. B. (11) LIPID-RICH OR LIPID-SECRETING CARCINOMA

Lipid-rich and lipid-secreting carcinoma are equally valid names for this tumour type. At present the writer uses the name in the sense used by van Bogaert and Maldague (1977) rather than in the more comprehensive sense of Fisher et al (1977a). It is important that this distinction be made since, in the more restricted sense, these tumours constitute only about 1.5 per cent of breast cancers, while, in the broader sense, they make up as much as 6 per cent of all breast cancers. There are also important morphological differences in routine preparations, and only further data can establish which definition is likely to be the more meaningful. The writer suspects that there is an overlap between apocrine and lipid-rich carcinoma, which is one reason for placing them in numerically adjacent categories: this still requires confirmation or refutation.

It should be noted here that 'lipid-rich carcinoma' is not to be equated with 'histiocytoid carcinoma', a point which will be amplified in Chapter Twelve.

II. B. (12) GLYCOGEN-RICH CARCINOMA

The glycogen-rich carcinoma is not usually separately identified. The writer has studied a few examples of this rare tumour type and has found them sufficiently distinctive to warrant considering whether they merit segregation. They are in general clear-cell carcinomas, often bulky and sometimes with extensive necrosis. The clear-cell appearance is sufficiently marked in most cases to make one pause and wonder about the possibility of metastatic carcinoma. They may have a superficial resemblance to renal carcinoma though they do not appear to be as vascular. An intraductal component is usually inconspicuous. Apart from the presence of abundant glycogen in well-fixed material and an absence of intracellular or extracellular mucin, some of these cancers are characterized by the presence of 'hyaline' intracytoplasmic globules which are strongly positive with PAS after diastase digestion and which contain lipoproteins: these globules are apparently identical to, and morphologically indistinguishable from, the globules which are so characteristic of some clear-cell renal carcinomas but which are not specific to them since they can be found more rarely in other types of carcinoma and also in certain sarcomas, e.g. liposarcomas. These clear-cell carcinomas usually have only a modest amount of stroma, elastosis is absent or inconspicuous, and they are composed of cellular sheet-like masses of neoplastic cells. They mostly are circumscribed and, if they are too rare or ill-defined to constitute a separate entity, they would best fit in the category of carcinoma NOS, multinodular type.

II. B. (13) JUVENILE (SECRETORY) CARCINOMA

Juvenile carcinoma is a distinct microscopic entity originally described, as the name implies, in childhood and early adolescence. Unfortunately, as happens so often with lesions given a name qualified by the prefix 'juvenile', they are frequently later recognized as occurring also in adult life. This happened for instance with the juvenile melanoma, later rechristened 'epithelioid and spindle-cell naevus' for at least two good reasons. Juvenile carcinoma has now been seen in 12 adult patients (including six merely referred to as a citation by Sullivan, Magee and Donald 1977). The six patients who have been specifically reported on were all aged below 30 years, having been selected in this way in the case of five of these six patients (Norris and Taylor, 1970). This occurrence of juvenile carcinoma in adults has naturally led to a search for another name, hence Norris and Taylor (1970) referred to them as carcinomas of the '*juvenile secretory type*' and Sullivan, Magee and Donald (1977) as '*secretory (juvenile) carcinoma*'. The name 'secretory carcinoma' adopted by Friedell et al (1973) presumably refers to the same entity. It is also not unlikely that eventually this type of carcinoma will be identified also in the fourth decade and the name 'juvenile' will appear even more inappropriate. However, in the search for a new name it is important that the partially inappropriate but at least distinctive name 'juvenile' should not be replaced by one like secretory carcinoma, which has already proven itself confusing. *Secretory, unqualified further, could be misunderstood* to be a reference to lipid-secreting carcinoma. Indeed when the writer found secretory carcinoma listed at the end of 'neoplasms of ductal epithelial origin' (Friedell et al, 1973), he understood it to mean lipid-secreting carcinoma, until further reading found a category of 'lipid-cell carcinoma'. The potential for confusion is even greater, for, in a recently circulated document of an international working party, the term 'secretory carcinoma' has been applied to a carcinoma found more frequently in children, which is said to be distinguished by having cells showing secretory activity of the type seen in pregnancy and lactation. While this is partly true, this description applies far more precisely to the third type of lipid-secreting carcinoma described by van Bogaert and Maldague (1977), an example of which is illustrated in Figure 12–18. If the name 'secretory carcinoma' were to replace juvenile carcinoma, there would be room for confusion with lipid-secreting carcinoma on these two counts.

It is suggested that the name 'juvenile carcinoma' be retained or, at most, *that it be modified only to juvenile (secretory) carcinoma* in order to avoid confusion. Besides, 'juvenile' has the additional merit that women in the third decade and perhaps approaching the fourth will mostly be flattered by the designation 'juvenile carcinoma' applied to their tumour. On a more serious note, they are more likely to be convinced of the excellent prognosis relating to this tumour if it is explained to them that it is a type of carcinoma which occurs mostly in young children, since even the lesser educated lay public is likely to be aware that carcinoma of the breast is not a disease which is known to kill children: the exceptions to this are so rare as barely to be known to the medical profession.

II. B. (14) CARCINOMAS WITH NOTEWORTHY CLINICAL MANIFESTATIONS OR THEIR PATHOLOGICAL EQUIVALENTS

This category of carcinomas exhibiting special clinical features is not strictly histopathological only, as with the other categories. It is composed of Paget's disease of the nipple and inflammatory carcinoma of the breast. Since the original clinical definitions were introduced, '*pathological equivalents*' have been found to exist even in the absence of the characteristic clinical findings. Thus, Paget's disease is sometimes found when a nipple block is examined microscopically as a routine procedure, in the absence of any clinical signs of it. This is frequently referred to as microscopic Paget's disease, as distinct from the clinically overt form.

Paget's Disease of the Nipple

Van Bogaert and Maldague (1978) argued that there was no real merit in reserving the name 'Paget's disease' for a peculiar type of spread of breast cancer which is not related to a particular histopathological type of cancer. While there is considerable logic in this, it can justifiably be argued that the mode of spread of a tumour is of some interest and that the circumstances in Paget's disease are unusual, to say the least. If the term is not universally accepted, it is certainly universally understood; indeed it is difficult to think of a name in breast cancer pathology which is less open to misunderstanding. Even some of the most commonly used names like scirrhous carcinoma and medullary carcinoma have different connotations for different workers. There is no single category from (1) to (13) which is totally devoid of the possibility of confusion, witness the problems which arise with adenoid cystic carcinoma, apocrine carcinoma, lipid-rich carcinoma, and the confusion revolving round the use of the term secretory carcinoma as a synonym for juvenile carcinoma.

Nevertheless, the basic tenet of van Bogaert and Maldague (1978), that Paget's disease of the nipple is not related to a special histopathological variant, is valid, and it could further be argued in their support that classification should depend on the nature of any invasive cancer present and, in the absence of this, that it will be classified as ductal carcinoma in situ. But the argument that appears to be overwhelmingly in favour of the opposite point of view is that *diagnostic pathology should not be practiced in a vacuum, that pathologists have to deal with clinicians and that, for these reasons alone, this specific term should be retained.* Invasive cancer accompanying Paget's disease should be classified as, say, carcinoma NOS (stellate)+Paget's disease, or infiltrating comedocarcinoma+Paget's disease, and so on, depending on the type of invasive cancer present. The first coding will satisfy those who lean towards the view of van Bogaert and Maldague (1978) while the second will satisfy those who wish to retain the name. The writer does not think he is being biased in his preference by any emotional attachment to the eponymous term.

Inflammatory Carcinoma: Dermal Lymphatic Carcinomatosis

Van Bogaert and Maldague (1978) argued for the abolition of the use of the term 'inflammatory carcinoma' in the classification of breast cancer. The main argument for the retention of the term 'Paget's disease' applies also, albeit with considerably less force, to the retention of the name 'inflammatory carcinoma'. It is true that, since the work of Saltzstein (1974), the presence of 'dermal lymphatic carcinomatosis' has achieved greater significance for pathologists, as it has become apparent that dermal lymphatic carcinomatosis is the pathological hallmark of surgical incurability of breast cancer. The finding of dermal lymphatic carcinomatosis appears to be more important than inflammatory appearances as a marker of surgical incurability (Ellis and Teitelbaum, 1974; Saltzstein, 1974). But there is still some doubt about the view of Ellis and Teitelbaum (1974) that inflammatory carcinoma, in the absence of dermal lymphatic carcinomatosis, may be amenable to surgical intervention. Other workers have, as will be explained in the relevant section, produced conflicting evidence. Until the matter is resolved, the name 'inflammatory carcinoma' had best be retained for pathological use, although it may well be deleted from the pathologist's vocabulary at a future date. The clinician will, of course, continue to use the term.

II. B. (15) MIXTURES OF TWO OR MORE OF THE TYPES OF IDC LISTED ABOVE (1 TO 14)

This category consists of *mixtures of any two or more of the types of IDC.* Thus, a carcinoma consisting of mucoid carcinoma+carcinoma NOS is catalogued here and the types of mixture noted; similarly with a mixture of, say, apocrine and lipid-rich carcinoma. On the other hand, Paget's disease with infiltrating carcinoma would not be placed here since Paget's disease per se is not an invasive carcinoma. Category 15 emphasizes the substantial limitations of tumour classifications and is a reminder that such classifications are only convenient but sometimes arbitrary man-made 'artefacts'. Carcinoma of the breast, in all its complexity, does not pay sufficient respect to our classifications!

A carcinoma should be categorized as of mixed ductal types only *if these are present within a single mass.* If there are two or more separate invasive carcinomas in a breast, they should be treated for purposes of classification as two distinct carcinomas, in the same way as one regards bilateral primary breast carcinomas as two tumours. Obviously with bilateral cancers it is usually easier to demonstrate that they are neither metastatic nor spatially connected. With two or more macroscopically discrete cancers in the same breast, it must be appreciated that, even when these are separated by several centimetres of apparently normal parenchyma, the two discrete nodules are sometimes found to be linked in continuity by in situ carcinoma. This is even more frequent when the apparently discrete carcinomas are situated close to each other. It is for this reason important that blocks be taken perpendicular to a line joining the centre of the two tumour nodules. This blocking procedure will demonstrate any connection present if the two invasive cancers are situated along the ramifications of the same major duct. If, however, the two cancers are based on different major branches of a segmental duct, blocks taken between the cancers and the nipple are in general more likely to demonstrate any continuity present.

III. INVASIVE CARCINOMA OF UNCERTAIN TYPE: DUCTAL OR LOBULAR

This category includes all cases of invasive carcinoma in which there is no certainty as to whether the carcinoma is of ductal or lobular type. There is a tendency to place these tumours with IDC because it is much the commoner tumour. The writer believes that the honest policy of admitting that one does not know is more rewarding and that it is wrong to force an invasive carcinoma into a ductal category when the basis for doing so either does not exist or is tenuous in the extreme. In practice I have been surprised at the relative frequency with which tumours need to be placed in Section III. This finding emerged in the course of trying to establish objective criteria for separating ILC from

IDC. At least *3 to 4 per cent of carcinomas were classifiable with certainty as invasive carcinoma but with no certainty as to whether of ductal or lobular,* or even of mixed ductal and lobular type. This is at variance with most of the literature, which suggests that there is little or no difficulty in separating IDC and ILC. Fisher and coworkers (e.g. Fisher et al, 1977b) are one of the few groups who have acknowledged experiencing similar difficulties.

Some of these problematical carcinomas will be mentioned briefly so that the reader can draw his own conclusions. In the first 100 consecutive carcinomas studied, there were two carcinomas with some structural and cytological features suggestive of the solid variant of infiltrating lobular carcinoma (Fechner, 1975). In the absence of independent corroborative evidence, the view that the tumours described by Fechner represent variants of ILC is still tentative; also, since our cases were not identical with those of Fechner (1975), it would be premature to classify them as ILC. But to place them with IDC at this stage of our knowledge would be equally wrong. One cannot judge the type of the invasive carcinoma from the type of the in situ component but, for what it is worth, one case had small foci of CLIS with minute foci of lobular cancerization also, while in the second case there were foci of lobular cancerization only. A third carcinoma in this series of 100 was a so-called lymphomatoid carcinoma: this tumour type has been regarded as both ILC and IDC in the literature, so again no conclusion could be drawn.

In another carcinoma, outside this series of 100, the tumour had features of both ductal and lobular carcinoma but these were not conclusive in either direction; we slightly favoured a ductal carcinoma, especially because of the presence of distinct tubular differentiation, but were already aware that focal tubular differentiation of a certain type could be found in ILC; after reading the work of Fisher et al (1977b) on 'tubulolobular carcinoma', we felt even less able to classify this case as IDC, though we still think it probably does belong there (Martinez and Azzopardi, 1979).

Signet-ring cell carcinomas sometimes represent variant forms of ILC, as previously discussed. However, I have seen one case of signet-ring cell carcinoma with widespread ductal involvement by tumour without detectable lobular involvement. It would be perverse in these circumstances to identify this case as a variant of ILC. In this carcinoma there was fairly extensive pagetoid spread by the signet-ring cells, so it is conceivable that it represents lobular carcinoma with dominantly ductal spread and no residual CLIS or so little that it was not detected. But since pagetoid spread can occur in ductal carcinoma also, and rarely can even be extensive (Toker, 1961), its presence does not rule out ductal carcinoma. And there is no a priori reason to believe that signet-ring cell carcinoma can never arise as a ductal type carcinoma. Indeed there is reasonable evidence that it can so arise. I have seen a few examples of colloid carcinoma mixed with signet-ring cell carcinoma and I have also seen a few instances of IDC accompanied by both colloid and signet-ring cell carcinoma. The former type of case suggests that some signet-ring cell carcinomas may represent a variant of IDC while the latter type of case suggests this possibility very strongly.

In view of these findings, it is almost certain that a category of signet-ring cell carcinoma should be separately recognized under Section II. Harris et al (1978) went further and concluded that signet-ring cell carcinomas are *all* variants of infiltrating ductal carcinoma on the basis of a similar ultrastructural pattern of mucin synthesis in colloid and signet-ring cell cancers. But while their study of the mechanism of mucin synthesis as it applies to various breast carcinomas is very valuable, it does not entirely resolve the question of the histogenesis of signet-ring cell carcinomas.

Harris et al (1978) reached their conclusion because they believed that other workers had identified signet-ring cells in lobular carcinoma merely on the basis of the finding of intracytoplasmic lumina. Steinbrecher and Silverberg (1976) appear to have identified signet-ring cells merely on this basis. Harris et al (1978) rightly regarded this as unjustifiable and indeed misleading. The writer agrees with Harris that neoplastic cells with intracytoplasmic lumina do not constitute signet-ring cells: the amount of mucin in signet-ring cells is vastly in excess of that present in cells containing intracytoplasmic lumina, and the morphological appearance of the two is different in H and E preparations and even more strikingly so in sections stained for mucin. The identification of signet-ring cells in invasive lobular carcinoma by the writer (Gad and Azzopardi, 1975; Martinez and Azzopardi, 1979) is based on the classical

well-known criteria. But the possibility remains that the signet-ring cells of lobular carcinoma contain mucin with a different localization from that of signet-ring cells in ductal carcinoma of the type illustrated by Harris et al (1978).

Pending further clarification of the origins of signet-ring cell carcinoma, it is best regarded as partly a variant of lobular and partly a variant of ductal carcinoma. It might be preferable to classify all signet-ring carcinomas together, following the course adopted by Friedell et al (1973), though this has the disadvantage that the recently discovered link between some signet-ring cell carcinomas and ILC is thereby lost sight of. If this course is, nevertheless, considered preferable these rare tumours could all be placed together in Section III, while recognizing that some belong in Section I, some in Section II, while others cannot yet be safely categorized. Further work, and ultrastructural study in particular, may enable one to identify differences between Section I and Section II signet-ring cell tumours, tumours which are indistinguishable, or virtually so, at light microscopic level.

There is also the problem of classification of the recently described *carcinoid tumours* (Cubilla and Woodruff, 1977). The little evidence to date indicates that they are more likely to be related to ductal than to lobular carcinoma but this is by no means certain in view of the question of a possible relationship between them and the so-called solid variant of ILC of Fechner (1975). In fact, Cubilla and Woodruff (1977) themselves reclassified two cases, previously diagnosed as ILC, as carcinoid tumours. In view of these doubts, carcinoid tumours should be categorized under Section III, pending further study. Eventually they will almost certainly require a category of their own, given their intrinsic interest and importance, their possibly distinct histogenesis and their potential metabolic activity (Kaneko et al, 1978).

IV. DEFINITE MIXTURES OF IDC AND ILC IN THE SAME TUMOUR MASS

Carcinomas composed in part of tumour with the definitive characters of IDC and in part of tumour with the definitive characters of ILC should be classified separately. One such carcinoma studied consisted partly of mucoid carcinoma with 'mucoid canceriza-tion' as well as more conventional types of lobular cancerization, and partly of signet-ring cell carcinoma with other features of invasive lobular carcinoma: a decidedly rare combination. Such a tumour can justifiably be classified as IDC (mucoid carcinoma)+ILC occurring within the same tumour mass. Another tumour consisted of tubular carci-noma and invasive lobular carcinoma, again meriting classification as IDC (tubular carcinoma)+ILC. Such carcinomas are un-common, or at least they can only rarely be so designated since, from what has been said under Section III, it is clear that the positive identification of IDC and ILC *within the same tumour mass* is only rarely possible. Thus, carcinomas will be classifiable in Section III considerably more frequently than in Section IV. There may, of course, be separate carcinomas within the same breast, some classifiable as IDC and some as ILC, but this does not represent a mixture of IDC and ILC within the one tumour mass.

V. CARCINOMA BORNE BY A FIBRO-ADENOMA OR CYSTOSARCOMA

This category includes *carcinoma of any type in a fibroadenoma or in benign cystosarcoma phyllodes*. It includes *only carcinoma in situ if it occurs in an overtly malignant cystosarcoma phyllodes* for reasons to be discussed.

There are two main problems here, an academic one and a more practical one. The academic one will be discussed first.

THE MORE ACADEMIC PROBLEM

Carcinoma of Any Type in a Fibroadenoma or Benign Cystosarcoma. Carcinoma, whether in situ or invasive and whether lobular or ductal, occurring in a fibroadenoma should be classified here; so also can any type of carcinoma occurring in a benign cystosarcoma phyllodes. There is no question of calling the latter a carcinosarcoma since the benign cystosarcoma phyllodes does not really qualify as a sarcoma in the accepted sense of this term. Hence the immense difficulties appertaining

to the nomenclature of this tumour, which are dealt with in Chapter Fourteen.

CLIS in a Malignant Cystosarcoma. The matter becomes rather more complex when one comes to consider carcinoma in a histologically overtly malignant cystosarcoma phyllodes. If CLIS is found in such a sarcoma, the combination might be regarded as meriting the name of carcinosarcoma even though the neoplastic epithelial ingredient is only in situ. But since there is still so much controversy over the essential nature of CLIS, and whether or not it should be elevated to the stature of a full carcinoma, CLIS in a setting of malignant cystosarcoma phyllodes does not justify a diagnosis of carcinosarcoma.

DCIS in a Malignant Cystosarcoma. A ductal type carcinoma in situ in a histologically overtly malignant cystosarcoma phyllodes is in a slightly different category since the carcinomatous nature of DCIS is not questioned by any authority. The finding of DCIS in a malignant cystosarcoma phyllodes is in fact extremely rare, especially if one includes only cases in which the malignancy of the epithelial component is not in any serious doubt and in which there is no room for concern that one is dealing merely with a very florid but non-malignant epithelial hyper-plasia. In this extremely rare situation a diagnosis of carcinosarcoma could be logically justified, but it is an accepted convention that tumours of this type are not labelled carcinosarcoma and the present writer agrees with the wisdom of this convention.

Invasive Carcinoma in Malignant Cysto-sarcoma is Not Classified Here. When invasive carcinoma is present in an overtly malignant cystosarcoma phyllodes, the criteria for the diagnosis of a true carcinosarcoma are fully satisfied and the tumour is placed in Section VI. Some workers wish to exclude even this type of tumour from the category of carcinosarcoma but I can see no reason for this, unless one has decided in advance either that carcinosarcoma does not exist at all or else that this name can be applied only to tumours arising de novo. The former position, though it is held by some very competent workers, is unjustified, as will be shown in the section on carcinosarcoma in Chapter Fourteen. The second alternative, that only carcinosarcomas arising de novo should be so labelled, is equally untenable. Such a policy would exclude five of the 15 acceptable carcinosarcomas of the breast reported since 1937, since these were considered to have originated in pre-existing cystosarcomas or fibroadenomas (see Chapter Fourteen), and some workers believe that more extensive study would have shown that an even greater proportion of carcinosarcomas than is indicated by these figures had actually originated in such a pre-existing tumour. The latter belief may or may not be realistic, but there is very little doubt that true carcinosarcomas exist and that they can originate in one of two ways. Both these types of genuine composite malignant tumour deserve the name carcinosarcoma in the strict histogenetic sense. But it remains to be said that carcinosarcomas of the breast are extremely rare and that if the genuine article is diluted by reports which lack the stamp of authenticity their very existence will continue to be denied.

In conclusion, carcinoma of any type in a fibroadenoma or in a benign cystosarcoma phyllodes is classified under Section V. In situ carcinoma, lobular or ductal, in malignant cystosarcoma phyllodes is also best placed in Section V. But invasive carcinoma within a malignant cystosarcoma phyllodes qualifies a tumour to be placed in Section VI.

THE MORE PRACTICAL PROBLEM

So far only the more academic problem has been dealt with, viz. when does a tumour in which carcinoma is contained within a cystosarcoma phyllodes qualify to be called a carcinosarcoma? *The more common problem in practice is the decision as to whether a carcinoma in a fibroadenoma or a cystosarcoma has originated there or has spread from without.*

There are three distinct possibilities. The commonest is the *invasion of the connective tissue of a fibroadenoma from without* by an invasive cancer. This is a not infrequent incidental finding during the examination of a mastectomy specimen containing an invasive carcinoma. This finding is of no special significance and requires no categorization.

The second possibility is *lobular neoplasia affecting the epithelium of a fibroadenoma or a cystosarcoma.* This most commonly takes the form of CLIS. This may or may not be accompanied by CLIS in the adjacent breast

tissue and, in the case of a fibroadenoma, there may be little or no tissue on which to assess the state of affairs in the neighbouring breast parenchyma. It will be shown later that CLIS is the type of neoplasm found most frequently restricted entirely or, at any rate, predominantly to the interior of a fibroadenoma. In some cases ILC will be found in the fibroadenoma or cystosarcoma, in others it can be found in the surrounding parenchyma. Fibroadenoma or cystosarcoma phyllodes bearing CLIS or ILC within its interior should be placed in Section V. The rare, fascinating, *argyrophilic endocrine-type tumours (?carcinoids)* contained within fibroadenomas, and described in Chapter Four, should also be classified in Section V. They are carcinoids or carcinoid-like tumours rather than CLIS or more conventional carcinomas. To allow for the recognition of such tumours in the future it might be desirable to alter the designation of Section V to 'Epithelial Neoplasms of all Types' rather than 'Carcinoma' arising secondarily in a fibroadenoma or cystosarcoma phyllodes.

The third possibility is the finding of *ductal type carcinoma in a fibroadenoma or cystosarcoma.* Ductal type carcinoma is found solely or even predominantly in the crevices of a fibroadenoma or cystosarcoma, very much less frequently than is CLIS. More usually there is carcinoma within the crevices of the fibroadenoma as well as in the adjacent tissues. In these cases the carcinoma may have originated outside the fibroadenoma and spread inwards, or it may have originated inside the fibroadenoma and spread outwards, or alternatively it may have had its origin simultaneously in both sites, as part of a wider field neoplastic change: these possibilities are discussed in the relevant section at the end of Chapter Twelve. Ductal type carcinoma in the epithelial crevices of a fibroadenoma, with or without invasion of the connective tissue, should, like lobular carcinoma, also be classified in Section V. It must be recognized, however, that with ductal carcinoma, as opposed to CLIS, the malignant tissue has in some (? many) cases probably extended from outside along the epithelial channels via the feeding ductules so that the involvement is not really a basic change in the fibroadenoma but only a secondary manifestation, dependent on changes occurring in the surrounding parenchyma. But since we cannot be certain in many of these cases, it is best to classify them in Section V.

VI. TRUE CARCINOSARCOMA

True carcinosarcoma must be diagnosed only after applying the most stringent criteria as described in Chapter Fourteen. Since this is both a carcinoma and a sarcoma it must be included in the classification of breast carcinomas as well as in the classification of sarcomas.

VII. UNCLASSIFIED CARCINOMAS AND POSSIBLE CARCINOMAS

An unclassified category should exist in any tumour classification, both because it is a practical and realistic necessity and also because it caters for future research. 'Unclassified' is preferable to 'unclassifiable' because a tumour which defies classification today may become classifiable in the light of further work.

In this category are *malignant tumours which it is not possible to classify with certainty as carcinomas rather than sarcomas*. If the differential diagnosis is between undifferentiated carcinoma and malignant lymphoma, electron microscopic study can sometimes provide the clinching evidence because of the absence of desmosomes in malignant lymphoma. Mucin stains can also be helpful in confirming a diagnosis of carcinoma. This is especially true of infiltrating lobular carcinomas and other carcinomas with prominent intracytoplasmic lumina. In the differentiation between carcinoma and sarcomas other than lymphoma, ultrastructural study should also sometimes provide an answer.

Tumours which cannot be categorized with certainty as carcinosarcomas, as opposed to carcinomas, should be placed here. This includes carcinomas with cartilaginous areas, in which an objective decision between metaplastic carcinoma and true carcinosarcoma is notoriously difficult and is not even a valid theoretical one according to Hamperl (1970) (see Chapter Fourteen).

A third group of tumours which cannot usually be classified with any ease is the *carcinomas which contain osteoclast-like giant cells in the absence of any osseous or cartilaginous metaplasia*. One such case of McDivitt, Stewart and Berg (1968) resembled a sarcoma closely but was finally traced to metaplastic change in a medullary carcinoma; the real nature of this lesion was only revealed to them after the study of numerous blocks of tissue. Epulis-like giant cells were also illustrated by McDivitt, Stewart and Berg (1968) in an infiltrating ductal carcinoma, but this must be a singularly rare event. In this last case the giant cells were regarded by these workers as fused cancer cells. Factor et al (1977), on the other hand, regarded the osteoclast-like giant cells in their carcinomas as stromal cells of histiocytic origin. The cancers of Factor et al (1977) and the so-called 'adeno-osteoclastoma' (Willis, 1967) studied by the writer certainly belong in the unclassified category.

A fourth group of tumours which is not easily classified consists of *the very rare mammary carcinomas which may simulate granular-cell 'myoblastoma' but run the course of a carcinoma* (McDivitt, Stewart and Berg, 1968). These are breast cancers which masquerade as granular-cell 'myoblastoma'. The myoblastoma-type cytological change remains almost as mysterious a phenomenon as it was 20 years ago. It is, however, certain that the identical or, at any rate, an indistinguishable cellular alteration can occur in a variety of tumours and lesions which are quite distinct from the granular-cell 'myoblastoma'. This is well exemplified by, for instance, the granular-cell ameloblastoma. McDivitt, Stewart and Berg (1968) mentioned that they had seen a very few instances of a breast carcinoma which was traced into an infiltrative granular cell pattern which cytologically resembled granular cell 'myoblastoma'. They warned against mistaking this extremely rare 'myoblastomatoid' carcinoma for the common or garden granular-cell 'myoblastoma', which does, of course, occur in the breast. The writer has not had the opportunity of examining an example of myoblastomatoid carcinoma.

Lastly, there are *the very rare but interesting cases in which even pseudotumour enters the differential diagnosis*. These are more likely to be confused with sarcomas, notably liposarcoma and fibroxanthosarcoma, than with carcinomas. In one such perplexing case, a largely fasciculated spindle-cell lesion contained a few small cystic spaces partially lined by very bland benign-looking squamous epithelium (? metaplastic, ? neoplastic). Originally diagnosed as a carcinosarcoma, the diagnosis was later revised to malignant fibrous histiocytoma by a leading North American pathologist. Another very competent pathologist regarded the lesion as a probable pseudotumour, a diagnosis considered very seriously by at least two other pathologists. The present writer and another surgical pathologist, on the other hand, regarded the tumour as a probable spindle-cell carcinoma which appeared to arise from the, admittedly seemingly innocuous, squamous epithelium present. The diagnostic problem in this case is outlined merely to emphasize how essential it is to have a category of unclassified tumours. Cases of this complexity and perplexity are not as rare in practice as one might gather from the literature. The diagnosable and classifiable is sometimes apt to receive more than its fair share of attention. Our attention needs to be directed to the undiagnosed and the unclassified cases since it is these which constitute the challenge for the future.

References

Cubilla, A. L. and Woodruff, J. M. (1977) Primary carcinoid tumor of the breast. A report of eight patients. *American Journal of Surgical Pathology*, **4**, 283–292.

Ellis, D. L. and Teitelbaum, S. L. (1974) Inflammatory carcinoma of the breast. A pathologic definition. *Cancer*, **33**, 1045–1047.

Factor, S. M., Biempica, L., Ratner, I., Ahuja, K. K. and Biempica, S. (1977) Carcinoma of the breast with multinucleated reactive stromal giant cells. A light and electron microscopic study of two cases. *Virchows Archiv A: Pathological Anatomy and Histology*, **374**, 1–12.

Fechner, R. E. (1972) Infiltrating lobular carcinoma without lobular carcinoma in situ. *Cancer*, **29**, 1539–1545.

Fechner, R. E. (1975) Histologic variants of infiltrating lobular carcinoma of the breast. *Human Pathology*, **6**, 373–378.

Fisher, E. R., Gregorio, R. M. and Fisher, B. (1975) The pathology of invasive breast cancer. *Cancer*, **36**, 1–263.

Fisher, E. R., Gregorio, R., Kim, W. S. and Redmond, C. (1977a) Lipid in invasive cancer of the breast. *American Journal of Clinical Pathology*, **68**, 558–561.

Fisher, E. R., Gregorio, R. M., Redmond, C. and Fisher, B. (1977b) Tubulolobular invasive breast cancer: a variant of lobular invasive cancer. *Human Pathology*, **8**, 679–683.

Foote, F. W., Jr and Stewart, F. W. (1941) Lobular carcinoma in situ. A rare form of mammary cancer. *American Journal of Pathology*, **17**, 491–496.

Friedell, G. H., Gallager, H. S., Hartmann, W. H., Hutter, R. V. P., Ozzello, L., Sommers, S. C. and Taylor, H. B. (1973) Standardized management of breast specimens. Recommended by Pathology Working Group, Breast Cancer Task Force. *American Journal of Clinical Pathology*, **60**, 789–798.

Gad, A. and Azzopardi, J. G. (1975) Lobular carcinoma of the breast: a special variant of mucin-secreting carcinoma. *Journal of Clinical Pathology*, **28**, 711–716.

Gallager, H. S. and Martin, J. E. (1969) Early phases in the development of breast cancer. *Cancer*, **24**, 1170–1178.

Gatchell, F. G., Dockerty, M. B. and Clagett, O. T. (1958) Intracystic carcinoma of the breast. *Surgery, Gynecology and Obstetrics*, **106**, 347–352.

Haagensen, C. D. (1971) *Diseases of the Breast.* Second edition — revised reprint. pp. 605–608. Philadelphia, London, Toronto: W. B. Saunders.

Hamperl, H. (1970) The myothelia (myoepithelial cells). In *Current Topics in Pathology*, Vol. 53. Berlin: Springer-Verlag.

Harris, M., Vasudev, K. S., Anfield, C. and Wells, S. (1978) Mucin-producing carcinomas of the breast: ultrastructural observations. *Histopathology*, **2**, 177–188.

Hood, C. I., Font, R. L. and Zimmerman, L. E. (1973) Metastatic mammary carcinoma in the eyelid with histiocytoid appearance. *Cancer*, **31**, 793–800.

International Union Against Cancer, Committee on Tumour Nomenclature and Statistics (1965) Berlin, Heidelberg, New York: Springer-Verlag.

Kaneko, H., Hōjō, H., Ishikawa, S., Yamanouchi, H., Sumida, T. and Saito, R. (1978) Norepinephrine-producing tumors of bilateral breasts. A case report. *Cancer*, **41**, 2002–2007.

Lane, N., Goksel, H., Salerno, R. A. and Haagensen, C. D. (1961) Clinicopathologic analysis of the surgical curability of breast cancers: a minimum ten-year study of a personal series. *Annals of Surgery*, **153**, 483–498.

Martinez, V. and Azzopardi, J. G. (1979) *Histopathology*, in press.

McDivitt, R. W., Stewart, F. W. and Berg, J. W. (1968) *Tumors of the Breast.* Atlas of Tumor Pathology, Second series, Fascicle 2. Washington, D.C.: Armed Forces Institute of Pathology.

Norris, H. J. and Taylor, H. B. (1970) Carcinoma of the breast in women less than thirty years old. *Cancer*, **26**, 953–959.

Ridolfi, R. L., Rosen, P. P., Port, A., Kinne, D. and Miké, V. (1977) Medullary carcinoma of the breast. A clinicopathologic study with 10 year follow-up. *Cancer*, **40**, 1365–1385.

Saltzstein, S. I. (1974) Clinically occult inflammatory carcinoma of the breast. *Cancer*, **34**, 382–388.

Silverberg, S. G. and Chitale, A. R. (1973) Assessment of significance of proportions of intraductal and infiltrating tumor growth in ductal carcinoma of the breast. *Cancer*, **32**, 830–837.

Steinbrecher, J. S. and Silverberg, S. G. (1976) Signet-ring cell carcinoma of the breast. The mucinous variant of infiltrating lobular carcinoma? *Cancer*, **37**, 828–840.

Sullivan, J. J., Magee, H. R. and Donald, K. J. (1977) Secrectory (juvenile) carcinoma of the breast. *Pathology*, **9**, 341–346.

Toker, C. (1961) Some observations on Paget's disease of the nipple. *Cancer*, **14**, 653–672.

Toker, C. and Goldberg, J. D. (1977) The small cell lesion of mammary ducts and lobules. In *Pathology Annual* (Ed.) Sommers, S. C. and Rosen P. P. Vol. 12, pp. 217–249. New York: Appleton-Century-Crofts.

van Bogaert, L.-J. and Maldague, P. (1977) Histologic variants of lipid-secreting carcinoma of the breast. *Virchows Archiv A: Pathological Anatomy and Histology*, **375**, 345–353.

van Bogaert, L.-J. and Maldague, P. (1978) Histologic classification of pure primary epithelial breast cancer. *Human Pathology*, **9**, 175–180.

Wellings, S. R., Jensen, H. M. and Marcum, R. G. (1975) An atlas of subgross pathology of the human breast with special reference to possible precancerous lesions. *Journal of the National Cancer Institute,* **55,** 231–273.

Wheeler, J. E. and Enterline, H. T. (1976) Lobular carcinoma of the breast in situ and infiltrating. In *Pathology Annual* (Ed.) Sommers, S. C. Vol. 11. New York: Appleton-Century-Crofts.

Willis, R. A. (1967) *The Pathology of Tumours.* Fourth edition. Figure 58, p. 216. London: Butterworth.

Chapter Twelve

Special Problems in Breast Pathology

1. GENESIS OF PAGET'S DISEASE OF THE NIPPLE

That Paget Cells are Altered Melanocytes

There are four main views requiring consideration. The first of these is the view that Paget cells represent altered melanocytes (Orr and Parrish, 1962); this hypothesis is partly based on the observation that Paget cells not infrequently are found to contain melanin. In deeply pigmented races melanin within Paget cells can be quite abundant, and this fact gave rise to the suspicion that Paget cells might represent altered melanocytes. In the view of the writer the melanin is derived from adjacent melanocytes. In support of their view Orr and Parrish claimed to have demonstrated dopa-oxidase activity within Paget cells. If the cells in question were indeed Paget cells, such enzyme activity was most likely the result of the ingestion of still functional melanosomes derived from melanocytes. The evidence against their view is so overwhelming that it need not be detailed here. Paget cells are not altered melanocytes.

That Paget's Disease is a Form of Squamous Carcinoma

The second view, championed especially by Willis (1967), is that Paget cells arise in situ from keratinocytes. Willis goes further and adduced evidence to suggest a transitional form between keratinizing in situ squamous carcinoma of the nipple and Paget's disease (Willis and Goldie, 1959). The latter case is not regarded as convincing by the writer. Nevertheless, the concept that in Paget's disease the epidermal changes *could* be primary and constitute part of a wide field of neoplastic change must be given serious consideration and will be returned to in considering the fourth view.

That Paget Cells are Adenocarcinomatous Cells

The third and fourth views have in common the belief that Paget cells are malignant cells of

258

adenocarcinomatous type lacking any relationship to Bowen's disease or to any other form of in situ squamous carcinoma. The third view is based on the fact that in almost all cases of adequately studied Paget's disease there is a ductal carcinoma involving one or more major ducts opening on to the nipple surface. Hence Paget cells are considered to be ductal carcinoma cells which migrate centrifugally within the nipple epidermis, i.e. Paget cells are held to be, as it were, 'foreign' neoplastic cells derived from a carcinoma of the galactophores, thus constituting a specialized type of epidermotropic cancer. *There are two main variants of this view,* depending on whether or not the more deeply situated carcinoma, often present in cases of Paget's disease at the time of clinical presentation, is regarded as usually of independent origin (Muir, 1939), or as a lesion continuous with the carcinoma in the large ducts of the nipple (Inglis, 1946, 1952). That these two lesions may be connected sometimes was admitted by Muir, and the fact that this can happen is suggested by the remarkable case of Toker (1961), who demonstrated continuity between the deep-seated lesion and the nipple lesion by single-cell permeation of a lactiferous duct — in other words a pagetoid spread in the ducts connected the deep cancer with the Paget changes of the nipple. But these variations on a theme do not alter all these workers' view that *the nipple lesion itself is caused by migration of cancer cells from the largest ducts.*

That Some Paget Cells have an In Situ Origin in the Epidermis

The fourth view proposes that Paget cells arise in situ (from keratinocytes or other cells) and differentiate into glandular malignant cells, with the ability, potential at any rate, to secrete mucin. It seems to the writer that the distinction between the third and fourth views is not as substantial as might appear at first sight. Tumours, especially glandular ones, are sometimes classified not according to the precise cells of origin, which are often unknown, but by their direction of differentiation. *It would not appear to matter materially, then, whether the stem cells of origin are in the last fraction of a millimetre of the galactophore, or 'round the corner' so to speak, just on the surface of the nipple* . Is it not reasonable to suppose that the last part of the galactophore (normally lined by keratinizing squamous epithelium),

as well as the epithelium on the nipple surface, may have a generative layer which is capable, in neoplastic conditions, of metaplastic change to adenocarcinomatous cells rather than giving rise to a squamous carcinoma? That the circumstances in Paget's disease are exceptional is not in any doubt. Most authors accept that there is an unusually wide field of tumour origin and that the vast majority of cases are associated with a cancer of a major duct opening on to the nipple. It seems a small step in conceptual thinking to conceive of the same process affecting the specialized epithelium of the nipple.

The Third and Fourth Views are Compatible with Each Other

The third view, tumour cell migration, has the widest support, but, from what has been said above, the fourth view is not a priori inconceivable. In fact the third and fourth views are quite compatible with each other. There is very strong evidence to support the migration view whilst there is a little evidence to support the possibility, at least, of an in situ origin of some Paget cells.

Other Evidence with a Bearing on Histogenesis

Two pieces of evidence which have come to light would seem, to varying degrees, to support the fourth and less popular mode of origin. *Firstly,* Toker (1970) described the remarkable finding of clear cells, sometimes in acinar formation, in 9 per cent of otherwise normal nipples examined routinely in breast cancer patients as well as in 12 per cent of nipples in a necropsy series. In fact, these benign clear cells have to be distinguished from Paget cells. So far the writer has failed to identify these cells but, if confirmation could be obtained, this would be a very important finding which, as Toker pointed out, could have an important bearing on the genesis of some cases of Paget's disease. *Secondly,* Sagebiel (1969) adduced interesting *ultrastructural evidence which might support an in situ origin of Paget cells.* He showed that neoplastic cells in the nipple epidermis which had clear desmosomal attachments to adjacent keratinocytes also showed microvillous differentiation on their surface. This observation, which was confirmed by Ozzello (1971), is suggestive of a local origin of Paget cells from cells of the keratinocyte series. The devil's advocate could still argue that the Paget cells migrated from elsewhere and established desmosomal attachments secondarily. If Sagebiel's finding is factually correct, and there is no reason to doubt it, there are two possible interpretations: firstly, that a cell of the keratinocyte population on the nipple surface has become neoplastic and, in the process, is showing evidence of glandular differentiation; or, alternatively, that migrating adenocarcinomatous cells, derived from a galactophore, secondarily established desmosomal attachments to keratinocytes of the nipple surface. The latter alternative would fit the most widely accepted view of the histogenesis of Paget's disease. The former alternative, which is just as easy to visualize, would lend support to the fourth and less popular view. *But the evidence remains inconclusive.*

The discovery that casein, or antigenically similar material, is produced by some mammary carcinoma cells may be significant in the present context. Bussolati and Pich (1975) demonstrated that, in 14 of 16 cases studied, casein was produced by Paget cells, and they imply that Paget cells produce casein more often than mammary cancer cells in general. Just as intriguing is these workers' claim to have identified casein in what they term 'pre-Paget' cells in the epidermis of the nipple, i.e. cells which on restaining, after photography in ultraviolet light, are not yet morphologically recognizable as Paget cells. It is too early to assess properly the significance of these fascinating findings. The apparent and unexpected presence of casein in sebaceous glands and other epidermal appendages is among the many features to be explained before the significance of these novel findings can be fully evaluated.

The present state of knowledge in relation to the histogenesis of Paget's disease of the nipple can be summarized as follows:

1. Epidermotropic carcinoma is now a well-established pathological concept.
2. That Paget's disease probably does represent a special variant of epidermotropic cancer must be accepted on general grounds and in view of the factual data as they apply to the breast.
3. The view that Paget's disease is a variant of Bowen's disease or any other form of squamous carcinoma must be completely rejected, as must also be the view that it is related to melanoma.
4. That Paget cells can *partly* arise in situ in the epidermis is not unlikely theoretically and has not been disproved. On the contrary, a few pieces of the evidence point to this *possibility* but conclusive proof is lacking. Such a mode of origin of Paget's disease would supplement the concept of epidermotropic spread and in no way supplants it.

2. ADENOMA OF THE NIPPLE

Synonyms

Papillary adenoma of the nipple, Florid papillomatosis of the nipple, Erosive adenomatosis of the nipple, Subareolar papillomatosis.

Historical Development of Knowledge and Correct Terminology

This rare but interesting condition was first formally described by Jones (1955) under the name of '*florid papillomatosis of the nipple ducts*'. He reported five cases as well as a sixth miniature lesion found incidentally, which he regarded as the preclinical form of the tumour.

Nichols, Dockerty and Judd (1958) described 16 cases and confirmed the findings of Jones (1955). Eleven of their patients were followed up for eight to 20 years and did not show any recurrence, thus demonstrating that the condition is essentially benign.

Handley and Thackray (1962) gave an excellent account of the condition, copiously illustrated both clinically and pathologically; of their nine patients, one had bilateral tumours. They questioned the designation of papillomatosis for this lesion on the grounds that while the tubules do show 'epithelial infoldings or even small stunted papillary ingrowths', in only two cases was there any intraduct papillary formation, and in neither of these was this more than a minor feature. Handley and Thackray (1962) suggested the name 'adenoma of the nipple' and this is certainly a more apt designation. Intraductal papillomas of the usual type may occur in a duct within the nipple itself and, rarely, these lesions may even extrude through the duct orifice (Figure 8–1). The term 'florid papillomatosis', apart from being descriptively inaccurate, has the additional disadvantage of causing confusion with true papillomas. Three of the five cases of Robert, De Brux and Winaver (1963) are conventional papillomas while their Cases 2 and 5 represent the entity described here. The over-use and abuse of the term 'papillary' in relation to epithelial hyperplasia in the breast in general has been discussed in Chapter Seven.

Taylor and Robertson (1965) also preferred the designation 'adenoma', while Perzin and Lattes (1972) compromised with the designation 'papillary adenoma'. In 12 of their 65 cases, including two cases sectioned serially, they found in addition a typical intraductal papilloma, usually deep to the adenoma. The association of these two lesions appeared more than fortuitous and they suggest, with some justification, that serial sections might well have revealed an intraductal papilloma in further cases. The term 'papillary adenoma' is a legitimate alternative to adenoma. However, Perzin and Lattes go on to stress that 'papillary adenoma of the nipple should be considered as a separate clinicopathologic entity as compared to intraductal papilloma' and emphasized that papillomas do not mimic Paget's disease clinically. They stressed that in papillary adenoma 'there is an active proliferation of new ducts and ductules growing into the stroma of the nipple', which is not seen in ductal papilloma.

To sum up, 'adenoma' and 'papillary adenoma' both characterize this distinctive lesion and both terms are descriptively accurate: the former term is regarded as the more appropriate. In contrast, the term 'florid papillomatosis' is not descriptively apt, and has the additional disadvantage of causing confusion with conventional ductal papilloma (Figure 8–1). 'Erosive adenomatosis' of the nipple is favoured by some workers because it alludes to the clinical as well as to the pathological features (Le Gal, Gros and Bader, 1959; Miller and Bernier, 1965; Smith, Kron and Gross, 1970).

Clinical Data

Adenoma of the nipple has been observed in teenagers as well as in elderly women but the condition usually affects women in middle age, with a peak incidence in the fourth and fifth decades. Nipple adenoma has even been described in a nine-year-old girl (Miller and Bernier, 1965). The most common clinical presentation is a nipple discharge, which is often blood-stained, associated with a crusted nipple which may be swollen or indurated, and may be accompanied by irritation, itching or burning sensations or actual pain. The latter symptoms were common in the series of Taylor and Robertson (1965) but rare in the series of Perzin and Lattes (1972). Pain was recorded by the latter authors in only one of 51 symptomatic patients, at any rate as a presenting symptom. The duration of symptoms varied between only a few weeks and many years, with an average in Handley and Thackray's (1962) series of five and one-half years.

Physical Examination and Usual Clinical Diagnosis Made

On examination the nipple may appear enlarged, firm and indurated. It may appear to be ulcerated (but see 'Pathology', below) or reddened and crusted and has been recorded as being fissured. A lump may be palpable either within the nipple or deep to it. Clinically, the lesion cannot be distinguished from Paget's disease with any certainty. All workers are agreed that the most common surgical diagnosis is Paget's disease and that the correct diagnosis can be established only by histological examination.

Pathology

The low-power impression is of a relatively well circumscribed nodule in the nipple region, which may reach the epidermal surface, replacing it over a small or even over a large area (Figure 12–1). This is the main reason for the clinical impression in many cases of ulceration or fissuring of the nipple surface. The 'ulcerated' area frequently represents exposed tumour covered by the same type of epithelium as is found in the tumour tubules (Handley and Thackray, 1962). However, if there has been trauma or

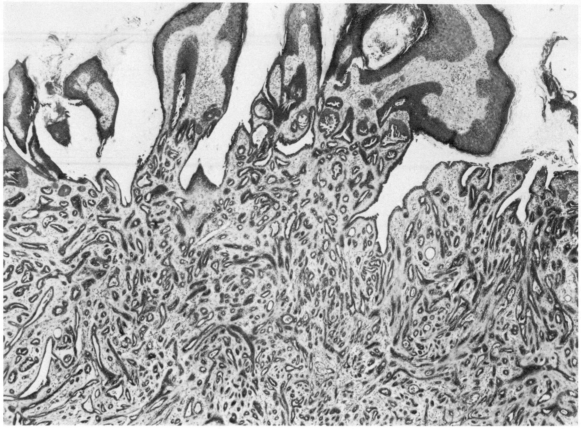

Figure 12–1 Adenoma of the nipple showing continuity with the stratified squamous epithelium on the surface. Intense adenomatous proliferation. H and E. ×40.

infection, a true ulcer with a granulation tissue floor may be present. The main ducts of the breast may traverse the tumour but are sometimes displaced to one side.

At a slightly higher magnification, it becomes evident that the lateral margins of the tumour may be somewhat ill-defined. The main bulk of the lesion has an oedematous structure but solid portions may make up a significant part of it. Basically there is an extensive proliferation of *two-layered tubules*, which ramify extensively in the nipple stroma (Figures 12–1 to 12–3). These have an outer, flattened to cuboidal layer of myoepithelial cells, and an inner layer of cuboidal or more usually tall columnar cells. Solid cellular areas were present in addition in 12/29 cases studied by Taylor and Robertson (1965). Tumours

with a prominent solid component are more likely to give rise to problems in the differential diagnosis from cancer. Jones (1955) described the solid component as consisting of polygonal cells interposed between the myoid cells and the tall columnar epithelial cells, while Taylor and Robertson (1965) regarded it as made up of a proliferation of the inner epithelial cells which fill the tubular lumina. Whatever the precise nature of these cells, their differentiation from malignant cells is of paramount importance. They are uniform in appearance, with little or no pleomorphism and no nuclear hyperchromasia (Figure 12–3). Their ovoid nuclei are also uniform, without heavy chromatin markings and with usually inconspicuous or small nucleoli (Figure 12–3). Occasionally

---

Figure 12–2 (*Opposite, above.*) Nipple adenoma. Dense proliferation of glands in connective tissue of nipple. Two cell types are variably conspicuous even within the same lesion. H and E. ×150.

Figure 12–3 (*Opposite, below.*) More solid parts of adenoma of nipple can be confused with an infiltrating carcinoma, especially on frozen section. H and E. ×400.

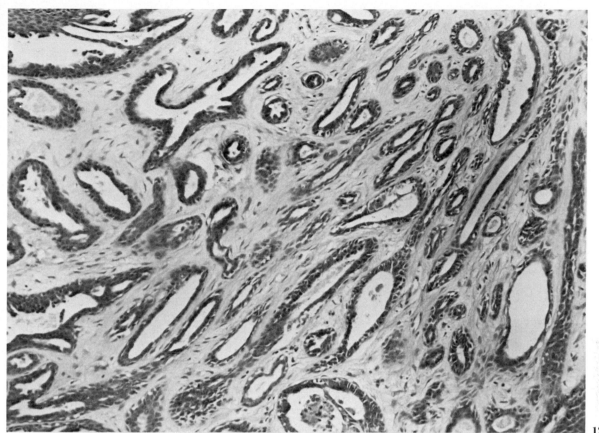

12-2

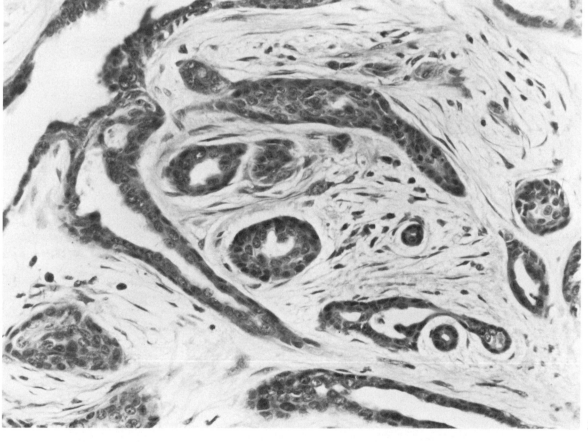

12-3

nucleoli can be prominent (Perzin and Lattes, 1972, and see Miller and Bernier, 1965). These solid areas, in association with a dense sclerotic stromal reaction which is frequently present, can mimic infiltrating carcinoma rather closely and this is especially true when the stromal reaction distorts the adenomatous and other epithelial structures. It should be stressed that papillary areas (strictly defined; see the introductory section on nomenclature) are usually inconspicuous. They were only a minor feature in 2/9 cases of Handley and Thackray (1962), and Perzin and Lattes (1972) found an associated ductal papilloma, usually deep to the main lesion, in 12/65 of their cases.

Other Epithelial Elements. Apocrine elements were described in 4/29 cases by Taylor and Robertson (1965) and in 15/65 cases collected by Perzin and Lattes (1972). These authors stressed that, when present at all, apocrine metaplasia is usually a focal and inconspicuous change. More common, and more conspicuous, is the presence of cysts lined by squamous cells or of foci of squamous epithelium. These features were present in 17/29 cases studied by Taylor and Robertson (1965) and in 21/65 in the series of Perzin and Lattes (1972). Squamous epithelium is most commonly observed in the superficial part of the lesion (Figures 12–1 and 12–2). It should be recalled, in this connection, that the last part of the galactophore is normally lined by keratinizing squamous epithelium and that the changes observed may sometimes represent merely an exaggeration of the normal features. There may in addition be squamous differentiation in newly formed adenomatous structures. Conversely, the nipple epidermis may be partly replaced by the glandular epithelium of the tumour (Figure 12–1). The relationship of the neoplastic tubules to the surface epithelium can be a complex one and it is well described and depicted by Handley and Thackray (1962).

Divergent Differentiation into Myoepithelial and Epithelial Tissue. The varied patterns seen in this tumour should be interpreted as representing divergent differentiation into myoepithelial and epithelial elements. The tumours bear a resemblance to hidradenomas, especially to syringadenoma papilliferum and to hidradenoma papilliferum. Taylor and Robertson (1965) outlined the histological differences and stressed how infrequently either of these skin appendage tumours involves the skin of the breast.

Distinction from Carcinoma. The most important distinction, however, is from carcinoma, and now that this rare entity is generally recognized, there is usually little difficulty in distinguishing it from a well-differentiated breast carcinoma. Necrosis is almost always absent, an important negative point. It was present in only a single tumour in the series of Taylor and Robertson (1965), occurring beneath an area of ulceration and infection and involving stroma as well as epithelium, i.e. necrosis was not an inherent attribute of the neoplastic epithelium but a mere consequence of ulceration. Necrosis was likewise noted only once in the huge series of 65 cases studied by Perzin and Lattes (1972) but its exact localization was not stated. Calcification has so far not been recorded in this tumour, and the lack of anaplasia and nuclear hyperchromasia have already been commented on. The only type of pleomorphism exhibited by the nipple adenoma is that of divergent differentiation and the most important single criterion in recognizing this feature is the presence of the two-cell-type differentiation in the glandular structures. This is often easily detected; in other cases, and especially in more solid areas, it may have to be searched for very diligently. The nature of the lesion must be judged on the overall pattern and not on isolated high-power fields.

Mitoses may be Numerous. A note of caution should be sounded regarding the presence of mitoses. Taylor and Robertson (1965) found them in 19/29 lesions and, though they were usually infrequent, they were fairly numerous in four of their cases. One should beware of attaching too much significance to abundant mitoses, particularly when present in the most superficial part of the lesion. In this region, in the presence of an inflammatory reaction, and in an area where columnar and squamous epithelium meet and one was possibly in the process of replacing the other, the writer has seen as many as five normal mitoses in a single high-power field in an otherwise perfectly orthodox adenoma of the nipple.

Behaviour of the Lesion

The vast majority of nipple adenomas are perfectly benign lesions. Nineteen out of 29 patients in the Taylor and Robertson (1965) series were treated by local excision. In only one patient was there recurrent or persistent tumour, which required two re-excisions; she was reported alive and well 17 months after the last operation. The writer has seen a similar recurrence, or persistence, 20 months after the first operation and the patient was well 24 months after a second local resection. Handley and Thackray (1962) advised excision of the nipple and areola, together with an underlying wedge of breast tissue, as the treatment of choice. They did not regard attempts at local resection, with preservation of the nipple, as a satisfactory procedure because the duct system is destroyed, the nipple is left deformed and there can be no certainty that the whole tumour has been excised. In Perzin and Lattes' (1972) series of 29 symptomatic cases, 14 were treated by local excision only while six were treated by partial and nine by total resection of the nipple. There was only one instance of local recurrence among the 14 patients treated by local excision. This 'recurrence', which was regarded as almost certainly persistent tumour rather than a true recurrence, was treated by a wider resection and the patient was well eight years later. These workers, unlike Handley and Thackray (1962), regarded simple local excision as an acceptable alternative to partial or total excision of the nipple. These are minor variations of operative technique which are best left for surgeons to debate.

Occurrence in Male Patients

The lesion also occurs in the male. Three cases of adenoma of the nipple in male patients were described by Taylor and Robertson (1965), and Waldo, Sidhu and Hu (1975) found three others in the literature and added a seventh; their patient developed the adenoma 10 years after starting treatment with diethylstilboestrol for carcinoma of the prostate. The writer has studied a further case of adenoma of the nipple in a man. It does not differ pathologically from the lesion as it affects women.

MALIGNANCY WITH ADENOMA OF THE NIPPLE

Rare Examples of Malignant Change. Up to 1971 it was generally accepted that the adenoma of the nipple is a completely innocuous lesion. While it remains true that the overwhelming majority of these tumours are innocent, very rare exceptions do occur. Gudjónsdóttir, Hägerstrand and Östberg (1971) reported the first case of malignant change in an adenoma of the nipple. This lesion proved fatal and at necropsy there were widespread metastases in axillary and other nodes, liver, vertebrae, spleen and kidney. The case is extremely well documented and the evidence presented is crisp and convincing. Bhagavan, Patchefsky and Koss (1973) reported two further cases of malignant change in nipple adenomas. Their two patients were treated by mastectomy but no nodal metastases were present; both in situ and infiltrating carcinoma were present in the nipple lesions. The reported cases of carcinomatous change in adenoma of the nipple are tabulated (Table 12–1).

Coexistence of Breast Carcinoma in Patients with Nipple Adenoma. An entirely different problem is the coexistence of breast carcinoma

Table 12–1   Carcinomatous change in nipple adenoma

Author and year	Age	Course of disease and comments
Gudjónsdóttir, Hägerstrand and Östberg (1971)	56 years	Fatal. Widespread metastases in lymph nodes, bones, liver, spleen, kidney
Bhagavan, Patchefsky and Koss (1973) (Case 1)	43 years	Mastectomy. Residual ductal and infiltrating carcinoma. Nodes negative
Bhagavan, Patchefsky and Koss (1973) (Case 2)	67 years	Mastectomy. Residual extensive ductal carcinoma, with infiltration at some distance from nipple adenoma. Nodes negative

in patients with a nipple adenoma. In the series of Jones (1955), Nichols, Dockerty and Judd (1958), Handley and Thackray (1962), Taylor and Robertson (1965) and Perzin and Lattes (1972) there were 0/5, 1/16, 1/9, 0/29 and 3/40 cases respectively of independent carcinoma, ipsilateral or contralateral (the last figure of 40 patients is derived from Perzin and Lattes by adding together their own 29 symptomatic cases and 11 cases seen in consultation in whom follow-up was obtained). Thus a total of five independent breast cancers were discovered in 99 patients with an adenoma of the nipple. Perzin and Lattes (1972) suggested that the incidence of independent breast cancer is no higher than one might expect in the population involved.

True, Jones (1955) found a miniature adenoma of the nipple as an incidental finding in a patient with carcinoma of the breast and Perzin and Lattes (1972) studied no fewer than nine such cases but, when it is appreciated that these were discovered 'in a series of several thousand carcinomas of the breast', one must agree with Perzin and Lattes (1972) that this may well be merely a coincidental association. At present the main dissenters are Fisher, Gregorio and Fisher (1975); this group of workers examined 967 nipples from patients with breast carcinoma and, rather surprisingly, found that as many as 12 (1.2 per cent) contained some degree of 'florid papillomatosis'. Further data are awaited.

3. PURE DUCTAL CARCINOMA IN SITU (DCIS)

Incidence of DCIS Among Breast Carcinomas. The diagnosis of pure in situ ductal carcinoma is a very satisfying one, since the cure rate at this stage of the disease is extremely high. The incidence of DCIS among mammary carcinomas as a whole varies somewhat in different series. These variations depend to some extent on the strictness of the criteria employed to make this diagnosis, but other, even more important factors are involved. Silverberg and Chitale (1973) found 14 cases of DCIS among 398 breast carcinomas, an incidence of 3.5 per cent comparable with the 3.3 per cent figure of Wulsin and Schreiber (1962) reported a decade previously. Farrow (1970) reported a 3.7 per cent incidence at the Memorial Hospital for the years 1964 to 1967. These incidence figures are a little lower than the 5.6 per cent found by Kouchoukos, Ackerman and Butcher (1967).

Rising Incidence of DCIS and its Causes. Millis and Thynne (1975) found that, with the increased use of mammography, *more cases of DCIS are being detected because of microcalcification.* This is borne out by the data of Lagios, Margolin and Rose (1977), in whose series 17 out of 25 cases of DCIS (68 per cent) were clinically occult, xeromammographically identified lesions. Lagios, Margolin and Rose (1977) had an incidence of DCIS of 25 cases among 249 of combined

DCIS and invasive carcinomas, an incidence of 10 per cent. These cases were collected over a three and one-half year period commencing in 1974. The incidence of DCIS reached a peak figure of 19.7 per cent during 1976, a very high figure indeed. This peak may be partly attributable to chance clustering but it could also be due in part to screening of a high-risk population, e.g. women with a strong family history of breast cancer. In the work of Moskowitz et al (1975), a preliminary report on 207 biopsies performed in 4128 volunteer screenees indicated that 33 per cent (12/36) of the carcinomas detected were non-invasive carcinomas of ductal type. It will be interesting to follow the reports from other centres with screening programmes over the next few years. It is predictable that there will be an increase of DCIS as a percentage of total breast carcinomas but it remains to be seen whether any increase is maintained over a long period or begins to drop after a few years of intensive screening. Collection of such information should provide a useful indication of the natural history of DCIS.

Is Radiologically Detected DCIS Clinically Important? With this increased identification of DCIS the problem arises as to whether more cases of ductal carcinoma, which would ordinarily have presented as clinical cancers, are being detected earlier or whether, possibly, these cases detected radiologically form a separate disease entity which would have remained in situ for a very long time, were it not for the radiological investigation that led to their identification and removal (Millis and Thynne, 1975). Silverberg and Chitale (1973) found no tendency towards a lower mean age for women with pure or predominantly intraductal growth, which might have suggested to them a slow natural evolution toward infiltrating ductal carcinoma. On the other hand, Lagios, Margolin and Rose (1977) found a mean age about six years lower than for invasive cancer. At least *three possibilities deserve consideration*: that DCIS, including radiologically detected DCIS, might, if left to itself, follow a rapid course to invasive cancer, a possibility consistent with the data of Silverberg and Chitale (1973): that DCIS has a natural history in terms of years if left to itself, as is perhaps suggested by the data of Lagios, Margolin and Rose (1977): or, thirdly, that it has such a long dormant in situ phase that, though it may represent a cancer biologically, it is of little clinical concern to most patients in whom it is detected. This last intriguing possibility is hinted at by Millis and Thynne (1975). *On present information, we should regard the first two possibilities as the more likely,* with the emphasis perhaps on the second. These alternatives are probably not mutually exclusive but we do not know whether, if two or all three are correct, each group forms a more or less distinct entity or represents part of a spectrum of disease with a corresponding spectrum of behaviour. Certainly, it would be wise at present to *regard all of it as cancer of potential clinical significance* until evidence to the contrary is forthcoming.

Comparison of Intraductal Carcinoma and Invasive Carcinoma: Patient Age and Duration of Symptoms. Westbrook and Gallager (1975), in an important study, compared 64 patients with intraductal carcinoma with a control group of 64 patients with invasive breast cancer. They compared the clinical characteristics of the patients, the clinical manifestations of the disease and other important features. The average age of the patients with intraductal carcinoma was 54.7 years and of those with invasive carcinoma 57.9 years ($0.1 < P < 0.2$). This difference of three years in mean patient age is intermediate between that found by Silverberg and Chitale (1973) and that found by Lagios, Margolin and Rose (1977). The difference did not reach statistical

significance. Westbrook and Gallager (1975), however, drew a different conclusion from that drawn by Silverberg and Chitale (1973). The former workers found that the duration of symptoms was longer in patients with intraductal carcinoma (14.1 *v.* 9.0 months, with $P < 0.05$). They stated that because the patient age distribution was similar and the duration of symptoms longer, these data imply that 'the lesions detected clinically before invasion were more slowly progressive and had longer pre-invasive periods'. This may well be true but the evidence is still conflicting, and their data are open to a number of interpretations. This very complex problem does not appear to be capable of resolution on the currently available information. There is more evidence to support the conclusion of Westbrook and Gallager (1975) that the time necessary for conversion of intraductal carcinoma to invasive tumour probably varies widely from patient to patient.

Lump, Localized Thickening and Nipple Discharge in DCIS. Millis and Thynne (1975) studied 28 patients with DCIS. Emphasis in the past has been mainly on presentation with a nipple discharge, but interestingly, in this series, no fewer than 24 patients presented with a clinical mass. Nevertheless, nipple discharge or bleeding was a symptom in eight patients. About one-quarter, or a little more, of all patients with DCIS have a nipple discharge which is usually bloodstained; this is frequently accompanied by localized thickening of the breast tissue or a more definite lump.

Comparison of Clinical Signs in Patients with Intraductal and Invasive Carcinoma. Westbrook and Gallager (1975) compared the clinical signs of intraductal and invasive carcinoma. A discrete or questionable mass was present in 75 per cent of the in situ cases compared with 96 per cent of the invasive tumours. The lesion was central (subareolar) in 52 per cent of the in situ and only 16 per cent of the invasive tumours. This suggests that symptoms are more likely to be produced prior to invasion when the lesion is centrally located. Another major difference was in the frequency of nipple abnormalities. Some nipple abnormality was present in 58 per cent of the in situ as opposed to 24 per cent of the invasive cancers. Nipple discharge was present in 28 per cent compared with 11 per cent, and Paget's disease was found in 25 per cent of

DCIS compared with a mere 1 per cent with invasive cancers. It should be noted that most of the patients in this series were seen *prior to the introduction of mammography as a screening procedure. This applies also to most other series.*

Contralateral Carcinoma. Two of the 28 patients of Millis and Thynne (1975) had bilateral DCIS. There was a 10 per cent incidence of contralateral invasive carcinoma in the series of Brown et al (1976). This included tumours removed both before (three) and after (one) the diagnosis of the intraductal carcinoma. Westbrook and Gallager (1975) found a *minimum* incidence of 12.5 per cent of contralateral cancer subsequent to the detection of the intraductal carcinoma (patients with previous or concurrent invasive carcinoma in the other breast were excluded in this study). This figure of 12.5 per cent is regarded by them as a minimum figure, since data regarding the contralateral breast were only fragmentary and no particular effort had been made to detect new contralateral carcinomas. Indeed the eight contralateral cancers, on which the figure of 12.5 per cent (8/64) is based, were detected among only 14 contralateral breast biopsies. Of these contralateral cancers five out of eight were in situ only. Thus, there was a 7.8 per cent incidence of subsequent development of contralateral in situ carcinoma, comparable to the 7 per cent incidence of Millis and Thynne (1975) in a smaller series, and a 4.7 per cent incidence of contralateral invasive cancer. Westbrook and Gallager (1975) stressed the relative frequency of contralateral carcinoma. In the series of Ashikari, Hajdu and Robbins (1971) there was prior, simultaneous or subsequent carcinoma in the contralateral breast in no fewer than 31.9 per cent of patients. This very high figure is not far short of the 36.5 per cent bilaterality quoted for LCIS (CLIS) in the same report. Though considerable weight must be attached to the report of Ashikari, Hajdu and Robbins (1971), if only because of the size of their series (112 patients), an element of selection cannot be entirely excluded.

FROZEN SECTION DIAGNOSIS

The diagnosis of DCIS on frozen sections can be very difficult and it was achieved in only 57 per cent of 112 patients at a specialized institute with a very major interest in this field (Ashikari, Hajdu and Robbins, 1971). This is, nevertheless, very much better than the accuracy of diagnosis in CLIS on frozen section: only 18 per cent accuracy for the latter as opposed to 55 per cent for DCIS in the later paper of Ashikari, Huvos and Snyder (1977). If there is any doubt about the malignancy of the lesion, paraffin sections should always be awaited before a definitive diagnosis of DCIS is made.

NUMBER OF BLOCKS NEEDED TO EXCLUDE INFILTRATION

Before a pathologist makes a diagnosis of pure DCIS, he has the problem of deciding in each case the number of blocks needed to exclude with reasonable confidence the presence of infiltration at one or more points. There are no hard and fast rules rules but six blocks are usually deemed to be the bare minimum required (McDivitt, Stewart and Berg, 1968). Silverberg and Chitale (1973) suggested that the eight to 10 or more blocks examined by them are at least desirable if not essential. This is especially true if treatment is going to be modified by the precise pathological report: it is only academic if the surgeon responsible treats DCIS as he would an invasive cancer. An average of 11 blocks was examined in the series of Ashikari, Huvos and Snyder (1977) but there is a limit to the sampling which can be undertaken in most laboratories and the practical limit should be determined by the increased yield of invasion which is likely to be detected through increased sampling, and by whether or not the treatment will be limited and tailored by the pathology report. The latter point can be determined easily enough by collaboration between pathologist and surgeon. The question of an increase in yield of invasive disease with more extensive sampling is more difficult to determine precisely but some data are available.

The necessity for fairly extensive sampling was shown by the work of Gillis, Dockerty and Clagett (1960). After selecting 50 cases of apparently pre-invasive carcinoma, 'many' further blocks were taken from the specimens and 14 out of the 50 lesions were found to be invasive at this second appraisal. Another informative study is that of Kouchoukos, Ackerman and Butcher (1967): when their diagnoses of DCIS were based on an average of only 3.2 sections per case, no fewer than three of 24 patients had nodal metastases in the presence of an *apparently* pure in situ carcinoma. On further sampling, however, two of these three patients were found to have stromal invasion in their primary tumours, giving a corrected incidence of nodal metastases of only one case among 22 patients with apparently pure DCIS. This does indicate that three or four blocks are inadequate for the purposes considered here. Empirically, *McDivitt, Stewart and Berg (1968) found that six blocks was an effective and practical number, but the eight or more recommended by Silverberg and Chitale (1973) are considered desirable*, especially if the surgeon is going to omit even low axillary dissection when faced with a diagnosis of pure DCIS. In any case it is essential that the surgeon understands that *the pathologist can never give an absolute guarantee* of the absence of microscopic stromal infiltration and, as will be seen later, this is even more true at the ultrastructural level.

RISK OF OCCULT INFILTRATION AND POSSIBILITY OF NODAL METASTASIS WITH DIAGNOSIS OF DCIS

If the pathologist makes a diagnosis of DCIS on the basis of examining, say, eight to 10 blocks, what advice should he give the surgeon in terms of the patient's prognosis in general and the possibility of axillary nodal metastases in particular? The incidence of nodal metastasis from apparently pure DCIS varies in different series from less than 1 per cent to as much as 7 per cent. Gillis, Dockerty and Clagett (1960) found only a solitary case with nodal metastases among 36 patients. Interestingly, only one slide was available for study in this case and it was also the only tumour which fell into their histological grade 4 category. This is an incidence of only 3 per cent and it is based on a case which was very inadequately sampled by any current standards. Ashikari, Hajdu and Robbins (1971) found axillary node involvement at level 1 in only one out of 113 specimens, an incidence of less than 1 per cent. On the other hand, Kouchoukos, Ackerman and Butcher (1967) had a 4.5 per cent incidence based on one patient among 22 with nodal metastases. The highest figure in the recent literature is that of Dossett (1976); he found nodal metastases in 7 per cent of 115 patients. Dossett referred exclusively to comedocancers and it is just possible that this selection influenced the results, a possibility discussed later. The discrepancy between 1

and 7 per cent is not easily explained but differences in the extent of sampling probably play a very large part.

Once there is stromal infiltration of even limited degree, the incidence of nodal metastases rises fairly sharply. Thus, none of the 12 patients of Silverberg and Chitale (1973) with pure DCIS who underwent radical mastectomy had axillary node involvement, contrasting with two out of 11 patients with node involvement among a group with dominant intraductal carcinoma and 'less than 10 per cent' of stromal infiltration.

Pooling the results of six series of patients with DCIS, only three patients among 184 were found to have node metastases, an incidence of only 1.6 per cent: in the individual series of Gillis, Dockerty and Clagett (1960), Wulsin and Schreiber (1962), Kouchoukos, Ackerman and Butcher (1967), Ashikari, Hajdu and Robbins (1971), Silverberg and Chitale (1973) and Millis and Thynne (1975) there were 1/26, 0/8, 1/22, 1/109, 0/12 and 0/7 respectively with axillary node involvement among patients eligible for analysis of nodal metastases by virtue of the operation performed. There are factors in all these series which could have affected the apparent as compared with the 'real' incidence of nodal metastases in a downward or upward direction. Thus, of the 28 patients studied by Millis and Thynne (1975), only the seven treated by some type of axillary dissection are eligible for analysis of nodal metastatic disease: yet, not only might these seven have been selected, but the results of follow-up in the overall study are so good as to suggest a very low incidence of nodal disease. On the other hand, the figure of one patient in 22 of Kouchoukos, Ackerman and Butcher (1967) was obtained only after it became clear from their study that an average of three sections per case was quite inadequate to exclude stromal invasion in the primary tumour. Initially three patients out of 24 with *apparent* DCIS were found to have node metastases. If one considers only the five series in the literature in which 20 patients or more are eligible for analysis of this point by virtue of having had a radical mastectomy or an axillary dissection, *lymph node metastases are present in 5 of 238 patients, an incidence of 2.1 per cent* (Table 12–2).

A word of caution is needed here about this relatively low figure of 2 per cent of nodal metastases. In most series it is evident that when a diagnosis of DCIS was made on biopsy

Table 12–2 The incidence of nodal metastases in patients with apparent ductal carcinoma in situ

Source and year	Number of patients with radical or modified radical mastectomy	Number of patients with positive axillary nodes
Gillis, Dockerty and Clagett (1960)	26	1
Kouchoukos, Ackerman and Butcher (1967)	22	1
Ashikari, Hajdu and Robbins (1971)	109	1
Westbrook and Gallager (1975)	60*	1
Brown et al (1976)	21	1

* Some had 'simple mastectomy' but it is not clear whether they had axillary dissection of some type also.

but invasive carcinoma was subsequently demonstrated at mastectomy, the case was excluded from the series of pure ductal carcinomas. Although this is logical, it can lead to an underestimation of *the danger of accepting a diagnosis of pure DCIS on the basis of a biopsy report.* Carter and Smith (1977) carried out a study with this problem in mind. There were 38 cases of apparently pure DCIS as assessed at biopsy. Only cases in which 'multiple' paraffin sections were available for study were included. At subsequent mastectomy no fewer than seven of the 38 cases were found to have invasive carcinoma, an incidence of 18 per cent. Equally disturbing is the fact that three of 29 patients with lymph node dissections had positive nodes; two of these were among the group of seven patients with invasive cancer at mastectomy. Unfortunately, because of the retrospective nature of this study, there is no information on the size of the lesions and other parameters which might have a bearing on the subsequent findings in this important group of seven cases. Nor can one be certain that the arbitrary minimum of six blocks or the highly desirable eight to 10 was examined in each case before a biopsy diagnosis of pure DCIS was made by the pathologist. Such extensive sampling is even more essential with a large lesion which extends to the resection margins and this probably applied to the bulk of the lesions in this series.

Despite these reservations, it is salutary to consider the findings obtained by Carter and Smith (1977) at a single institution over a 15-year period. Residual intraductal car-cinoma was present in 32 of 38 mastectomy specimens, presumably reflecting the size and extent of the lesions and the probable involvement of resection margins in much of the material. In 25 patients, only residual intraductal carcinoma was found, while in another seven both invasive and intraductal carcinoma were present. In only six out of 38 patients (16 per cent) did the biopsy apparently remove all of the neoplastic tissue. Two of the seven patients with invasive carcinoma detected only at mastectomy died of their disease.

Equally important is the behaviour of the tumour in the 25 patients who had only residual intraductal carcinoma at mastectomy. One patient (4 per cent) had a positive node dissection but was alive without evidence of disease almost 13 years later. Another patient, in whom no node dissection was carried out, died of her disease. Thus two out of 25 cases diagnosed as pure DCIS even at the time of mastectomy must have had undetected infiltration as judged by nodal metastases in one case and distant dissemination in another. This is a somewhat higher incidence of occult infiltration than has been reported in most other series. There is a wealth of other useful information in the paper of Carter and Smith (1977), which is valuable to pathologists and surgeons interested in this increasingly important topic. It should be pointed out that the *DCIS in this study, as in most others, refers to clinically detected disease* which is presumably more extensive, larger or 'later' than disease detected radiographically. This distinction will become increasingly important in future studies (Lagios, Margolin and Rose, 1977).

Conclusion on Nodal Metastasis with a Diagnosis of DCIS

It can be concluded that, *with adequate sampling as defined, nodal metastases with DCIS are found in not less than 1 per cent and not more than about 4 per cent* of patients.

RECURRENCE, BEHAVIOUR AND PROGNOSIS

Of nine patients in the series of Millis and Thynne (1975) treated initially by wide local excision only, there was local recurrence in only two: in one this occurred six months postoperatively and was treated by radical mastectomy; in the second patient, a recurrence at seven years was again treated by wide local excision, but a further recurrence at eight years was treated by simple mastectomy.

Of their total 28 patients, the only one known to have died of her disease was a patient who received radiotherapy only. Eighteen patients were alive and well: 11 were followed for over 10 years and the remaining seven for over five years. Three patients died of other causes before the 10-year follow-up period, and two others died between 10 and 14 years also of other causes. A further two patients were lost to follow-up after 15 years but were well and without recurrence when last seen. These data of Millis and Thynne (1975) justify an optimistic prognosis.

Westbrook and Gallager (1975) also found that the *prognosis* with intraductal carcinoma was *excellent*. Only one of 64 patients had positive axillary nodes, and only two had local or distant recurrences. The patient who had a local recurrence was the same patient who had positive axillary nodes. This exceptional patient presented with an axillary mass as the only symptom; subserial whole organ studies of the breast revealed only intraductal carcinoma without evidence of invasion. The only other patient to develop tumour recurrence had distant metastases. Thus, 62 of 64 patients with intraductal carcinoma remained free of recurrent disease, though apparently some patients may have had a follow-up period of only about four years, since the patients reviewed extended to 1970 and the presentation on which this paper is based was given in April 1975. It would have been valuable to know the mean follow-up period in this large series of patients, second in size only to that of Ashikari, Hajdu and Robbins (1971).

TREATMENT

Westbrook and Gallager (1975) regarded mastectomy with removal of the regional lymph nodes as adequate treatment. Radical mastectomy constitutes overtreatment since it seems possible to control this disease with a lesser procedure. Brown *et al* (1976) suggested that total mastectomy is adequate treatment because of the 'minimal' incidence of axillary node involvement. On the available evidence, simple mastectomy will remove all the regional tumour in 96 to 99 per cent of apparently pure ductal cancers provided that these have been adequately sampled. Partial or total axillary dissection should be carried out if a potential but very slight increase in the cure rate is considered to outweigh any resulting increase in morbidity; whether such a dissection results in a very slightly higher cure rate is debatable but it does extirpate the regional tumour in a further 2 to 3 per cent of patients. In the predominantly comedo pattern of carcinoma the case for axillary dissection would be stronger than with other tumour types if the findings of Dossett (1976) are confirmed. There is need for information as to whether this particular histological type is more likely to be associated with occult invasion and hence a greater likelihood of nodal metastasis. If this were true, there would be a good case for classifying the comedo type cancers separately, a policy which has not been followed in the classification adopted here. Unless there is confirmatory evidence, it is not regarded as proven that comedocancers are more likely to be associated with occult infiltration than other types of DCIS. The higher incidence of nodal metastases noted by Dossett (1976) is probably mainly due to sampling differences. Further data are necessary. With ductal carcinoma in situ in general, the surgeon's judgement and the patient's attitude should determine what must be a finely balanced decision; at least a partial axillary dissection is probably desirable.

Millis and Thynne (1975) suggested that patients between 35 and 70 years are probably best treated by simple mastectomy and low axillary node dissection. These workers tcntatively suggested that it might be justifiable to treat patients under 35 years and those over 70 years by wide local excision and careful follow-up study.

Radiotherapy. Data on the value of radiotherapy are very scanty. Four patients of Westbrook and Gallager (1975) received radiotherapy only, because they refused surgery or were medically unacceptable for surgery. No specific details of these patients are available. Two patients, in the series of Wulsin and Schreiber (1962) and Millis and Thynne (1975), who died with metastatic disease had had radiotherapy only as their definitive treatment.

The correct treatment of intraductal carcinoma is clearly going to become of increasing importance as the incidence among breast cancers rises from the mere 3 or 4 per cent it has been in the past to the 10 per cent and even much higher figures reported more recently (Moskowitz et al, 1975; Lagios, Margolin and Rose, 1977).

DEATHS FROM DISEASE

Wulsin and Schreiber (1962) reported one patient dead of cancer, at seven years after treatment, in their series of 13 patients, and Millis and Thynne (1975) similarly had a patient who succumbed with skeletal deposits seven years after treatment: pertinently, in both cases radiotherapy was the only treatment given. There were no deaths due to cancer in the series of Kouchoukos, Ackerman and Butcher (1967) and none is mentioned in the series of Gillis, Dockerty and Clagett (1960). Among the 112 patients of Ashikari, Hajdu and Robbins (1971) there was a single patient whose death was attributable to metastases from a breast carcinoma which was judged to be entirely intraductal. This is the exception to the general rule. In the two patients with recurrent tumour among the 64 studied by Westbrook and Gallager (1975), the patient with distant metastases is presumably a candidate for death from her disease and the patient with local recurrence might be, but no patient had yet died of her disease within the period of observation; there is the slight reservation that a few patients appear to have had relatively short follow-up periods of as little as four years, though the number in this category is unlikely to have affected the overall good prognosis appreciably. In the series of Brown et al (1976), of the 30 patients without contralateral breast cancer and suitable for five-year follow-up, none developed recurrent or metastatic disease. The only patient in this series to die of breast cancer died from a contralateral invasive carcinoma nine years after mastectomy for intraductal carcinoma.

ULTRASTRUCTURAL STUDIES AND OCCULT INVASION

The studies of Ozzello have a bearing on *the rare cases with nodal metastases in the absence of demonstrable invasion of the stroma at the light microscopic level.* It is difficult if not impossible to exclude microscopic foci of invasion in these cases without complete serial sections, and these have rarely been carried out. But Ozzello's work (1959) offers another alternative. Using histochemical techniques he studied the basement membranes of ducts containing carcinoma. In nearly all specimens he showed thinning, focal disruption or even absence of the basement membrane, deficiencies which were not discernible with conventional stains. Ozzello and Sanpitak (1970) and Ozzello (1971) found in their elegant studies that, in ducts apparently intact by light microscopy, there were *ultrastructural gaps in the basal laminae*; pseudopodal cytoplasmic projections or even whole cells protruded through these breaches to abut on the stroma. Ozzello (1971) found this to be true of both ductal and lobular carcinomas. Such breaches of the basal lamina are quite common at the ultrastructural level. But *to translate this into surgical practice would be imprudent.* Considering the doubt that exists about the behaviour of unselected cases of CLIS studied prospectively and the resulting arguments about the correct treatment of every newly diagnosed patient, the translation of academic advances into radical surgery would be premature and wholly unjustified. Even with ductal carcinomas, judged to be exclusively in situ after adequate study, only one of 113 specimens was found to have axillary node involvement by Ashikari, Hajdu and Robbins (1971). One should rather conclude that, despite the remarkable ultrastructural findings, therapy should be based on adequate sampling at the light microscope level and that prognosis and treatment can, on the whole, be best correlated with and related to these findings. Academic advances and practical strategy in the management of patients do not always blend easily.

MICROSCOPIC DUCTAL CARCINOMA IN SITU

All the foregoing data apply to DCIS diagnosed by conventional clinical and mammographic techniques. Equally important for diverse reasons are the tumours of microscopic dimensions, often incidentally discovered by the pathologist when breast tissue is excised for some other reason. Up to very recently, no studies of this type had been reported. The study of Betsill et al (1978) is thus of unique importance.

Betsill et al (1978) identified 25 women with ductal carcinoma between 1940 and 1950 whose lesions were only locally excised because they were either overlooked or not interpreted as carcinoma. Follow-up information was obtained on 10 patients, ranging from seven to 30 years with an average of 21.6 years. Seven of the 10 patients were found to have carcinoma at a later date, after an average interval of 9.7 years. Six of the seven, subsequently developing, carcinomas were invasive and lymph node involvement was present in five patients. Each of the subsequent carcinomas occurred in the breast in which the original biopsy showed intraductal carcinoma. Furthermore it was usually situated in the same breast quadrant.

Four of the seven patients with subsequent carcinoma died of metastatic mammary cancer or were alive with known metastases. The remaining three were free of disease after mastectomy.

In all this group of 10 patients, the carcinomas were 'low-grade, papillary intraductal carcinoma of microscopic size'.

Betsill et al (1978) contrasted their findings with those of patients with CLIS. The risk of subsequent carcinoma is substantially higher in the group under consideration here; the cancer occurs almost invariably in the same breast as the original neoplastic lesion, usually in or near the same site. The average interval before the appearance of the second cancer was considerably shorter than in patients with CLIS.

Even if one were to assume that no breast carcinoma developed in any of the 15 women lost to follow-up, a *minimum* figure for the later appearance of additional carcinoma would be 7/25 (28 per cent). Among the 10 patients with complete follow-up, seven (70 per cent) had subsequent carcinoma. From an analysis of the literature, these workers calculated that there was a 39 per cent risk of subsequent breast cancer development.

Betsill et al (1978) stressed that their series did not include instances of comedocarcinoma and other more easily recognizable varieties. Thus, while their results apply directly only to the 'histologically appearing low-grade intraductal lesions', one might reasonably expect a behaviour at least as bad with the other variants of ductal carcinoma.

Betsill et al (1978) justifiably concluded that lesions of the type they identified histologically as non-invasive ductal carcinoma represent a pre-invasive stage of malignant neoplasia. The type of lesion studied by these workers corresponds to those studied by the present writer and described in Chapter Six in the section on 'early cancer'.

4. THE PATHOLOGY OF BREAST CARCINOMA IN SCREENED POPULATIONS AND THE PATHOLOGY OF CLINICALLY OCCULT VERSUS PALPABLE CARCINOMAS

THE DIFFERENCE IN PATHOLOGY OF PALPABLE AND NON-PALPABLE LESIONS

Leaving aside the vexed issue of the benefits as opposed to the risks of mammography, there have been some important studies on the pathology of the clinically occult, non-palpable lesions. Patchefsky et al (1977) screened 17 526 asymptomatic women aged 45 to 64 years by mammography, thermography and physical examination. Breast cancer was detected in 156 women (8.9/1000) and 149 of these were reviewed pathologically. Of the 149, *62 tumours were not clinically palpable* (42 per cent) while *87 tumours were palpable* (58 per cent). One of the many interesting findings in this work is *the difference in the pathology of the two groups*, which can be summarized as follows:

1. Fully 65 per cent of the non-palpable carcinomas consisted of in situ, 'minimally invasive' and tubular carcinomas; only 16 per cent of the palpable tumours belonged in these categories ($P<0.01$).

2. Only 8 per cent (5/62) of the non-palpable tumours were associated with involved axillary nodes whereas 39 per cent (34/87) of the palpable tumours were associated with such nodal metastases ($P<0.01$).

3. Of the invasive carcinomas which were not detected clinically, only 23 per cent (5/22) were associated with nodal metastases, compared with 47 per cent (34/73) for those which were palpable. Perhaps more importantly, of the five patients with nodal involvement in the group of patients with impalpable carcinomas, four had only a single lymph node involved and the fifth woman only two nodes. By contrast, in the group of patients with palpable carcinomas, as many as 38 per cent (13/34) of those with nodal metastases had involvement of more than three lymph nodes.

These differences in the pathology of the cancers detected by different modalities are striking and important.

THE PATHOLOGY OF BREAST CARCINOMA IN A SCREENED POPULATION

If the whole 149 reviewed cancer cases in this screened population are considered, only 26 per cent were associated with axillary lymph node metastases. Even more noteworthy is the fact that 15 per cent (22) of patients had in situ carcinoma only, DCIS constituting 9 per cent (13) and CLIS 6 per cent (9). A further 21 per cent of patients had invasive tumours with a favourable prognosis: 12 per cent (18 cases) had 'minimally invasive' cancer while 9 per cent (14 cases) had a tubular carcinoma. Thus, 36 per cent of the total number (54 of the 149 patients) had carcinomas of a prognostically favourable type.

An Incidence of DCIS of 33 Per Cent of Cancers in a Screened Population: 'The Cost'. Moskowitz

et al (1975) reviewed 36 carcinomas found among 207 biopsies performed in 4128 'volunteer screenees'. Fourteen of the 36 cancers were in situ only and of these 12 were of ductal and two of lobular type. Thus 12 out of 36 cancers were DCIS, *an incidence of DCIS of 33 per cent among all cancers*: this is probably the highest figure of DCIS as a proportion of all cancers recorded to date. An additional five patients had microinvasive cancer only, making 19 patients in all or 53 per cent of the whole group with only minimal breast cancer.

In a later paper, Moskowitz et al (1976) reviewed 67 breast cancers found in screening 8100 consecutive volunteers. A total of 466 biopsies was performed representing 6 per cent of all the women seen. Thus, the 67 cancers detected represented only 14 per cent of the biopsies performed, so that a considerable financial, medical and emotional cost is involved, a factor which must be taken into account in assessing the value of screening procedures in general, as well as in comparing the total yield of cancers and the proportion of 'minimal cancer' in different series.

Higher Incidence of Minimal Cancer with an Aggressive Screeening Approach. Of the 67 patients with carcinoma, 32 or 48 per cent had only minimal cancers. Of these, 22 patients or one-third of the whole group had in situ carcinoma only, though we are not told the proportion of ductal to lobular tumours. In the earlier paper of these workers (Moskowitz et al, 1975), DCIS by itself accounted for one-third of all cancers detected and a diagnosis of DCIS has a somewhat different significance from a diagnosis of LCIS. These figures of 48 per cent for minimal cancer and 33 per cent for in situ cancer (Moskowitz et al, 1976) should be compared with the lower figures of 27 per cent and 15 per cent respectively in the data of Patchefsky et al (1977).

Reasons for the Differences Between Different Workers. There are at least two important reasons for the differences between the findings in the studies of these two groups of workers. Firstly, Moskowitz et al (1976) included young women aged 35 to 44 years in their screened group while Patchefsky et al (1977) did not. In this age group, the yield of malignant tumours/biopsy was low, only 6 per cent compared with 14 per cent for all ages: on the other hand, the 10 cancers in this age group represented 15 per cent of the total cancers detected and, an important point in making comparisons with other series, 80 per cent of the cancers in this young age group were minimal cancers. In fact Moskowitz et al (1976) noted that the incidence of minimal cancer decreases sharply with the three successive decades 35 to 44, 45 to 54 and 55 to 64 years. Thus the inclusion of women in the 35 to 44 year bracket automatically increases the proportion of minimal cancer.

The second important difference is the proportion of negative biopsies in the different series. One out of every three biopsy specimens was found to contain cancer in the Patchefsky series (1977) but only one out of seven in the Moskowitz series (1976), though the overall cancer yield was almost identical: 9 and 8/1000 women screened respectively. The failure of Moskowitz et al (1976) to find a higher cancer yield overall was probably largely attributable to the inclusion of 3272 screenees aged 35 to 44 years in their series. Moskowitz et al (1976) adopted an 'aggressive screening' approach. They carried out biopsies on 6 per cent of all women screened while Patchefsky et al (1977) performed biopsies on less than 3 per cent. Still more significant is the ratio of cancers found to total biopsies performed in the two series. Moskowitz et al (1976) justified the aggressive approach by obtaining a 48 per cent figure for minimal cancer compared with 27 per cent for the less aggressive approach. There is much that could be said in support of both sides and the question cannot be separated from the wider issue of the risks as against the benefits of mammography.

Relative Roles of Clinical Examination and Mammography. The relative roles of physical examination and mammography in the detection of carcinoma are indicated by a 60 per cent detection rate for the clinical examination and 76 per cent for the mammographic of the total cancers detected (Moskowitz et al, 1976). It is just as important to know that the physical and mammographic examinations detected 41 and 81 per cent of *minimal* cancers respectively. Mammography was responsible for detecting the majority of in situ and other minimal cancers, 60 per cent having been detected by this modality *alone*. On the other hand, while clinical examination detected less than one-half of all minimal cancers found, it did pick up 41 per cent, a not inconsiderable figure for so innocuous a procedure. Moreover, a significant minority, 19 per cent, were detected by physical examination *alone*. Thus the value of clinical examination as a screening procedure should not be underestimated. In general it remains true, however, that mammography is at least as good, and usually rather better, at detecting breast cancer in 'well women' and this is even more true of the minimal cancers (Moskowitz et al, 1976). There is a good deal of other valuable information in the work of Patchefsky et al (1977) (mainly histopathological) and in that of Moskowitz et al (1976) (mainly on the procedure of screening and the roles of different modalities).

5. CONSIDERATIONS RELATING TO THE COMMONER TYPES OF INVASIVE BREAST CARCINOMA

IS INFILTRATING DUCTAL CARCINOMA A MYOEPITHELIAL CELL CANCER?

Since infiltrating ductal carcinoma of no special type or carcinoma NOS constitutes the bulk of infiltrating cancer of the breast, it is important to take stock of current views about the nature of this tumour. Murad and Scarpelli (1967), while conceding that medullary carcinomas are epithelial tumours, put forward the interesting and revolutionary concept that the common 'scirrhous' carcinoma represents a myoepithelial cancer. This conclusion was based on ultrastructural studies which showed that in medullary carcinoma there was a production of microvilli on the surface of the cells, and that these microvilli frequently abutted directly on to the surrounding stroma. This and other features led these authors to the conclusion that medullary carcinoma showed definite evidence of epithelial differentiation. In the writer's opinion, the microvillous surfaces they described are probably not recognizable with a PAS and other mucin stains because of the complete lack of any mucin secretion in medullary carcinoma, as outlined later in this chapter. There is general agreement with the conclusion of Murad and Scarpelli (1967) about the epithelial nature of medullary carcinomas. Medullary carcinoma and mucoid carcinoma can justifiably be regarded as reflecting the opposite poles of differentiation, with the former showing almost exclusively absorptive surfaces and the latter demonstrating exaggerated secretory properties.

Murad and Scarpelli (1967) *went on further to conclude that 'scirrhous' carcinoma was a myoepithelial cancer,* basing this view mainly on their finding of basal lamina material around the clumps of infiltrating cancer cells. At first sight this appeared to be a very attractive hypothesis, especially if their findings were to receive independent confirmation. Unfortunately, these authors failed to consider all the existing evidence, including the formation of ducts with the presence of mucinous luminal secretion in these carcinomas, features which are hardly compatible with a *purely* myoepithelial type of tumour. Even the trabecular formations in infiltrating ductal carcinoma are much more suggestive of epithelial than of myoepithelial differentiation. There is no real question that there exists ample evidence of epithelial differentiation in infiltrating ductal carcinoma and that this tumour is most definitely *not a pure* myoepithelial cancer on well-established structural and histochemical grounds.

The Possibility of Dual Differentiation. Nevertheless, the possibility remains that 'scirrhous' carcinoma might show differentiation towards both epithelial and myoepithelial cells because there is no reason to assume that one type of differentiation necessarily excludes the other. There is a great diversity of opinion in regard to the cell of origin of mammary carcinomas. It should be pointed out here that the evidence for the cells of origin is scanty. As Ozzello (1971) emphasized, epithelial and myoepithelial cells probably share the same ancestry and hence they may represent different forms of differentiation of the same parent cell. Likewise, the same cell type, or 'stem cell', may give rise to most or almost all mammary carcinomas, the different tumour varieties representing different lines of differentiation. In other words it is

the direction of differentiation which can best be assessed and analysed; the actual cell of origin is frequently speculative and may be very similar, if not identical, in different tumour types. This is an important point with more general applicability to tumour pathology even outside the breast.

The Significance of Cytoplasmic Filaments. The question to be resolved is, therefore, whether carcinoma NOS shows myoepithelial differentiation, in addition to its proven and well-established epithelial line of differentiation. Some authors have seen a link between the cytoplasmic filaments of tumour cells and those of myoepithelial cells and have suggested that ductal carcinomas may arise from myoepithelium (Haguenau, 1959; Wellings and Roberts, 1963; Busch and Merker, 1968). In contrast, other workers have concluded that there is no evidence that the cytoplasmic filaments, present in breast cancer cells, are an indication of myoepithelial derivation (or rather, one should say, differentiation for the reasons just outlined). According to these other workers, cytoplasmic filaments with similar features can be found in numerous neoplastic and non-neoplastic cells unrelated to myoepithelium (Murad and Scarpelli, 1967; Goldenberg, Goldenberg and Sommers, 1969). Some of the coarser filaments have been regarded by these two groups of workers as indicative of squamous metaplasia. Goldenberg, Goldenberg and Sommers (1969), in one of the best early ultrastructural studies, emphasized that the presence in breast carcinomas of cells rich in cytoplasmic filaments does not necessarily guarantee their myoepithelial origin. However, they did feel that the more loosely arranged filaments they had observed were at least suggestive of myoepithelial differentiation. This is particularly suggested by their Figure 11, which depicted loosely arranged filaments showing 'the characteristic pale and dark zones'. In view of what is now known about myofibroblasts in the stroma of certain breast carcinomas (Harris and Ahmed, 1977), one may have to reappraise whether this cell type could not have been stromal rather than neoplastic. Goldenberg, Goldenberg and Sommers (1969) concluded that 'the coexistence in the same tumour of cells with abundant filaments and cells with secretory granules, and such surface membrane specializations as microvilli and canaliculi, would indicate that both cell types participate', i.e.

both epithelial and myoepithelial cells. Like Ozzello (1971), Goldenberg, Goldenberg and Sommers (1969) found evidence to suggest that these two cell types have a common histogenetic lineage. The nature of the commoner finer, as opposed to the coarser, filaments has not been conclusively settled but Ozzello (1971), after careful analysis, concluded that *'none of these filaments have the characteristics of those seen in myoepithelial cells'*. No new facts have emerged since then to challenge the conclusions of Ozzello (1971) about the significance of cytoplasmic filaments in breast cancer cells.

The Significance of Basal Laminae Around Infiltrating Tumour Cells. Murad and Scarpelli (1967) based their argument, however, not on the presence of cytoplasmic filaments, but on their finding that, in infiltrating ductal carcinoma, basal laminae are always present around the neoplastic cells. Carter, Yardley and Shelley (1969) were unable to confirm this. Ozzello (1971) found that most of the clusters of neoplastic cells in infiltrating ductal carcinomas were devoid of basal laminae. Only infrequently did he find basal lamina material surrounding partially or entirely a group of tumour cells. Goldenberg, Goldenberg and Sommers (1969) also found that, in some instances, infiltrating breast carcinoma cells are partially invested by and capable of producing basement-membrane-type material, thus partially confirming the findings of Murad and Scarpelli (1967). But they differed significantly in their interpretation of this finding. They recalled that in experimental systems it has long been accepted that malignant epithelial cells are indeed capable of basement membrane synthesis, and they referred especially to the work of Pierce and co-workers (1962, 1963, 1964). Goldenberg, Goldenberg and Sommers (1969) regarded their findings as contradicting the widely held view that neoplastic epithelium loses its ability to synthesize basement membrane. They did not relate the presence of basement membranes to myoepithelial differentiation in the tumour. Ozzello (1971), in his discussion of breast carcinoma, concluded that *'no convincing evidence was found to correlate mammary tumour cells with myoepithelium'*. Thus, other workers, while partially confirming one of the main findings of Murad and Scarpelli (1967), differed considerably from them in the interpretation of the observation which formed the main plank of their hypothesis. Most of the evidence points away from the ingenious Murad–Scarpelli (1967) hypothesis.

The Significance of ATPase Activity on the Surface of Cancer Cells. The concept of a myoepithelial cancer has, however, maintained its advocates. On the basis of enzymatic patterns, Murad (1970) postulated that most infiltrating ductal ('scirrhous') cancers are of myoepithelial nature. This conclusion was largely based on *the remarkable finding of abundant ATPase activity on the surface of the cancer cells,* a finding which boosted this hypothesis. In 1971 Murad put forward a tentative new classification of breast carcinoma based on enzymatic reactions. He recognized three groups: 'ductal epithelial' (medullary) cancer, 'ductular' carcinoma (LCIS or CLIS) and 'myoepithelial cell carcinoma'. Murad proposed that 'scirrhous' (infiltrating duct) carcinoma be renamed a myoepithelial carcinoma on the grounds of the presence of ATPase on the surface of the carcinoma cells. His findings were of great interest but to identify infiltrating ductal carcinoma as a myoepithelial cancer constituted a big leap which did not take the whole range of evidence into account. Ahmed (1974) was the first worker to demonstrate convincingly that *ATPase is localized to the plasma membrane of breast cancer cells which showed unequivocal evidence of epithelial differentiation* on other well-established grounds. Murad (1975) identified both intraductal and papillary carcinoma as myoepithelial, again based mainly on surface localization of ATPase activity. The ultrastructural evidence he put forward at this time was, however, inconclusive and unacceptable.

ATPase Not an Exclusive Marker for Myoepithelial Cells. Buell, Tremblay and Rowden (1976) investigated the distribution of adenosine triphosphatase in infiltrating ductal carcinoma as well as in the non-neoplastic breast. Discussing discrepancies in the literature they stressed that, for technical and other reasons, the histochemical identification of ATPase is not an entirely reliable method for differentiating myoepithelial from epithelial cells in the breast. They found that *the majority of infiltrating ductal carcinomas do not possess uniform ATPase activity* and they therefore doubted the validity of the proposed new classification of Murad (1971), unless an additional category of tumours with variable ATPase activity was added. Furthermore, Buell, Tremblay and Rowden (1976) confirmed Ahmed's (1974) finding that mucin-producing tumour cells were ATPase-positive, and also found marked ATPase activity in an apocrine carcinoma. They justifiably concluded that *ATPase is not an exclusive marker for myoepithelial cells,* and that data resulting from the use of this enzymatic pattern to study the role of the myoepithelium in mammary carcinoma must be interpreted with caution. Like Ozzello (1971), Buell, Tremblay and Rowden (1976) emphasized the shared ancestry of, and close relationship between, epithelial and myoepithelial cells. These workers suggested that the presence of ATPase activity on some neoplastic epithelial cells may reflect this close relationship between the cell types, may indicate an increased metabolic activity of the cells or may be a reflection of both these factors. Indeed these workers suggested a possible third alternative: Moynahan, Sethi and Brooks (1972) found that in developing foetal rat skin the basal epithelial layer is transiently ATPase-positive, a property which disappears after birth. It has yet to be established whether an analogous situation exists in the breast, whereby undifferentiated cells may be transiently ATPase-positive. In the absence of this knowledge, as Buell, Tremblay and Rowden (1976) rightly maintained, the possibility exists that ATPase activity in breast carcinomas simply mimics the pattern shown by the less differentiated cells in the developing ducts of the foetal breast. Only histochemical investigation of foetal breast tissue will provide the answer to this particular problem. One has to agree with Buell, Tremblay and Rowden (1976) that, on several grounds, *the significance of ATPase in breast carcinomas in different circumstances is far from clear* and that it is premature to draw sweeping conclusions from the data currently available.

In a subsequent communication, Murad, Swaid and Pritchett (1977) again identified papillary carcinoma with myoepithelial cells, a view which is a priori so unlikely that it is surprising that it should be reiterated so forcefully without stronger evidence to support it, and without any reference to prior work which puts the opposite viewpoint so well. They appear to have based their conclusion solely on the ultrastructural findings in the 1975 work but these are, as already indicated, quite inconclusive.

As far as infiltrating ductal carcinoma is concerned, Ozzello (1971) should have the last authoritative word: in answer to the question which forms the heading of this section, *infiltrating duct carcinoma is not, on the best evidence available, a myoepithelial cell cancer.* This concept is rejected since it is confusing in practice as well as being largely erroneous at the theoretical level. If there is an element of myoepithelial differentiation, it is either a rare or a very partial phenomenon and even this has not been proven to the satisfaction of most workers. Murad's work has stimulated a great deal of work in this field but the central tenet of his hypothesis must be rejected.

INVASIVE LOBULAR CARCINOMA

Incidence. It is now 12 years or more since this tumour type was accurately defined (Newman, 1966), yet there is a distinct suspicion that it is not as generally recognized or as frequently diagnosed as it ought to be. The incidence given in the literature varies very widely between less than 1 per cent and about 20 per cent. Some of the very low figures in the older literature on this subject (pre-1960) are fairly easy to understand but it is considerably more difficult to explain some of the low incidences cited since 1965 or thereabouts. Newman (1966) established an incidence of 5.2 per cent, which he regarded as a minimum figure since he excluded another 5 per cent of carcinomas which were considered to be partly but not wholly of lobular type. Newman (1966) gave one of the first indications that there is a considerable element of difficulty in differentiating between ILC and IDC, a difficulty only rarely mentioned in the literature. Newman's (1966) findings indicated an incidence of ILC of at least 5 per cent and, perhaps, between 5 and 10 per cent. McDivitt, Stewart and Berg (1968) found an incidence of 8.7 per cent in a series of 1458 infiltrating breast carcinomas treated by radical mastectomy.

Racial and Possible Geographical Variations. The incidence rates of 2.5 per cent reported by Warner (1969) and of 0.7 per cent reported by Donegan and Perez-Mesa (1972) are very low. It is possible that some of these discrepancies in the incidence are attributable to genetic or environmental factors. Thus, for instance, it is known that Negroes have a substantially lower incidence of lobular carcinoma than Caucasians (Ashikari et al, 1973). This must be taken into account when considering reports from different centres in the USA and when comparisons are made between the USA and other countries. To date, the vast majority of the work in this field has been carried out in the USA and there is an urgent need for comparative geographical studies.

Is the Incidence in the UK Higher? Wheeler and Enterline (1976) found an incidence of 4 per cent of ILC, based on a series of 499 very carefully studied cancers. They came to the conclusion that about 4 to 6 per cent of all breast carcinomas are infiltrating lobular tumours and that 'incidence rates widely divergent from this should be scrutinized carefully'. We have found that, in our material in Britain, the incidence of ILC is as high as 14 per cent in a smaller series of 203 cases (Martinez and Azzopardi, 1979). We concluded that, unless there is an incidence of 8 per cent or more of infiltrating lobular carcinoma among invasive breast cancers, the criteria for diagnosis may need revising. This applies only to the UK, and there are no data from this country with which to compare our figures.

INHERENT DIFFICULTIES IN DIAGNOSIS AND CLASSIFICATION

While geographical and racial differences may go some way towards explaining the reported differences in frequency, we think that there are inherent difficulties in diagnosis and classification which are probably largely responsible. When we started our study to establish the frequency of this tumour type in the UK, we were aware of certain difficulties in classification both on the basis of the literature and our own experience. We were not expecting to find, however, that in about 4 per cent of cases we could not classify invasive carcinoma as ductal or lobular with any certainty and that in a few other cases there appeared to be a mixture of ILC and IDC in the same tumour mass. Hence the necessity for having categories III and IV in the classification of breast carcinomas (page 241). Infiltrating ductal and infiltrating lobular carcinoma cannot be separated quite as easily as is implied by much of the literature.

Newman (1966) gave the first real indica-tion of this difficulty. Fechner (1975) described a variant form of ILC which, remarkably, had a solid pattern. Fisher et al (1977b) described a tubulolobular variant of invasive carcinoma. These variants, as their very names imply, obviously differ radically from the classical variety of ILC described and illustrated by McDivitt, Stewart and Berg (1968).

Features in Identification Stressed by Different Workers

In the identification of ILC, some workers have laid stress on the importance of certain patterns of infiltration while others have emphasized the importance of cytological parameters. Fechner (1975) stressed *the significance of bland, homogeneous, cytological appearances* in the recognition of the solid variant of ILC. Toker and Goldberg (1977) emphasized *the importance of 'small-cell neoplasia'* in the identification of lobular carcinoma, in situ or infiltrating. They rightly pointed out that the mere anatomical location of the in situ component did not have the value it was previously considered to have in respect of the separation of ductal from lobular carcinoma. Fisher et al (1977b) laid stress on *the importance of a targetoid pattern of infiltration* in making a diagnosis of ILC. The cytological criteria laid down by Fechner (1975) and by Toker and Goldberg (1977) are in general both valid and useful. The criterion of cell size adopted by Toker and Goldberg (1977) is not, however, universally applicable because in the cribriform duct carcinomas especially there is an overlap in cell size with lobular carcinomas. Thus, this criterion, although generally useful, has to be interpreted cautiously and in the context of the whole picture, and exceptions must be allowed for. Similarly, the classical targetoid pattern, with single cells orientated around pre-existing normal structures, is certainly typical of infiltrating lobular carcinoma. However, this pattern of infiltration is also seen less commonly with infiltrating ductal carcinoma and cannot be relied upon entirely in the diagnosis of ILC, unless it is accompanied by the correct structural and cytological features.

Personal Observations

Because of these difficulties in the diagnosis of ILC, and in an attempt to identify any variants, we studied prototype IDC and ILC in an endeavour to establish which parameters are the most reliable in the diagnosis of either tumour and which features are shared to some extent by both tumour types. The features assessed included: a targetoid pattern; the presence of cohesive cell clumps, sheets and plexiform masses; the presence of tubules and their characteristics; the presence and character of trabeculae, with particular reference to their width and degree of cell cohesion; the presence of dissociated cells arranged randomly or in thread-like or Indian file fashion; the presence of signet-ring cells; and the presence of a 'loose alveolar' pattern. In addition, cell size and homogeneity, as opposed to pleomorphism, of the tumour cell population was assessed.

The Absence of a Single Uniformly Valid Criterion. By so doing, we were able to confirm *the usefulness to varying degree of all the criteria laid down by recent workers* as well as of a newly observed one, but our somewhat unexpected finding was that *there was no single criterion which was uniformly valid in the differential diagnosis between ILC and IDC.* Several criteria have to be considered together and the overall structure and cytology accorded more importance than any particular fields of tissue. Because of this absence of a single completely reliable diagnostic criterion, there is an irreducible minimum of about 3 to 4 per cent of carcinomas which cannot be classified with any certainty. This is perhaps not unexpected if one reflects on the overlap in the site or sites of origin of lobular and ductal carcinoma, and the overlap in the lines of differentiation seen in adjacent lobules of a breast and even within the same lobule. These unclassified tumours represent carcinomas in which objective separation between IDC and ILC is not possible on the basis of the criteria currently in use or, put another way, they may be genuinely transitional tumours in which differentiation is in both directions or in an intermediate direction. If this is true of the in situ forms, is it not also likely to be true of the invasive varieties?

CLASSICAL TYPE

The classical type of infiltrating lobular carcinoma with dissociated cells dispersed in linear threads and having a targetoid arrangement and consisting of small, relatively uniform and rather monotonous, almost bland neoplastic cells, sometimes slightly compressed by the fibrous tissue reaction, is easily identified. But other patterns and appearances are also seen.

That *focal signet-ring cell differentiation* is frequent in ILC is in need of emphasis. It is generally easily recognizable even in routine sections but much more easily appreciated if sections stained for mucin are examined. The histiocytoid carcinoma is only a variation on the theme of classical ILC but, for reasons considered elsewhere, it is a descriptive term worth retaining (Figure 12–15). The cells are a little larger than in the more classical variety and have a rather clear cytoplasm.

VARIANT TYPES

Signet-ring Cell Carcinoma. More extensive signet-ring cell differentiation is much less frequent and as a dominant feature, constituting 50 per cent or more of a carcinoma, it is decidedly rare (Figure 12–4). Signet-ring cell carcinoma probably constitutes no more than 0.2 or 0.3 per cent of invasive breast carcinomas. Most signet-ring cell carcinomas are probably variants of invasive lobular carcinoma but some are probably more closely related to ductal carcinoma.

Closely Aggregated Cells with Non-solid Pattern. Most invasive lobular carcinomas contain neoplastic cells which are widely dispersed, but there are exceptions to this. Much more closely aggregated cells may be seen in small or larger foci and it is in the latter case that the tumours may easily be confused with IDC (Figure 12–5). The neoplastic cells are closely aggregated but yet are dissociated one from another. This pattern is not sheet-like in the accepted sense of that term

---

Figure 12–4 (*Opposite, above.*) Dominant signet-ring cell differentiation in an infiltrating lobular carcinoma. Alcian blue followed by diastase–PAS. ×150.

Figure 12–5 (*Opposite, below.*) Closely aggregated but dissociated cells of invasive lobular carcinoma. Intracytoplasmic lumina are visible. This must not be confused with sheet-like growth. H and E. ×400.

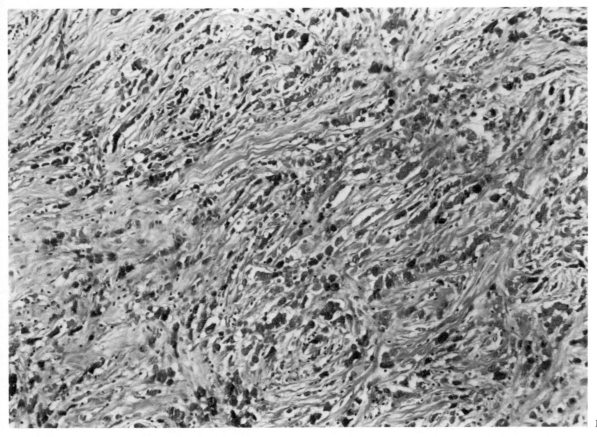

12–4

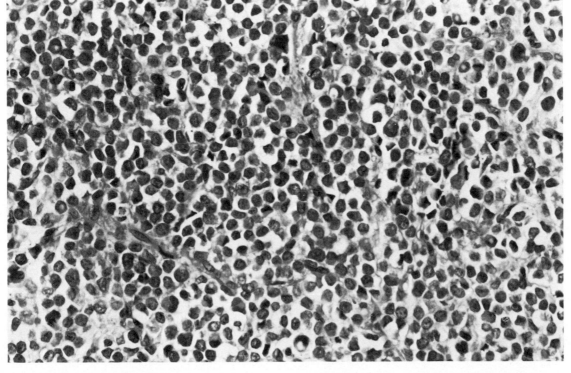

12–5

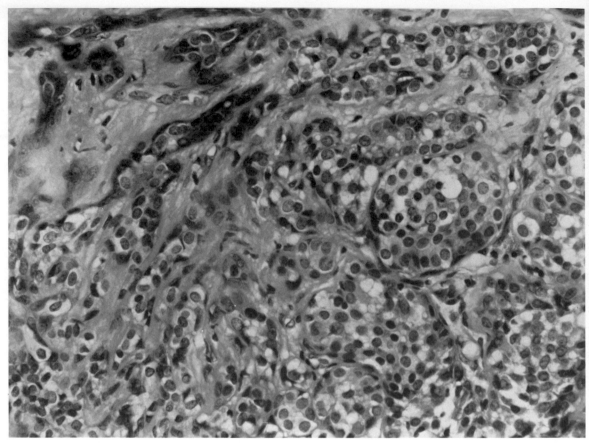

Figure 12–6 A solid growth pattern with small clumps and nests. Narrow trabeculae are also present. H and E. ×400.

nor should it be confused with the solid pattern of Fechner (1975). Closely aggregated yet dissociated neoplastic cells, mimicking the sheet-like growth found in some cases of IDC, are found both in primary carcinomas of the breast and in their distant metastases. The different growth pattern of ILC when situated in lymph nodes, as compared with the pattern of the primary tumour in the breast, is already a well-recognized phenomenon, though no less remarkable for being well recognized.

Solid Pattern. The solid pattern of Fechner (1975) has only been identified by the writer in small and limited foci of invasive lobular carcinoma (Figure 12–6). I have not seen it as the exclusive or even predominant pattern of growth as described by Fechner (1975). And yet it is true that this worker's illustrations and description are suggestive of a special type of carcinoma. Whether or not these carcinomas represent a variant of ILC is a problem which has been additionally complicated by the

recent description by Cubilla and Woodruff (1977) of primary carcinoid tumours of the breast. These can be confused with, or alternatively they may even be related to, invasive lobular carcinomas.

Trabecular Pattern. A trabecular pattern, as defined in Chapter Seven, is responsible for some of the difficulties in distinguishing between ILC and IDC. An extensive trabecular pattern is much more typical of IDC, but limited trabecular differentiation is found even in ILC (Figure 12–6). It is true that the trabeculae in ILC are largely of the one-cell width variety and, therefore, narrow and less easily detected. It is also true that the cells in the narrow trabeculae of ILC are in general less cohesive and indeed merge with and melt into the 'linear threads' of classical ILC. It is impossible to separate the less cohesive trabeculae from the linear threads because the distinction is entirely arbitrary. Trabeculae of one-cell width are present in approximately

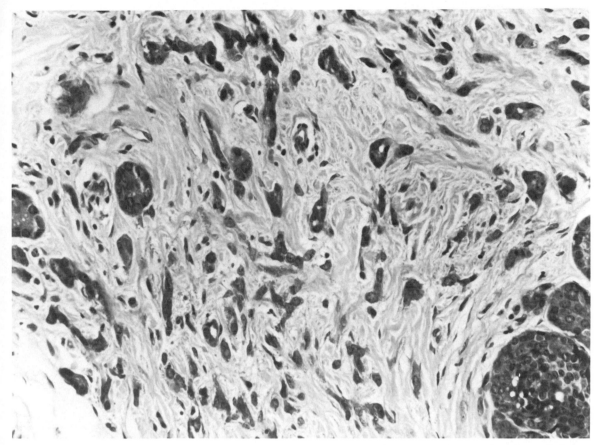

Figure 12–7   CLIS is present in one corner. The infiltrative lobular carcinoma includes tubular growth of the small 'closed' or 'tight' variety. H and E. ×375.

one-half of cases of ILC, trabeculae of two-cell width in one-third of cases, while trabeculae of three-cell width are rare.

Tubular Pattern. The tubular pattern of ILC is another one which has been recognized only recently (Fisher et al, 1977b). In our material it was present in about one-quarter of cases of ILC but it was neither prominent nor easy to identify in most of these cases. The tubular pattern is only reasonably prominent in about one-tenth of tumours and even then it is present only in limited areas. But the fact that it occurs at all is important. The tubules are mostly small with very small lumina, which is one reason for the failure to recognize them up to recently. Usually they mostly take the form of 'closed' or 'almost closed' tubules with a hypothetical or absent lumen in the former case and a minute lumen in the latter (Figure 12–7). The 'closed tubule' is one in which the cells are arranged around a hypothetical or very rudimentary lumen but show evidence of

orientation by virtue of a basal or marginal position of their nuclei (Figure 12–7).

Loose Alveolar Pattern. A pattern not previously recognized is the one we have called 'loose alveolar' (Figure 12–8), in which there is a loose alveolar grouping of the tumour cells (Martinez and Azzopardi, 1979). Where this grouping is rounded, as it frequently is, there is distinct mimicry of lobular carcinoma in situ. Indeed, though the suspicion that this represented invasive tumour has been with us for some time, we were still influenced against its possibility by the traditional teaching that ILC does not show evidence of any structural as opposed to cytological differentiation when it is invasive. Our suspicion was unequivocally confirmed, however, when we found tumour of this type which had destructively invaded the erectile muscle of the nipple, the pectoralis major muscle and was finally even detected in an ovarian metastasis. The loose alveolar pattern

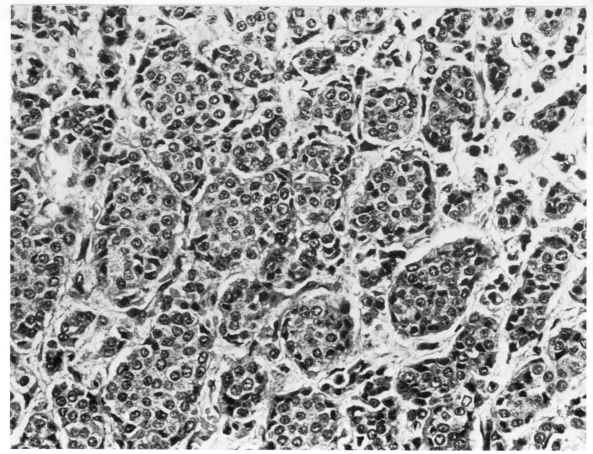

Figure 12–8 An alveolar pattern in a tumour which, in most other areas, showed classical features of an invasive lobular carcinoma. The two patterns merged indefinably and there was no suggestion that these represented two distinct tumours which had become inextricably mixed. The alveolar pattern shown here is unusually cohesive. The alveolar grouping is in most cases a much looser one and best appreciated at low magnification. H and E. ×400.

is present in about one-third of tumours but it usually constitutes only a small percentage of the total bulk of a given tumour. This pattern is unfortunately not specific to, or pathognomonic of, ILC: it is also seen occasionally in tumours which have definite structural traits of IDC.

Spindle-cell Chains. A final pattern sometimes seen in ILC is one consisting of spindle-cell chains of cells, in which short elongated columns are composed of spindle-shaped cells orientated longitudinally, an appearance one associates usually with sclerosing adenosis (Figure 12–9). Because this pattern is seen focally only, and in quite a different context, there is no possibility of confusion with sclerosing adenosis. This pattern has been seen mainly in areas of fibroelastosis and it is possible that the stromal component has influenced the shape of the

neoplastic cells and the appearance of the chains of cells. But this is unlikely to be the total explanation since the same appearance has been noted also in areas without significant elastosis or fibrosis. It is a feature which has been identified mainly in small foci of 'incipient' infiltration in a setting of extensive CLIS (Figure 12–9). It is an intriguing possibility that the shape of the cells is related to their invasive properties and that there is a relationship between a spindled neoplastic cell and invasion of the stroma.

Practical Implications of the Variant Forms

Prognosis. The newly identified variants of ILC, apart from their innate theoretical interest, may have practical implications also. Fechner (1975) and Fisher et al (1977b) suggested that they may be associated with a

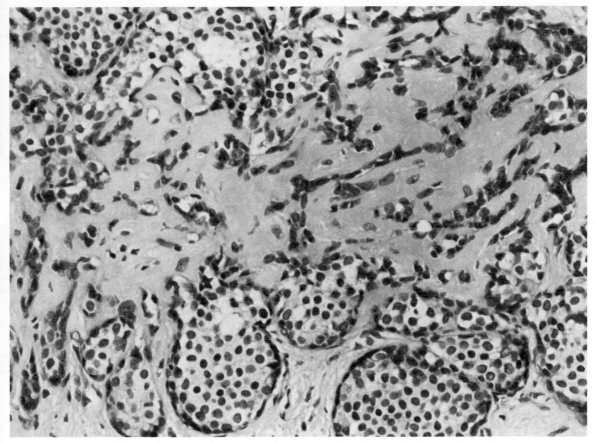

Figure 12–9 Spindle-cell chains of neoplastic cells in ILC. Here they are present in an elastotic stroma but this is not invariable. In the CLIS present along one margin, persistent myoepithelial cells are clearly identifiable. H and E. ×400.

lesser incidence of nodal metastases and that there was a trend towards a lesser incidence of short-term treatment failures in their two respective series.

RELEVANCE OF PRECISE DIAGNOSIS TO TREATMENT AND OTHER CORRELATIONS

It has been shown that lobular carcinomas have a much higher incidence of oestrogen receptor proteins compared with ductal carcinomas (Eusebi et al, 1977). Thus, categorizing a tumour as lobular rather than ductal *may have a bearing on determining treatment by endocrine manipulations*, especially if tissue has not been kept aside for the assay of oestrogen receptor protein. Similarly, casein-like and other milk protein synthesis is far more pronounced in lobular carcinomas than in ductal tumours (Eusebi et al, 1977). Such correlations will require as precise an identification of lobular carcinomas as possible, to match refinements in the specificity of the methods for detecting casein and other milk proteins in the tissues.

Future Work

There is clearly a lot more we need to know about the incidence of lobular carcinoma in different parts of the globe and in different racial groups. Much more data is required also on the variant forms of invasive lobular carcinoma and their clinical and other associations. There is a great need for information on the relationship of the carcinoid-like tumour of the breast to invasive lobular carcinoma. The new information already available has made the task of the histopathologist a more complex one from a diagnostic point of view but this is more than balanced by the fascination of the new aspects it has revealed.

6. PROBLEMS RELATING TO CERTAIN HISTOLOGICAL TYPES OF CARCINOMA

MEDULLARY CARCINOMA AND RELATED TUMOURS

The Incidence in Relation to Criteria for Identification. Since Moore and Foote (1949) described this tumour type (Figure 12–10) and it became generally accepted as an entity (Richardson, 1956), certain problems have developed in connection with its diagnostic features, prognosis and other aspects. What are the criteria for its recognition and what is its frequency? The answers to these two questions are closely interrelated. Moore and Foote found an incidence of 5.2 per cent, Richardson (1956) a slightly higher incidence of 7 per cent. Most workers are agreed that this tumour has a better prognosis than the ordinary infiltrating ductal carcinoma, but just how good it is depends to some extent on the pathologist's diagnostic criteria. In their classical work, Moore and Foote (1949) cited an 82.7 per cent survival rate at five years, with only six patients (11.5 per cent) dying of tumour. McDivitt, Stewart and Berg (1968), using somewhat different diagnostic criteria, gave actuarial survival rates of 69 per cent, 68 per cent and 62 per cent at 5, 10 and 20 years respectively.

Prognosis Related to Strict Definition. There are two important points to which attention should be drawn at the start. *The very good prognosis in this group applies only if one adopts stringent diagnostic criteria.* The incidence of medullary carcinoma was 4.3 per cent in the

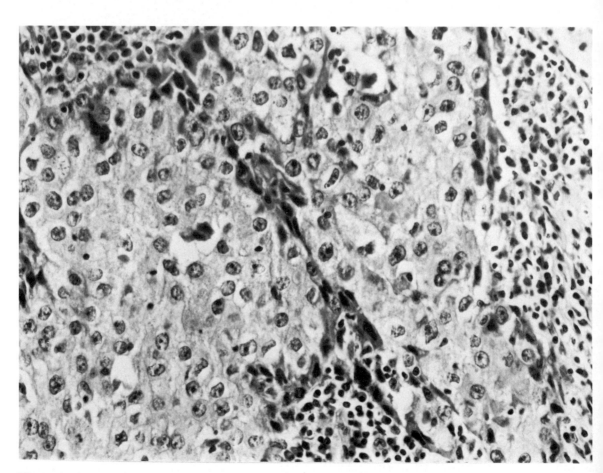

Figure 12–10   Medullary carcinoma with lymphoid infiltration. H and E. ×400.

work of McDivitt, Stewart and Berg (1968) and, with the much stricter criteria demanded by Ridolfi et al (1977), the incidence is probably lower, though no figure is given by these workers.

If It Kills, It Kills More Rapidly. Tumours that prove fatal usually result in death within five years of operation, and there are very few or no tumour deaths after 10 years (Richardson, 1956). In the series of Ridolfi et al (1977), 27 of 29 patients in their 'typical' and 'atypical' medullary carcinoma groups who died of this disease did so within five years of initial treatment and no patient died of disease after seven years. Medullary carcinoma, if it kills, kills faster than other types of breast carcinoma. This may imply that it is inherently either a more malignant or a more rapidly growing tumour. Presumably the better prognosis is due to the tumour being entirely, or almost entirely, restricted to the breast at the time of operation in a greater proportion of patients. This may be attributable to the cellular reaction of the host but it could also be due in part to greater cohesion of the tumour cells and a relative lack of infiltrative properties leading to a circumscribed type of expansile growth. Both factors probably play a part and the two factors may well be independent of each other.

Racial Difference in Incidence. Medullary carcinoma has a relatively high frequency in native, as opposed to expatriate, *Japanese women* (MacMahon et al, 1973; Rosen et al, 1977), a finding for which no satisfactory explanation has been proffered. It was observed by these workers that the proportion of premenopausal women with breast carcinoma was substantially greater in Japan than in the USA. A possible link between these two observations is found in the work of those who, like Schwartz (1969), noted that 66 per cent of women with 'solid circumscribed' carcinoma were in the less than 50-year-old age group. However, no such predilection of medullary carcinoma for younger or premenopausal women appears in the data of McDivitt, Stewart and Berg (1968), Ridolfi et al (1977) and those of most other workers. The relatively high frequency of medullary carcinoma among the Japanese cannot apparently be explained on this basis.

Clinical, Mammographic and Gross Findings. Clinically these tumours are often mobile and may mimic fibroadenomas and other benign lesions. Mammographically they appear as a circumscribed density which lacks most of the other characteristics of malignancy. In particular they do not show radiological calcification or skin thickening although abnormal vessels may be present. Even at operation the nature of the lesion may be in doubt. The inexperienced pathologist may confuse the lesion macroscopically with a fibroadenoma, but close inspection of the cut face will show none of the trabeculation or whorling of a fibroadenoma.

Bilaterality. Bilaterality of breast carcinoma occurred in 18 per cent (10/57) of patients with medullary carcinoma in the series of Ridolfi et al (1977), an incidence of bilaterality not significantly different from that seen in breast cancer in general. The contralateral carcinomas were largely infiltrating ductal lesions, the medullary carcinomas tending to be the second tumour to develop in these cases, and the interval between the breast carcinomas making their appearance being nearly twice as long with medullary as with the non-medullary tumours (8.8 *v.* 4.6 years) (Ridolfi et al, 1977).

Bilaterality and Family History. Bilateral tumours are more common when a family history is present: 42 per cent *v.* 16 per cent for the entire group of 185 patients in whom analysis of this relationship was possible (Ridolfi et al, 1977). For patients with both typical and atypical medullary carcinoma such a relationship was demonstrable only in regard to first degree relatives.

Tumour Size. The question of the average size of these tumours is in need of clarification. Moore and Foote (1949) mentioned that this tumour type had been referred to at the Memorial Hospital for many years as 'bulky carcinoma'. This report was based on a series of tumours identified prior to 1944. Later, McDivitt, Stewart and Berg (1968) concurred that the tumours are commonly quite bulky, with an average diameter of 3.4 cm, significantly but not very much more than the 3.1 cm recorded for ordinary infiltrating ductal carcinomas. Ridolfi et al (1977), reporting from the same hospital for the period 1955 to 1965, found an average diameter of 2.9 cm for both typical and atypical medullary carcinomas. It appears possible, however, that if the volume rather than the diameter were calculated, the difference in actual size between medullary carcinoma and carcinoma NOS would be appreciably greater than when expressed merely, as it usually is, in terms of the maximum diameter. The *clinical, radiological and macroscopic impressions*, based as they are on volume, *may be actually more realistic than an accurate measurement of only one dimension.*

HISTOPATHOLOGY

Dominant Growth Pattern

The growth pattern is a *predominantly syncytial solid, sheet-like* one with broad, anastomosing, plexiform masses. This syncytial-type pattern should constitute 75 per cent or more of the growth pattern for a tumour to be included in the medullary category. Smaller, more rounded nests of cells and even some trabecular growth may be present, but the more conspicuous the latter pattern, the greater the care necessary to make sure of the correct identity of the tumour. The cells are generally large with large nuclei and indistinct cytoplasmic margins (Figure 12–10), except where autolysis, which is sometimes marked, leads to separation of the cells. The large ovoid or rounded nuclei are not always particularly hyperchromatic: they vary between hyperchromatic and vesicular with a punctate chromatin pattern. More constant is the fact that they have prominent and frequently large or multiple nucleoli. The cytoplasm sometimes has a suggestion of granularity or reticulation and may be slightly amphophilic.

Less Well Known Features

Delineation of Tumour Clumps by Smaller Cells. A noteworthy feature is the frequency with which *sheets and clumps of tumour cells are delineated at their margins by smaller, more elongated cells with denser cytoplasm and sometimes denser nuclei* (Figure 12–10). It is not at present clear whether there is an element of artefactual squeeze which might be responsible even in part for this appearance. The alternative view, that they might represent myoepithelial cells, is superficially attractive but there is scant evidence to support it.

Gould, Miller and Jao (1975) found rare elongated cells with prominent bundles of cytoplasmic filaments with alternating pale and dark zones; hemidesmosomes and a basal lamina accompanied these cells. Since these findings conflict with those of Murad and Scarpelli (1967) and of Michaud and Morin (1971), further investigation is needed.

Microglandular Differentiation. We have observed that *small tubular lumina* may occasionally be found within the tumour nests, though in general they are of course uncommon. These lumina are devoid of any secretion but are lined by epithelial cells possessing microvilli. This finding is in agreement with the observation of Murad and Scarpelli (1967) that, at the ultrastructural level, the tumour cells have microvilli which may even abut directly on the stroma. Thus, medullary carcinoma would appear to be a tumour which, insofar as it exhibits any differentiation at all, differentiates exclusively towards epithelial cells with characteristics of absorptive cells but lacking any trace of secretory activity. Mucin secretion not being a feature, the detection of epithelial mucin in a breast carcinoma effectively negates a diagnosis of medullary carcinoma. Microglandular differentiation was observed also by Ridolfi et al (1977) but they regarded such tumours as atypical medullary carcinomas. They did, however, state that 'we suspect that focal microglandular differentiation . . . had no appreciable effect on survival'.

Abnormal Mitoses and Tumour Giant Cells. At the cytological level, it is generally agreed that mitoses are numerous, but the fact that abnormal mitoses are often also prominent needs stressing. Another feature, which is not generally recognized, is the presence of tumour giant cells. These may take a number of forms. In some 10 per cent of tumours there are varying numbers of mononuclear or multinuclear giant cells with cytoplasmic characteristics which are similar to those of the rest of the tumour; these are easily recognizable as neoplastic cells. These cells merge with tumour giant cells of more grotesque and bizarre appearances, even simulating syncytial trophoblast on very rare occasions. Another type of giant cell, encountered less frequently, is an osteoclast-like cell, with multiple small uniform nuclei. The nature of this cell type is debatable. It may be a modified tumour cell or it may represent a reactive stromal cell; further study is needed. Ridolfi et al (1977) noted an association between the presence of tumour giant cells and concurrent pregnancy. They also detected a trend towards a poorer prognosis in the presence of such cells.

Squamous Metaplasia. Squamous metaplasia is said to occur in 16 per cent of medullary carcinomas (Ridolfi et al, 1977). It is not at all clear, however, that a strict definition of 'squamous' has been adhered to in arriving at this figure.

Papillary Differentiation. This pattern of differentiation has frequently been recorded as occurring in these tumours, but this is probably based on loose usage of the term 'papillary', as elaborated elsewhere. The writer has not seen papillary differentiation in medullary carcinoma. If it occurs, it is extremely rare.

Necrosis, Liquefaction and Absence of Calcification. Necrosis is a frequent feature of this tumour both grossly and histologically. On rare occasions it may be so extensive as to give rise to a central cyst within the tumour as a result of liquefaction. It is a curious fact that, despite the extensive necrosis, this tumour does not calcify and *the absence of calcification is an important negative finding at mammography.* Necrosis in medullary carcinoma tends to leave little behind in the way of nuclear debris, DNA or recognizable cytoplasmic structures, and the absence of mucin has already been mentioned. Calcification in other tumour types often occurs around a nidus of DNA, cell membranes and mucinous secretion. The absence of such material in medullary carcinoma is perhaps responsible for the absence of calcification in areas of necrosis. Other factors, like the absence of casein in the tumour cells, may also contribute to this conspicuous absence of calcification.

Rarity of Distinct In Situ Component. One of the more curious aspects of medullary carcinoma is the rarity of a distinct in situ component. It is one of the few breast cancers in which such a component is very difficult or frankly impossible to detect even with the most extensive sampling (McDivitt, Stewart and Berg, 1968). Ordinarily, if a patient with a breast cancer develops a tumour in the contralateral breast, the latter is regarded as a definite second primary cancer, as opposed to a metastasis, only if it contains an in situ component to confirm its primary nature. Medullary carcinoma is an exception to this rule, the second tumour being acceptable as a new primary tumour in the absence of in situ cancer.

The reasons for this rarity of detection of an in situ component are obscure. One possible explanation is that most tumours break out of their confines when still very small and, since the in situ component will then constitute only a very small fraction of the total tumour volume, it will be correspondingly more difficult to find. A second possibility is that the tumour has essentially the same morphological appearances whether it is in situ or infiltrating. It will be recalled that in most breast cancers the in situ and the invasive components are morphologically different in a number of ways, as pathologists will have noted either consciously or otherwise. For this reason, non-invasive and invasive tumour are frequently already easily distinguishable at a low magnification in most types of cancer. *That medullary cancers have the same structural and other traits, whether in situ or infiltrating, is suggested by the work of Ridolfi et al* (1977). These workers noted that the in situ component was accompanied by the prominent mononuclear infiltrate present elsewhere in the tumour mass. Growth within lobules can lead to 'cancerization' of lobules (q.v.), and this will lead to distension by tumour and an appearance very similar to that seen in the infiltrating portion.

Originally Ridolfi et al (1977) placed all tumours with an in situ component in their atypical group, since like McDivitt, Stewart and Berg (1968) they had been impressed prior to their study by the virtual absence of any in situ component in characteristic medullary carcinomas. They found in the course of their study that the presence of this feature did not affect survival and rightly decided that there was no justification in excluding a lesion from the typical medullary carcinoma category solely because of the presence of an intraductal component. Accordingly they transferred seven tumours from the atypical to the typical medullary category. In all but one of these seven tumours intraductal carcinoma was limited to a single microscopic field. All seven patients were alive without recurrence after 10 years of follow-up. It should, however, be noted that the good survival figures they reported for patients with typical medullary carcinoma were calculated before this transfer was carried out, so that there is no question of any manipulation of data to obtain a possibly preconceived result.

On the basis of these adjusted figures, Ridolfi et al (1977) found *an in situ component in 11 per cent of otherwise typical medullary carcinomas* (7/64 tumours). This still represents only one in nine of these tumours and the intraductal component was very limited in extent in almost all cases. Nevertheless, if this finding is confirmed, it could explain the presence of the myoepithelial cells detected by Gould, Miller and Jao (1975), for these might represent residual cells in an in situ part of the tumour.

PROGNOSIS

Is the Mononuclear Stromal Infiltrate of Prognostic Significance? It has sometimes been suggested that, since circumscription of a mammary carcinoma is a good prognostic indicator independent of histological type, the lymphoid infiltrate may be of little or no importance in determining the favourable prognosis. Some workers have even questioned whether medullary carcinoma represents a specific morphological entity and expressed grave doubts about or frankly denied the good prognosis attributed to this lesion (Schwartz, 1969; Flores et al, 1974). Schwartz (1969) introduced the term 'solid circumscribed' to describe medullary carcinoma, but the use of this term is a potential source of confusion. More than 95 per cent of all mammary carcinomas are solid, i.e. non-cystic, so that the designation 'solid' adds little to the identification of a medullary carcinoma. Furthermore, as already pointed out, occasionally medullary carcinoma can be cystic. Admittedly Schwartz (1969) was apparently referring to the solid growth pattern, i.e. syncytial pattern, at the *microscopic* level, but even workers as experienced as Ridolfi et al (1977) understood the term 'solid' as a reference to the gross appearance of the lesion. Little purpose is served by attempting to replace the acceptable and generally used designation 'medullary' by a slightly more cumbersome name which has no real advantage. In addition, Lane et al (1961) had already shown that many carcinomas with rounded, well-delimited contours are not medullary carcinomas. Indeed, medullary carcinomas accounted for less than one-third of all such tumours in Lane's series. It was Lane et al (1961) who made the important observation that circumscription, regardless of specific histological type, is a favourable prognostic indicator. But this does not answer the question whether medullary carcinoma constitutes a specific entity nor whether the mononuclear stromal infiltrate is of any special prognostic significance.

Ridolfi et al (1977) applied themselves to this problem. They divided their three groups of medullary, atypical medullary and non-medullary cancers according to whether the mononuclear infiltrate was modest or severe. A better 10-year survival was found to correlate in each group with a more intense infiltrate. The 10-year survival figures were 71 and 91 per cent for the typical medullary group ($P<0.03$), 66 and 82 per cent for the atypical medullary group ($P<0.07$) and 56 and 86 per cent for the non-medullary group ($P<0.10$). The trend is the same in all groups, with the result statistically significant in the medullary group and nearly reaching this level in the atypical medullary group. As far as it is possible to do so, these data would seem to dispose of the argument that the lymphoid infiltrate is not of itself of prognostic significance. *These results also underscore the importance of a substantial mononuclear cell infiltration in the definition of medullary carcinoma.*

Ridolfi et al (1977) drew two conclusions of major importance. They emphasized, after a very careful analysis of conflicting data, that, as strictly defined by them, *medullary carcinoma is a distinct entity with a very favourable prognosis and a 10-year survival rate of 84 per cent.* It should be remembered that a 10-year survival rate is virtually the equivalent of a cure rate in the case of medullary carcinoma, since with this tumour type a fatal outcome, if it occurs, may be expected within seven years of treatment. Interestingly, this 10-year survival rate of 84 per cent is very similar to the original observation by Moore and Foote (1949). In some subsequent work this excellent prognosis was somewhat obscured because of a less precise definition of the concept of medullary carcinoma. Thus even McDivitt, Stewart and Berg (1968), from the same institute as Ridolfi et al (1977), reported a 10-year survival of 68 per cent, which compares unfavourably with the original work of Moore and Foote (1949).

Schwartz (1969) found that, despite a lower incidence of axillary metastases in the 'solid circumscribed' carcinomas, the 10-year survival was no better in comparison with a series of breast carcinomas of all types. This is completely at variance with most other workers. Unfortunately the composition of the control non-medullary carcinoma group was not defined and, as hinted at by Ridolfi et al (1977), appears to have included special types of breast carcinoma with a favourable prognosis. The present writer considers that the illustrations of Schwartz (1969) do not reassure the reader that the group of tumours analysed compares at all strictly with medullary carcinomas as the term is generally employed by pathologists. Probably the use of the term 'solid circumscribed' has contributed to this misunderstanding.

Flores et al (1974) also found no demonstrable improvement in 10-year survival rates in patients with medullary carcinoma of the breast. Their illustrations show tumours which are perfectly acceptable as medullary carcinomas though one cannot be sure that this would apply to all their cases. Ridolfi et al (1977) found and detailed a number of inconsistencies in the data of Flores et al (1974) in view of which they felt unable to draw any conclusions regarding survival from this report.

It seems to the writer that the conclusions of Schwartz (1969) are based on an inadequate understanding of what constitutes a medullary carcinoma. Many of the tumours on which his conclusions are based appear to be circumscribed carcinomas, as opposed to stellate carcinomas, with an element of solid growth pattern microscopically. This is of course not the definition of medullary carcinoma adopted by Moore and Foote (1949) and more recently delineated even more precisely by Ridolfi and coworkers (1977). In the intervening period between these two key papers, the definition has been obscured, only partially by some workers, but more or less completely by some others.

The *second major conclusion of Ridolfi et al* (1977) was that only 21 per cent of patients with typical medullary carcinoma had axillary nodal metastases, compared with 42 per cent for a control group with infiltrating ductal carcinoma. Of those with node involvement, two-thirds had only one to three involved nodes and only one-third, or 7 per cent of the whole, had four or more positive nodes. Of interest is the fact that no patient with typical medullary carcinoma with axillary metastases died of this disease when not more than three axillary nodes were involved by carcinoma. Ridolfi et al (1977) were at pains to point out that *more important perhaps than the difference in the incidence of axillary node metastases is the more favourable prognosis in the presence of such nodal metastases.*

DIFFICULTY OF MAKING THIS DIAGNOSIS

The writer has found that in practice one of the most difficult assessments with invasive carcinoma can be in deciding whether or not a particular tumour should be included in the medullary carcinoma group (Figures 12–10 and 12–11). McDivitt, Stewart and Berg (1968) required an 'embryonal–carcinoma-like' and delicate quality of the cell (Figure 12–10); but whereas this feature is present in typical cases, it is not a characteristic which lends itself at all easily to objective definition. It would appear that the latter authors did not regard lymphoid and plasma cell (LP) infiltration as an essential criterion for defining this tumour type. Fisher, Gregorio and Fisher (1975) insisted on a moderate or marked lymphoid infiltrate with a scant fibrous component, in addition to the histological circumscription demanded by all workers (Figures 12–10 and 12–11). This definition is commendable, and the necessity for at least a moderate lymphoid infiltrate is insisted upon also by Ridolfi et al (1977) (Figures 12–10 and 12–11). There is every reason to agree with Fisher, Gregorio and Fisher (1975) that tumours which lack even a moderate LP infiltrate should be excluded. The failure to insist on this requirement is responsible for some of the dissension which has arisen in relation to the prognosis of this tumour even among those who accept it as an identifiable entity.

Peripheral Extension into Adjacent Tissue. A problem arises in relation to tumours which fulfil all the other criteria but which, while having a very sharply circumscribed margin for the most part, show some degree of peripheral extension into the adjacent tissue. If multiple microscopic fields show such extension, the tumour should not be classified

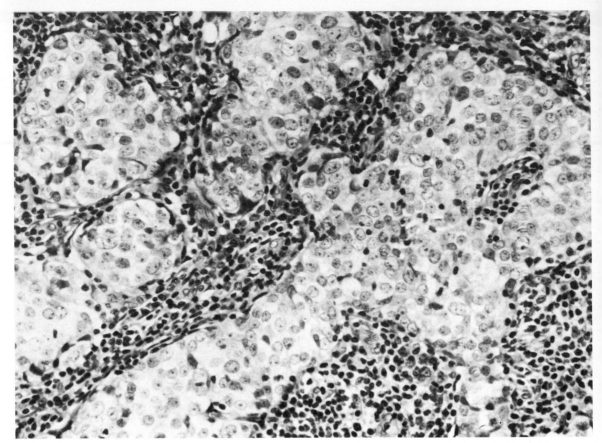

Figure 12–11 A well-circumscribed tumour with sheet-like growth of tumour cells and a heavy mononuclear cell infiltration. The tumour cells are smaller and paler-staining than those of a typical medullary carcinoma and have a less heavy chromatin structure. H and E. ×400.

as a typical medullary carcinoma and the same applies if there is infiltration of surrounding tissue at a number of points. If the infiltration is categorized as minimal (or focal), in the sense that it occupies only one low-power field (×10), there may well be a case for accepting the tumour as a medullary carcinoma. This is based on the finding of Ridolfi et al (1977) that focal infiltration, as defined, at the periphery of an otherwise typical medullary carcinoma did not appear to affect the outcome, although their data did not allow for certainty on this point. It could of course be argued that if any extension at all is present, further foci could be found with more extensive sampling. Nevertheless, the suggestion of Ridolfi et al (1977) is a very reasonable one and a basis for further study.

Quantity of Fibrous Stroma. The amount of fibrous stroma can pose something of a dilemma. Tumours are occasionally seen which fit largely into the medullary pattern but which are endowed with moderate amounts of fibrous stroma in some parts. It does seem likely that the necrotic portions of a medullary carcinoma may be replaced by fibrous tissue and it is perhaps a little unreasonable to exclude a tumour from the medullary category solely on this basis. But it must be admitted that it has not yet been proven that medullary carcinoma undergoes post-necrotic fibrosis, for the necrotic tissue sometimes liquefies with little or no sign of fibrous replacement. For the present the insistence of Fisher, Gregorio and Fisher (1975) that there must be only a scant fibrous component is to be commended.

Difficulty of Classifying 'Circumscribed Carcinomas'. From all that has been said it will be abundantly clear that the statement of

Haagensen (1971) that 'circumscribed carcinomas . . . are among the easiest of breast carcinomas to classify' cannot be accepted as applicable to medullary carcinoma. Herein lies perhaps the most important single cause of discrepancy in the literature. The term 'circumscribed carcinoma' is not really useful to indicate a specific *histological* entity with a very good prognosis. It can be used in the sense of Lane et al (1961) to indicate a *heterogeneous* group of tumours with a better than average prognosis. The use of the term should be discontinued in the histopathological diagnosis of individual tumours.

CRITERIA FOR MAKING THIS DIAGNOSIS

A diagnosis of typical medullary carcinoma should be made only when the following criteria are satisfied. A syncytial growth pattern must constitute at least 75 per cent of the tumour sampled. The tumour must be not only well delineated grossly but also sharply and completely circumscribed microscopically: the only possible exception is the presence of extension at the margin which occupies only one low-power field, but even this is still questionable. There must be a mononuclear stromal infiltrate which is both substantial and diffuse. A mere sprinkling of lymphoid cells or their patchy presence is inadequate. So also is the presence of an infiltrate at the margins of the tumour only, with little or none in the interior of the mass. The neoplastic cells should be large, larger in general than in most types of mammary carcinoma (compare Figures 12–10 and 12–11). The nuclei may vary considerably in appearance in different tumours and, to a lesser extent, in the same tumour, but in general they should correspond to nuclear grade 1 or 2 to allow a diagnosis of medullary carcinoma. An extensive intraductal component is rarely present in medullary carcinoma and, in its presence, a tumour will hardly ever qualify as medullary carcinoma. A very small in situ component was found by Ridolfi et al (1977) in a minority of otherwise typical cases (9 per cent only) so that, while a small in situ component does not entirely exclude a typical medullary carcinoma, the presence of any in situ component should lead to extreme caution in making this diagnosis. These criteria are based, with minor modifications, on those carefully laid down by Ridolfi et al

(1977). Even utilizing all these criteria, difficulties will still arise, but they will be reduced. If there is reasonable doubt about the inclusion of a tumour after consideration of all these features, it should be excluded. Only in this way will the entity 'medullary carcinoma with lymphoid infiltration' retain its identity.

Atypical Medullary Carcinoma

Fisher, Gregorio and Fisher (1975) hinted that tumours which fall into the atypical medullary group require segregation, for the time being, until more is learned about them, and that eventually they may require separate recognition for a number of reasons (Figure 12–11). Atypical medullary carcinoma was the name adopted also by Ridolfi et al (1977); 79 of the carcinomas with medullary features they studied fell into this subgroup, compared with 57 in the typical medullary category. It is worth noting that axillary node involvement was present in 30 per cent of the atypical cases compared with 21 per cent in the typical medullary group. The 10-year survival for atypical medullary carcinoma was 74 per cent, a figure not as good as for typical tumours but considerably better than for carcinoma NOS. Ridolfi et al (1977) concluded that the tumours they categorized as atypical medullary carcinomas probably represented a heterogeneous group which should more appropriately be classified as infiltrating ductal carcinomas. While it is true that they probably constitutute a heterogeneous group, the suggestion of Fisher et al (1975) that they should be segregated provisionally is a reasonable compromise which may or may not prove to be justified by further studies.

The paper by Ridolfi et al (1977) constitutes *a classical milestone* in the study of medullary carcinoma.

INFILTRATING DUCTAL CARCINOMA WITH CIRCUMSCRIPTION AND PLASMA CELL INFILTRATION

McDivitt, Stewart and Berg (1968) drew attention to the problem of infiltrating ductal carcinoma which has circumscribed rather than the more usual infiltrative margins and which is also associated with lymphoid and plasma cell infiltration. This subgroup constituted about 11 per cent of their infiltrating duct-cancer group; it was selected on the basis of two pathological criteria which quite possibly are of independent significance. The prognosis lay between that of the ordinary infiltrating ductal carcinoma and the medullary carcinoma group. For this reason alone, it is a useful subgroup to recognize, but it must be admitted that it is not always easy to decide whether a given tumour should be placed in this category. If there is doubt about a particular tumour it should not be placed in this subgroup.

Ridolfi's 'non-medullary' group corresponds roughly to McDivitt's under consideration here, as it was selected from tumours with 'medullary features' which did not satisfy the criteria for inclusion in either the medullary or the atypical medullary varieties. Their non-medullary carcinomas 'generally appeared to be grossly circumscribed infiltrating duct carcinomas with areas of syncytial growth or prominent mononuclear infiltrates'. This definition, while not identical with that of McDivitt, Stewart and Berg (1968), does indicate a considerable overlap. Interestingly enough, they found a 63 per cent 10-year survival in this group comparable with the 56 per cent of McDivitt, Stewart and Berg (1968). LP infiltration per se appeared to be a factor affecting prognosis, those with the heavier infiltrate having an 86 per cent compared with a 56 per cent 10-year survival, though the figures were not statistically significant ($P<0.10$). Similarly there was a trend to a better prognosis when plasma cells, as distinct from lymphocytes, were abundant: 75 per cent as opposed to 51 per cent 10-year survival. It is pertinent that McDivitt, Stewart and Berg (1968) found that if the plasma cell reaction completely surrounded the tumour, there was less axillary nodal involvement and a better chance of survival. When the plasma cell response around the margins was incomplete, the frequency of nodal involvement was not reduced but survival rates were much improved both with and without nodal involvement. It is remarkable that McDivitt, Stewart and Berg (1968) and Ridolfi et al (1977) reached conclusions which are so similar despite their different starting points. The McDivitt fascicle is more conclusive about the significance of a plasma cell infiltrate, as would be expected from the way their material was selected.

MUCOID OR COLLOID CARCINOMA

Synonyms. Another circumscribed carcinoma of distinctive microscopic type goes by the name of mucoid carcinoma: synonyms are colloid carcinoma, gelatinous carcinoma, mucinous carcinoma and mucin-producing carcinoma. Gelatinous and colloid carcinoma are names which reflect the macroscopic appearances, the former possibly doing so better than the latter. However, in order to conform with the practice of classifying carcinomas primarily, as far as possible, by their microscopic rather than their macroscopic characteristics, the alternative names are slightly to be preferred. 'Mucoid', 'mucinous' and 'mucin-producing' carcinoma all reflect the most striking microscopic feature of this tumour. 'Mucin-producing' has no particular advantage over 'mucoid' and 'mucinous', and the latter two names have the advantage of brevity. Mucoid carcinoma is one of the terms in most frequent use and is used here. 'Mucinous' is an equally acceptable alternative.

None of these terms is perfect. All three names which denote mucin production could imply that all mucin-secreting carcinomas are classified here, but this is not true. *The signet-ring cell carcinoma, specifically, must be excluded.* But it is true that these mucoid carcinomas have a more copious *extracellular* mucin secretion than any other type. Intracellular mucin is also present but it is relatively scanty, though the neoplastic cells are the source of the copious extracellular mucin.

'Colloid' carcinoma rivals 'mucoid' carcinoma in the frequency with which it is used. Literally it means 'gluey', which does not seem particularly appropriate even as a macroscopic descriptive term, but presumably it has gained vogue because it is a term used in other organs also. 'Colloid' carcinoma, as applied to breast cancer, also suffers from having unfortunate overtones of the time when the mucin content was regarded as a stromal degenerative product.

But all the five synonyms listed are reasonably acceptable. The two which refer to the macroscopic features exclusively are clearly understood by all. The three which refer predominantly to microscopic characteristics are preferable for reasons already stated and 'mucoid', because it is probably least likely to be misunderstood, is perhaps marginally the best of the three.

Largely because they are not open to misinterpretation, the terms mucoid and colloid carcinoma have, therefore, been selected to head this section.

PURE AND IMPURE MUCOID CARCINOMA

Incidence of Pure Mucoid Carcinoma. The main point requiring emphasis in the diagnosis of this entity (Figure 12–12) is the sharp separation which must be made between pure tumours and impure tumours, i.e. those which have an additional component of ordinary infiltrating ductal carcinoma. The more clearly this distinction is made, the more evident the clinicopathological differences between mucoid carcinoma and carcinoma NOS become. The incidence of pure mucoid carcinoma varies only slightly in most of the larger series between 1.8 per cent (Veronesi and Gennari, 1960) and 2.6 per cent (McDivitt, Stewart and Berg, 1968), with an average of 2.4 per cent or approximately 1 in

40 of operable breast cancers. A higher incidence of 5.3 per cent is reported by Silverberg et al (1971) but the reasons for this are not clear.

COMPARISON OF MUCOID CARCINOMA WITH CARCINOMA NOS

Patient Age and Tumour Size. There is no agreement on whether these tumours tend to be more frequent in older age groups. Silverberg et al (1971) found a mean age among 28 patients of 68.6 years as compared with 54.3 years for NOS cancer. McDivitt, Stewart and Berg (1968) found no age difference. The higher incidence of larger tumours reported by McDivitt, Stewart and Berg (1968) was confirmed by Silverberg et al (1971). An average size of 3.8 cm compares with an average of 3.1 cm for carcinoma NOS.

In Situ Component Usually Inconspicuous. In most cases, ductal carcinoma in situ is not

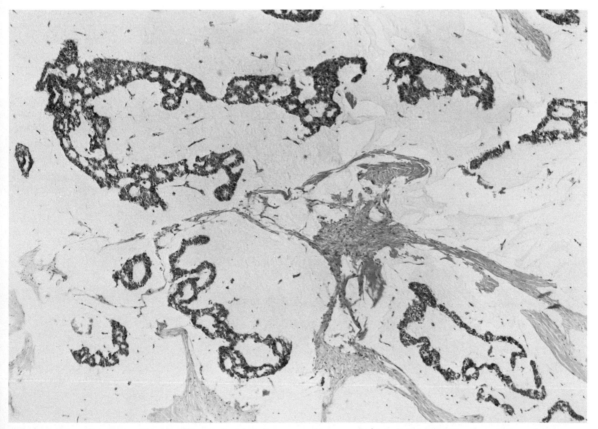

Figure 12–12 Mucoid carcinoma. The copious mucinous matrix may stain so palely in routine preparations that its very presence can be missed. H and E. ×60.

found in these tumours and, when it is detected, it is usually not extensive. The in situ phase may exhibit little or no mucin secretion or it may display a copious extracellular mucin production.

INCIDENCE OF NODAL METASTASIS, PROGNOSIS AND TREATMENT

The generally favourable prognosis of this tumour type is now widely, if not universally, accepted. *The more stringent the criteria in defining a pure mucoid carcinoma, the more favourable is the prognosis.* There is some discrepancy regarding the frequency of axillary node involvement, though all observers are agreed that the incidence is lower than in carcinoma NOS. The earlier cited figure of 36 per cent nodal involvement had dropped marginally to 32 per cent and 28.6 per cent by 1971 (Veronesi and Gennari, 1960; Melamed, Robbins and Foote, 1961; McDivitt, Stewart and Berg, 1968; Silverberg et al, 1971). Norris and Taylor (1965) provided a striking contrast of only 4 per cent nodal involvement (one of 27 patients). This difference needs explaining, and it is probably not entirely due to chance or to the relatively small size of the series. Norris and Taylor (1965) laid great stress on the importance of the purity of a mucoid carcinoma and, because of the enormous material they were dealing with, they were probably able to apply very stringent criteria in their case selection. Only 10 per cent of patients with pure colloid carcinomas in their series were known to have died of their tumours, compared with 29 per cent of those with 'mixed colloid carcinomas'. And they imply that acceptance of only cases with very adequate sampling as pure tumours would show that the lethal potential was even less. Indeed, Norris and Taylor (1965) advocated a somewhat conservative approach in treatment. If, after excisional biopsy with thorough study of adequate samples, a given tumour is shown to be pure and there is no palpable axillary node enlargement, they cautiously advocated that a simple mastectomy be performed. There is probably some risk in adopting this course, and it is not standard procedure in most centres, but it is an interesting point of departure for further discussion. It must, however, be stated that Haagensen (1971) has criticized this recommendation and states boldly that 'any surgeon who performs less than a thorough and meticulous radical mastectomy for them [mucoid carcinomas] is risking his patient's life unnecessarily'. Reconciling these two views is not easy. As with ductal carcinoma in situ, the pathologist can provide the surgeon with the most credible data available in the literature, and as accurate a diagnosis as he can possibly give in an individual case. There his task stops and, in the final analysis, the surgeon must decide on the best treatment in the individual patient. He is not thereby prevented from holding a view but he sometimes best keeps his own counsel.

DIFFICULT 'BORDERLINE' OF TUMOUR ENTITIES

The difficulty with all classification is the placing of tumours which show *transitional features* between two tumour groups and those which show variable *mixtures* of two or more distinct entities. With the former, they should be placed according to the observer's interpretation of which features should determine the nosological position of a given tumour, as has been discussed for medullary carcinoma. With mixtures of entities, they can be categorized according to the dominant tumour type or, better perhaps, according to the tumour type which is considered to have the worse prognosis; perhaps it is best to categorize such a neoplasm as an 'impure' tumour consisting of A+B or B+C+D and so on. Up to 10 years ago especially, most of the emphasis was on delineating new entities and new subtypes, and the 'borderline' types of tumour were understandably, but regrettably, swept under the carpet and conveniently ignored. This trend has now been reversed (see, for instance, Fisher, Gregorio and Fisher, 1975). Pathologists, while always endeavouring to delineate tumour types more accurately, have increasingly appreciated that mixtures of tumour types may be found in the same breast, in the same area of the same quadrant of a breast and, very much less frequently, even in the same lobule (see the section on lobular cancerization).

PAPILLARY CARCINOMA

Papillary carcinoma, retaining a papillary structure in its invasive portion, is a very rare tumour. The figure of about 0.3 per cent given by Fisher, Gregorio and Fisher (1975) conforms with the writer's findings and views. Almost certainly the use of the term 'papillomatosis' for what is more correctly termed 'epitheliosis' (Chapter Seven) has contributed to the abuse of the designation 'papillary carcinoma' for certain invasive tumours where there is nothing to justify it. Fisher et al (1975) are one of the few groups of workers to recognize and point out the rarity of papillary structure in invasive breast carcinoma.

SQUAMOUS CARCINOMA

'Partially Apocrine' and Medullary Carcinomas Misdiagnosed. Squamous metaplasia may be present focally in carcinomas of the breast but it is not a common finding. *Pure squamous carcinomas are extremely rare.* Some tumours are erroneously regarded as squamous neoplasms because of one of two main reasons. There is a lingering tendency to call large-polygonal-cell tumours squamoid or even squamous, even when there is no convincing evidence by modern standards that the tumours exhibit any distinct evidence of squamous differentiation. Some of these tumours are in fact showing *partial* apocrine differentiation, which accounts for their eosinophilia and slight to moderate cytoplasmic granularity, nucleolar prominence and nuclear staining variability. Others probably belong in the category of medullary carcinomas, in which squamous differentiation has been reported to occur with a somewhat higher frequency than that found by the present writer. Aside from the question of the precise incidence of squamous metaplasia in medullary carcinomas, when such true squamous metaplasia is present focally in a medullary carcinoma, the tumour is occasionally mistaken for a pure squamous carcinoma and the fact that it is essentially a medullary carcinoma can be missed altogether. Thus, partially apocrine carcinomas and medullary carcinomas are among the types of breast cancer which are, for different reasons, sometimes mistaken for pure squamous carcinomas.

Squamous Metaplasia in Adenocarcinoma. The second reason for the overdiagnosis of pure squamous carcinoma is a lack of adequate sampling, which would have shown that most cases so labelled are instances of ordinary carcinoma with squamous metaplastic alteration. There is a natural tendency for pathologists to diagnose a rather exotic 'squamous carcinoma of the breast' rather than a more prosaic, if more truthful, adenocarcinoma with squamous metaplasia.

LITERATURE SURVEY

Arffmann and Højgaard (1965) reviewed the literature and found that pure squamous carcinoma of the breast parenchyma, not involving the epidermis or nipple region, was excessively rare. Stewart (1950) had not encountered such a case. McDivitt, Stewart and Berg (1968) also implied, though they did not categorically state, that they had never seen a case. Haagensen (1971) had never seen it, though he had found 20 cases of breast carcinoma with squamous metaplasia over 50 years. Haagensen (1971) is a valuable source of references to the earlier reports in the German, French, American and British literature between 1921 and 1955. Arffmann and Højgaard (1965) reported a solitary convincing example of pure squamous carcinoma originating in the glandular tissue of the breast.

Cornog et al (1971) reviewed the literature with a bearing on this problem in an attempt to explain the discrepancies in the reports on the incidence of squamous carcinoma. They found that only three out of 24 tumours in their own material diagnosed as squamous carcinoma could be regarded as genuinely pure squamous carcinomas; in no fewer than two of these three cases an epidermal origin could not be excluded. The solitary case of pure squamous carcinoma with a definite origin in the breast parenchyma arose in a cystosarcoma phyllodes.

PERSONAL CONCLUSIONS

From a study of the literature and my own experience, it is my distinct impression that most of the tumours which are candidates for serious consideration as pure squamous carcinomas of the mamma are those which exhibit marked spindle-cell metaplasia and which are considered in the next section on

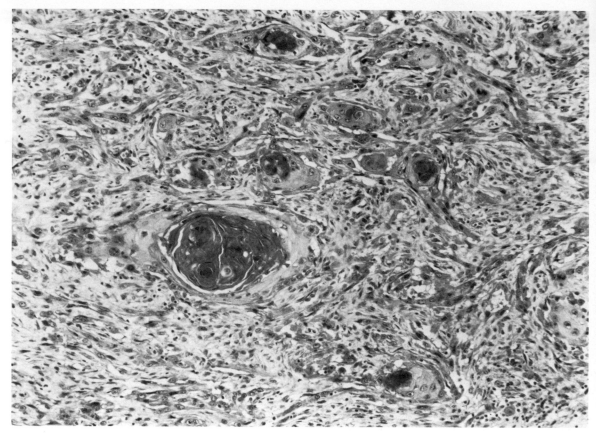

Figure 12–13   Keratinizing squamous carcinoma with marked spindle-cell metaplasia and merger with fasciculated areas mimicking fibrosarcoma. H and E. ×150.

pseudofibrosarcoma and pseudocarcinosarcoma. I have seen four cases of the latter type, but in only one was the material available in its entirety so that I could be reasonably convinced of its purity because of the absence of any neoplastic glandular elements (Figures 12–13 and 12–14). The only other case of possibly pure squamous carcinoma I have seen was situated in a cystosarcoma phyllodes, but, since the material was not available in its entirety, there is no proof that adenocarcinomatous elements were completely lacking. Nevertheless, this keratinizing squamous carcinoma in a cystosarcoma phyllodes is of interest in that it is similar to the only definite case of pure squamous carcinoma of the breast in the detailed study of Cornog et al (1971).

If one excludes tumours of the nipple region and of the skin and its appendages, pure squamous carcinoma of the mamma is very rare. One should remember that *appendage tumours, especially those of the hair sheath,* can mimic squamous carcinomas very closely and, as they are situated deep to the epidermis, they *can be confused with a tumour of the breast parenchyma.* The writer has seen a pilar tumour of the axillary skin mistaken for a squamous carcinoma of the axillary tail of the breast, a compounded error since the pilar tumour is for practical purposes always benign. After exclusion of such errors, squamous carcinoma of the breast falls into four categories; these are, in descending order of frequency:

1. The vast majority are adenocarcinomas of various types showing different degrees of squamous metaplasia: even these are less common than is sometimes implied. Only 20 were seen at the Presbyterian Hospital, New York, over a 50-year period (Haagensen, 1971).
2. Squamous carcinomas with extensive spindle-cell metaplasia and sometimes marked desmoplasia with varying degrees of mimicry of fibrosarcoma and of carcinosarcoma (Figures 12–13 and 12–14).

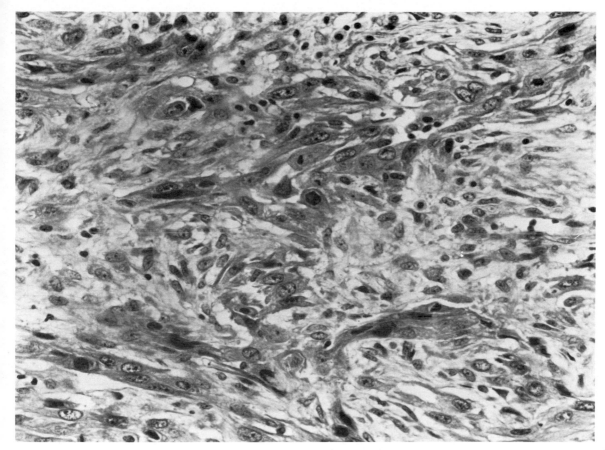

Figure 12–14   Same tumour as shown in Figure 12–13. There is the beginning of a sarcomatoid aspect. H and E. ×400.

3. Extremely rare squamous carcinomas occurring in cystosarcoma phyllodes, as described by Cornog et al (1971) and seen in a personally studied case.
4. Extremely rare pure squamous carcinoma without spindle-cell metaplasia, and not arising in a pre-existing tumour, of the type described by Arffmann and Højgaard (1965). Authentic tumours of this type are so rare that any case detected in the future deserves the most thorough study and documentation.

RECORDED DISCREPANCIES ON PATIENT AGE AND PROGNOSIS

Squamous metaplasia in breast carcinomas is said to be more common in elderly women (McDivitt, Stewart and Berg, 1968) but the average age of the patients was only 50 years in the series of Haagensen (1971), and these tumours did not have any distinctive clinical characteristics. Carcinomas with squamous metaplasia can metastasize to regional lymph nodes and other sites and can cause death. Pure squamous carcinoma or carcinoma of combined spindle-cell and squamous type may be present in the metastases.

These squamous metaplastic breast carcinomas have sometimes been said to have a hopeless prognosis, but the prognosis was found to be about average by Haagensen (1971). Other workers have implied a better prognosis for squamous carcinoma of the breast. These discrepancies in the average age of the patients with, and in the behaviour of, this tumour bedevil the literature on this subject.

There is a need to separate squamous carcinomas of the breast into the four categories listed above, apart from making certain in the first place that the tumour shows unequivocal squamous differentiation. Having separated carcinomas with genuinely squamous differentiation into the four categories, tumours in the first group, which is the largest, deserve further analysis. Small foci of widely scattered squamous differentiation may have a different significance from a substantial element of squamous differentiation, and very extensive or dominant squamous metaplasia may have a greater significance still. Until attention is paid to these categories of squamous carcinoma and to the extent of the squamous differentiation, the widely discordant findings about the clinical aspects and the behaviour of this tumour type are likely to go on repeating themselves. Because of the rarity of these carcinomas, *probably only one of the multicentre studies will be able to produce any really meaningful data in this respect.*

For the moment, the available information is sufficient to enable one to conclude that:

1. It is not true that the prognosis of patients with this tumour is as hopeless as has sometimes been suggested, witness the eight 10-year survivors among 13 patients of Haagensen (1971) treated by radical mastectomy more than 10 years previously.
2. It is true, on the other hand, that these tumours can metastasize and kill and there is no reason to treat them any more conservatively than other breast carcinomas, unless there are purely clinical reasons for so doing.

PSEUDOCARCINOSARCOMA AND PSEUDO-FIBROSARCOMA

Carcinosarcoma of the breast is a very rare tumour and one is only allowed the luxury of this diagnosis when a tumour has been very thoroughly sampled and studied. This applies also to organs other than the breast, though there are sites like the endometrium, and more rarely the ovary, in which a diagnosis of true carcinosarcoma is more easily established. This applies particularly to the mixed mesodermal uterine tumours in which heterologous elements like striated muscle are frequently demonstrable.

In the case of the breast, a malignant spindle-cell fasciculated tumour, in the presence of foci of carcinoma (which may themselves require a careful search before their presence and identity can be established), should not be considered sarcomatous until an exhaustive search has failed to show any evidence of transition from the carcinomatous foci to the spindle-cell tumour (Figures 12–13 and 12–14). The evidence of transition may be restricted to small areas and often takes the form of a 'splintering off' or fraying out of the peripheral cells of carcinomatous foci and their imperceptible merging with and gentle fading into an apparently sarcomatous tumour (Figures 12–13 and 12–14). Step or even serial sections through carcinomatous foci are frequently essential to establish this point with reasonable confidence. The problem is analogous to that encountered with the polypoid squamous carcinomas of the upper alimentary and respiratory tracts: very extensive sampling and searching is often necessary to establish the presence of continuity between squamous carcinoma foci and malignant spindle cells in the tumour core. In the case of the breast, the carcinomatous foci may be glandular, squamous or both. Robb and MacFarlane (1958) cautioned against a diagnosis of carcinosarcoma when the sarcomatoid component of a breast tumour may in fact represent spindle-cell metaplasia in a carcinoma, as in their Case 1. Willis (1958) drew attention to the danger of a diagnosis of primary fibrosarcoma of the breast in cases of this type when the obviously carcinomatous component is difficult to detect, or of a diagnosis of true carcinosarcoma when two apparently distinct elements are found. In his case, several pathologists had fallen into the trap of diagnosing a carcinosarcoma but Willis (1958) demonstrated unequivocal evidence of transition between the squamous carcinomatous foci and the spindle-cell malignant tumour. The spindle-cell carcinoma was associated with marked desmoplasia and was indistinguishable in many areas from fibrosarcoma. I have studied three similar cases, two by courtesy of Professor H. Schornagel and of Professors A. Arrigoni and P. Lampertico respectively, in which a spindle-cell tumour merged indefinably into fusiform-cell tumour, which in turn merged with nests of carcinoma cells, which in their turn could be traced into keratinizing squamous carcinoma (Figures 12–13 and 12–14). Jones (1969) described a similar case and the writer has studied yet another one very recently. The latter mimicked a pure sarcoma, as the carcinomatous elements were few, scattered and difficult to pick out even in selected sections. In many of these sarcomatoid carcinomas, the tumour is a squamous carcinoma which has the ability, as in some other sites, to show extensive spindle-cell metaplasia (Figures 12–13 and 12–14).

In conclusion, before diagnosing a primary fibrosarcoma of the breast or a true carcinosarcoma, one has the duty to exclude spindle-cell metaplasia in a carcinoma, usually of the squamous type, by all available means. Of course, apparent primary fibrosarcoma of the breast has also to be distinguished from malignant cystosarcoma phyllodes, but that is not the problem under consideration here.

7. RECENTLY RECOGNIZED TYPES OF CARCINOMA AND ONES ON WHICH NEW DATA ARE AVAILABLE

HISTIOCYTOID CARCINOMA

This pathological variant of breast carcinoma is well worth recognition because of the diagnostic problems it raises (Figure 12–15). The apt term 'histiocytoid carcinoma' was coined by Hood, Font and Zimmerman (1973). These authors studied a group of 13 cases with metastatic mammary cancer in the eyelid. These metastases were often the first clinical sign of cancer or else the first detected metastasis in a patient previously subjected to mastectomy for carcinoma; this applied to nine of their 13 patients. These clinical features themselves would present a diagnostic challenge but particularly so when combined with a 'histiocytoid' microscopic appearance in eight of the 13 cases (Figure 12–15).

Differential Diagnosis. The differential diagnostic misinterpretations included xanthelasma, xanthoma, histiocytosis, and granular-cell 'myoblastoma', reflecting the histiocytic appearance of these mucus-secreting adenocarcinomas (Figure 12–15). All eight cases in which mucin stains were carried out contained variable amounts of intracytoplasmic, hyaluronidase-resistant, alcianophilic material, which also stained with the PAS technique. Fat stains were negative on three tumours in which suitable material was available for study, though the authors could not be certain that storage in alcohol may not have been responsible for the negative results. Hood, Font and Zimmerman (1973) suggested a similarity with and a relationship to the lipid-secreting breast cancers considered in the next section but, apart from the negative fat stains, the writer believes that the two groups are not closely related, except by virtue of cytoplasmic vacuolation in both types of tumour. The 'Indian file' arrangement in most tumours and the mucinous cytoplasmic vacuolation (Gad and Azzopardi, 1975) leave little room for doubt that most of these tumours belong to the infiltrating lobular carcinoma group (Figure 12–15); at least eight, and perhaps 10, of these 13 carcinomas appear to fall into this category.

LIPID-RICH CARCINOMA

Lipid-secreting breast cancer was described by Aboumrad, Horn and Fine in 1963. Ramos and Taylor (1974) carried out a detailed study of 13 cases of lipid-rich carcinoma of the breast (Figures 12–16 and 12–17). These tumours are characterized by an abundant foamy cytoplasm which contains a large amount of neutral lipid. The cells do not contain mucin. The lipid material is not degenerative in origin (Figures 12–16 and 12–17). Nodes are involved in a 'sinusoidal fashion' and this mode of involvement together with the appearance of the cytoplasmic content combine to mimic some form of histiocytosis or reticuloendotheliosis (Ramos and Taylor, 1974). The presence of intramitochondrial crystals in a case studied ultrastructurally has not been noted in other types of breast cancer studied to date. These tumours can be associated with either ductal or lobular carcinoma in situ. Three examples of lipid-rich carcinoma studied by the writer were all associated with ductal carcinoma patterns, in situ or infiltrating.

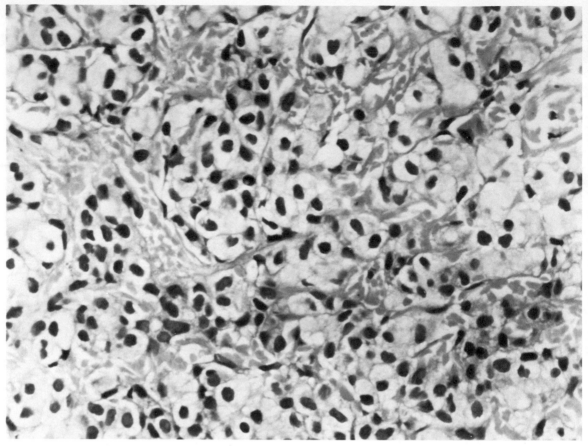

Figure 12–15 Histiocytoid carcinoma with small cell clumps and single cells. The pale cytoplasm and relatively small nuclei may lead superficially to confusion with a conglomerate of histiocytes. H and E. ×600.

Histiocytoid Carcinoma is Not a Lipid-Rich Carcinoma. Ramos and Taylor (1974) equated their tumours with the histiocytoid carcinomas of Hood, Font and Zimmerman (1973), which Ramos and Taylor (1974) refer to as 'lipid cell carcinomas', despite the fact that Hood et al (1973) found negative reactions for fat and positive reactions for mucin. One cannot state that there is no overlap at all but, on present evidence, these two entities appear to be distinct. The incidence of lipid-secreting breast cancer was found to be of the order of 1.4 per cent of all breast carcinomas.

Incidence. Van Bogaert and Maldague (1977) described 10 lipid-secreting car-cinomas found in a review of 600 cases of breast cancer, an incidence of 1.6 per cent, comparable with the 1.4 per cent of Ramos and Taylor (1974). Their review of the literature yielded only 15 other well-documented cases. Like the writer, van Bogaert and Maldague (1977) were puzzled by the suggestion of Hood, Font and Zimmerman (1973) that their histiocytoid carcinomas are related to the lipid-rich carcinomas, for the reasons stated previously.

Varieties of Lipid-secreting Carcinoma. Van Bogaert and Maldague (1977) divided their cases of lipid-secreting breast cancer (Figures 12–16 to 12–18) into three varieties: a histiocytoid type (five cases), a sebaceous type

Figure 12–16 (*Opposite, above.*) Lipid-rich carcinoma with foamy cytoplasm of neoplastic cells. Contrast with histiocytoid carcinoma in Figure 12–15. H and E. ×400.

Figure 12–17 (*Opposite, below.*) Higher magnification of part of field shown in Figure 12–16. The cytoplasm is grossly vacuolated and foamy and the appearance resembles that of the so-called sebaceous type of lipid-secreting carcinoma. H and E. ×600.

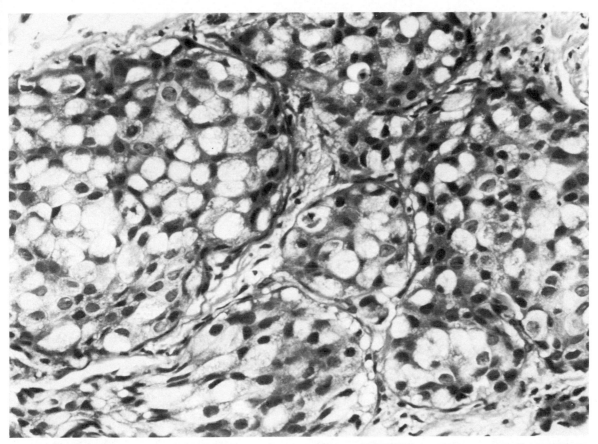

12–16

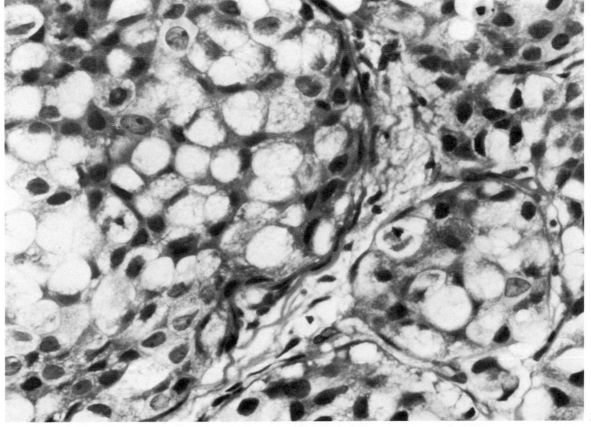

12–17

303

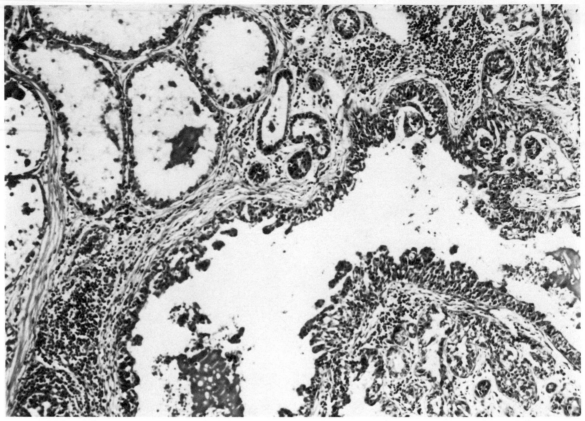

Figure 12–18   Lipid-rich carcinoma of a rare variety. There is apocrine protrusion of the nuclei. The inflammatory response and cytological atypia help distinguish it from the 'McFarland type' change (see Figure 16–3). H and E. ×120.

(three cases) and a type with 'apocrine extrusion of nuclei' (two cases). Their 'sebaceous' type differed from their 'histiocytoid' type by virtue of exhibiting greater nuclear pleomorphism and a more grossly vacuolated and bubbly cytoplasm. It seems to the writer that these two subtypes may merely represent gradations of the same entity, 'lipid-rich carcinoma', and that separate designations are probably undesirable. In any case the designation 'histiocytoid' is unfortunate since it would appear on current evidence that lipid-rich carcinomas and histiocytoid carcinomas are, for the most part at least, distinct entities. The common denominator of lipid-rich carcinomas is the presence of abundant intracytoplasmic neutral fat demonstrable by oil red 0 staining.

Nomenclature. Since Ramos and Taylor (1974) showed that the lipids are not of degenerative origin but represent a true secretory product, van Bogaert and Maldague (1977) argued that it is justifiable to call them

'lipid-secreting', as originally suggested by Aboumrad, Horn and Fine (1963), rather than 'lipid-rich', a term introduced by Ramos and Taylor (1974).

Carcinoma with 'Apocrine Extrusion of Nuclei'. The third type of lipid-secreting breast cancer recognized by van Bogaert and Maldague (1977) is the 'carcinoma with apocrine extrusion of nuclei' (Figure 12–18). Two of their 10 cases belonged in this category. This tumour type corresponds to the very rare variant of lipid-secreting breast carcinoma described by Hamperl (1977) (Figure 12–18). This variant is characterized by a hobnail appearance of the neoplastic cells lining glandular lumina, brought about by protrusion towards the lumen of the apically-orientated, pleomorphic nuclei. In the case reported on by Hamperl (1977) the patient had received exogenous hormonal stimulation with oestrogen–progestogen preparations. This exceptional variant, of which the writer has seen one example, merits separate recognition because of its distinctive characteristics (Figure 12–18). But it still belongs to the category of lipid-secreting carcinoma.

Different Method of Identifying Lipid-rich Carcinoma. Fisher et al (1977a) studied 87 consecutive breast cancers for fat content. They demonstrated intracytoplasmic lipid with oil red 0 in viable tumour cells in 65 of 87 tumours (75 per cent). The quantity of lipid was graded as moderate or marked in 30 per cent, while in 70 per cent it was absent or only slight. Lipid content was marked in five of the 87 tumours (6 per cent). This 6 per cent is considerably higher than that given by other workers, a difference probably accounted for by the method of selection. Other workers identified their tumours on morphological grounds and confirmed the presence of fat with oil red 0. By contrast, Fisher et al (1977a) identified their cases by fat stains primarily, irrespective of the morphology in routine preparations. Fisher et al stated that 'cancers that contained marked lipid showed quantities comparable to or even greater than those depicted as representative of so-called "lipid-rich" carcinoma'. None of the neoplasms in their study 'had unusual morphologic features, except for the occurrence of foci of clear cells in a few, which might prompt their recognition as a unique histologic type of mammary cancer'. While Fisher et al (1977a) appear to be suggesting that lipid-rich cancer of the breast may not represent a distinct clinicopathological entity, they agree that intracytoplasmic lipid may represent a useful histological discriminant in mammary cancer.

Prognosis. Ramos and Taylor (1974) reported a 50 per cent mortality rate during the two years following the diagnosis of lipid-rich carcinoma. Because of this, van Bogaert and Maldague (1977) tentatively suggested that secretory carcinomas may have a bad prognosis compared with other types. Several aspects of lipid-rich carcinoma are clearly still in need of elucidation by further studies.

SIGNET-RING CELL CARCINOMA

The histogenesis of signet-ring cell carcinoma is complex and has been discussed in Chapter Eleven. That some cases might well represent a variant of infiltrating lobular carcinoma was suggested by Gad and Azzopardi (1975). That this is almost certainly true has been established recently by Martinez and Azzopardi (1979). Harris et al (1978) have demonstrated that some cases are probably variants of infiltrating ductal carcinoma. Indeed, as indicated in Chapter Eleven, it is becoming apparent that there may be two histogenetic variants of signet-ring cell carcinoma.

It should be stressed that signet-ring cell carcinoma must in no way be confused with colloid carcinoma. The fact that mixtures of the two types can be found, as indicated in Chapter Eleven, stems from the shared histogenesis of colloid carcinoma and one type of signet-ring cell carcinoma. Signet-ring cell carcinoma and colloid carcinoma are distinct morphologically, prognostically and, as we now know, sometimes even histogenetically.

It is to be regretted that the A.F.I.P. fascicle (1968) lists the signet-ring cell tumour as synonymous with colloid carcinoma. The fascicle has inherited the long-standing tradition of listing synonyms and unfortunately, in the process, the enthusiastic desire to be comprehensive has occasionally taken precedence over accuracy and the overriding importance of not misleading the reader. If for historical reasons it is felt necessary to list signet-ring cell carcinoma and colloid carcinoma as synonyms, it is absolutely imperative to stress that no pathologist would regard them as synonymous nowadays.

CARCINOMA WITH OSTEOCLAST-LIKE GIANT CELLS

Factor et al (1977) described two cases of breast carcinoma with multinucleated osteoclast-like stromal giant cells believed to be of histiocytic origin. They found only two similar tumours in a review of the literature. The case of McDivitt, Stewart and Berg (1968) with epulis-type giant cells traceable to a medullary carcinoma after extensive sampling could represent a related tumour. One of my own cases with osteoclast-like cells mixed with mammary adenocarcinoma has many features in common with the tumours described by Factor et al. Factor et al (1977) divided tumours of the breast resembling giant-cell tumour of bone or containing osteoclast-like cells into three distinct categories, each of which is rare: (1) metaplastic carcinoma of the type described by Huvos, Lucas and Foote (1973), described on page 340; (2) the extraskeletal 'osteoclastoma' or giant-cell tumour of soft tissues (Salm and Sissons, 1972), of which McDivitt, Stewart and Berg (1968) had two possible examples and I have seen another by courtesy of Dr R. Salm; and (3) infiltrating carcinoma with reactive stromal giant cells, the type of tumour they described. Differentiation between these apparently distinct groups is not always easy, particularly between groups 2 and 3. The latter distinction depends mainly on the identification of definite carcinomatous areas in the tumours falling into the last category.

PRIMARY CARCINOID-LIKE TUMOUR

Cubilla and Woodruff (1977) recently identified a new entity which they believe represents a primary carcinoid tumour of the breast. They studied 10 patients with 12 tumours (including two patients mentioned in an addendum to their paper). The mean age of the patients was 54 years. *No carcinoid syndrome* was present, even in the presence of widely disseminated disease.

PATHOLOGY

The tumours were well circumscribed, mostly solid, firm and pale tan in colour. Remarkably, three of the tumours were identified by one of the authors at frozen section among 110 consecutive breast biopsies examined during a 12-month period.

The predominant pattern was one of solid nests and cords of small cells embedded in a vascularized stroma. The tumours had a distinctly organoid appearance. A ribbon pattern was present focally in one tumour and a glandular pattern in three others. Intraductal carcinoma was identified at the margins of three tumours. In two cases, in addition to nests, tumour cells exhibited focally an infiltrative pattern simulating an infiltrating lobular carcinoma.

The cytoplasm of the tumour cells varied from amphophilic to lightly eosinophilic and cell margins were poorly defined. Mitoses were generally rare, with a solitary exception containing five to 10 per high-power field.

The stroma was usually dense and fibrous. Elastic tissue and calcification were each noted in only one case.

Argyrophilia. Argyrophilic granules were present in each tumour examined and argyrophilia was considered essential to the diagnosis. Argyrophilic granules were abundant and widespread in most cases. These workers utilized a new modification of the Grimelius technique.

Focal intra- and extracellular mucin was detected in two of six cases studied, a finding which in no way invalidates the diagnosis, as these workers stressed. No argyrophilia was found in 40 control breast carcinomas of all types, in 10 control normal breast specimens, in the normal breast tissue present in about one-half of the 40 control carcinomas, and in single specimens of sclerosing adenosis, fibrocystic mastopathy, lactating breast and apocrine papillomatosis. Vogler (1947), using the Gross–Schultz method, studied 18 benign breast specimens and identified argyrophilia in ductal cells in one case with fibrocystic disease. This finding was regarded by Cubilla and Woodruff (1977) as having a bearing on the possible histogenesis of their group of tumours.

Ultrastructure. Three tumours were examined ultrastructurally and they all contained dense-core neurosecretory granules, varying in diameter between 120 and 350 nm and averaging 250 nm. These granules were uniformly round and their dense cores were separated by a narrow, clear halo from the encasing membrane. Two of the cases contained abundant granules in most cells while they were scanty in the third case.

Size of Tumours and Behaviour. Four of the tumours in their older material (1940 to 1943) were 3 cm or larger in greatest diameter. They were associated with nodal and distant metastases. Three patients had died of metastatic disease 1, 2.5 and 16 years after diagnosis. The fourth patient was alive with disseminated disease 14 years after the diagnosis.

The four more recent patients all had smaller tumours between 1 and 2 cm in diameter. None had nodal metastases and the patients are alive without evidence of disease, but the periods of follow-up are very short, between 6 months and 3.5 years after surgery.

Identity of this Tumour Type

Cubilla and Woodruff (1977) made out a very strong case for the identity of this tumour entity. It is an argyrophilic, endocrine-type tumour with dense-core granules of the type seen in other tumours of endocrine cells. There is an undoubted similarity with extra-intestinal carcinoids as pointed out by Cubilla and Woodruff (1977). Whether mammary carcinoid is the most desirable or accurate designation may be debatable at this stage, but probably no more so than in the case of other non-argentaffin carcinoids identified in organs like the thymus and cervix uteri in the last few years. Certainly the tumours described by Cubilla and Woodruff (1977) are primary breast tumours and not metastatic deposits from occult primaries in other organs.

Differentiation From and Possible Relationship to Infiltrating Lobular Carcinoma. Cubilla and Woodruff (1977) rightly suggested that these tumours must have been mistaken for other types of carcinoma in the past. Indeed, two of their own cases had been originally interpreted as infiltrating lobular carcinomas and they speculated that some of the tumours which Fechner (1975) identified as solid variants of infiltrating lobular carcinoma may have been carcinoid tumours. This interesting notion is still speculative and must be confirmed or rebutted by further studies.

In Chapter Four it was noted that the present writer had found argyrophilic cells in three fibroadenomas, a new manifestation perhaps of 'lobular neoplasia'. Time alone will tell whether or not these argyrophilic cells are related in any way to those identified by Cubilla and Woodruff (1977).

No Authentic Argentaffin Carcinoid. Devitt (1978) reported on a reputed case of an argentaffin carcinoid tumour of the breast. Though this is claimed to be a typical carcinoid tumour, the illustration provided is non-contributory, no reference is made to the staining methods employed to demonstrate argentaffinity and, just as surprising, no reference is made to the pathologist who made this unique diagnosis. The authenticity of this tumour is obviously highly questionable. If it is indeed the first recognized case of a genuinely argentaffin primary carcinoid tumour of the breast, proper documentation by a pathologist of what is, after all, a pathological entity is the minimum that a reader is entitled to expect.

'Carcinoid' with Possible Hormonal Secretion

In quite a different category are the bilateral breast tumours in a 78-year-old man reported on by Kaneko et al (1978). The tumour of the left breast was considered to be a carcinoid tumour. At necropsy, intraductal tumour was also found in the large lactiferous ducts of the right nipple. Argyrophilic granules were demonstrated in both tumours by the Bodian and Sevier–Munger methods. There was a negative argentaffin reaction in the surgically removed left breast tumour. Ultrastructurally both tumours contained dense, round, membrane-bound granules with an average diameter of 250 nm. Carcinoid tumour was not found at necropsy in any organ other than the residual right breast. Kaneko and co-workers (1978) made out a very good case for accepting this as a bilateral carcinoid-like tumour of the breast or, at the very least, an argyrophilic endocrine-type tumour with dense-core granules.

Possible Hormonal Secretion. The patient of Kaneko et al (1978) is unique also because of the moderately raised norepinephrine detected in the urine. They considered the possibility that the tumours in their patient may have represented ordinary carcinomas with ectopic hormone production, but justifiably concluded that they probably represented carcinoid-like tumours. The norepinephrine was thought to be derived from the right nipple tumour, though unfortunately direct biochemical proof was lacking since the unusual nature of the tumours was unsuspected at both surgery and necropsy and the opportunity of obtaining such proof was missed.

Importance of This Case. The case of Kaneko et al (1978) is important in that it provides independent confirmation of the existence of the new entity described by Cubilla and Woodruff (1977). It is also the first case to be recorded in a male patient. It further introduces a new dimension by providing indirect evidence that this type of tumour may be hormonally active and that the evidence for this may, as in their case, be biochemical only without overt clinical manifestations. None of the patients documented to date presented the carcinoid syndrome and this applies even to those patients with widely disseminated disease (Cubilla and Woodruff, 1977). Thus any hormone or hormones potentially or actually produced or secreted by these tumours will have to be searched for systematically when a tumour of this type is suspected in the future. Cubilla and Woodruff (1977) and Kaneko and co-workers (1978) may well have opened the way to some fascinating discoveries. Further studies are eagerly awaited.

INFLAMMATORY CARCINOMA: DERMAL LYMPHATIC CARCINOMATOSIS

Incidence. Age Contrast Between Old and New Series. Inflammatory carcinoma of the breast represented 1 per cent of patients with untreated breast cancer in the series of Robbins et al (1974) and about 2 per cent in that of Stocks and Simmons Patterson (1976). The median age of 55 years was the same as for the breast cancer patients in general (Robbins et al, 1974). Stocks and Simmons Patterson (1976) found an average age of 48 years, also similar to their breast cancer patients in general. This is in contradistinction to the older series in the literature, which indicated that patients with inflammatory carcinoma were younger than average and that the disease was frequently associated with late pregnancy or lactation: these findings do not apply to more recent series (Saltzstein, 1974). In fact 53 per cent of patients were postmenopausal in one series (Stocks and Simmons Patterson, 1976) and as many as 69 per cent in another (Robbins et al, 1974).

Men and Children. Treves (1953) described inflammatory carcinoma in three male patients among 131 men with breast cancer. Nichini et al (1972) described inflammatory carcinoma in a 12-year-old girl.

CLINICAL SIGNS. IS RADICAL SURGERY CONTRA-INDICATED?

In the series of 83 cases of inflammatory carcinoma, probably the largest recorded series, reported on by Robbins et al (1974), all patients had increased warmth with associated redness in 85 per cent of cases. An erysipeloid edge was always evident. Two-thirds of their patients had a definite palpable mass, with the remainder showing diffuse breast involvement. Robbins et al considered inflammatory carcinoma to be an absolute contraindication to the performance of a radical mastectomy, either initially or following radiation therapy. McDivitt, Stewart and Berg (1968) also stated that this type of disease is not amenable to radical surgery. Stocks and Simmons Patterson (1976) stated that no radical mastectomy has been performed for this disease at their medical centre since 1965. They quoted an array of the best surgical opinions to support the view that radical mastectomy in this condition is to no avail and is indeed contraindicated. A few workers only believed that it can and should be so treated, and they advocated a bolder approach to therapy (Meyer, Dockerty and Harrington, 1948; Barber, Dockerty and Clagett, 1961). Rogers and Fitts (1956) also believed that radical mastectomy is justified in selected patients.

PATHOLOGICAL APPROACH TO THE DEFINITION

These slightly conflicting views on therapy can perhaps be reconciled if one adopts a pathological rather than a clinical approach to the definition of inflammatory carcinoma (Ellis and Teitelbaum, 1974). The crucial histopathological criterion is the presence or absence of dermal lymphatic carcinomatosis as shown by biopsy. Most, but not all, patients with inflammatory carcinomas show dermal lymphatic carcinomatosis. Ellis and Teitelbaum (1974) examined the pathological material and/or reports of all but one patient reported free of disease at least five years following radical mastectomy for inflammatory carcinoma: none of these patients had dermal lymphatic metastases. In addition, no patient with erythema of the breast or clinical inflammatory carcinoma who survived five years without recurrence following radical mastectomy at Barnes Hospital, St Louis, Missouri, over a 10-year period had dermal lymphatic metastases. Ellis and Teitelbaum concluded that the histological hallmark of surgically incurable breast carcinoma is *tumour emboli in the dermal lymphatics.* They proposed the name '*dermal lymphatic carcinomatosis of the breast*' for this entity and stressed the necessity of a palliative approach towards patients with this pathologically defined disease. Radiation therapy offers the best palliation.

On the other hand, if inflammatory carcinoma is not accompanied by dermal lymphatic invasion, Ellis and Teitelbaum (1974) believed that definitive surgery is indicated. In the two Mayo Clinic series, which accounted for seven of eight patients of this type reviewed by these authors, in addition to their own case, as many as 20 per cent of all patients with inflammatory carcinoma of the breast did not have dermal lymphatic metastases. This could explain why five of the 50 Mayo Clinic patients survived at least five years following surgery (Barber, Dockerty and Clagett, 1961). The overall prognosis of inflammatory carcinoma is, nonetheless, extremely gloomy. Only two out of 63 patients, treated prior to 1967, were clinically free of disease longer than five years in the Memorial Hospital series, a five-year salvage rate of only 3 per cent (Robbins et al, 1974); Stocks and Simmons Patterson (1976) had two out of 30 patients surviving five years, only 6.7 per cent of the whole series. The five-year survival of five out of 50 patients reported by Barber, Dockerty and Clagett (1961), or 10 per cent, is the best figure recorded in the literature.

The value of Ellis and Teitelbaum's (1974) work is in pinpointing the small number of patients with inflammatory carcinoma, clinically defined, who *may* be eligible for surgery and in confirming pathologically, unfortunately in a big majority, that dermal lymphatic carcinomatosis is present and that surgery is contraindicated. One patient of Stocks and Simmons Patterson (1976) represents an exception to the Ellis–Teitelbaum rule. This patient with inflammatory carcinoma had invasion of the dermal lymphatic system, despite which she survived for 11 years, then developed osseous and hepatic metastases, for which she was still receiving treatment at the time of reporting. This exceptional patient serves to demonstrate that every patient is in a sense unique.

'Clinically Occult Inflammatory Carcinoma'. Saltzstein (1974) looked particularly at the other end of the spectrum of inflammatory carcinoma and considered the 'clinically occult inflammatory carcinoma of the breast'. He summarized the literature on the subject succinctly since the entity was described by

Klotz in 1869 under the heading of 'mastitis carcinomatosa'. Bryant in 1889 pointed out the association with tumour in the dermal lymphatics. Since then most authors have used the clinical appearance to define the entity. A few authors have pointed out that infiltration of the dermal lymphatics by tumour cells is a distinctive histological finding and some, like Ackerman and Butcher (1968), have stressed that packing of the dermal lymphatics with tumour must be present before the pathologist can *confirm* a clinical diagnosis of inflammatory carcinoma. Saltzstein (1974) states that it is fair to conclude that 'most authors do not even raise the question of dermal lymphatic invasion in the absence of clinical evidence of inflammatory carcinoma'.

In the majority or, at any rate, a substantial proportion of cases, a cellulitis-like clinical picture and the presence of dermal lymphatic carcinomatosis coincide (Figure 12–19). However, two other populations of undetermined size also exist and it is to these populations that these workers have directed their attention. The first population, represented by the left-hand crescent in Figure 12–19, consists of women with breast carcinoma and a clinical appearance of cellulitis who, however, do not have dermal lymphatic carcinomatosis. Logic would dictate, Saltzstein (1974) said, that these

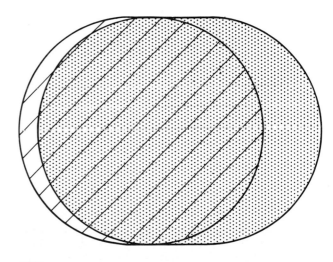

◪ inflammatory carcinoma

▦ dermal lymphatic carcinomatosis

Figure 12–19 Modified Venn diagram showing the degree of overlap between patients with inflammatory carcinoma and those with dermal lymphatic carcinomatosis. There are three populations to be considered.

women would follow the course of breast carcinoma without cellulitis but, he went on to state, 'there is no evidence to support this'. At about the same time, Ellis and Teitelbaum (1974) presented precisely such evidence, suggesting that breast cancers in these women did not share the fulminant course of the vast majority of inflammatory carcinomas. The second population, represented by the right-hand crescent in Figure 12–19, consists of women whose carcinomas involve the dermal lymphatics but who do not present the clinical picture of a cellulitis, i.e. patients with 'clinically occult inflammatory carcinoma'. This population is exemplified by four patients reported on in detail by Saltzstein (1974). Though clinically they did not have inflammatory carcinoma, the course of their disease was entirely typical of it. Saltzstein (1974) was careful to point out that conclusions drawn from so small a group of patients are hazardous and that confirmation of his findings was necessary. Should this be forthcoming, he suggested that a pathological diagnosis may have to supersede the clinical one in the recognition of inflammatory carcinoma, especially since the latter diagnosis implies a different method of treating the patient.

As a corollary to this line of reasoning, Saltzstein (1974) suggested that perhaps the term 'inflammatory carcinoma' should be discarded by pathologists. Instead, one could state that the finding of tumour in the dermal lymphatics is an absolute contraindication to radical mastectomy.

The Validity of the Two Hypotheses. The sizes of the populations considered by Ellis and Teitelbaum (1974) and by Saltzstein (1974) have yet to be established. The concepts put forward by both groups of workers are interesting and the fact that they reached very similar conclusions by starting from opposite poles of the problem lends support to their findings. The Saltzstein (1974) hypothesis is acceptable. The Ellis–Teitelbaum (1974) hypothesis still requires corroboration. The clinician is unlikely to stop using the term 'inflammatory carcinoma' in the accepted conventional sense, but he should realize that possibly a very small fraction of such cases *may* not be inoperable (Ellis and Teitelbaum, 1974)

and, conversely, that patients without inflammatory cancer but with dermal lymphatic carcinomatosis will probably respond in the same way as patients who do have inflammatory cancer (Saltzstein, 1974).

Lucas and Perez-Mesa (1978) examined the questions raised by Ellis and Teitelbaum (1974) and by Saltzstein (1974) in relation to the definition of inflammatory carcinoma of the breast. They studied 58 patients with 'clinical' inflammatory carcinoma and 15 patients with 'occult' inflammatory cancer (i.e. dermal lymphatic carcinomatosis without inflammation). Of the 58 patients, 39 demonstrated tumour in the dermal lymphatics (their Group I) while 19 patients with the clinical stigmata lacked such microscopic evidence (their Group II). These two groups, with 'clinical' inflammatory carcinoma, constituted 2.2 per cent of all breast malignancies seen between 1940 and 1975. The 15 cases of 'occult inflammatory cancer' in Group III formed 1.8 per cent of breast malignancies in patients on whom mastectomies were performed between 1967 and 1974. Thus the three groups constituted approximately 4 per cent of all primary breast cancers.

Saltzstein Hypothesis Largely Confirmed. Lucas and Perez-Mesa (1978) concluded that the occult inflammatory cancers delineated by Saltzstein (1974) have almost as fulminant a clinical course as the clinical inflammatory cancers and, to this extent, are in agreement with Saltzstein. They doubted, however, whether skin biopsy for evaluation of operability was justified as a routine procedure.

Ellis–Teitelbaum Hypothesis Still in Doubt. Lucas and Perez-Mesa (1978) further concluded that the diagnosis of clinical inflammatory carcinoma stands on its own, even in the absence of dermal lymphatic carcinomatosis. In this sense they cast some doubt on the validity of Ellis and Teitelbaum's (1974) contention. Lucas and Perez-Mesa (1978) believed that either clinical or pathological findings justify use of the term 'inflammatory carcinoma' to indicate a bad short-term prognosis despite the forms of treatment currently available.

8. METASTATIC CARCINOMA AND OTHER TUMOURS IN THE BREAST

Sandison (1959) was one of the earlier workers to study the problem of metastatic tumours in the breast. He is a valuable source of the earlier references, including those of Charache (cited by Sandison), who studied 10 cases.

CLINICAL SERIES

Ratio of Metastatic to Primary Malignancy. Sandison (1959) separated his cases into nine which were detected clinically and 40 found in a necropsy series. The former are clearly of more interest and importance to the surgical pathologist. Of the nine clinically detected cases, eight were found during an 11-year period in a single large teaching hospital. During the same period there were over 1300 specimens of primary malignant tumour of the breast studied in the laboratory, a ratio of metastatic to primary malignancy in the breast of 1:165. If two of the cases, which are considered to be of dubious origin, are excluded (his Cases 7 and 8), the corrected ratio becomes 1:220. Metastatic tumour to the breast presenting as a clinical mass in the breast, as opposed to a mere necropsy finding, is not, by any standard, common.

High Proportion of Leukaemia–Lymphoma Cases. Of the eight cases in the series of Sandison (1959), three had leukaemic or lymphomatous masses while five had carcinomatous or sarcomatous deposits, a relatively high proportion of leukaemia–lymphoma cases, an observation made also in the necropsy series. In the two leukaemic patients a breast mass was the first indication of disease and in the third patient, with reticulosarcoma found at mastectomy, it was discovered only later that the patient had had an orbital tumour of similar histological appearance removed previously. Of the other five patients, there is doubt in Cases 7 and 8 about the real seat of the primary tumour. The remaining three patients had metastatic oat cell carcinoma of the bronchus, metastatic melanoma and metastatic leiomyosarcoma respectively. Of these three patients, only in the patient with oat cell carcinoma of the bronchus was the breast mass the presenting symptom, in the absence of any other signs of metastases. In the patient with a malignant melanoma of the skin removed 18 months previously, a solitary metastatic mass was found in the breast and the patient was well 42 months after her breast surgery. In a further selected case, outside the consecutive series of eight, the patient presented clinically with a breast lump which was treated by mastectomy; the specimen contained a metastatic deposit from a renal carcinoma. This patient later developed cutaneous and osseous metastases and the renal carcinoma was revealed at necropsy.

Spectrum of Clinical Modes of Presentation. This small but informative series of Sandison (1959) illustrates the spectrum of the clinical modes of presentation. Sometimes the metastasis in the breast is the first indication of disease, as in the two leukaemic patients and in the patients with bronchial oat cell carcinoma and with renal carcinoma; sometimes the breast lump is apparently the first indication of disease because of an unavailable history, as in the patient with reticulosarcoma; or, alternatively, despite the history of a previous malignancy, the breast mass may be judged clinically to be a possible second primary tumour, as in the patient with a malignant melanoma — indeed in this patient the solitary metastasis in the breast was still the only indication of metastatic disease 42 months after breast surgery. At the other end of the spectrum are the cases in which the patient already has fairly obvious metastatic disease in additional sites, as in the patient with leiomyosarcoma.

NECROPSY SERIES

By contrast, in the necropsy series of 357 patients, no less than 21 of 40 patients with metastatic tumour in the breast had developed metastasis from a contralateral carcinoma of the breast (Sandison, 1959). Admittedly it is possible that some of these might well have been bilateral primary carcinomas of the breast, since the incidence of bilaterality of primary breast cancer was not as fully appreciated 20 years ago as it is today. Carcinoma metastatic from the contralateral breast was regarded by Sandison (1959) as the commonest form of secondary tumour in the female breast detected at necropsy, usually as a result of transthoracic lymphatic spread.

Incidence in Leukaemia and Lymphoma at Necropsy. In the 357 patients studied by Sandison (1959) at necropsy, metastases in the breast were found in 13.8 per cent (30/218) of women and in 7.2 per cent (10/139) of men. The fact that metastases were found in women with only twice the frequency found in men is somewhat surprising and mainly attributable to an interesting finding emerging from this study, viz. the high incidence of deposits in the breast in cases of leukaemia and lymphoma in both sexes. This incidence was 29 per cent in the lymphoma group and 47 per cent in patients with leukaemia, an incidence which was similar in both sexes, a finding which the writer finds a little difficult to understand. Four of the six cases with malignant lymphoma involving the breast were patients with Hodgkin's disease. These very high incidences of breast involvement in patients, both male and female, with malignant lymphoma require confirmation from other studies.

Metastases from Contralateral Breast Carcinoma. If patients with leukaemia and lymphoma are excluded, women have metastatic disease in their breast at necropsy with a frequency some six or seven times greater than that found in men. But this difference is largely if not entirely attributed by Sandison (1959) to metastasis from contralateral breast carcinoma occurring in the female patients: this was present in 30 per cent (21/70) of necropsies in women with breast carcinoma, with the reservation previously made about possible dual primary tumours in both breasts.

Relative Rarity of Metastases from Other Malignancies. If cases of breast carcinoma are excluded, metastases in the breast were found in only 2.3 per cent (3/128) and 1.8 per cent (2/113) of women and men respectively with malignant disease other than lymphoma and leukaemia. This incidence, as expected, is low. There is no real suggestion of a marked difference between men and women (although the positive findings are much too scanty to draw any definite conclusions), which possibly is an indication that the necropsy findings might be based on microscopic rather than gross pathology, a point which could be verified in future studies.

Female: Male Ratio in Clinical Series. Certainly in clinical, as opposed to necropsy, studies the female:male ratio of metastatic tumour in the breast from primary tumours other than breast carcinoma is about 10:1 (McIntosh et al, 1976) or 7:1 (Hajdu and Urban, 1972).

MORE RECENT STUDIES

The Frequency in Perspective. McIntosh et al (1976) discussed the problem of metastatic carcinoma in the breast based on a study of 29 of their own patients and a review of 105 others from the literature. Metastatic carcinoma within the breast was seen once to every 370 new cases of primary breast cancer, a figure which puts the problem in perspective. Also dual primaries, consisting of a breast carcinoma and a primary carcinoma in another organ, are distinctly more common than a primary tumour elsewhere that metastasizes to the breast, in a ratio of about 6:1.

Frequency of Oat Cell Bronchial Carcinoma and Melanoma. McIntosh et al (1976) found 13 instances of bronchial carcinoma, 10 of them of the oat cell variety, among their 29 cancers metastatic to the breast. Melanoma was second in frequency, constituting the primary source in four patients. In their review of the literature, melanoma headed the list (29), with bronchial carcinoma second (17). These two sources alone thus accounted for 46/105 of the cases reviewed and for 17/29 in the series of McIntosh et al (1976). Of the remaining 59 cases in the literature reviewed, 10 had a prostatic, seven a gastric, seven an ovarian, eight a uterine cervical and five a renal origin. The remaining 22 cases had miscellaneous primary sites of origin.

Absence of Calcification. Calcification was not demonstrated pathologically or radiologically in tumours metastatic to the breast in the series of McIntosh et al (1976). Their paper is a source of much valuable information.

Metastases from Unusual Primary Sites

Harrist and Kalisher (1977) reported on a patient with a metastasis to the breast from a *bronchial carcinoid.* The lesion was mistaken clinically and pathologically for a primary breast carcinoma. They found reports of five other definite cases of carcinoid tumour metastatic to the breast and in four of these, as well as in their own patient, the metastasis presented as an isolated breast mass. The patients were subjected to radical mastectomy, partly because of an absence of information about the history of a primary carcinoid tumour elsewhere and partly because of an inability to make the correct diagnosis on frozen section.

Other tumours which extremely rarely have metastasized to the breast include *uterine leiomyosarcoma* and *carcinoma of the endometrium, thyroid and liver* (Sandison, 1959). Even *angioblastic meningioma* has been known to metastasize to the breast (Lowden and Taylor, 1974).

PROSTATIC CARCINOMA IN PATIENTS ON STILBOESTROL

Relative Frequency of Prostatic Metastases in the Breast. In the male, there is a different problem which must be considered. Men with prostatic carcinoma can certainly develop metastatic disease in one or both breasts, usually late in the disease and generally not long before the patient succumbs to it. These patients almost invariably have gynaecomastia associated with stilboestrol therapy. Salyer and Salyer (1973) found *a minimum incidence of 5 per cent with metastatic disease in the breast* among 221 consecutive autopsy cases of carcinoma of the prostate with metastases. *In the past many cases with such metastatic disease were erroneously diagnosed as primary carcinoma of the male breast and this was attributed to stilboestrol treatment.* The main question is whether such treatment, in conventional dosage, does give rise to breast cancer in the male. One of the best-documented examples of such an occurrence is that reported by O'Grady and McDivitt (1969). In the two patients reported on by Symmers (1968), large doses of oestrogens were administered in men whose primary and secondary sexual characteristics were being deliberately altered. If there are a substantial number of other such cases they have escaped the writer's attention.

Fortuitous Association of Prostatic and Breast Carcinoma. Since prostatic carcinoma is a common disease, one would expect it to coexist with breast carcinoma on very rare occasions, if only by chance. Such a chance association is mentioned by McDivitt, Stewart and Berg (1968). Pertinently, Salyer and Salyer (1973) found no instance of primary breast cancer in their large autopsy series of oestrogen-treated prostatic cancer. At present the matter must be regarded as not proven either way but, if carcinoma of the male breast can be induced by stilboestrol in the moderate dosage now used for the treatment of prostatic cancer, the sequence of events must be a very rare one.

METASTASES, OTHER THAN PROSTATIC, IN THE MALE BREAST

The fact that emphasis has been put on prostatic cancer metastatic to the breast and on the problem of whether exogenous oestrogens can cause breast cancer in men reflects the relative frequency and the importance of these issues. It is not, however, meant to imply that cancers, other than prostatic ones, do not metastasize to the male breast. Seven of 51 cases of cancer metastatic to the breast in both sexes studied by Hajdu and Urban (1972) were in male patients and a prostatic source is not listed for any of them. The same is true of the three male patients in the series of McIntosh et al (1976).

PERSONAL OBSERVATIONS

Metastatic deposits in the breast from primary tumours elsewhere assume their greatest importance when they present to the clinician or the pathologist as tumours which mimic primary breast cancer and may be erroneously diagnosed and unnecessarily treated as such. In Britain, two of the tumours which most commonly metastasize to the breast and present in this way are bronchial carcinoma, especially of the oat cell variety, and malignant melanoma of the skin. The relative frequency with which oat cell carcinoma metastasizes to the breast in this country is partly a reflection of the greater incidence of oat cell cancer in the UK compared with the USA and some other countries. The characteristic histological patterns and cytological features of oat cell carcinoma minimize problems in differential diagnosis. With amelanotic or poorly pigmented melanoma, a high degree of alertness is needed to suspect the correct diagnosis and sometimes the clinical setting will help clarify it. Melanoma will hardly ever mimic the typical 'scirrhous' or 'stellate' carcinoma but it can be confused with the more cellular and undifferentiated varieties of multinodular breast cancer. The writer has seen this mistake made even with a moderately pigmented tumour in which there was no reason to suspect melanoma and in which the pigment was assumed to be iron; the clinical story, though highly relevant, had been suppressed; a 'mole' had been previously removed from the face and a histopathological diagnosis had not been clearly established. In these circumstances two very experienced pathologists assumed the pigment to be iron associated with haemorrhage into necrotic tumour; it was in fact melanin.

Usual Absence of Elastosis. It is worthy of note that elastosis has not yet been documented with metastatic disease in the breast and its presence is probably useful as a confirmatory sign of a primary as opposed to a metastatic tumour. This is not meant to indicate that other types of malignancy do not induce elastosis since observations on large bowel and other cancers have shown that they may do (page 387). Nevertheless, breast cancer usually has greater desmoplastic and elastosis-inducing properties than, say, most cases of melanoma or oat cell carcinoma. Also, in general, primary breast tumours are likely to have been present for considerably longer periods of time than metastatic deposits, and elastosis is, to some extent, a function of time (Azzopardi and Laurini, 1974). The presence of elastosis, but not its absence, is therefore potentially useful in the differentiation of a primary breast cancer from a metastatic tumour in the breast.

IDENTIFICATION OF METASTATIC DEPOSITS

Mucin Stains and Ultrastructure in Differentiation of Lymphoma and Carcinoma. Malignant lymphoma and leukaemic deposits in the breast are high on the list of metastatic lesions which must be distinguished from primary carcinoma (Sandison, 1959). These can pose substantial problems. The differential diagnosis between an undifferentiated malignant lymphoma and an undifferentiated carcinoma can be as difficult here as in other organs. In the differentiation between lymphoma and carcinoma, especially of the invasive lobular variety, both mucin stains and ultrastructural studies can be of diagnostic value.

Distinctive Histological Appearances of Renal and Prostatic Carcinomas. Other carcinomas, e.g. of the female genital tract, have been known to cause diagnostic problems, and even renal and other carcinomas may do so very rarely (Hajdu and Urban, 1972). The renal, prostatic, gastric and some other types of carcinoma which metastasize to the breast with relative frequency have histological appearances which are often sufficiently distinctive to arouse suspicion in the mind of an alert pathologist that he is dealing with metastatic rather than primary breast disease.

MAMMARY METASTASIS AS THE FIRST MANIFESTATION OF DISEASE

It is important to remember that in about a quarter of all patients, both female and male, the mammary lesion represents the first clinical manifestation of an occult extramammary primary tumour. Recognition by the pathologist that the tumour is metastatic will prevent unnecessary and mutilating radical surgery and allow for the commencement of the appropriate forms of systemic therapy.

9. EFFECTS OF HORMONAL MEDICATION ON BREAST TISSUE AND BREAST DISEASES

ORAL CONTRACEPTIVE TREATMENT

With the enormous use of oral steroid preparations as anti-ovulatory (contraceptive) agents, it is obviously important to know what effects such agents may have in health and disease. This knowledge is important in general terms to determine what disorders can be attributed to contraceptive agents and it is important to the pathologist in particular so that any potential drug effects can be interpreted correctly on frozen or paraffin section.

Oral Contraceptives and Breast Cancer. Concern that oral contraceptives may be carcinogenic for the breast is based upon experimental observations in lower animals. As far as the human is concerned, the evidence to date indicates that in therapeutic dosage there is no increased risk of breast cancer (Vessey, Doll and Sutton, 1972). Some workers have suggested that atypical features in mammary carcinoma can be attributed to oral steroids (e.g. Goldenberg, Wiegenstein and Wolff, 1968) and Penman (1970) attributed secretory changes in a carcinoma to such treatment. The writer is in agreement with other workers that most carcinomas discovered while women are taking oral contraceptives are indistinguishable from carcinoma in women not having such medication (Fechner, 1970c). Secretory changes of the type described by Penman can be seen in the absence of exogenous hormone administration. Taylor (1971) stressed the importance of examining a large number of age-matched controls in studies of this type. Taylor concluded that when large groups of lesions are compared with control groups, no differences are found (Fechner, 1970c).

Oral Contraceptives and Cystic Disease. Another problem is whether oral contraceptive treatment affects cystic disease in any way. Fechner (1970b) found no difference in the incidence of this disorder or in its age of occurrence. There were no specific histological features that could be attributed to the medication. Vessey, Doll and Sutton (1972) provided evidence that oral progestogens actually protect against benign breast disease. Sartwell, Arthes and Tonascia (1973) concluded that there is no association between the use of oral progestogens and benign breast disease.

Oral Contraceptives and Fibroadenomas. Epithelial hyperplasia in fibroadenomas, with unusual patterns, has been reported by Goldenberg, Wiegenstein and Mottet (1968) and by Brown (1970) in women taking contraceptive medication. Again, Fechner (1970a), in a carefully controlled investigation of a large series of tumours, concluded that there were no significant differences in the degree and type of epithelial hyperplasia in the tumour or in the surrounding non-neoplastic tissue. The only definite, and perhaps predictable, difference in women taking contraceptive medication was acinar formation with secretory changes in the fibroadenomas of four of the 54 women, i.e. changes analogous to those seen in fibroadenomas in some pregnant or lactating women. None of the 54 women with 'control' fibroadenomas showed these changes. Interestingly, two of these four women receiving medication showed lactational changes in the excised non-neoplastic tissue also, presumably the morphological and functional counterpart of galactorrhoea, a well-recognized complication of this type of treatment.

OESTROGEN ADMINISTRATION

A slightly different problem is the effect of pure oestrogenic substances on patients with benign breast disease. The increasing use of oestrogen therapy at the menopause or postmenopausally as hormone replacement therapy is likely to make this an important problem in the future. Fechner (1972) found no qualitative differences in patients receiving this treatment. A slightly increased incidence of hyperplasia in the specimens examined, 39 per cent compared with 32 per cent in untreated controls, was not considered to be significant.

10. AXILLARY LYMPH NODAL METASTASIS WITH OCCULT PRIMARY TUMOUR IN THE BREAST

The presence in a woman of an axillary node containing tissue which resembles breast carcinoma is almost always indicative of an occult primary carcinoma of the breast, no matter how difficult or impossible it is to detect this clinically. On pathological examination, the proportion of patients in whom the primary tumour is found is closely related to the care with which the breast is examined, the extent of sampling and the determination, tenacity and technical resources of the pathologist. Rarely, an in situ ductal carcinoma will be found without evidence of infiltration; the obvious inference that must be drawn in such cases is that the infiltrative portion of the carcinoma is minute and has not been detected.

Ashikari et al (1976) reviewed 34 patients who presented with enlarged axillary lymph nodes that were found to contain metastatic adenocarcinoma. There were no significant physical findings in the ipsilateral breast. Radical mastectomy revealed 23 occult ipsilateral breast carcinomas, 20 of which were invasive and three in situ only. Two-thirds of these occult primary cancers were less than 2 cm in diameter. In 11 of the whole group of 34 patients (32 per cent) no primary tumour in the breast was detected even after mastectomy. With current radiological techniques an increased detection rate of the primary cancers is to be expected both prior to and after operation.

For an axillary nodal metastasis with the features of a breast carcinoma but in the absence of an apparent breast primary, the assumption must be that there is an occult carcinoma in the breast. The onus of proof that it is otherwise rests squarely on the clinician and pathologist. In these circumstances, after thorough consultation between clinician and pathologist and the exclusion of other primary sites as potential sources of the axillary metastases, mastectomy is indicated. Interestingly, in the series of Ashikari et al (1976), 10-year post-mastectomy survival rates were the same (79 per cent), regardless of whether or not a primary tumour in the breast was found on pathological examination.

With metastatic tumour presentations of this type, the pathologist should direct his attention particularly to the axillary tail of the breast. The writer has twice found small cancers in this situation after an initial examination of the breast had failed to reveal any carcinoma. In one of these cases, the 5 mm primary tumour was intimately associated with the axillary lymph nodes and had, unknowingly, been blocked by the dissector along with the axillary lymph nodes. On microscopic examination it had initially been regarded as a totally replaced lymph node, although its stellate configuration made this unlikely. The fact that it was indeed the primary tumour was confirmed by the abundant elastosis in it, quite unlike anything seen in metastatic nodal deposits even when they have extended beyond the confines of the nodes; the correctness of this interpretation was further supported by the presence of a small amount of non-neoplastic mammary tissue immediately adjacent to the small primary cancer.

There is no acceptable documentation of carcinoma of breast tissue arising primarily in lymph nodes. However, in view of the extremely rare presence of benign epithelial tissue, probably mammary, in axillary lymph nodes, the *theoretical* possibility of such an occurrence is just conceivable.

11. NAEVUS CELLS IN AXILLARY LYMPH NODES: BENIGN MAMMARY TISSUE IN AXILLARY LYMPH NODES

NAEVUS CELLS IN AXILLARY LYMPH NODES

Johnson and Helwig (1969) reported the extraordinary finding of naevus cells in the capsule of lymph nodes of six patients aged between 40 and 82 years. In five of the six cases axillary lymph nodes were involved. The writer has seen a similar case with naevus cells in the capsule of an axillary node from a woman who had a radical mastectomy for infiltrating carcinoma of the breast. In these circumstances, the naevus cells are easily mistaken for metastatic carcinoma, especially if one is unaware of the existence of this condition. Naevus cells in nodal capsules have been found mostly in axillary nodes, rarely in cervical and inguinal nodes (Johnson and Helwig, 1969; McCarthy et al, 1974). This makes it particularly important to pathologists with an interest in breast disease. McCarthy et al (1974) described 24 examples of this condition, 22 of them detected in block dissections of lymph nodes draining sites of overt or suspected malignant tumours. Four cases were in women with carcinoma of the breast. In a deliberate search through material from 362 patients, 10 cases were discovered for an overall incidence of almost 2.8 per cent. When axillary lymph nodes only were considered, the incidence was no less than eight in 129 cases or 6.2 per cent. It should be stressed that, although numerous nodes were examined in 20 of the cases, foci of benign naevus cells were found in only one or two, and rarely in three, of the lymph nodes in each patient. This, combined with the fact that melanin pigment was present in only two of the 24 cases, doubtless partly explains why these lesions have escaped recognition for so long. The reader is referred to McCarthy et al (1974) for a discussion of the probable histogenesis of the naevus cell lesion. Here, the main concern is that the lesion should not be confused with metastatic carcinoma of the breast. The usual, but not invariable, presence of the naevus cells in the capsule and trabeculae, as opposed to the sinuses of the lymph node, aids in this differentiation. In addition to ordinary naevus cells, even blue naevi are very rarely observed in the capsule of lymph nodes (Azzopardi, Ross and Frizzera, 1977), but these should not be confused with metastatic breast carcinoma.

BENIGN MAMMARY TISSUE IN LYMPH NODES

The occurrence of benign mammary epithelium in axillary lymph nodes was reported by McDivitt, Stewart and Berg (1968). It is an exceptionally rare phenomenon in need of further thorough documentation. McDivitt, Stewart and Berg (1968) referred to a lesion in an axillary node 'completely similar to a benign breast papilloma'; it would appear that this is the same lesion referred to on their page 139 in association with subareolar duct papillomatosis. McDivitt, Stewart and Berg (1968) believed that this represented benign nodal transport of breast tissue; a similar structure in the lymph node had undergone carcinomatous change. At the time of their writing, the occurrence of malignant change

in subareolar papillomatosis had not yet been recognized and it is just possible that this case might have been interpreted differently in the light of subsequent knowledge. This remarkable case of McDivitt, Stewart and Berg (1968) remains sub judice. Embolization to lymph nodes of benign epithelial structures, as envisaged by these workers, is now a well-recognized phenomenon in association with certain organs and diseases and there is no reason to doubt that such a phenomenon could occur in relation to the breast.

McDivitt, Stewart and Berg (1968) also described two cases in which axillary nodes contained structures looking like normal breast ducts and possessing a normal double-layered epithelium 'with readily identifiable myoid'. Both instances showed 'epidermoidization' of the glands with cyst formation; in one case similar structures were present also in the breast itself, additional circumstantial evidence that the epithelium was of mammary origin.

Edlow and Carter (1973) reported on a woman who had bilateral mastectomies for cystic disease and in whom 10 axillary lymph nodes were removed incidentally. Five of these nodes contained a variety of epithelial tubules and apocrine and squamous cysts. Cogent reasons are given for considering these heterotopic structures mammary, rather than cutaneous, in derivation. They found only five similar cases in a comprehensive review of the literature, including the two cases of McDivitt, Stewart and Berg (1968) already referred to. In two patients, the cystic epithelial structures in the nodes had led to a remarkable presentation with an axillary mass. In the patient reported on by Edlow and Carter (1973), both breasts were examined histologically in their entirety and malignancy was very convincingly excluded. Edlow and Carter (1973) gave guidelines for distinguishing these benign ectopic structures from metastatic carcinoma in axillary nodes. There is a complete lack of the cytological features of malignancy and the patterns seen do not correspond with those of any type of breast cancer. Secondly, there is a striking heterogeneity of structure with apocrine cysts, squamous cysts and a variety of glandular structures. Thirdly, some of the glands possess two discernible cell layers, epithelial and myoepithelial in type respectively. Indeed the structure illustrated in Figures 1 and 2 of Edlow and Carter (1973) is indistinguishable from a normal breast lobule, except for its situation in the cortex of a lymph node. The two main hypotheses considered in histogenesis are embryological admixture and lymphatic embolization. Further cases of this exceptional type need documentation before any firm conclusions can be drawn about its precise histogenesis. In view of what is known of the invasive potential of sclerosing adenosis, it is perhaps surprising that benign mammary epithelium is not found more often than it is in axillary nodes. Presumably the tissue in sclerosing adenosis hardly ever invades the lumen of lymphatics and breaks away to form emboli to the lymph nodes or, if it does so, the nodal environment must be inimical to its survival.

12. MELANOCYTE COLONIZATION OF BREAST CARCINOMA

Rarely, when a breast carcinoma invades the skin it can become secondarily pigmented to such an extent that the observer may seriously contemplate a diagnosis of malignant melanoma. This pigmentation is attributable to melanocyte colonization of the mammary carcinoma. In this florid form, the writer has seen it only twice in 20 years, once in my own material and once in consultation. But the phenomenon is seen frequently at the histological level. In a recent study (Azzopardi and Eusebi, 1977), we found melanocyte colonization of breast carcinoma in 14 of 20 cases in which there was cutaneous invasion with breaching of the basement membrane of the epidermis by the tumour. The phenomenon is analogous to the colonization of skin tumours by melanocytes with transfer of melanin pigment to cells unable to synthesize it themselves. It is seen also in the well-known pigmentation of Paget cells by melanin, referred to elsewhere in this chapter. Melanocytes from the epidermis 'descend into' and are found amongst carcinoma cells in the upper dermis. It is remarkable that melanocytes should migrate into a breast carcinoma in this manner. The writer has observed similar colonization only twice in a hidradenoma; pigmentation of hidradenomas appears to be rare even in Negroes, though further study of this point is indicated. Perhaps most curious is the fact that melanocyte colonization of mammary carcinoma is usually accompanied by depigmentation and loss of melanocytes from the overlying epidermis. Why the melanocytes should choose to inhabit the carcinoma at the expense of their normal habitat is a considerable mystery.

From a practical point of view, the melanin-containing breast carcinoma behaves like its conventional non-pigmented counterpart. It should not be mistaken for malignant melanoma, as long as one is aware of this fascinating phenomenon.

13. DISEASES OF THE ADOLESCENT FEMALE BREAST

Incidence. Girls aged 21 years or less are affected by breast disease or attend a breast clinic more frequently than is often realized. Most of these girls present with physiological problems. Sometimes breast development is regarded as precocious: at other times unilateral breast development is the cause of concern for the patient or her family. In most cases reassurance is all that is necessary. Girls of this age may constitute up to 10 per cent of patients seen clinically but usually provide only about 3 per cent of specimens that are seen by the pathologist.

FREQUENCY OF DIFFERENT DISEASES

Frequency of Tumours and Cystic Disease. *Fibroadenoma* is the commonest lesion of the breast below the age of 21 years. There were

114 fibroadenomas among 124 tumours in the series of Sandison and Walker (1968). There were an additional five cases of rather diffuse fibroadenomatosis, one of them associated with bilateral hypertrophy. *Ductal papillomas* are rare in adolescent girls: there were only three examples in the large Sandison–Walker (1968) series. There were only four patients with *cystic disease* and epithelial hyperplasia, a low incidence of cystic mastopathy as might be expected. These four patients were aged 20 or 21 years.

Frequency of Inflammatory Disease. Inflammatory disease was diagnosed 20 times among 151 specimens. This included two cases of proven *tuberculosis,* four of *lactational abscess* and four of *duct ectasia.* There is a good deal of useful information on breast pathology in adolescent girls in the paper by Sandison and Walker (1968).

BENIGN TUMOURS

Daniel and Mathews (1968) reported on a study of 95 adolescent females with breast tumours. The patients were aged 12 to 21 years. They were studied over a ten-year period. This report comes from a special 'adolescent unit' where there is a complete medical examination for every patient at her first clinic visit for any complaint. This no doubt partly explains the large number of girls in whom breast tumours were discovered. Ninety of the patients had *fibroadenomas.* There was a sharp increase in the incidence at 16 years and above. Caucasian and Negro girls were equally affected, but see page 45 for some possibly conflicting evidence about the racial incidence of fibroadenomas in all age groups. A striking finding was the observation that 25 per cent of all patients had multiple tumours and this applied to both races. Only one girl, aged 12 years, had a *ductal papilloma*: she presented with a bloody nipple discharge.

'Juvenile Type' of Fibroadenoma

Ashikari, Farrow and O'Hara (1971) discussed the question of fibroadenoma in the breast of juvenile patients. Of 181 fibroadenomas in adolescent female breasts, 169 were of the ordinary 'adult' type while 12 belonged to what they called the 'juvenile type'. They found a further six patients with this tumour type in the period preceding the main study, making a total of 18 fibroadenomas of the juvenile variety. These tumours are described on page 46.

Giant Fibroadenoma

Nambiar and Kannan Kutty (1974) reported on 25 adolescent girls with giant fibroadenoma and reviewed another 61 collected from the literature. These tumours are apparently not too rare in Malaysia and Singapore and may be commoner in Chinese girls than in some other races. These workers discussed the dangers of using the term 'cystosarcoma' synonymously with 'giant fibroadenoma' and emphasized that local excision is adequate treatment for the latter lesion and that the breast tissue should be conserved whenever possible.

'CYSTOSARCOMA' OF ADOLESCENCE

Amerson (1970), in a report on seven cases of benign cystosarcoma phyllodes in Negro adolescents aged 10 to 17 years, made the very important point that *'cystosarcomas' in this age group may well have a better behaviour than those seen in older patients.* This was the experience also of Nambiar and Kannan Kutty (1974), whose tabulated cases from the literature included cystosarcomas as well as giant fibroadenomas, and the prognosis in this age group was uniformly favourable.

Malignant Cystosarcoma is a Great Rarity At This Age. Cystosarcoma is rare below the age of 21 years and the great majority of these rare tumours are of the benign variety, as assessed by the Norris and Taylor (1967) criteria (Amerson, 1970). Clinically malignant cystosarcoma in children (q.v.) is an exceptional rarity and a diagnosis of malignant cystosarcoma should be made with very great caution in this age group.

CARCINOMA AND OTHER MALIGNANT DISEASES

These are discussed in the following section dealing with tumours in childhood.

14. CARCINOMA AND OTHER MALIGNANT DISEASE IN CHILDHOOD: BENIGN TUMOURS IN CHILDREN

'JUVENILE' CARCINOMA: JUVENILE TYPE 'SECRETORY' CARCINOMA IN CHILDREN AND ADULTS

This is a very rare tumour of which there are probably no more than 25 cases documented. It has naturally excited considerable interest because of the youth of the patients (McDivitt and Stewart, 1966). The tumours have a distinctive microscopic pattern (Figures 12–20 and 12–21) which is tubuloalveolar, hypernephroid, with eosinophilic PAS-positive secretory material in the neoplastic lumina (Figures 12–20 and 12–21). The tumour cells usually have a bland appearance with a copious lightly-staining cytoplasm (Figure 12–21). Mitoses and

necrosis are usually absent. The prognosis is much better than with the conventional carcinomas of adults and wide local excision may constitute adequate therapy. Local recurrence has been recorded after as long an interval as 21 years (Oberman and Stephens, 1972). There are now three possibly authentic cases on record with solitary axillary nodal metastases (Byrne, Fahey and Gooselaw, 1973), a fact which these authors regarded as supporting radical mastectomy as the treatment of choice for this type of carcinoma in children. It should, however, be noted that the patient of Kraus and Kline, reported on in 1926, almost certainly had a different type of carcinoma which was papillary and affected both breasts at the ages of 16 and 17½ years

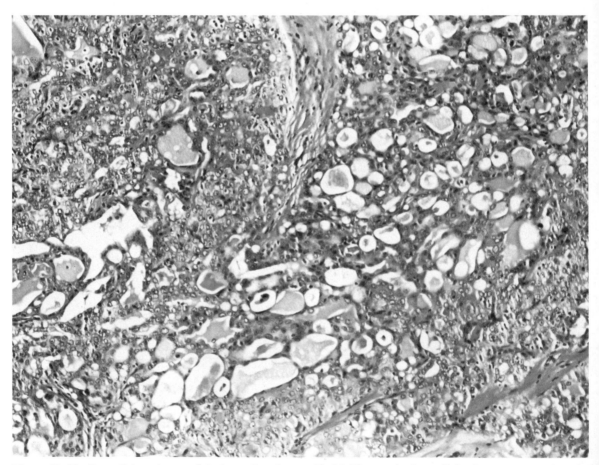

Figure 12–20 'Juvenile' carcinoma of the breast in a 5-year-old girl. The tumour has a distinctive structure and can be identified with reasonable certainty without knowledge of the patient's age. Rarely this type is found also in young adults. H and E. ×150.

respectively. The tumour in the case of Hartman and Magrish (1955) does not appear to be identical with those more recently reported: only one of 21 lymph nodes was involved. The best treatment for this distinctive type of juvenile carcinoma or 'secretory' carcinoma of childhood has yet to be determined.

This disease has been documented in a three-year-old girl (McDivitt and Stewart, 1966) and in a four-year-old girl (Oberman and Stephens, 1972). It has even been reported in a five-year-old boy (Simpson and Barson, 1969) and in a six-year-old boy (Hartman and Magrish, 1955). No deaths have as yet been attributable to these distinctive secretory tumours.

At first this unusual type of adenocarcinoma was regarded as a tumour of children exclusively, with an age range of three to 15 years in the first six cases reported by McDivitt and Stewart (1966). It has, however, become apparent that tumours with the same morphology and the same indolent clinical behaviour may rarely be found also in adult women. In a survey of 5000 cases of breast carcinoma from the A.F.I.P., Norris and Taylor (1970) found that 135 were in women less than 30 years old; six of these 135 carcinomas were of the juvenile secretory type, an incidence of only 4 per cent even in this highly selected group. Apart from one 10-year-old child, all the patients were aged between 20 and 30 years. This in fact constituted a report of five cases of 'juvenile carcinoma' occurring in adult patients. None had axillary nodal metastases. McDivitt is cited (Sullivan, Magee and Donald, 1977) as stating that he had seen six tumours of this distinctive type in adult patients. They were all nulliparous women who had received no hormone therapy. The behaviour of the tumours appeared to compare with the indolent behaviour seen in childhood.

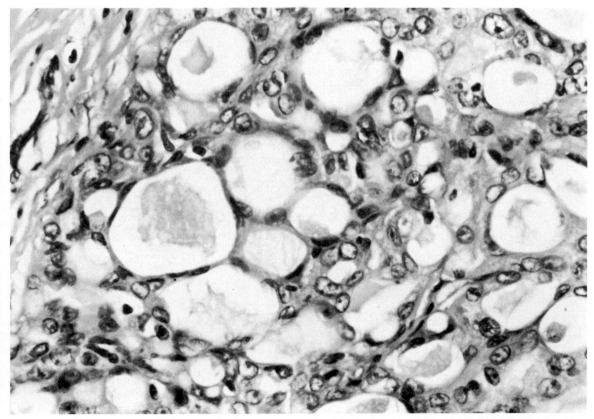

Figure 12–21   Higher magnification of juvenile carcinoma. The tubular or follicular pattern is characteristic. Nucleoli may be prominent but mitoses are very sparse and the cytological features are not those of an aggressive tumour. H and E. ×600.

Sullivan, Magee and Donald (1977) reported on a 'secretory (juvenile) carcinoma' in a 26-year-old multiparous woman. This case is unusual in that eight months after local resection there was tumour recurrence in the scar and, following radical mastectomy, three lymph nodes were found to contain metastatic deposits. This is a somewhat more aggressive behaviour than previously recorded for this tumour. Sullivan, Magee and Donald (1977) cited McDivitt as expressing the opinion that this tumour should probably not be treated by a procedure less than simple mastectomy with low axillary dissection. Other authorities favour a more conservative approach.

MORE AGGRESSIVE TUMOURS IN YOUTH

Apart from the juvenile secretory carcinomas with a distinctive microscopic appearance, there are reports in the literature of breast carcinoma in children which pursued an evil and aggressive course. The child aged 11 years reported on by Ramirez and Ansfield (1968) died quickly of her tumour; the illustrations, however, are more suggestive of malignant lymphoma than of carcinoma. The two girls reported on by Close and Maximov (1965) also died of tumour: in the girl with bilateral mammary tumours at age 17 and 20 years respectively, malignant lymphoma is again suggested by the illustrations: the other postpubertal girl, aged 14 years, did indeed appear to have a very poorly differentiated type of carcinoma. Even inflammatory carcinoma has been recorded in a 12-year-old girl (Nichini et al, 1972). These must be exceptionally rare tumours. Nevertheless, they illustrate that even aggressive and lethal mammary tumours, be they epithelial or not, can occur very exceptionally in children. But they must be clearly separated from the quasi-benign tumours with the distinctive secretory, tubuloalveolar pattern.

OTHER TUMOURS IN CHILDREN AND INFANTS

The rarity of breast tumours in children is illustrated by the fact that only nine cases were seen during a 40-year period at the Hospital for Sick Children, Toronto (Simpson and Barson, 1969). Two of the nine tumours were common or garden dermal capillary haemangiomas close to the nipple: after excluding these, we are left with only seven tumours. Five were fibroadenomas in girls aged between 10 and 16 years. One was the extremely rare juvenile type of carcinoma present in a boy aged five years. The seventh case was a three-month-old North American Indian boy with ductal papilloma. Fibroadenoma is far and away the commonest breast tumour occurring in childhood. Fibroadenoma was the diagnosis in 90 of 95 cases of breast tumour in females aged 12 to 21 years (Daniel and Mathews, 1968). Ductal papillomas are much less common but have been diagnosed even in young children aged four, 10 and 12 years (Simpson and Barson, 1969), apart from the infant boy already referred to.

15. CARCINOMA OF THE MALE BREAST

The salient points relating to carcinoma of the male breast can be enumerated as follows:

1. It accounts for about 1 per cent of breast cancers in both sexes. The *female: male ratio*, in other words, *is about 100:1.*
2. Men tend to develop breast cancer at an *older age than women.* In the series of Norris and Taylor (1969) the median age in male patients was 59 years.
3. The lesions are *generally located centrally* about the nipple.
4. *Skin involvement* by fixation, ulceration and microscopic Paget's disease is much *more common* than in women.
5. Axillary *nodal metastases* occur with slightly *greater frequency* than in women.
6. *The tumour types found are similar in both sexes.* Papillary carcinoma is said to be relatively common in men (Norris and Taylor, 1969). Lobular carcinoma had not been reported at all until recently, as might have been expected on theoretical grounds. Giffler and Kay (1976) documented two cases with the appearance of an infiltrating lobular carcinoma in the male breast. In one case there was a

suggestion of accompanying in situ lobular carcinoma but they did not regard the evidence for this as conclusive. These authors reinterpreted two other cases in the English-language literature as possible examples of infiltrating lobular carcinoma in the male. Giffler and Kay (1976) made a detailed analysis of the types of breast cancer in men reported in the larger series in the literature. They summarized the available data in a useful table. There is *a good deal of scope for further investigation* in this field because some of the data are taken from the older literature and the criteria for classification have altered considerably during that time. Yogore and Sahgal (1977) reported a case of small cell carcinoma of the male breast which they interpreted as an infiltrating lobular carcinoma.

7. Men with breast carcinoma tolerate *symptoms for a slightly longer time* before seeking medical advice.

8. The most conspicuous difference between the sexes is the *slightly worse prognosis* in men. Norris and Taylor (1969) attributed this in part to the central location of the tumours, for it is known that even in women cancers in the central areas of the breast have a worse prognosis. The male breast lacks sufficient substance to encompass the tumour so that even a 2 cm tumour may have ready access to dermal and subareolar lymphatic channels and to the pectoral fascia. Metastases to the internal mammary nodes are therefore probably more frequent. All the same, the commonly held opinion that the prognosis in men is much worse than in women has been exaggerated by the use of crude survival statistics, because these do not take into account the fact that men have a worse survival outlook than women of the same age and, secondly, that men with breast cancer tend to be older than women with breast cancer (Norris and Taylor, 1969).

9. *The relationship of gynaecomastia to breast cancer* is an obscure and complex issue. In the majority of series of patients with gynaecomastia there is no evidence that carcinoma develops with any increased frequency (Sirtori and Veronesi, 1957). Conversely, in carcinoma of the male breast there is practically never coexistent, or a history of preceding, gynaecomastia (Treves and Holleb, 1955),

although Scheike and Visfeldt (1973) are not completely in agreement with this.

If one defines gynaecomastia histologically rather than clinically, then the ductal changes of gynaecomastia may be seen sometimes accompanying carcinoma, according to McDivitt, Stewart and Berg (1968). However, one does not encounter the periductal accumulation of acid mucopolysaccharide which is characteristic of 'active' gynaecomastia and this has led Norris and Taylor (1969) to conclude that most mammary cancer develops in men with 'either non-existent or quiescent gynaecomastia'. Scheike and Visfeldt (1973) found an incidence of histological gynaecomastia of 27 per cent in men with breast cancer (21 of 79 cases). These workers admitted, however, that some control series report even higher incidences of histological gynaecomastia, findings which clearly render interpretation of their own data extremely difficult. Scheike and Visfeldt (1973) put forward additional epidemiological and other data to support a possible relationship between gynaecomastia and breast cancer but concluded that they were unable to prove it. They nevertheless asserted that 'certain facts appear to support the theory that gynaecomastia may be a premalignant state'. This assertion is not borne out by other workers' data. McDivitt, Stewart and Berg (1968) saw breast cancer only once in a breast with the classical changes of gynaecomastia, indicating that this must be a very exceptional event.

In a study of 351 patients with gynaecomastia, four patients are said to have had intraductal carcinoma, a surprisingly high incidence of more than 1 per cent (Bannayan and Hajdu, 1972). Moreover, the gynaecomastias are said to have been of 'the florid or intermediate types'. It is a pity that no details are given of the specific four cases and that no illustrations are provided of the type of histological changes on which these diagnoses of intraductal carcinoma were based. The statements of these authors conflict with those of the McDivitt fascicle from the same institution. Credence must be given to McDivitt, Stewart and Berg (1968) and to Norris and Taylor (1969) unless and until convincing pathological evidence to the contrary is presented.

It is noteworthy that *the incidence of mammary cancer is increased in men with Klinefelter's syndrome* (Jackson et al, 1965) but the precise degree of this increase has still to be established (Cuenca and Becker, 1968). While Jackson et al (1965) calculated that the incidence of carcinoma of the breast in patients with Klinefelter's syndrome was of the same order as that found in women, Scheike, Visfeldt and Petersen (1973) concluded in a careful analysis that the increased incidence of breast carcinoma in men with chromatin-positive Klinefelter's syndrome is *of the order of × 20.* They found that, though the incidence was much higher than in normal males, it was still considerably lower than in women. Interestingly, though gynaecomastia is frequent in patients with Klinefelter's syndrome, these workers noted that only four of the 13 documented patients with Klinefelter's syndrome and breast carcinoma had gynaecomastia; their own patient also had no clinical signs of gynaecomastia.

Cole (1976) came to the same conclusion as Scheike, Visfeldt and Petersen (1973). Nine out of 242 male breast cancer patients were found to be chromatin-positive. The estimated frequency of Klinefelter's syndrome in males with breast cancer is therefore 3.7 per cent. The frequency of Klinefelter's syndrome in the male population is 0.2 per cent. Thus the risk of getting breast cancer in a man with Klinefelter's syndrome is increased 18 to 19-fold. The mechanism of this relationship is still speculative.

As far as the writer is aware, breast cancer has not been reported in persons with testicular feminization.

10. The problem of *the true nature of a cancer situated in the breast in patients with prostatic carcinoma* receiving oestrogen therapy is considered on page 313.

REVIEWS OF MALIGNANT DISEASE OF THE MALE BREAST

Useful data on breast cancer in the male are found in the papers by Crichlow, Kaplan and Kearney (1972), Crichlow (1972), Visfeldt and Scheike (1973) and Cole (1976). Sarcomas of the male breast are considered by Visfeldt and Scheike (1973), though Crichlow (1972) argued that these are tumours 'in and not of the breast' and that they bear no relation to the breast as a special organ. There is something to be said for both points of view. Crichlow's (1972) collective review of over 2000 men with breast carcinoma is a mine of information and a very valuable source of references. Epidemiological factors and aetiological aspects are considered in detail. The relationship to exogenous oestrogens and to gynaecomastia is critically examined and the role of ionizing radiation as a cause of breast carcinoma in both sexes is critically evaluated. Fortunately the practice of radiation therapy for gynaecomastia in the young has now been abandoned.

NIPPLE DISCHARGE IN THE MALE

This question is discussed in detail by Treves, Robbins and Amoroso (1956). In their own material, only 2 per cent of 577 men with benign breast disease had a nipple discharge. On the other hand, nearly 14 per cent of 131 male patients with carcinoma of the breast had a nipple discharge and the discharge was blood-stained in 80 per cent of the malignant cases. Conversely, a bloody discharge was rare with benign disease in the male and was confined to patients with ductal papilloma.

PAGET'S DISEASE OF THE MALE BREAST

Twenty cases of Paget's disease of the male breast in the English-language literature were collected and tabulated by Nehme (1976). This included five cases reported by Coley and Kuehn (1972) including the first documented case of bilateral Paget's disease in a man. Two cases each were reported by Treves (1954) and by Crichlow and Czernobilsky (1967) respectively, while the remainder consisted of single case reports. In addition Nehme (1976) also collected 11 cases from the non-English literature: these were not all histologically documented.

16. MALIGNANCY IN FIBROADENOMA

CARCINOMA INVOLVING A FIBROADENOMA

We are not concerned here with the development of cystosarcoma phyllodes. Statements in the literature to the effect that malignant alteration in a fibroadenoma usually takes the form of a sarcoma (Evans, 1966) are true if cystosarcoma phyllodes is considered also. The extremely rare and exotic sarcomas of the type described by Rottino and Howley (1945), which sometimes originate in a fibroadenoma, are much more lethal than most cystosarcomas of whatever origin. Carcinoma restricted to a fibroadenoma, on the other hand, is usually an eminently curable disease.

CARCINOMA INFILTRATING THE STROMA OF A FIBROADENOMA FROM WITHOUT

While carcinoma, or at least an epithelial neoplasm, can certainly arise in and even be restricted to a fibroadenoma, it is a rare event for carcinoma of any type to have its origin in a fibroadenoma. The most frequent event by far is for an adjacent carcinoma to infiltrate around and engulf a pre-existing fibroadenoma. The carcinoma may infiltrate the fibroadenoma, from without, to varying degrees. This does not pose any serious diagnostic problem for the pathologist.

CARCINOMA IN THE CREVICES OF A FIBROADENOMA AS WELL AS THE ADJACENT TISSUE

Distinctly less frequently, in situ carcinoma is found within a fibroadenoma as well as in the adjacent breast tissue. The carcinoma may be infiltrative in the fibroadenoma, the adjacent tissue or in both sites. In these circumstances, the carcinoma may have originated in both sites simultaneously, it may have started in the fibroadenoma and extended outwards or it may have originated in the adjacent breast parenchyma and spread into the fibroadenoma secondarily, via the feeding ductule or ductules. The latter probably explains most cases and the situation is then analogous to cancerization of previously normal lobules. It should be recalled that the fibroadenoma represents a tumour of breast lobules. In these cases, the architecture and cytology of the tumour is that of a ductal carcinoma, even to the extent that necrosis and calcification in necrotic debris may be found in the epithelial crevices of the fibroadenoma.

CARCINOMA RESTRICTED ENTIRELY OR AT LEAST DOMINANTLY TO A FIBROADENOMA

Carcinoma arising in a fibroadenoma and restricted to it was regarded about 10 to 12 years ago as an extremely rare entity, perhaps even a non-existent one. The first definitive paper on the subject was that of McDivitt, Stewart and Farrow (1967), who reported on 26 patients. They were all women with an age range of 23 to 62 years. The average age was 41 years for patients with a non-infiltrating cancer and 46 years for those with infiltrating cancer. This is about 20 years older than the peak incidence of fibroadenoma in the general population (Goldman and Friedman, 1969). The symptoms are those of a fibroadenoma and this is the usual preoperative diagnosis. The diagnosis can be established only by pathological examination, generally of randomly selected blocks, as there is usually nothing to arouse suspicion macroscopically.

Types of Carcinoma

Sixteen of the 26 cancers (62 per cent) in the series of McDivitt, Stewart and Farrow (1967) were of lobular and 10 of ductal type. The dominance of the lobular type is to be expected from what is known of the origin of fibroadenoma, viz. that it is a lobular tumour. Of the 16 lobular carcinomas, nine were limited exclusively to the fibroadenoma while seven showed involvement also of the immediately adjacent breast tissue; in six of these seven, the fibroadenoma was predominantly involved. Of the nine lobular carcinomas restricted to the fibroadenoma, seven were in situ and two infiltrative. Of the 10 additional carcinomas of ductal type, eight (six in situ, two infiltrative) were entirely confined to the fibroadenoma while two involved adjacent breast tissue. These ductal type carcinomas were of solid, comedo and papillary types.

Lobular Carcinoma Restricted Entirely to Fibroadenoma

Four of the five patients with CLIS limited to the fibroadenoma and treated by local excision only were well at three to nine years: the fifth developed a recurrence at the same site after five years and, on excision, CLIS was found with foci of probable early stromal invasion. At the time of the report, this patient had recently had a radical mastectomy and no further disease was found in the mastectomy specimen. The other two patients with CLIS limited to the fibroadenoma were treated by simple mastectomy initially and remained free of disease. Both patients with infiltrating carcinoma confined to the fibroadenoma had a radical mastectomy and were free of disease at five and eight years.

Lobular Carcinoma Restricted Dominantly to Fibroadenoma

Of the six patients with CLIS in the fibroadenoma as well as in the adjacent tissue, five were treated by simple or radical mastectomy: no residual disease was present in three, while in two patients there was residual disease in two quadrants and four quadrants respectively. The sixth tumour was removed by wide local excision only (CLIS was erroneously thought to be limited to the fibroadenoma at that time) and a recurrent mass of infiltrating lobular carcinoma developed at the same site three years later. On review of the original material it was realized that CLIS had originally involved the adjacent tissue as well as the fibroadenoma. Radical mastectomy was curative in this patient at 10 years.

Evidence of Multifocal, Residual or Recurrent Lobular Neoplasia

It is pertinent to note that two patients returned later with infiltrating carcinoma at sites where, initially, CLIS was considered to be confined to a fibroadenoma. Also, of the patients treated by mastectomy, two were found to have additional CLIS in quadrants other than that containing the fibroadenoma.

Results of Treatment of Lobular Carcinoma In Situ in a Fibroadenoma

Looked at somewhat differently, of a total of 29 patients with lobular carcinoma arising in fibroadenomas documented in the literature, 23 had CLIS alone, two had CLIS and ILC combined, while four had ILC alone (Bosincu and Eusebi, 1972; Buzanowsky-Konakry, Harrison and Payne, 1975). While 16 of the patients with CLIS alone underwent mastectomy, seven had only a local excision. Six of these seven were living and well up to nine years later; the seventh was the patient of McDivitt, Stewart and Farrow (1967), already mentioned, who developed a recurrence five years later with 'probable early stromal invasion'; this patient had a radical mastectomy and no further disease was found.

Ductal Type Carcinoma in Fibroadenoma

Five of the 10 patients with 'ductal type' carcinoma in the series of McDivitt, Stewart and Farrow (1967) had a radical mastectomy: no evidence of residual disease was found.

Treatment

McDivitt, Stewart and Farrow (1967) recommended some form of mastectomy on the basis of their evidence. If CLIS is found, some authors, e.g. Goldman and Friedman (1969), recommended simple mastectomy and a biopsy of the contralateral breast, but treatment is bound to be affected by the most modern views on the treatment of CLIS in general, i.e. when CLIS is unrelated to a fibroadenoma (see Fisher and Fisher, 1977). With an infiltrative lesion of either lobular or ductal type, standard mastectomy is said to be the treatment of choice. Non-invasive ductal type lesions pose a difficult problem: simple mastectomy and partial axillary dissection are considered to be the best treatment by Goldman and Friedman (1969). The whole question of the correct treatment of carcinoma restricted or largely restricted to a fibroadenoma is in need of further study.

PROGNOSIS

The prognosis of carcinoma limited exclusively, or almost exclusively, to a fibroadenoma is very favourable, possibly because the lesions present at an early stage because of the setting in which they occur. Of the 17 patients reported on by McDivitt, Stewart and Farrow (1967), with carcinoma limited exclusively to the fibroadenoma, only one is known to have died of metastatic breast cancer, and this was probably from a contralateral infiltrating ductal carcinoma treated simultaneously. *The development of CLIS or other type of carcinoma in a fibroadenoma may be no more than a chance occurrence which benefits the patient by acting as a vehicle for clinical presentation of an otherwise microscopic disease.*

LOBULAR CARCINOMA IS THE DOMINANT TYPE TO ARISE IN A FIBROADENOMA

Bosincu and Eusebi (1972) tabulated the data in the literature and reported a case of their own in a young girl of 15 years of age. They maintained that only carcinomas of lobular type arose primarily in fibroadenomas. The concept that carcinoma, primary in a fibroadenoma, is almost always of the lobular variety is an intellectually satisfying one. The five examples in my collection are all of this type (Figure 12–22).

INTERPRETATION OF FLORID EPITHELIAL HYPER-PLASIA OF 'DUCTAL TYPE' IN FIBROADENOMA

If Bosincu and Eusebi (1972) are correct, then even extreme degrees of epithelial hyperplasia of 'ductal type' which can very rarely be found in fibroadenomas should be disregarded as of little consequence. In practice, this is certainly almost always true. The epithelial hyperplasia in fibroadenoma is sometimes of the exuberant type seen also in gynaecomastia and in cystosarcomas. Very rarely a gross epithelial hyperplasia is seen filling some of the epithelial crevices of a fibroadenoma. This is usually solid, with

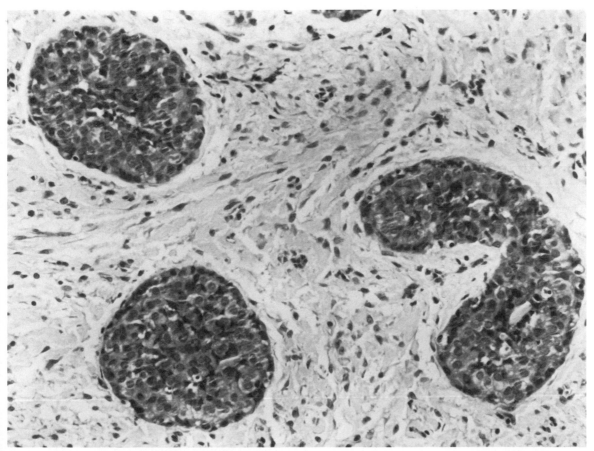

Figure 12–22 CLIS in a fibroadenoma. H and E. ×375.

uniform cytology and regular ovoid vesicular nuclei with inconspicuous nucleoli, but mitoses of normal type may be numerous in areas. The writer has seen a case of this type, very similar to the one illustrated by Fisher, Gregorio and Fisher (1975) in their Figures 35 and 36, but even more florid. The patient has had no further trouble five years after a simple enucleation procedure. Like Fisher, Gregorio and Fisher (1975) the writer interpreted this as benign. There.is a need for further study of cases of this type.

'DUCTAL TYPE' CARCINOMA CAN ARISE VERY RARELY IN A FIBROADENOMA

One must, however, allow for the possibility that carcinomas of ductal type can, very rarely, arise in fibroadenomas, e.g. eight cases of McDivitt, Stewart and Farrow (1967) and at least one case of Goldman and Friedman (1969). The case of Austin and Fidler (1953) may also belong in this category, but it is difficult to categorize the interesting case of More and Sandison (1973). The writer has recently been shown a case of probable ductal carcinoma, of cribriform type, limited to the crevices of an intracanalicular fibroadenoma. Such cases are extremely rare but their existence raises the possibility, discussed on page 210, that so-called cancerization of lobules may sometimes have its origin within the lobule and its neoplastic equivalent, viz. the fibroadenoma. There is a need for careful documentation of cases of carcinoma of whatever type arising in a fibroadenoma, especially those restricted solely to its interior.

INCIDENCE OF CARCINOMA IN FIBROADENOMA

Bosincu and Eusebi (1972) gave an incidence of 0.6 per cent for lobular carcinoma arising in a fibroadenoma but the incidence in unselected material is almost certainly considerably lower, since their solitary case was presumably the reason for their report. Buzanowski-Konakry, Harrison and Payne (1975) reported on five cases of fibroadenoma with carcinoma arising in them. They were all examples of CLIS. The five cases were found in a review of 4000 instances of fibroadenoma, an incidence of a little more than 0.1 per cent.

CONCLUSION

Carcinoma arising in a fibroadenoma is very rare. The incidence is probably little more than 1 in 1000 fibroadenomas. The carcinoma is usually, perhaps almost always, of the lobular variety, especially if one is strict in defining what is truly primary in the fibroadenoma. Ductal type carcinoma can, however, extremely rarely arise in a fibro-adenoma.

The prognosis of carcinoma limited exclusively, or almost exclusively, to a fibro-adenoma is excellent. The correct treatment has yet to be decided and will necessarily be influenced by current views on the treatment of CLIS when unrelated to the presence of a fibroadenoma.

SARCOMA AND CARCINOSARCOMA

Cystosarcoma, arising in a fibroadenoma, is considered in Chapter Fourteen. Extremely rarely, bizarre sarcomas including *osteosar-comas* (Rottino and Howley, 1945) can develop in a fibroadenoma. Because of the character of these tumours, they have attracted consider-able attention in the literature. They are described on page 366. True *carcinosarcomas* are extremely rare and are also considered in Chapter Fourteen. There is evidence that some carcinosarcomas may originate in a pre-existing fibroadenoma or cystosarcoma (Harris and Persaud, 1974).

References

Aboumrad, M. H., Horn, R. C., Jr and Fine, G. (1963) Lipid secreting mammary carcinoma. *Cancer,* **16,** 521–525.

Ackerman, L. V. and Butcher, H. R. (1968) *Surgical Pathology.* Fourth edition, pp. 741–743. St Louis: C. V. Mosby.

Ahmed, A. (1974) The myoepithelium in human breast carcinoma. *Journal of Pathology,* **113,** 129–135.

Amerson, J. R. (1970) Cystosarcoma phyllodes in adolescent females. A report of seven patients. *Annals of Surgery,* **171,** 849–858.

Arffmann, E. and Højgaard, K. (1965) Squamous carcinoma of the breast. Report of a case. *Journal of Pathology and Bacteriology,* **90,** 319–320.

Ashikari, R., Farrow, J. H. and O'Hara, J. (1971) Fibroadenomas in the breast of juveniles. *Surgery, Gynecology and Obstetrics,* **132,** 259–262.

Ashikari, R., Hajdu, S. I. and Robbins, G. F. (1971)

Intraductal carcinoma of the breast (1960–1969). *Cancer,* **28,** 1182–1187.

Ashikari, R., Huvos, A. G. and Snyder, R. E. (1977) Prospective study of non-infiltrating carcinoma of the breast. *Cancer,* **39,** 435–439.

Ashikari, R., Huvos, A. G., Urban, J. A. and Robbins, G. F. (1973) Infiltrating lobular carcinoma of the breast. *Cancer,* **31,** 110–116.

Ashikari, R., Rosen, P. P., Urban, J. A. and Senoo, T. (1976) Breast cancer presenting as an axillary mass. *Annals of Surgery,* **183,** 415–417.

Austin, W. E. and Fidler, H. K. (1953) Carcinoma developing in fibroadenoma of the breast. *American Journal of Clinical Pathology,* **23,** 688–690.

Azzopardi, J. G. and Eusebi, V. (1977) Melanocyte colonization and pigmentation of breast carcinoma. *Histopathology,* **1,** 21–30.

Azzopardi, J. G. and Laurini, R. N. (1974) Elastosis in breast cancer. *Cancer,* **33,** 174–183.

Azzopardi, J. G., Ross, C. M. D. and Frizzera, G. (1977) Blue naevi of lymph node capsule. *Histopathology,* **1,** 451–461.

Bannayan, G. A. and Hajdu, S. I. (1972) Gynecomastia: clinicopathologic study of 351 cases. *American Journal of Clinical Pathology,* **57,** 431–437.

Barber, K. W., Jr, Dockerty, M. B. and Clagett, O. T. (1961) Inflammatory carcinoma of the breast. *Surgery, Gynecology and Obstetrics,* **112,** 406–410.

Betsill, W. L., Jr, Rosen, P. P., Lieberman, P. H. and Robbins, G. F. (1978) Intraductal carcinoma: long-term follow-up after treatment by biopsy alone. *Journal of the American Medical Association,* **239,** 1863 1867.

Bhagavan, B. S., Patchefsky, A. and Koss, L. G. (1973) Florid subareolar duct papillomatosis (nipple adenoma) and mammary carcinoma: report of three cases. *Human Pathology,* **4,** 289–295.

Bosincu, L. and Eusebi, V. (1972) Carcinoma della mammella insorto in fibroadenoma. *Tumori,* **58,** 195–202.

Brown, J. M. (1970) Histological modification of fibroadenoma of the breast associated with oral hormonal contraceptives. *Medical Journal of Australia,* **1,** 276–277.

Brown, P. W., Silverman, J., Owens, E., Tabor, D. C., Terz, J. J. and Lawrence, W., Jr (1976) Intraductal 'noninfiltrating' carcinoma of the breast. *Archives of Surgery,* **111,** 1063–1067.

Buell, R. H., Tremblay, G. and Rowden, G. (1976) Distribution of adenosine triphosphatase in infiltrating ductal carcinoma and non-neoplastic breast. *Cancer,* **38,** 875–887.

Busch, W. and Merker, H. J. (1968) Elektronenmikroskopische Untersuchungen an menschlichen Mammacarcinomen. *Virchows Archiv A: Pathologische Anatomie,* **344,** 356–371.

Bussolati, G. and Pich, A. (1975) Mammary and extramammary Paget's disease. An immunocytochemical study. *American Journal of Pathology,* **80,** 117–128.

Buzanowski-Konakry, K., Harrison, E. G., Jr and Payne, W. S. (1975) Lobular carcinoma arising in fibroadenoma of the breast. *Cancer,* **35,** 450–456.

Byrne, M. P., Fahey, M. M. and Gooselaw, J. G. (1973) Breast cancer with axillary metastasis in an eight and one-half-year-old girl. *Cancer,* **31,** 726–728.

Carter, D. and Smith, R. R. L. (1977) Carcinoma in situ of the breast. *Cancer,* **40,** 1189–1193.

Carter, D., Yardley, J. H. and Shelley, W. M. (1969) Lobular carcinoma of the breast: an ultrastructural comparison with certain duct carcinomas and benign lesions. *Johns Hopkins Medical Journal,* **125,** 25–43.

Close, M. B. and Maximov, N. G. (1965) Carcinoma of breast in young girls. *Archives of Surgery,* **91,** 386–389.

Cole, E. W. (1976) Klinefelter syndrome and breast cancer. *Johns Hopkins Medical Journal,* **138,** 102–108.

Coley, G. M. and Kuehn, P. G. (1972) Paget's disease of male breast. *American Journal of Surgery,* **123,** 445–450.

Cornog, J. L., Mobini, J., Steiger, E. and Enterline, H. T. (1971) Squamous carcinoma of the breast. *American Journal of Clinical Pathology,* **55,** 410–417.

Crichlow, R. W. (1972) Carcinoma of the male breast. *Surgery, Gynecology and Obstetrics,* **134,** 1011–1019.

Crichlow, R. W. and Czernobilsky, B. (1967) Paget's disease of the male breast. *Cancer,* **20,** 1617–1624.

Crichlow, R. W., Kaplan, E. L. and Kearney, W. H. (1972) Male mammary cancer: an analysis of 32 cases. *Annals of Surgery,* **175,** 489–494.

Cubilla, A. L. and Woodruff, J. M. (1977) Primary carcinoid tumor of the breast. A report of eight patients. *American Journal of Surgical Pathology,* **4,** 283–292.

Cuenca, C. R. and Becker, K. L. (1968) Klinefelter's syndrome and cancer of the breast. *Archives of Internal Medicine,* **121,** 159–162.

Daniel, W. A., Jr and Mathews, M. D. (1968) Tumors of the breast in adolescent females. *Pediatrics,* **41,** 743–749.

Devitt, P. G. (1978) Carcinoid tumour of the breast. *British Medical Journal,* **ii,** 397.

Donegan, W. L. and Perez-Mesa, C. M. (1972) Lobular carcinoma — An indication for elective biopsy of the second breast. *Annals of Surgery,* **176,** 178–187.

Dossett, J. A. (1976) Malignant potential of breast lesions. In *Risk Factors in Breast Cancer* (Ed.) Stoll, B. A. Chapter 3, pp. 54–66. London: Heinemann Medical.

Edlow, D. W. and Carter, D. (1973) Heterotopic epithelium in axillary lymph nodes: report of a case and review of the literature. *American Journal of Clinical Pathology,* **59,** 666–673.

Ellis, D. L. and Teitelbaum, S. L. (1974) Inflammatory carcinoma of the breast. A pathologic definition. *Cancer,* **33,** 1045–1047.

Eusebi, V., Pich, A., Macchiorlatti, E. and Bussolati, G. (1977) Morpho-functional differentiation in lobular carcinoma of the breast. *Histopathology,* **1,** 301–314.

Evans, R. W. (1966) *Histological Appearances of Tumours.* Second edition. London: E. & S. Livingstone.

Factor, S. M., Biempica, L., Ratner, I., Ahuja, K. K. and Biempica, S. (1977) Carcinoma of the breast with multinucleated reactive stromal giant cells. A light and electron microscopic study of two cases. *Virchows Archiv A: Pathological Anatomy and Histology,* **374,** 1–12.

Farrow, J. H. (1970) Current concepts in the detection and treatment of the earliest of the early breast cancers. *Cancer,* **25,** 468–477.

Fechner, R. E. (1970a) Fibroadenomas in patients receiving oral contraceptives. *American Journal of Clinical Pathology,* **53,** 857–864.

Fechner, R. E. (1970b) Fibrocystic disease in women receiving oral contraceptive hormones. *Cancer,* **25,** 1332–1339.

Fechner, R. E. (1970c) Breast cancer during oral contraceptive therapy. *Cancer,* **26,** 1204–1211.

Fechner, R. E. (1972) Benign breast disease in women on estrogen therapy. *Cancer,* **29,** 273–279.

Fechner, R. E. (1975) Histologic variants of infiltrating lobular carcinoma of the breast. *Human Pathology,* **6,** 373–378.

Fisher, E. R. and Fisher, B. (1977) Lobular carcinoma of the breast: an overview. *Annals of Surgery,* **185,** 377–385.

Fisher, E. R., Gregorio, R. M. and Fisher, B. (1975) The pathology of invasive breast cancer. *Cancer,* **36,** 1–263.

Fisher, E. R., Gregorio, R., Kim, W. S. and Redmond, C. (1977a) Lipid in invasive cancer of the breast. *American Journal of Clinical Pathology,* **68,** 558–561.

Fisher, E. R., Gregorio, R. M., Redmond, C. and Fisher, B. (1977b) Tubulolobular invasive breast cancer: a variant of lobular invasive cancer. *Human Pathology,* **8,** 679–683.

Flores, L., Arlen, M., Elguezabal, A., Livingston, S. F. and Levowitz, B. S. (1974) Host tumor relationships in medullary carcinoma of the breast. *Surgery, Gynecology and Obstetrics,* **139,** 683–688.

Gad, A. and Azzopardi, J. G. (1975) Lobular carcinoma of the breast: a special variant of mucin-secreting carcinoma. *Journal of Clinical Pathology,* **28,** 711–716.

Giffler, R. F. and Kay, S. (1976) Small-cell carcinoma of the male mammary gland. A tumor resembling infiltrating lobular carcinoma. *American Journal of Clinical Pathology,* **66,** 715–722.

Gillis, D. A., Dockerty, M. B. and Clagett, O. T. (1960) Preinvasive intraductal carcinoma of the breast. *Surgery, Gynecology and Obstetrics.,* **110,** 555–562.

Goldenberg, V. E., Goldenberg, N. S. and Sommers, S. C. (1969) Comparative ultrastructure of atypical ductal hyperplasia, intraductal carcinoma, and infiltrating ductal carcinoma of the breast. *Cancer,* **24,** 1152–1169.

Goldenberg, V. E., Wiegenstein, L. and Mottet, N. K. (1968) Florid breast fibroadenomas in patients taking hormonal oral contraceptives. *American Journal of Clinical Pathology,* **49,** 52–59.

Goldenberg, V. E., Wiegenstein, L. and Wolff, M. (1968) Atypical features in breast carcinomas in patients on oral contraceptives. (Abstract.) *American Journal of Clinical Pathology,* **50,** 635.

Goldman, R. L. and Friedman, N. B.(1969) Carcinoma of the breast arising in fibroadenomas with emphasis on lobular carcinoma. A clinicopathologic study. *Cancer,* **23,** 544–550.

Gould, V. E., Miller, J. and Jao, W. (1975) Ultrastructure of medullary, intraductal, tubular and adenocystic breast carcinomas. Comparative patterns of myoepithelial differentiation and basal lamina deposition. *American Journal of Pathology,* **78,** 401–407.

Gudjónsdóttir, A., Hägerstrand, I. and Östberg, G. (1971) Adenoma of the nipple with carcinomatous development. *Acta Pathologica et Microbiologica Scandinavica, Section A,* **79,** 676–680.

Haagensen, C. D. (1971) *Diseases of the Breast.* Second edition — revised reprint, pp. 574, 594, 600–601. Philadelphia, London, Toronto: W. B. Saunders.

Haguenau, F. (1959) Le cancer du sein chez la femme. Étude comparative au microscope électronique et au microscope optique. *Bulletin de l'Association Française pour l'Étude du Cancer,* **46,** 177–211.

Hajdu, S. I. and Urban, J. A. (1972) Cancers metastatic to the breast. *Cancer,* **29,** 1691–1696.

Hamperl, H. (1977) Das sogenannte Schweissdrüsencarcinom der Mamma. *Zeitschrift für Krebsforschung,* **88,** 105–119.

Handley, R. S. and Thackray, A. C. (1962) Adenoma of nipple. *British Journal of Cancer,* **16,** 187–194.

Harris, M. and Ahmed, A. (1977) The ultrastructure of tubular carcinoma of the breast. *Journal of Pathology,* **123,** 79–83.

Harris, M. and Persaud, V. (1974) Carcinosarcoma of the breast. *Journal of Pathology,* **112,** 99–105.

Harris, M., Vasudev, K. S., Anfield, C. and Wells, S. (1978) Mucin-producing carcinomas of the breast: ultrastructural observations. *Histopathology,* **2,** 177–188.

Harrist, T. J. and Kalisher, L. (1977) Breast metastasis: an unusual manifestation of a malignant carcinoid tumor. *Cancer,* **40,** 3102–3106.

Hartman, A. W. and Magrish, P. (1955) Carcinoma of breast in children. Case report. Six-year-old boy with adenocarcinoma. *Annals of Surgery,* **141,** 792–798.

Hood, C. I., Font, R. L. and Zimmerman, L. E. (1973) Metastatic mammary carcinoma in the eyelid with histiocytoid appearance. *Cancer,* **31,** 793–800.

Huvos, A. G., Lucas, J. C., Jr and Foote, F. W., Jr (1973) Metaplastic breast carcinoma. Rare form of mammary cancer. *New York State Journal of Medicine,* **73,** 1078–1082.

Inglis, K. (1946) Paget's disease of the nipple. *American Journal of Pathology,* **22,** 1–33.

Inglis, K. (1952) The essential difference between 'the epidermal' changes in Paget's disease of the nipple and those in Bowen's 'precancerous dermatosis'. *Journal of Pathology and Bacteriology,* **64,** 637–643.

Jackson, A. W., Muldal, S., Ockey, C. H. and O'Connor, P. J. (1965) Carcinoma of male breast in association with the Klinefelter syndrome. *British Medical Journal,* **i,** 223–225.

Johnson, W. T. and Helwig, E. B. (1969) Benign nevus cells in the capsule of lymph nodes. *Cancer,* **23,** 747–753.

Jones, D. B. (1955) Florid papillomatosis of the nipple ducts. *Cancer,* **8,** 315–319.

Jones, E. L. (1969) Primary squamous-cell carcinoma of breast with pseudo-sarcomatous stroma. *Journal of Pathology,* **97,** 383–385.

Kaneko, H., Hōjō, H., Ishikawa, S., Yamanouchi, H., Sumida, T. and Saito, R. (1978) Norepinephrine-producing tumors of bilateral breasts. A case report. *Cancer,* **41,** 2002–2007.

Kouchoukos, N. T., Ackerman, L. V. and Butcher, H. R., Jr (1967) Prediction of axillary nodal metastases from the morphology of primary mammary carcinomas. *Cancer,* **20,** 948–960.

Kraus, L. W. and Kline, B. X. (1926) Carcinoma of both breasts in a woman under 20 years of age. *American Journal of Surgery,* **1,** 277–280.

Lagios, M. D., Margolin, F. R. and Rose, M. R. (1977) Personal communication.

Lane, N., Goksel, H., Salerno, R. A. and Haagensen, C. D. (1961) Clinicopathologic analysis of the surgical curability of breast cancers: a minimum ten-year study of a personal series. *Annals of Surgery,* **153,** 483–498.

Le Gal, Y., Gros, C.-M. and Bader, P. (1959) L'adénomatose erosive du mamelon. *Annales d'Anatomie Pathologique,* **4,** 292–304.

Lowden, R. G. and Taylor, H. B. (1974) Angioblastic meningioma with metastasis to the breast. *Archives of Pathology,* **98,** 373–375.

Lucas, F. V. and Perez-Mesa, C. (1978) Inflammatory carcinoma of the breast. *Cancer,* **41,** 1595–1605.

MacMahon, B., Morrison, A. S., Ackerman, L. V., Lattes,

R., Taylor, H. B. and Yuasa, S. (1973) Histologic characteristics of breast cancer in Boston and Tokyo. *International Journal of Cancer,* **11,** 338–344.

Martinez, V. and Azzopardi, J. G. (1979) *Histopathology,* in press.

McCarthy, S. W., Palmer, A. A., Bale, P. M. and Hirst, E. (1974) Nevus cells in lymph nodes. *Pathology,* **6,** 351–358.

McDivitt, R. W. and Stewart, F. W. (1966) Breast carcinoma in children. *Journal of the American Medical Association,* **195,** 388–390.

McDivitt, R. W., Stewart, F. W. and Berg, J. W. (1968) *Tumors of the Breast.* Atlas of Tumor Pathology, Second series, Fascicle 2. Washington, D.C.: Armed Forces Institute of Pathology.

McDivitt, R. W., Stewart, F. W. and Farrow, J. H. (1967) Breast carcinoma arising in solitary fibroadenomas. *Surgery, Gynecology and Obstetrics,* **125,** 572–576.

McIntosh, I. H., Hooper, A. A., Millis, R. R. and Greening, W. P. (1976) Metastatic carcinoma within the breast. *Clinical Oncology,* **2,** 393–401.

Melamed, M. R., Robbins, G. F. and Foote, F. W., Jr (1961) Prognostic significance of gelatinous mammary carcinoma. *Cancer,* **14,** 699–704.

Meyer, A. C., Dockerty, M. B. and Harrington, S. W. (1948) Inflammatory carcinoma of the breast. *Surgery, Gynecology and Obstetrics,* **87,** 417–424.

Michaud, J. and Morin, J. (1971) Ultrastructure d'un épithélioma médullaire de la glande mammaire. *Laval Médical,* **42,** 496–507.

Miller, G. and Bernier, L. (1965) Adénomatose erosive du mamelon. *Canadian Journal of Surgery,* **8,** 261–266.

Millis, R. R. and Thynne, G. S. J. (1975) In situ intraduct carcinoma of the breast: a long term follow-up study. *British Journal of Surgery,* **62,** 957–962.

Moore, O. S., Jr and Foote, F. W., Jr (1949) The relatively favorable prognosis of medullary carcinoma of the breast. *Cancer,* **2,** 635–642.

More, I. A. R. and Sandison, A. T. (1973) Triple carcinoma of the breast, one arising within a fibro-adenoma. *Journal of Pathology,* **109,** 263–265.

Moskowitz, M., Russell, P., Fidler, J., Sutorius, D., Law, E. J. and Holle, J. (1975) Breast cancer screening. Preliminary report of 207 biopsies performed in 4128 volunteer screenees. *Cancer,* **36,** 2245–2250.

Moskowitz, M., Pemmaraju, S., Fidler, J. A., Sutorius, D. J., Russell, P., Scheinok, P. and Holle, J. (1976) On the diagnosis of minimal breast cancer in screenee population. *Cancer,* **37,** 2543–2552.

Moynahan, E. J., Sethi, N. C. and Brooks, M. (1972) Histochemical observations on developing rat skin. *Journal of Anatomy,* **111,** 427–435.

Muir, R. (1939) Further observations on Paget's disease of the nipple. *Journal of Pathology and Bacteriology,* **49,** 299–312.

Murad, T. M. (1970) Histochemical differentiation of human breast cancers. *Proceedings 67th Annual Meeting American Association Pathologists Bacteriologists,* Abstract 81.

Murad, T. M. (1971) A proposed histochemical and electron microscopic classification of human breast cancer according to cell of origin. *Cancer,* **27,** 288–299.

Murad, T. M. (1975) Evaluation of the different techniques utilized in diagnosing breast lesions. *Acta Cytologica,* **19,** 499–508.

Murad, T. M. and Scarpelli, D. G. (1967) The ultrastructure of medullary and scirrhous mammary duct carcinoma. *American Journal of Pathology,* **50,** 335–360.

Murad, T. M., Swaid, S. and Pritchett, P. (1977) Malignant and benign papillary lesions of the breast. *Human Pathology,* **8,** 379–390.

Nambiar, R. and Kannan Kutty, M. (1974) Giant fibroadenoma (cystosarcoma phyllodes) in adolescent females — A clinicopathological study. *British Journal of Surgery,* **61,** 113–117.

Nehme, A. E. (1976) Paget's disease of the male breast: a collective review and case report. *American Surgeon,* **42,** 289–295.

Newman, W. (1966) Lobular carcinoma of the female breast. Report of 73 cases. *Annals of Surgery,* **164,** 305–314.

Nichini, F. M., Goldman, L., Lapayowker, M. S., Levy, W. M., Maier, W. and Rosemond, G. P. (1972) Inflammatory carcinoma of the breast in a 12-year-old girl. *Archives of Surgery,* **105,** 505–508.

Nichols, F. C., Dockerty, M. B. and Judd, E. S. (1958) Florid papillomatosis of nipple. *Surgery, Gynecology and Obstetrics,* **107,** 474–480.

Norris, H. J. and Taylor, H. B. (1965) Prognosis of mucinous (gelatinous) carcinoma of the breast. *Cancer,* **18,** 879–885.

Norris, H. J. and Taylor, H. B. (1967) Relationship of histologic features to behavior of cystosarcoma phyllodes. Analysis of ninety-four cases. *Cancer,* **20,** 2090–2099.

Norris, H. J. and Taylor, H. B. (1969) Carcinoma of the male breast. *Cancer,* **23,** 1428–1435.

Norris, H. J. and Taylor, H. B. (1970) Carcinoma of the breast in women less than thirty years old. *Cancer,* **26,** 953–959.

Oberman, H. A. and Stephens, P. J. (1972) Carcinoma of the breast in childhood. *Cancer,* **30,** 470–474.

O'Grady, W. P. and McDivitt, R. W. (1969) Breast cancer in a man treated with diethylstilbestrol. *Archives of Pathology,* **88,** 162–165.

Orr, J. W. and Parrish, D. J. (1962) The nature of the nipple changes in Paget's disease. *Journal of Pathology and Bacteriology,* **84,** 201–208.

Ozzello, L. (1959) The behavior of basement membranes in intraductal carcinoma of the breast. *American Journal of Pathology,* **35,** 887–899.

Ozzello, L. (1971) Ultrastructure of the human mammary gland. In *Pathology Annual* (Ed.) Sommers, S. C. Volume 6, pp. 1–59. London: Butterworth.

Ozzello, L. and Sanpitak, P. (1970) Epithelial–stromal junction of intraductal carcinoma of the breast. *Cancer,* **26,** 1186–1198.

Patchefsky, A. S., Shaber, G. S., Schwartz, G. F., Feig, S. A. and Nerlinger, R. E. (1977) The pathology of breast cancer detected by mass population screening. *Cancer,* **40,** 1659–1670.

Penman, H. G. (1970) The effect of oral contraceptives on the histology of carcinoma of the breast. *Journal of Pathology,* **101,** 66–69.

Perzin, K. H. and Lattes, R. (1972) Papillary adenoma of the nipple (florid papillomatosis, adenoma, adenomatosis). *Cancer,* **29,** 996–1009.

Pierce, G. B., Jr, Midgley, A. R., Jr and Sri Ram, J. (1963) The histogenesis of basement membranes. *Journal of Experimental Medicine,* **117,** 339–348.

Pierce, G. B., Jr, Midgley, A. R., Jr, Sri Ram, J. and Feldman, J. D. (1962) Parietal yolk sac carcinoma: clue to the histogenesis of Reichert's membrane of the mouse embryo. *American Journal of Pathology,* **41,** 549–566.

Pierce, G. B., Jr, Beals, T. F., Sri Ram, J. and Midgley, A. R., Jr (1964) Basement membranes. IV. Epithelial origin and immunologic cross reactions. *American Journal of Pathology*, **45**, 929–961.

Ramirez, G. and Ansfield, F. J. (1968) Carcinoma of the breast in children. *Archives of Surgery*, **96**, 222–225.

Ramos, C. V. and Taylor, H. B. (1974) Lipid-rich carcinoma of the breast. A clinicopathologic analysis of 13 examples. *Cancer*, **33**, 812–819.

Richardson, W. W. (1956) Medullary carcinoma of the breast: a distinctive tumour type with a relatively good prognosis following radical mastectomy. *British Journal of Cancer*, **10**, 415–423.

Ridolfi, R. L., Rosen, P. P., Port, A., Kinne, D. and Miké, V. (1977) Medullary carcinoma of the breast. A clinicopathologic study with 10 year follow-up. *Cancer*, **40**, 1365–1385.

Robb, P. M. and McFarlane, A. (1958) Two rare breast tumours. *Journal of Pathology and Bacteriology*, **75**, 293–298.

Robbins, G. F., Shah, J., Rosen, P., Chu, F. and Taylor, J. (1974) Inflammatory carcinoma of the breast. *Surgical Clinics of North America*, **54**, 801–810.

Robert, H., De Brux, J. and Winaver, D. (1963) La papillomatose bénigne du mamelon. *Presse Médicale*, **71**, 2713–2715.

Rogers, C. S. and Fitts, W. T., Jr (1956) Inflammatory carcinoma of the breast; a critique of therapy. *Surgery*, **39**, 367–370.

Rosen, P. P., Ashikari, R., Thaler, H., Ishikawa, S., Hirota, T., Abe, O., Yamamoto, H., Beattie, E. J., Jr, Urban, J. A. and Miké, V. (1977) A comparative study of some pathologic features of mammary carcinoma in Tokyo, Japan and New York, USA. *Cancer*, **39**, 429–434.

Rottino, A. and Howley, C. P. (1945) Osteoid sarcoma of the breast: a complication of fibroadenoma. *Archives of Pathology*, **40**, 44–50.

Sagebiel, R. W. (1969) Ultrastructural observations on epidermal cells in Paget's disease of the breast. *American Journal of Pathology*, **57**, 49–64.

Salm, R. and Sissons, H. A. (1972) Giant-cell tumours of soft tissues. *Journal of Pathology*, **107**, 27–39.

Saltzstein, S. I. (1974) Clinically occult inflammatory carcinoma of the breast. *Cancer*, **34**, 382–388.

Salyer, W. R. and Salyer, D. C. (1973) Metastases of prostatic carcinoma to the breast. *Journal of Urology*, **109**, 671–675.

Sandison, A. T. (1959) Metastatic tumours in the breast. *British Journal of Surgery*, **47**, 54–58.

Sandison, A. T. and Walker, J. C. (1968) Diseases of the adolescent female breast. A clinico-pathological study. *British Journal of Surgery*, **55**, 443–448.

Sartwell, P. E., Arthes, F. G. and Tonascia, J. A. (1973) Epidemiology of benign breast lesions: lack of association with oral contraceptive use. *New England Journal of Medicine*, **288**, 551–554.

Scheike, O. and Visfeldt, J. (1973) Male breast cancer. 4. Gynecomastia in patients with breast cancer. *Acta Pathologica et Microbiologica Scandinavica*, Section A, **81**, 359–365.

Scheike, O., Visfeldt, J. and Petersen, B. (1973) Male breast cancer. 3. Breast carcinoma in association with the Klinefelter syndrome. *Acta Pathologica et Microbiologica Scandinavica*, Section A, **81**, 352–358.

Schwartz, G. F. (1969) Solid circumscribed carcinoma of the breast. *Annals of Surgery*, **169**, 165–173.

Silverberg, S. G. and Chitale, A. R. (1973) Assessment of significance of proportions of intraductal and infiltrating tumor growth in ductal carcinoma of the breast. *Cancer*, **32**, 830–837.

Silverberg, S. G., Kay, S., Chitale, A. R. and Levitt, S. H. (1971) Colloid carcinoma of the breast. *American Journal of Clinical Pathology*, **55**, 355–363.

Simpson, J. S. and Barson, A. J. (1969) Breast tumours in infants and children. *Canadian Medical Association Journal*, **101**, 100–102.

Sirtori, C. and Veronesi, U. (1957) Gynecomastia. A review of 218 cases. *Cancer*, **10**, 645–654.

Smith, E. J., Kron, S. D. and Gross, P. R. (1970) Erosive adenomatosis of the nipple. *Archives of Dermatology*, **102**, 330–332.

Stewart, F. W. (1950) *Tumors of the Breast*. Atlas of Tumor Pathology, Section 9, Fascicle 34, p. 58. Washington, D.C.: Armed Forces Institute of Pathology.

Stocks, L. H. and Simmons Patterson, F. M. (1976) Inflammatory carcinoma of the breast. *Surgery, Gynecology and Obstetrics*, **143**, 885–889.

Sullivan, J. J., Magee, H. R. and Donald, K. J. (1977) Secretory (juvenile) carcinoma of the breast. *Pathology*, **9**, 341–346.

Symmers, W. S. (1968) Carcinoma of breast in transsexual individuals after surgical and hormonal interference with the primary and secondary sex characteristics. *British Medical Journal*, **ii**, 83–85.

Taylor, H. B. (1971) Oral contraceptives and pathologic changes in the breast. *Cancer*, **28**, 1388–1390.

Taylor, H. B. and Robertson, A. G. (1965) Adenomas of the nipple. *Cancer*, **18**, 995–1002.

Toker, C. (1961) Some observations on Paget's disease of the nipple. *Cancer*, **14**, 653–672.

Toker, C. (1970) Clear cells of the nipple epidermis. *Cancer*, **25**, 601–610.

Toker, C. and Goldberg, J. D. (1977) The small cell lesion of mammary ducts and lobules. In *Pathology Annual* (Ed.) Sommers, S. C. and Rosen, P. P. Vol. 12, pp. 217–249. New York: Appleton-Century-Crofts.

Treves, N. (1953) Inflammatory carcinoma of the breast in the male patient. *Surgery*, **34**, 810–820.

Treves, N. (1954) Paget's disease of the male mamma; a report of 2 cases. *Cancer*, **7**, 325–330.

Treves, N. and Holleb, A. I. (1955) Cancer of the male breast. A report of 146 cases. *Cancer*, **8**, 1239–1250.

Treves, N., Robbins, G. F. and Amoroso, W. L., Jr (1956) Serous and serosanguineous discharge from the male nipple. *Archives of Surgery*, **73**, 319–329.

van Bogaert, L.-J. and Maldague, P. (1977) Histologic variants of lipid-secreting carcinoma of the breast. *Virchows Archiv A: Pathological Anatomy and Histology*, **375**, 345–353.

Veronesi, U. and Gennari, L. (1960) Il carcinoma gelatinoso della mammella. *Tumori*, **46**, 119–155.

Vessey, M. P., Doll, R. and Sutton, P. M. (1972) Oral contraceptives and breast neoplasia: a retrospective study. *British Medical Journal*, **iii**, 719–724.

Visfeldt, J. and Scheike, O. (1973) Male breast cancer. Histologic typing and grading of 187 Danish cases. *Cancer*, **32**, 985–990.

Vogler, E. (1947) Über das basilare Helle-Zellen-Organ der menschlichen Brustdrüse. *Klinische Medizin*, **2**, 159–168.

Waldo, E. D., Sidhu, G. S. and Hu, A. W. (1975) Florid papillomatosis of male nipple after diethylstilbestrol therapy. *Archives of Pathology*, **99**, 364–366.

Warner, N. E. (1969) Lobular carcinoma of the breast. *Cancer*, **23**, 840–846.

Wellings, S. R. and Roberts, P. (1963) Electron microscopy of sclerosing adenosis and infiltrating duct carcinoma of the human mammary gland. *Journal of the National Cancer Institute,* **30,** 269–287.

Westbrook, K. C. and Gallager, H. S. (1975) Intraductal carcinoma of the breast. A comparative study. *American Journal of Surgery,* **130,** 667–670.

Wheeler, J. E. and Enterline, H. T. (1976) Lobular carcinoma of the breast in situ and infiltrating. In *Pathology Annual* (Ed.) Sommers, S. C. Vol. 11. New York: Appleton-Century-Crofts.

Willis, R. A. (1958) Squamous-cell mammary carcinoma of predominantly fibrosarcoma-like structure. *Journal of Pathology and Bacteriology,* **76,** 511–515.

Willis, R. A. (1967) *The Pathology of Tumours.* Fourth edition, pp. 246–251. London: Butterworth.

Willis, R. A. and Goldie, W. (1959) Papillary intraepidermal carcinoma of the nipple and skin of the male breast. *Journal of Pathology and Bacteriology,* **78,** 565–567.

Wulsin, J. H. and Schreiber, J. T. (1962) Improved prognosis in certain patterns of carcinoma of the breast. Colloid, medullary with lymphoid stroma, and intraductal. *Archives of Surgery,* **85,** 791–800.

Yogore, M. G. and Sahgal, S. (1977) Small cell carcinoma of the male breast. Report of a case. *Cancer,* **39,** 1748–1751.

Chapter Thirteen

Tumours Analogous with Tumours of the Salivary and Sweat Glands

These can be categorized following Hamperl (1970) into:

- A. 'Mixed' Tumour of Salivary Gland Type
- B. Adenoid Cystic Carcinoma
- C. Adenomyoepithelioma

To which the writer would add:

- D. Eccrine Spiradenoma-like Tumour

One must first concede with Hamperl (1970) that, although these types of tumour occur in all three organs (breast, salivary gland and skin), they are *not necessarily identical in the different sites*; differences of morphology and behaviour are found according to the site. Secondly, *rare transitional forms between these tumour types must be allowed for.*

MIXED SALIVARY TYPE TUMOUR

The benign 'mixed' tumour of salivary type is a very rare tumour in the breast. It is not significantly different morphologically from the tumour as it occurs in the salivary glands. The role of the myoepithelium is seen even in the presence of elastic tissue as an integral component of these tumours (Azzopardi and Zayid, 1972). In the human breast these tumours have to date all been benign. A possible malignant example was reported by Wald and Kakulas (1964); lymph nodes were not involved and there is no record of follow-up. The interesting 'mixed tumours' described by Smith and Taylor (1969) fall into a different category altogether, though the authors described them as 'similar in appearance to mixed tumours of salivary gland origin'. Their tumours had a mixture of epithelial and mesenchymal elements without apparent transition between the two components. The chondroid and osseous tissue was regarded as metaplastic in the stroma of lesions which were otherwise ductal papillomas. This is of course quite different from the origin of chondroid and cartilage as seen commonly in the 'mixed' tumour of salivary glands (Azzopardi and Smith, 1959).

The first historical report is attributed to Lecène in 1906, cited by Nabert, Kermanach and Saout (1968). Sheth, Hathway and Petrelli (1978) reviewed and tabulated the cases of pleomorphic adenoma ('mixed' salivary type

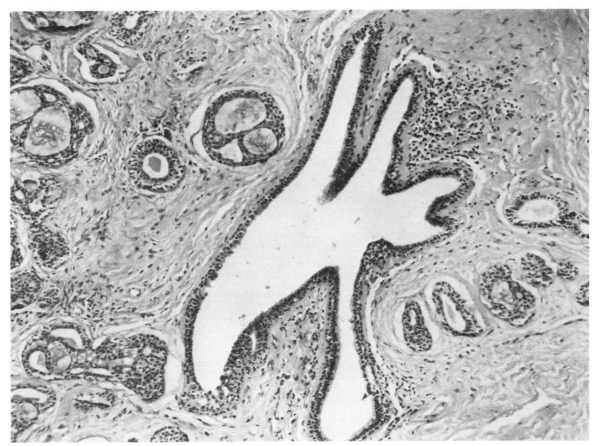

Figure 13–1   Adenoid cystic carcinoma of the breast with a relatively normal lactiferous sinus in the centre. H and E.×150.

tumour) reported since 1968. They found only six cases, including their own, apart from the nine cases reported on by Smith and Taylor (1969). It is not at all clear that the latter cases belong in the same category; they were regarded by Smith and Taylor (1969) as intraductal papillomas with chondroid and osseous metaplasia of the stroma. The case reported by Sheth, Hathway and Petrelli (1978) mimicked a carcinoma clinically and radiologically and was treated by simple mastectomy because a definitive diagnosis was not possible at frozen section.

The histogenesis of this rare tumour is apparently similar to that of the same tumour in the salivary glands. Only one tumour is known to have recurred after three years, and this was still regarded as benign (Sheth, Hathway and Petrelli, 1978).

ADENOID CYSTIC CARCINOMA

The adenoid cystic carcinoma of the breast resembles closely the cribriform tumour seen most commonly in the major and minor salivary glands and the mucous and muco-serous glands of other sites (Figures 13–1 and 13–2). For reasons which are unknown, this type of tumour has a much better prognosis when situated in the breast than the equivalent tumour of the salivary glands.

Older Studies. Adenoid cystic carcinoma of the breast is a very rare tumour. In the older literature single case reports predominate, but Galloway, Woolner and Clagett (1966) described nine cases from the Mayo Clinic and Cavanzo and Taylor (1969) reported on 21 cases. A good review of the subject is given by Friedman and Oberman (1970), who added five cases. Lusted (1970) reported on three new cases and included a long-term follow-up on a previously reported case. By 1970, there were about 54 reasonably documented cases in the English and Italian languages though there is doubt about the authenticity of a few (e.g. Case 4 of Lusted, 1970).

Clinical Features. Some interesting clinical

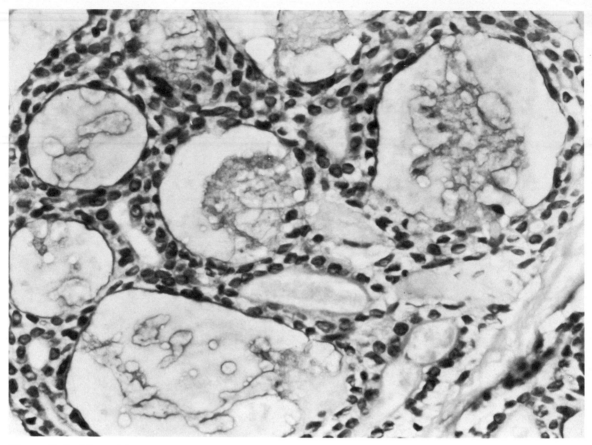

Figure 13–2   Dimorphic pattern necessary to identify adenoid cystic carcinoma with certainty. At least four ducts are visible in a background of basaloid cells surrounding larger, more rounded, mucin-containing spaces. This very rare tumour must be distinguished from ordinary ductal carcinoma exhibiting the so-called 'adenocystic' pattern (see Figure 7–25). H and E. ×600.

features emerge from an analysis of the literature. In 13 of 27 cases in which the location of the tumour was stated, it was either subareolar or adjacent to the areola (Figure 13–1). The second point of interest is the duration of symptoms. While in some cases this was only 'days' or 'weeks', three of the nine cases studied by Galloway, Woolner and Clagett (1966) had histories of 12, 13 and 15 years. There was a history of five years' duration or more in eight of 26 cases collected by Friedman and Oberman (1970), though in their own five cases symptoms did not exceed six months. In seven of the eight cases with long histories the duration was actually 10 years or more. Further data on this point are required. Another moot point is the question of whether pain or tenderness is more frequent than would appear from the older literature. Four out of nine of the patients of Galloway, Woolner and Clagett (1966) had a painful or tender mass; two of the five patients

of Friedman and Oberman (1970) presented with painful nodules and Lusted (1970) reported a painful mass in one case and a tender recurrence in another, with two others asymptomatic. Two of the three cases reported on by Hopkins and Tullis (1972) were tender, as were two of the three cases of Anthony and James (1975).

Pathology. Most tumours are solid but six have, somewhat unexpectedly, been described as cystic.

In order to identify a tumour as an adenoid cystic carcinoma, it is essential that it shows a distinct *biphasic cellular pattern,* in some part at least (Figure 13–2), and that it has the structural features that characterize these tumours when they affect other organs (Azzopardi and Smith, 1959; Tandler, 1971). The main differential diagnosis is from ductal carcinoma with a cribriform pattern and this distinction is not always an easy one. The pathologist must be familiar with the appearance and significance of the true glandular lumina lined by epithelial cells and the pseudocysts of the cribriform areas of adenoid cystic carcinoma (Figure 13–2), i.e. the divergent differentiation into two cell types which characterizes this tumour and separates it objectively from cribriform ductal carcinoma. Other features of the type mentioned by Friedman and Oberman (1970) can serve as subsidiary pointers in the differential diagnosis but there are many exceptions and the writer agrees with Anthony and James (1975) that a biphasic cellular pattern is essential for unequivocal identification. Identification of the *two distinctive types of mucin* can also be very useful in recognition of the entity (Azzopardi and Smith, 1959).

Strict Definition and Frequency. If one does not adopt these stringent criteria, the diagnosis of adenoid cystic carcinoma of the breast will lose much of its significance. Hence Fisher, Gregorio and Fisher (1975) found an incidence of 0.4 per cent among breast cancers (4 in 1000), almost certainly too high a figure and based on a wider and less precise definition of the term. These authors even recognized 'mixed' forms of the tumour, constituting an additional 1.8 per cent of the total breast cancers. The writer agrees with Anthony and James (1975) that this is a tumour type with an incidence of only about 0.1 per cent or, possibly, fractionally more (three cases of 2700 in their material). Cammoun, Contesso and Rouëssé (1972) found eight cases of adenoid cystic carcinoma among two series of breast cancers from different sources totalling 3950, an incidence of 0.2 per cent. This is rather higher than the 0.1 per cent of Anthony and James (1975). One cannot be sure that all cases included are authentic since there is no mention of a dimorphic pattern with dual ductal and pseudocyst differentiation or of two types of mucin secretion. At the time of this report, the difficulty of differentiation from certain cribriform ductal carcinomas was not as fully appreciated as it should be today. The figure of 0.2 per cent might therefore be legitimately regarded as a maximum figure.

It is particularly important that the view of Fisher, Gregorio and Fisher (1975), which fails to distinguish adenoid cystic carcinoma from cribriform ductal carcinoma, be rejected. Otherwise the features of true adenoid cystic carcinoma will be obscured altogether. A good illustration of this is seen in Case 2 of Verani and van der Bel-Kahn (1973). These authors reported what is said to be the first case of adenoid cystic carcinoma of the breast with metastases to axillary lymph nodes. Figure 2 of these authors does not, in the writer's opinion, show adenoid cystic carcinoma but ordinary infiltrating ductal cancer. The lesion that developed in the lung 14 years later was regarded as metastatic but the illustrations do not show any of the diagnostic features of adenoid cystic carcinoma: psammoma bodies, which were a striking feature, have not, on the authors' own admission, been previously recorded in this tumour type. Clearly this case cannot be accepted as the first instance of adenoid cystic carcinoma of the breast metastasizing to lymph nodes. Acceptable nodal metastases from this tumour have not yet been documented. Case 1 of Qizilbash, Patterson and Oliveira (1977) is also a little suspect while their Case 2 is convincing. The two cases of adenoid cystic carcinoma of the male breast reported by Ferlito and DiBonito (1974) are also rejected. Harris (1977) also cautioned against confusion of adenoid cystic carcinoma with cribriform ductal carcinoma. He called his tumour a '*pseudoadenoid cystic carcinoma*', a descriptively apt term. The writer does not, however, agree that the diagnosis of adenoid cystic carcinoma cannot be safely made by conventional techniques aided, perhaps, by mucin histochemistry. Ultrastructural studies complement but do not replace other diagnostic methods in the diagnosis of this lesion.

Prognosis. Strictly defined, this tumour has a very good prognosis. Seven patients had a local recurrence but five had been treated by local excision of the tumour only (Cavanzo and Taylor, 1969; Woyke, Domagala and Olszewski, 1970; Cammoun, Contesso and Rouëssé, 1972). The other two recurrences occurred after excisional biopsy (Lusted, 1970) and after simple mastectomy (Wilson and Spell, 1967). Both these patients were alive, without evidence of tumour, after 39 and 16 years respectively. The recurrences did not appear to alter the survival prospects even in the patient who had two recurrences (Wilson and Spell, 1967). Case 1 of Lusted (1970) was unusual in a number of respects including recurrence, as three neoplastic foci, $22\frac{1}{2}$ years after excision biopsy (Table 13–1).

Table 13–1   Cases with recurrent tumour from adenoid cystic carcinoma of breast

Author	Year	Treatment	Course	Outcome and other information
1. Wilson and Spell	1967	Simple mastectomy	Recurrence in scar Pectoral muscles and axillary contents removed en bloc 10 years later: 2nd recurrence, necessitating removal ribs and adjacent soft tissue	Alive 16 years
2. Lusted	1970	Excisional biopsy	Recurrence at $22\frac{1}{2}$ years Simple mastectomy and node dissection	Alive 39 years (after discovery mass and 2 years post-mastectomy)
3. Cavanzo and Taylor	1969	Simple excision	Local recurrence 3 years later Simple mastectomy	
4. Cavanzo and Taylor	1969	Simple excision	Local recurrence 7 years later Simple mastectomy	
5. Woyke, Domagala and Olszewski	1970	Local excision	Recurrence as 4 nodules 5 years postoperatively Recurrence as deposit in 'armpit' at 7 years	Male patient

Cammoun, Contesso and Rouëssé (1972) reported on two cases which were already recurrent at the time of their study (their cases 6 and 7).

Metastases. Two patients died of disseminated malignant disease, mainly pulmonary, after radical mastectomy for adenoid cystic carcinoma of the breast (Nayer, 1957; O'Kell, 1964) (Table 13–2). Regrettably, the documentation in both cases is not as perfect as one would wish. A third case (Elsner, 1970) developed asymptomatic lung metastases six years after mastectomy. Elsner (1970) rightly maintained that better follow-up studies are necessary. Since recurrences can be delayed for as long as 10 to 20 years and lung metastases have appeared in two cases six years and nine years postoperatively, there is *need for longer follow-up studies* than are mostly available (Hjorth, Magnusson and Blomquist, 1977).

Absence of Nodal Metastases and Bearing on Treatment. It should be stressed that there is no genuine case with proven lymph node metastases despite the many cases treated by radical mastectomy or axillary dissection. Cammoun, Contesso and Rouëssé (1972) found no nodal involvement in their six patients in whom lymph nodes were available

for study; a total of 83 axillary nodes were examined by them (Table 13–3). Whereas many authors advise radical mastectomy, the writer is in complete agreement with Cavanzo and Taylor (1969) that simple mastectomy is, on present evidence, the treatment of choice and that radical mastectomy is an unnecessary mutilation. Cammoun, Contesso and Rouëssé (1972) also recommended a simple mastectomy and, on the basis of their data, rightly regarded radical mastectomy as too drastic a procedure for treating this disease. Future data might show this to be incorrect but this seems unlikely.

More Recent Studies. Almost a hundred cases were collected from the literature by Anthony and James (1975) and by Hjorth, Magnusson and Blomquist (1977). Anthony and James (1975) demonstrated the *presence of actomyosin* in all three of their tumours, supporting the concept of rudimentary myoepithelial cell differentiation in this tumour. These workers stressed the importance of not confusing cribriform ductal carcinoma with adenocystic carcinoma: significantly, no immunofluo-

Table 13–2   Cases with fatal metastases or metastases from adenoid cystic carcinoma

Author	Year	Treatment	Evidence of metastases	Necropsy
1. Nayer	1957	Radical mastectomy	Pulmonary opacities x-ray 9 years later. Death 13 years post-mastectomy Pleural fluid aspirated shortly before death contained cell clusters suggestive of ACC	None[a]
2. O'Kell	1964	Radical mastectomy	Records mastectomy and pathology not available[a] Biopsy scar 3 years postoperatively revealed ACC	Yes Tumour in anterior thoracic wall, lungs, inferior vena cava
3. Elsner	1970	Radical mastectomy	Asymptomatic lung metastases 6 years postoperatively	

[a] Cases very probably genuine, although documentation not complete.

Table 13–3   Cases with proven nodal metastases from adenoid cystic carcinoma

None

rescent staining was obtained with anti-actomyosin serum in cases of cribriform ductal carcinoma. This underlines again the importance of distinguishing between adenoid cystic carcinoma and cribriform ductal carcinoma, a mistake seen in the figures of those who claim an incidence of this tumour of 0.4 per cent and even more.

Male Breast. Woyke, Domagala and Olszewski (1970) recorded the first example of adenoid cystic carcinoma of the male breast. It recurred as four tender nodules five years postoperatively. Two years later a further deposit appeared in the armpit but, from the illustrations, it does not appear as if this tumour was in a lymph node. The patient was treated by radical mastectomy; there is no record of subsequent follow-up. Case 1 of Verani and van der Bel-Kahn (1973) is probably another case of adenoid cystic carcinoma of the male breast. This man died of metastatic disease but there was no necropsy; a polypoid bladder tumour was found during investigation of haematuria but it was not possible to obtain a biopsy; there is no proof that this man died of metastatic disease derived from the breast tumour, though such a claim has been made. A third case in a man was reported by Hjorth,

Magnusson and Blomquist (1977). It presented in a 21-year-old, as a tender lump dating from puberty. The two other cases reported in men (Ferlito and DiBonito, 1974) are not acceptable for the reasons already indicated.

Ultrastructure. The ultrastructural features of adenoid cystic carcinoma of the breast are well described and illustrated by Koss, Brannan and Ashikari (1970) and by Gould, Miller and Jao (1975). They are similar to those of adenoid cystic carcinoma in the salivary glands and other sites. Myoepithelial cell differentiation and basal lamina production are characteristic features. Pseudocysts and true ductal lumina are easily distinguished, as indeed they are on light microscopy (Azzopardi and Smith, 1959).

Van Bogaert et al (1975) in a histochemical study stressed the role of the myoepithelial cell in the production of the major mucopolysaccharide component.

CLEAR-CELL HIDRADENOMA AND RELATED TUMOURS

The *adenomyoepithelioma* of the breast is a very rare tumour of which the writer has seen only a single example by courtesy of Hamperl (1975). More common is the '*clear-cell hidradenoma*' of the breast described by Finck, Schwinn and Keasbey (1968). Hamperl (1970) thought it likely that the latter is a variant of the adenomyothelioma, but it would be wise to reserve judgement on this point. The 'clear-cell hidradenoma' of the breast, whatever its precise nature, is benign. Hertel, Zaloudek and Kempson (1976) mentioned briefly a case of '*eccrine acrospiroma*', a basically similar tumour, which was however only focally clear-celled. Toth (1977) described a virtually pure benign myoepithelioma, a leiomyoma-like multifocal neoplasm.

ECCRINE SPIRADENOMA-LIKE TUMOUR

The eccrine spiradenoma-like lesion is so called from the close resemblance to the dermal tumour (Kersting and Helwig, 1956). It was first described in the breast by Draheim, Neubecker and Sprinz (1959) and recently another case was mentioned by Hertel, Zaloudek and Kempson (1976) in a comprehensive survey of breast adenomas. It is extremely rare and benign.

Under the heading of '*Malignant Tumours Containing Myothelia*', Hamperl (1970) placed:

A. Malignant 'Mixed' Tumours of the Salivary Gland Type (Carcinomas with Cartilaginous and Osseous Metaplasia)
B. Malignant Adenomyotheliomas
C. Certain Sarcomas and Carcinosarcomas.

CARCINOMA WITH CARTILAGINOUS AND OSSEOUS METAPLASIA

Malignant 'Mixed' Tumours, in the strict sense, are very rare in both the breast and the salivary glands as opposed to 'carcinoma ex mixed tumour', which is, of course, well known in the salivary glands. In the human mammary gland, malignant 'mixed' tumours have been documented by Stewart (1950) under the heading of 'carcinoma with cartilaginous and osseous metaplasia'. Smith and Taylor (1969) described 10 cases of this somewhat exotic condition. Cartilage was present in all 10 and bone in seven of the cases.

Transitions from the carcinoma to the heterotopic elements were noted in all. These are aggressive tumours with six out of the 10 patients dead of tumour at the time of follow-up. Huvos, Lucas and Foote (1973) gave a good account of these tumours in a paper entitled 'Metaplastic Breast Carcinoma': carcinomas with chondroid and osseous metaplasia constitute group II of the metaplastic carcinomas and number 16 cases. The *rarity* of these tumours is emphasized by the fact that Huvos, Lucas and Foote (1973) found only 16 cases over a 50-year period in an institute dealing with nearly 400 new patients with breast cancer annually. The lesions tended to be large, averaging 5.5 cm. Axillary node metastases were seen in only 19 per cent. Despite this, the five-year survival rate was only 38 per cent compared with 59 per cent for carcinoma NOS. It seems that these patients exhibit primarily a blood-borne type of spread. The *bad prognosis* with this type of carcinoma is in agreement with the findings of Smith and Taylor (1969). Certainly, in the human, these tumours do not have the good prognosis associated with the corresponding tumours in the bitch.

Kahn et al (1978) studied two examples of breast carcinoma with chondroid metaplasia and demonstrated convincing *transitions between the carcinomatous and chondrosarcomatous areas* at both light and electron microscopic levels.

In the bitch, of course, this type of tumour is commoner and widely recognized (von Bomhard and von Sandersleben, 1974, 1975).

MALIGNANT ADENOMYOEPITHELIOMA

The malignant adenomyoepithelioma is an exceptionally rare tumour in all three sites: skin, salivary glands and breast, in descending order of frequency. One in the parotid is illustrated in Figure 13–3. Cameron, Hamperl and Warambo (1974) described a leiomyosarcoma of the breast of myothelial origin, the counterpart of the benign leiomyoma-like tumour of Toth (1977). This tumour, which is so far unique, forms a natural link with Hamperl's (1970) next group.

VERY RARE SARCOMAS AND SOME SO-CALLED CARCINOSARCOMAS

Hamperl (1970) summarized the evidence for regarding some, at least, of these tumours

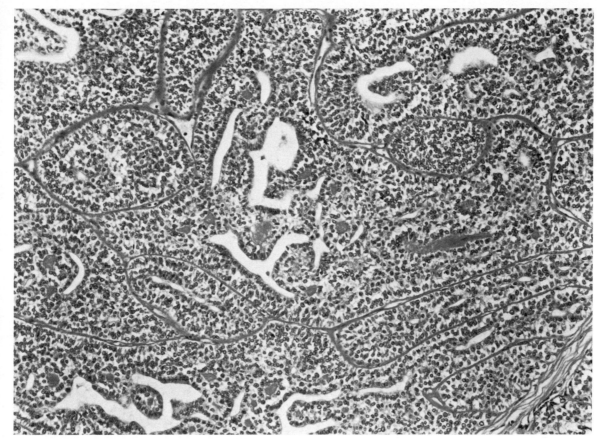

Figure 13–3 Malignant adenomyoepithelioma of the parotid gland. This is an insufficiently recognized entity. H and E. ×150.

as malignant tumours showing the metaplastic potential of both epithelial cells and myoepithelial cells, without the necessity of postulating a dual epithelial and connective tissue origin. There is something to commend this view in certain special cases but the writer believes, nevertheless, that it is not possible to explain the majority of pure sarcomas on this basis; nor can rhabdomyosarcomatous differentiation be accounted for on this histogenetic view. Equally, some cases of carcinosarcoma are probably genuine (page 374), and are generally held to have a dual epithelial and connective tissue origin.

APOCRINE CARCINOMA

Apocrine carcinoma has a rare counterpart in the skin but there is no known tumour of salivary glands which is strictly analogous. A malignant tumour of the breast composed entirely of easily recognizable apocrine type epithelium is a considerable rarity, probably consituting no more than 0.3 to 0.4 per cent of cancers, depending on the strictness of one's criteria (Figures 13–4 to 13–6). By 'easily recognizable apocrine-type epithelium' is meant here epithelium which, though neoplastic, has some of the specific cytological features of apocrine epithelium, as it is most commonly seen in cystic disease of the breast or, focally, in papillomas of the ducts. The cytoplasm is copious, variably granular and acidophilic (Figures 13–4 and 13–5) but these features are not enough to label a carcinoma 'apocrine' with certainty. In addition, where there is glandular differentiation, the luminal margin of the cells is not always clean-cut but in parts it exhibits the convex, bulbous, gasolene-pump edge that is seen in benign apocrine metaplasia. Naturally, the extent and prominence of this appearance will depend on the degree of differentiation of the tumour and it may vary within the same tumour. Nuclei are often deeply staining in some parts and vesicular in other parts; in either case the nucleoli are frequently prominent (Figure 13–5). Most characteristic, if present, are 'inclusions' of the type seen in apocrine metaplasia as found in cysts. Rarely vacuoles containing eosinophilic lipoprotein 'inclusions' or even brownish-yellow pigment may be found. The highly refractile, eosinophilic,

341

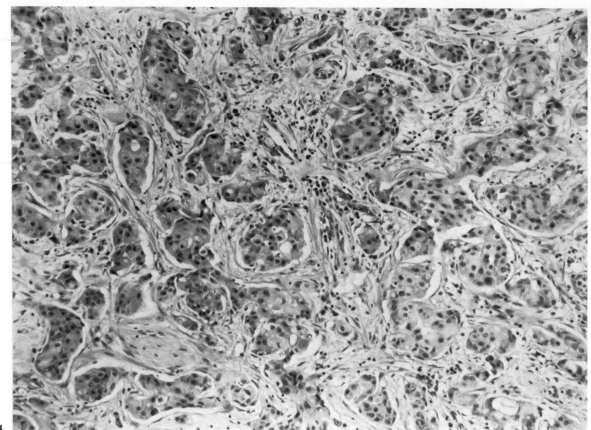

13–4

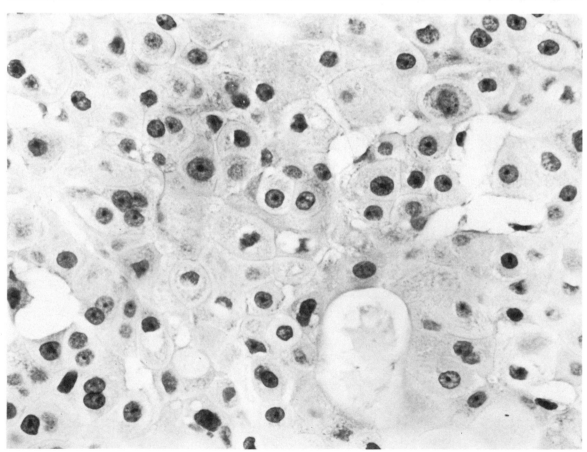

13–5

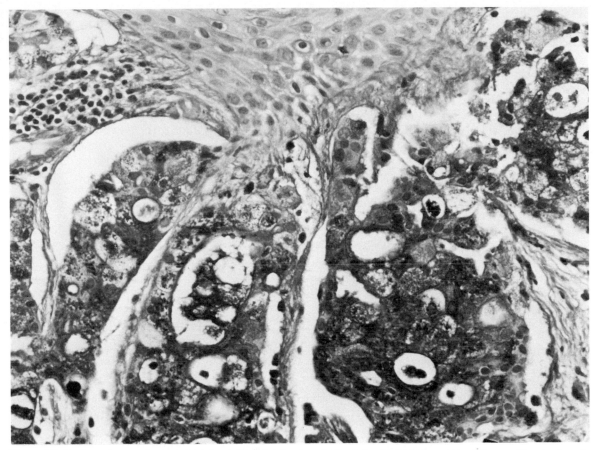

Figure 13–6   Apocrine carcinoma which has infiltrated the dermis. Part of epidermis seen at top. The specific cytoplasmic granules are unusually abundant in this case and stain deeply with PAS. Diastase–PAS. ×400.

PAS-positive granules with a high lipid content described on page 70 can usually be found in these tumours but a careful search for them is often required (Figure 13–6). These granules may even occasionally be found to occupy a crescentic area of the cytoplasm, as in the corresponding benign epithelium.

Incidence According to Different Definitions. If one includes carcinomas which show distinct apocrine differentiation in focal parts of the tumour only, the incidence of apocrine carcinoma is nearly 1 per cent, the figure given by Stewart (1950) and by Frable and Kay (1968). If, by apocrine carcinoma, one merely means tumours with a copious, acidophilic cytoplasm, then the incidence rises to anything between 2.2 per cent (Fisher, Gregorio and Fisher, 1975) and 14.5 per cent (Bonser, Dossett and Jull, 1961).

Prognosis. There is nearly general agree-ment that apocrine differentiation does not alter the ultimate prognosis, though the median survival may be longer (Frable and Kay, 1968). Bonser, Dossett and Jull (1961) implied that there may be some prognostic difference but Lee, Pack and Scharnagel (1933), whom they quoted, did not support this contention.

Correct Designation. Bonser, Dossett and Jull (1961) called these tumours by the colourful name of 'pink cell carcinomas'; they chose this term partly because they were not convinced that the epithelial change could be equated with apocrine metaplasia. The writer would argue that the similarities of the benign equivalent seen in cystic disease to apocrine epithelium far outweigh the subtle differ-ences: the similarities include light structural, histochemical and ultrastructural ones. Pier, Garancis and Kuzma (1970) are quoted by Fisher, Gregorio and Fisher (1975) as

Figure 13–4   (*Opposite, above.*)   Panoramic view of apocrine carcinoma. H and E. ×150.

Figure 13–5   (*Opposite, below.*)   Apocrine carcinoma. Neoplastic cells have copious eosinophilic and granular cytoplasm. H and E. ×600.

disclaiming the apocrine nature of this epithelium: Pier, Garancis and Kuzma (1970) actually pointed out the ultrastructural identity with the epithelium of apocrine glands: it is only the occurrence of 'apocrine' secretion (i.e. decapitation secretion) which is in question, as it is in fact for the baseline apocrine glands of the skin, with which comparison was being made.

Two Main Forms. From the point of view of recording and documentation, it is probably more meaningful to restrict the term 'apocrine carcinoma' to the 1 per cent or so of *tumours in which differentiation of this type is unequivocal,* even if it affects only parts of a given carcinoma. Defined in this way, apocrine carcinoma takes *two main forms.* Sometimes the macroscopic appearance is indistinguishable from the common run of carcinomas and its apocrine nature is *detected only on microscopic examination.* In other cases, one finds a rather sharply demarcated tumour which may be occupying the cavity of a cyst detectable macroscopically, or else the origin in a tension cyst lined in part by attenuated benign apocrine epithelium is discovered histologically. Sometimes with a tumour of this sort, origin in a cyst may be presumptive rather than based on clear-cut unequivocal evidence. In the first group, apocrine metaplasia may take place pari passu with neoplasia while, in the second group, apocrine carcinoma may take *origin in a tension cyst* already lined by benign apocrine epithelium. Bonser, Dossett and Jull (1961) claimed that such a cystic origin was still discernible in 12 of 220 unselected infiltrating cancers but independent confirmation of this high figure is needed before it can be accepted. *Origin of carcinoma in an apocrine cyst does not automatically mean that the carcinoma will show apocrine differentiation.* Of the last four cases studied by the writer, three in referred material, one was a typical apocrine carcinoma, another showed probable apocrine differentiation of the type discussed below, while the remaining two showed little or no evidence of apocrine differentiation and were carcinomas NOS type.

Other Possibly Apocrine Carcinomas. The foregoing is not meant to imply that incidences of 2.2 per cent and more of apocrine differentiation given by some workers are necessarily too high. It is merely felt that complete proof of the apocrine nature of such tumours is lacking and that they are in need of further investigation; my own view is that they probably do represent tumours with a partial degree of apocrine metaplasia and that they certainly should not be termed 'squamoid', an error prevalent in some of the literature. Nevertheless, for the present, it seems better to segregate as definite apocrine carcinomas those tumours in which all, most or at least a substantial part of a given tumour shows unequivocal evidence of such differentiation (Figure 13–6). For the others a less definitive and uncommitted term seems preferable.

Hamperl (1977) reviewed the subject of apocrine carcinomas of the breast. He made a plea for the use of the term 'oncocytic carcinoma', believing that these neoplastic cells and their benign counterpart in the breast showed oncocytic metaplasia rather than apocrine differentiation. For reasons already stated, however, the term 'apocrine' is regarded as largely tenable. Hamperl's review of the subject is extensive and has a very valuable bibliography.

APOCRINE ADENOMA

A *benign apocrine cell neoplasm* of the type described by Costa (1974) must be one of the rarest of breast tumours. A 14-year-old girl was affected in the solitary case reported to date.

References

Anthony, P. P. and James, P. D. (1975) Adenoid cystic carcinoma of the breast: prevalence, diagnostic criteria, and histogenesis. *Journal of Clinical Pathology,* **28,** 647–655.

Azzopardi, J. G. and Smith, O. D. (1959) Salivary gland tumours and their mucins. *Journal of Pathology and Bacteriology,* **77,** 131–140.

Azzopardi, J. G. and Zayid, I. (1972) Elastic tissue in tumours of salivary glands. *Journal of Pathology,* **107,** 149–156.

Bonser, G. M., Dossett, J. A. and Jull, J. W. (1961) *Human and Experimental Breast Cancer.* London: Pitman Medical.

Cameron, H. M., Hamperl, H. and Warambo, W. (1974) Leiomyosarcoma of the breast originating from myothelium (myoepithelium). *Journal of Pathology,* **114,** 89–92.

Cammoun, H., Contesso, G. and Rouëssé, J. (1972) Les adénocarcinomes cylindromateux du sein. *Annales d'Anatomie pathologique, Paris,* **17,** 143–154.

Cavanzo, F. J. and Taylor, H. B. (1969) Adenoid cystic carcinoma of the breast. An analysis of 21 cases. *Cancer,* **24,** 740–745.

Costa, A. (1974) Una variante non conosciuta di adenoma puro della ghiandola mammaria: l'adenoma puro a cellule apocrine. *Archivio Di Vecchi: per l'Anatomia patologica e la Medicina clinica,* **60,** 393–401.

Draheim, J. H., Neubecker, R. D. and Sprinz, H. (1959) An unusual tumor of the breast resembling eccrine spiradenoma. *American Journal of Clinical Pathology,* **31,** 511–516.

Elsner, B. (1970) Adenoid cystic carcinoma of the breast. A review of the literature and clinico-pathologic study of seven patients. *Pathologia Europaea,* **5,** 357–364.

Ferlito, A. and DiBonito, L. (1974) Adenoid cystic carcinoma of the male breast. Report of a case. *American Surgeon,* **40,** 72–76.

Finck, F. M., Schwinn, C. P. and Keasbey, L. E. (1968) Clear cell hidradenoma of the breast. *Cancer,* **22,** 125–135.

Fisher, E. R., Gregorio, R. M. and Fisher, B. (1975) The pathology of invasive breast cancer. *Cancer,* **36,** 1–263.

Frable, W. J. and Kay, S. (1968) Carcinoma of the breast: histologic and clinical features of apocrine tumors. *Cancer,* **21,** 756–763.

Friedman, B. A. and Oberman, H. A. (1970) Adenoid cystic carcinoma of the breast. *American Journal of Clinical Pathology,* **54,** 1–14.

Galloway, J. R., Woolner, L. B. and Clagett, O. T. (1966) Adenoid cystic carcinoma of the breast. *Surgery, Gynecology and Obstetrics,* **122,** 1289–1294.

Gould, V. E., Miller, J. and Jao, W. (1975) Ultrastructure of medullary, intraductal, tubular and adenocystic breast carcinomas. Comparative patterns of myoepithelial differentiation and basal lamina deposition. *American Journal of Pathology,* **78,** 401–407.

Hamperl, H. (1970) The myothelia (myoepithelial cells). In *Current Topics in Pathology,* Vol. 53. Berlin: Springer-Verlag.

Hamperl, H. (1977) Das sogenannte Schweissdrüsencarcinom der Mamma. *Zeitschrift für Krebsforschung,* **88,** 105–119.

Harris, M. (1977) Pseudoadenoid cystic carcinoma of the breast. *Archives of Pathology and Laboratory Medicine,* **101,** 307–309.

Hertel, B. F., Zaloudek, C. and Kempson, R. L. (1976) Breast adenomas. *Cancer,* **37,** 2891–2905.

Hjorth, S., Magnusson, P. H. and Blomquist, P. (1977) Adenoid cystic carcinoma of the breast. Report of a case in a male and review of the literature. *Acta Chirurgica Scandinavica,* **143,** 155–158.

Hopkins, G. B. and Tullis, R. H. (1972) Adenoid cystic carcinoma of the breast. *California Medicine,* **117,** 9–11.

Huvos, A. G., Lucas, J. C., Jr and Foote, F. W., Jr (1973) Metaplastic breast carcinoma. Rare form of mammary cancer. *New York State Journal of Medicine,* **73,** 1078–1082.

Kahn, L. B., Uys, C. J., Dale, J. and Rutherfoord, F. (1978) Carcinoma of the breast with metaplasia to chondrosarcoma: a light and electron microscopic study. *Histopathology,* **2,** 93–106.

Kersting, D. W. and Helwig, E. B. (1956) Eccrine spiradenoma. *Archives of Dermatology,* **73,** 199–227.

Koss, L. G., Brannan, C. D. and Ashikari, R. (1970) Histologic and ultrastructural features of adenoid cystic carcinoma of the breast. *Cancer,* **26,** 1271–1279.

Lee, B. J., Pack, G. T. and Scharnagel, I. (1933) Sweat gland cancer of the breast. *Surgery, Gynecology and Obstetrics,* **56,** 975–996.

Lusted, D. (1970) Structural and growth patterns of adenoid cystic carcinoma of the breast. *American Journal of Clinical Pathology,* **54,** 419–425.

Nabert, C., Kermanach, G. and Saout, J. (1968) Épithelioma à stroma remanie ou tumeur mixte du sein: a propos d'une observation. *Journal des Sciences Médicales de Lille,* **86,** 507–510.

Nayer, H. R. (1957) Cylindroma of the breast with pulmonary metastases. *Diseases of the Chest,* **31,** 324–327.

O'Kell, R. T. (1964) Adenoid cystic carcinoma of the breast. *Missouri Medicine,* **61,** 855–858.

Pier, W. J., Garancis, J. C. and Kuzma, J. F. (1970) The ultrastructure of apocrine cells. In intracystic papilloma and fibrocystic disease of the breast. *Archives of Pathology,* **89,** 446–452.

Qizilbash, A. H., Patterson, M. C. and Oliveira, K. F. (1977) Adenoid cystic carcinoma of the breast. Light and electron microscopy and a brief review of the literature. *Archives of Pathology and Laboratory Medicine,* **101,** 302–306.

Sheth, M. T., Hathway, D. and Petrelli, M. (1978) Pleomorphic adenoma ('mixed' tumor) of human female breast mimicking carcinoma clinicoradiologically. *Cancer,* **41,** 659–665.

Smith, B. G. and Taylor, H. B. (1969) The occurrence of bone and cartilage in mammary tumors. *American Journal of Clinical Pathology,* **51,** 610–618.

Stewart, F. W. (1950) *Tumors of the Breast.* Atlas of Tumor Pathology, Section 9, Fascicle 34, pp. 53, 66. Washington, D.C.: Armed Forces Institute of Pathology.

Tandler, B. (1971) Ultrastructure of adenoid cystic carcinoma of salivary gland origin. *Laboratory Investigation,* **24,** 504–512.

Toth, J. (1977) Benign human mammary myoepithelioma. *Virchows Archiv A: Pathological Anatomy and Histology,* **374,** 263–269.

van Bogaert, L.-J., Maldague, P., Pham-Maldague, H. and Staquet, J.-P. (1975) Le cylindrome mammaire. Étude histochimique et histogénétique. *Virchows Archiv A: Pathological Anatomy and Histology,* **368,** 157–165.

Verani, R. R. and van der Bel-Kahn, J. (1973) Mammary adenoid cystic carcinoma with unusual features. *American Journal of Clinical Pathology,* **59,** 653–658.

von Bomhard, D. and von Sandersleben, J. (1974) Über die Feinstruktur von Mammamischtumoren der Hündin. II. Das Vorkommen von Myoepithelzellen in chondroiden Arealen. *Virchows Archiv A. Pathological Anatomy and Histology,* **362,** 157–167.

von Bomhard, D. and von Sandersleben, J. (1975) Über die Feinstruktur von Mammamischtumoren der Hündin. III. Die Anfangsstadien der myoepithelialen Proliferation. *Virchows Archiv A: Pathological Anatomy and Histology,* **367,** 219–229.

Wald, M. and Kakulas, B. A. (1964) Apocrine gland carcinoma (sweat gland carcinoma) of the breast. *Australian and New Zealand Journal of Surgery,* **33,** 200–204.

Wilson, W. B. and Spell, J. P. (1967) Adenoid cystic carcinoma of breast: a case with recurrence and regional metastasis. *Annals of Surgery,* **166,** 861–864.

Woyke, S., Domagala, W. and Olszewski, W. (1970) Fine structure of mammary adenoid cystic carcinoma. *Polish Medical Journal,* **9,** 1140–1148.

Chapter Fourteen

Sarcomas of the Breast

CYSTOSARCOMA PHYLLODES

This is one of the most difficult tumours of the breast on which to make pronouncements. Perhaps the only definite assertion one can safely make is that it is a distinctive fibro-epithelial tumour of the breast without a counterpart in any other organ. One could also say that practically any generalization about it needs to be qualified.

Designation. The definition and appropriate designation of this distinctive tumour are both problematical. The alternative name *'giant fibroadenoma'*, frequently used as a synonym, reflects the problem. Neither term is entirely satisfactory. 'Giant fibroadenoma' implies that the lesion is identical with ordinary fibro-adenoma except for its size; however, not only is this not the case, but this designation underrates the malignant potential of the tumour. The term *'cystosarcoma phyllodes'* suffers from several defects. It is a cumbersome name which is not self-explanatory; it could imply a relationship to cystic disease or, at least, that the lesion always contains macroscopically visible cysts, but this is not always the case; perhaps worst of all, the name overstates the malignant potential of the vast majority of these lesions and may therefore be unduly alarming to surgeon and patient alike. Despite all these faults, 'cystosarcoma phyllodes' is still the name most frequently used and, until an obviously better one is adopted, we will have to learn to live with it.

The term 'cystosarcoma' is not too objectionable when it refers to the malignant and borderline malignant varieties. But it is certainly *difficult to justify the appellation 'benign cystosarcoma'* (Figure 14–1). It is quite erroneous to call these tumours 'giant fibroadenomas' for a number of reasons, clinical and pathological, and yet this term is almost easier to justify in many ways than 'benign cystosarcoma'. There is clearly a great need for a term which is distinct from fibroadenoma and which does not include the word 'sarcoma' in the name. *'Cellular intracanalicular fibroadenoma'* was adopted by Scarff and Torloni (1968) on behalf of the W.H.O. Though rather lengthy, this is a reasonable name except perhaps that it lacks a distinctive quality. *'Fibroadenoma phyllodes'* is

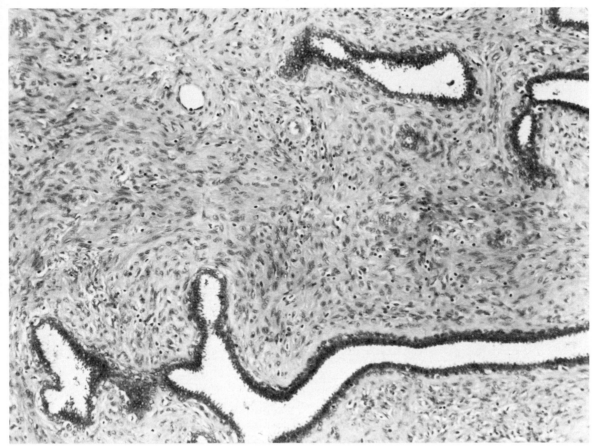

Figure 14–1 'Benign cystosarcoma phyllodes' (fibroadenoma phyllodes). This formed a 4 cm mass in a 33-year-old woman. If a tumour has this appearance throughout and is sharply delineated at the histological level, it will not metastasize. H and E. ×150.

possibly appropriate, especially if applied only to those tumours which are deemed, after careful study, to be almost certainly benign. It has the merit of alerting the surgeon to the fact that he is dealing with an unusual tumour, without at the same time alarming him unduly. If this term is used for tumours which have a recurrence rate of nearly 20 per cent (Hajdu, Espinosa and Robbins, 1976), but which rarely undergo malignant alteration and still more rarely show an unexpectedly aggressive behaviour, a reasonable compromise will have been struck. If this, or a similar term, eventually replaces the abominable 'benign cystosarcoma', it will have to be made clear that 'fibroadenoma phyllodes' needs to be treated differently from ordinary fibroadenoma. As will be seen, the 'borderline' category of tumour in which behaviour is more unpredictable poses a problem of nomenclature and, for this reason, some workers may prefer to retain the term 'cystosarcoma' for the whole group and qualify this as necessary: but there is no doubting the serious disadvantages of this course.

Perhaps the ideal solution would be to call this lesion a *phyllodes tumour* and to qualify this according to the pathologist's assessment of the microscopical appearances and likely behaviour. This term has the merit of keeping all the tumours together under a single heading, a procedure the value of which will be appreciated when the separation of benign from malignant tumours is considered. Secondly, its introduction conforms with some already accepted practice on the European mainland, especially in France. Thirdly, adoption of this name introduces no entirely new terminology: what it effectively does is to abstract from the name 'cystosarcoma phyllodes' the most desirable component of the three elements included in this traditional name. An alteration along the lines indicated is highly desirable though it would be foolish to underestimate the difficulties involved in bringing about such a change.

Definition and Distinction from Fibroadenoma. Cystosarcoma phyllodes resembles fibro- adenoma in being a *fibroepithelial tumour.* It differs in being usually larger and in its possession of a *different type of connective tissue element*; it is the latter which constitutes the essential difference. A tumour which looks microscopically like a conventional fibro- adenoma but which is large, measuring more than 4 or 5 cm in diameter, should still be classed as a fibroadenoma. On the other hand, a tumour which is only 2.5 or 3 cm in diameter but which has a more cellular, more pleomorphic or mitotically more active connective tissue component should be classed as cystosarcoma phyllodes. It is the cellularity of the connective tissue which is the most important distinguishing point in a difficult case. This method of distinguishing between the two lesions is *theoretically justifiable* and its *practical value* is borne out by the behaviour of the respective tumours. Thus the true 'giant fibroadenoma', which is uncom- mon, is not an aggressive tumour. Conversely, a cystosarcoma of modest proportions fre- quently recurs if enucleated and may behave aggressively if not treated adequately. *An enucleated fibroadenoma does not recur. An enucleated cystosarcoma will recur frequently.* It may do this because of surface projections from the tumour which are cut through and unknowingly left behind, as with a pleomor- phic adenoma of salivary glands, or because even microscopic foci of cells left behind have sufficient autonomy of growth to form the nidus of a recurrent tumour. Probably both explanations are valid but, irrespective of the reasons, there is no doubt about the facts.

Histogenesis. What proportion of cystosar- comas *arises from pre-existing fibroadenomas* and how many *arise de novo* has not been clarified by any of the more recent studies. Extreme views favouring one or other mode of origin have been expressed but the evidence is not always as crisp and convincing as one might wish. Pathological and clinical evidence favouring the first view is present in many, perhaps one-half of the cases, but an origin de novo in other cases is not excluded.

Age Incidence. The mean age of patients with cystosarcoma phyllodes (CSP) is about 45 years at the time of diagnosis; this is some 20 years older than for fibroadenoma. But averages mean little in individual patients and there is a wide range extending from the teenager to the later decades. Patients with malignant, as opposed to benign, CSP are on average three years older, and those who die of metastatic disease have a median age seven years older than all patients together (McDivitt, Urban and Farrow, 1967; Norris and Taylor, 1967).

Clinical Data. It has been noted that patients are often surprisingly fit even in the presence of metastatic disease (Cooper and Ackerman, 1943). There is an interesting *difference in the histories of patients with benign and malignant CSP.* McDivitt, Urban and Farrow (1967) found that only 15 per cent of patients with benign lesions had a one-year or longer history of a breast mass, while 35 per cent of patients with malignant CSP gave such a history (the text in their paper gives a figure of five years but this is an error, see their Table II). Also, a period of apparent acceleration following initially slow tumour growth was recorded in more than one-third of patients with malignant CSP but not at all in patients with benign CSP. Despite reservations because of the notorious unreliability of histories on points of this sort, their data are at least suggestive of alterations with time in the nature of a tumour in a given patient. This has important implications for the possible pathogenesis of some of the more malignant lesions and also for therapy.

Tumour Size and Relationship to Histological Malignancy and Clinical Aggressiveness. The average diameter of the benign tumours was 4.6 cm and that of the malignant ones 6.2 cm in the series of McDivitt, Urban and Farrow (1967). The average size of tumours which metastasized was 11.8 cm (Kessinger et al, 1972). But there is *a very large overlap.* Huge tumours, 30 or 40 cm in diameter or more, may be benign. At the other end of the scale, tumours as small as 2 cm in diameter have been known to metastasize (Oberman, 1965), but this is the exception which proves the rule. Among the 94 patients studied by Norris and Taylor (1967), *no tumour smaller than 4 cm proved fatal.* In Haagensen's (1971) four fatal cases, the smallest tumour measured 8 cm. But seven of the 14 malignant tumours in the series of McDivitt, Urban and Farrow (1967) measured 4 cm or less and two of six which killed the patient in the series of Rix, Tredwell and Forward (1971) measured only 4 cm.

Growth Rate and Mobility. When they grow to a large size, these tumours characteristically do so rapidly, frequently over a period of only a few weeks or months. This very *rapid growth does not necessarily imply malignancy.* The shiny, stretched and attenuated skin with prominent veins over a massive tumour is a well-known clinical manifestation. In these circumstances, skin ulceration also does not necessarily indicate malignancy. It is a sign of extreme distension of the skin with pressure ulceration. Even large tumours remain mobile and unattached to the skin. It is arguable whether a benign CSP can become attached to the pectoral fascia and lose some of its mobility (Hafner, Mezcer and Wylie, 1962).

Axillary Lymphadenopathy. Axillary lymph node enlargement occurred in 17 per cent of the series of patients studied by Norris and Taylor (1967) (15 of 94 patients) but it is important to recognize that this is *not usually due to metastatic disease.* Necrotic tumour or infected, ulcerated tumour are among the more common non-metastatic causes of regional lymphadenopathy. Unless one appreciates that regional lymphadenopathy is rarely caused by metastatic tumour, one may erroneously consider axillary dissection a necessary part of the surgical treatment.

Macroscopic Appearances. The macroscopic appearances are too well known to need reiteration and nothing of note has been added in the last three decades. Most lesions are reasonably well circumscribed in the gross but McDivitt, Urban and Farrow (1967) rightly stressed that *irregular surface projections* may be cut through during surgical excision and that this will predispose to local recurrence. It is these sometimes barely visible protrusions and finger-like projections which are largely responsible for the high recurrence rate when these tumours are enucleated or closely dissected.

Degrees of Aggressiveness and Histological Malignancy. The aggressiveness of cystosarcoma phyllodes can be either overrated or underrated by both pathologists and surgeons and the treatment can consequently be inappropriate in either direction. Its behaviour is unpredictable and various attempts to assess the degree of aggressiveness by mitotic counts, estimates of cellularity, pleomorphism and similar features have met with only partial success. It is therefore surprising to read authoritative statements recommending that 'malignant cystosarcoma' (Figure 14–2) be distinguished sharply from 'benign cystosarcoma' (Figure 14–1) without any guidance as to how this eminently desirable objective should be achieved. True, a small number of these tumours shows frank evidence of histological malignancy as witnessed by gross cellular and nuclear pleomorphism, numerous and atypical mitoses, tumour giant cells, etc. This type of tumour should be labelled 'cystosarcoma phyllodes, malignant' (Figures 14–3 and 14–4); its incidence has varied in different series between 19.5 per cent and as little as 2.8 per cent (Treves, 1964). In *unselected material* this histologically frankly malignant variant probably represents less than 10 per cent of all cystosarcomas. Frankly malignant cystosarcomas (Figures 14–3 and 14–4) clearly deserve segregation and the clinician must be alerted to the true situation. However, the vast majority of cystosarcomas are not of this type.

Also it must be appreciated that while cystosarcomas frequently look malignant microscopically, they are fortunately less frequently malignant clinically than one would be led to believe at the purely cytological level. *Their bark is usually worse than their bite* and histologically malignant tumours are sometimes cured by a mere wide local excision. But, rather less frequently, the converse is true: a seemingly benign CSP unexpectedly metastasizes and kills, and only retrospectively, and with some difficulty, can an area of histologically malignant tissue be identified in the primary tumour. This was the sequence of events in Case 1 of Haagensen (1971). *This unexpected type of behaviour in both directions* is the reason for the controversies over the classification of these tumours and the need for flexibility in attaching labels to them.

MICROSCOPICAL APPEARANCES

Fibrosarcoma-like Appearances. Most cystosarcomas have a structure which could be described as a *caricature of a very cellular, usually variable, intracanalicular type of fibroadenoma* (Figures 14–1 and 14–2). The more cellular parts generally have the aspect of a variably differentiated fibrosarcoma with bundles of long, plump cells with fairly plump nuclei,

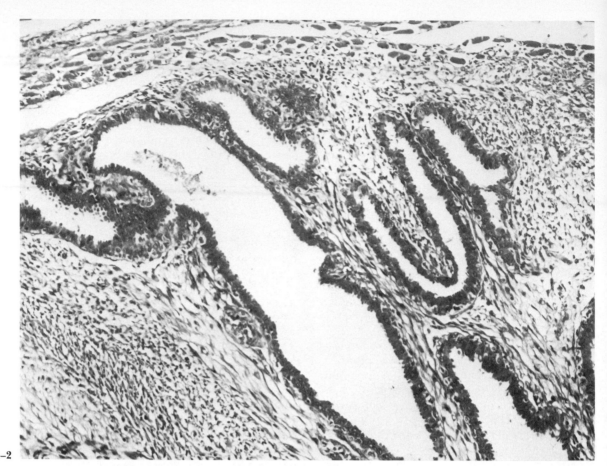

14–2

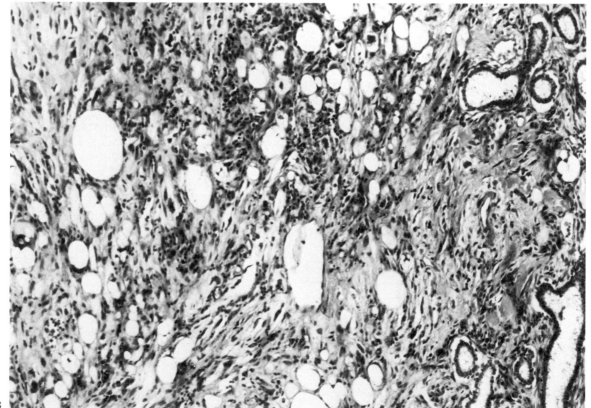

14–3

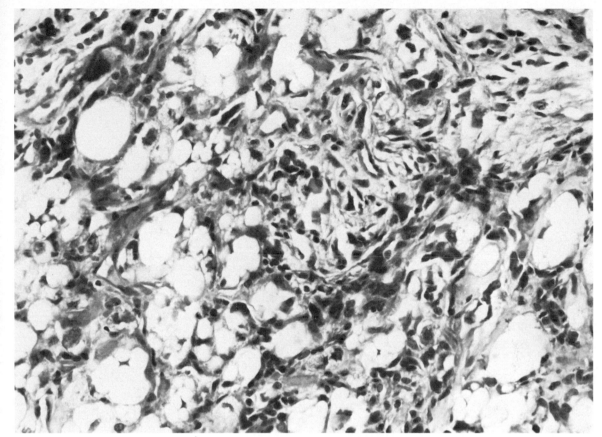

Figure 14–4 From same tissue as Figure 14–3. Liposarcomatous differentiation in cystosarcoma. H and E. ×400.

accompanied by little collagen, forming parallel, sinuous or interlacing bands. The nuclei are sometimes markedly hyperchromatic and frequently have heavy chromatin markings. But the precise nuclear details, the plumpness of the nuclei, the amount of collagen will depend on whether one is dealing with a benign (Figure 14–1) or a malignant (Figure 14–2) cystosarcoma. Mitotic figures vary similarly from occasional or even sparse to five, 10 or many more/10 high-power fields (HPF). Some tumours are composed largely of *fibrosarcoma-like tissue* of varying degrees of differentiation (Figure 14–2) but in most tumours there are areas of *oedematous and myxomatous tissue* which are sparsely cellular. In addition, tumours frequently contain densely *fibrous· and even hyalinized zones*, especially occupying the broad polypoid processes which frequently project into the epithelial crevices of the tumour. Such fibrous zones and the more cellular fibrosarcoma-like zones either merge imperceptibly or abut on one another.

In some tumours *the more densely fibrous parts* appear localized to a certain area with a vaguely or distinctly ovoid outline, an appearance which has been interpreted, probably correctly in certain cases, as representing *the residue of a benign fibroadenoma* which constituted the nidus which gave origin to the cystosarcoma. But where the more fibrous areas are more dispersed and blend gently with the more cellular tissue, they represent *an integral part of the cystosarcoma.*

Myxosarcoma and Liposarcoma. In some tumours, especially the more malignant ones,

Figure 14–2 (*Opposite, above.*)   An apparently well delimited cystosarcoma phyllodes showed subtle signs of infiltration between striated muscle fibres as seen in the upper part of this illustration. The connective tissue element of the tumour showed only a moderate degree of atypia. After three local recurrences, this tumour metastasized at 10 years and killed the patient. H and E. ×150.

Figure 14–3 (*Opposite, below.*)   Malignant cystosarcoma. Fibrosarcomatous and liposarcomatous elements are present. H and E. ×60.

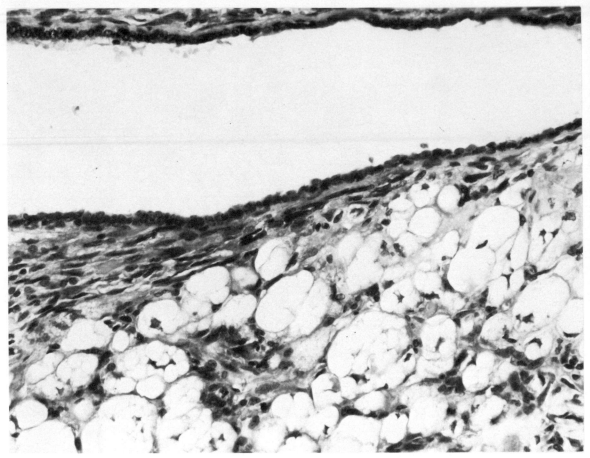

Figure 14–5   From same tissue as the two preceding illustrations. Cuff of liposarcoma around a glandular space. H and E. ×400.

a myxoid pattern can be prominent or even dominant, myxosarcoma alternating with fibrosarcoma. Some of the myxosarcomatous component may represent liposarcomatous differentiation. After fibrosarcoma, liposarcoma represents the second most frequent line of differentiation in the more malignant variety of CSP (Figures 14–3 to 14–5). Liposarcomatous differentiation is well discussed by Qizilbash (1976). These two main lines of differentiation are to be expected from the structure of the normal breast stroma. The tumour is replicating, in bizarre fashion, the cell types present in normal and involuting breast stroma.

Anaplastic Sarcoma. Less frequently there is frankly anaplastic sarcoma, which on rare occasions has even been confused with an undifferentiated carcinoma. This is much more likely to happen with frozen than with paraffin sections, both because they are inherently more difficult to interpret and

because the pathologist does not have the benefit of the gross appearances to alert him to the distinct possibility that he is dealing with a CSP. Although a fibroadenoma and a CSP cannot be distinguished by macroscopic examination in many cases, a CSP and a carcinoma can be so distinguished in the vast majority of cases. *The use of frozen sections can, therefore, lead to unnecessary radical mastectomy,* as in Case 4 of Haagensen (1971). But frozen section diagnosis is recommended by Haagensen (1971) as a means of identifying CSP at the time of surgery so as to perform a wide rather than a close excision as a primary surgical procedure. This recommendation is made in an attempt to eliminate the high local recurrence rate of CSP when it is treated in the manner of a fibroadenoma. Apart from the chore of this procedure, and the increase in time and money spent on performing frozen sections on apparent fibroadenomas, there is the additional snag that this method of management can lead to an occasional unnecessarily radical procedure because of a mistaken diagnosis of carcinoma. The alternative is presumably to perform a wider excision after a definitive diagnosis has been made on paraffin sections. As a pathologist, I am not qualified to decide on the technical feasibility of this course of action but, if it is feasible, would it not be a more practical policy?

Neoplastic Cartilage and Bone. Cystosarcomas, rarely, may even contain neoplastic cartilage or bone (Smith and Taylor, 1969), but the numbers studied were too small for any conclusion as to whether such differentiation per se alters the behaviour of the tumour. McDivitt, Urban and Farrow (1967) commented that 'focal calcification was observed in both benign and malignant cystosarcoma as was osseous and cartilagenous metaplasia'. Later McDivitt, Stewart and Berg (1968) referred to osseous and cartilaginous metaplasia in the section on malignant cystosarcoma only, but did not specify whether it has prognostic significance. Haagensen (1971) reported that 'several' of the tumours in his series of 84 cases contained cartilage or osteoid but that 'they were not the tumours that metastasized': this is not entirely clear since the tumour in his fatal Case 3 was described as an osteosarcoma-like tumour which contained osteoid. Pietruszka and Barnes (1978) made a plea for the identification of the type or types of sarcomatous tissue present in each case since they may have variable significance.

Neoplastic Smooth and Striated Muscle. One of the rarest types of differentiation in a CSP is smooth muscle development, analogous to the same rare development in a fibroadenoma. Rhabdomyosarcomatous differentiation was found in one of the 42 cases of Pietruszka and Barnes (1978).

In order of frequency, the types of differentiation found are fibrosarcoma, liposarcoma, chondrosarcoma, osteosarcoma and muscle sarcoma. The occurrence of haemangiopericytoma (Pietruszka and Barnes, 1978) is in need of further documentation.

The Distribution of the Connective Tissue Cells. There are certain features about the distribution of the fibroblastic cells which deserve attention. In some tumours there is a hint or a distinct tendency to *cellular aggregation around the epithelial canaliculi and sometimes around the blood vessels.* The greater cellularity, often with increased mitotic activity, around blood vessels may be related to the good blood supply but the greater cellularity around the epithelial spaces is not so obviously explained. It is possible that it represents an inductive effect of the neoplastic epithelium upon the fibroblastic tissue; if this is the explanation it would represent a retention by the neoplastic epithelium of a function possessed by the normal breast epithelium. Others have also noted increased cellularity and atypia surrounding canaliculi (McDivitt, Stewart and Berg, 1968). These authors found that all tumours with this appearance behaved in a benign fashion. The writer has studied a case with this change in which, after three local recurrences, the tumour metastasized to the skull, and then to other bones and to the lungs, with a fatal outcome. This illustrates just one of the many controversial issues surrounding this tumour. If the finding of McDivitt, Stewart and Berg (1968) is the rule, this case is a good illustration of the exception, and the whole subject of cystosarcoma phyllodes seems to abound with exceptions.

The fibroblasts around epithelial structures usually follow a parallel or concentric course, depending on the plane of section. Quite frequently there is, however, an unusual arrangement which does not appear to have been previously noted, although it is also frequently present in fibroadenoma: in such areas the fibroblasts are orientated perpendicularly to the epithelial channels with a palisaded effect. The significance of, or reason for, this orientation is not clear.

The Site of Origin of Cystosarcoma. What little is known about the genesis and site of origin of cystosarcoma is derived by implication from the tumours that have their origin in or are associated with a fibroadenoma. Fibroadenoma is demonstrably a tumour of lobular derivation. Cystosarcoma has hardly been investigated from this point of view, presumably because of its relative rarity, the greater size of most lesions and because microscopic tumours and incidentally discovered small tumours are so rare, and it is the latter types which would lend themselves to the study of the histogenesis.

We recently had the opportunity of studying a tumour which, in addition to a main mass, consisted of several outlying unconnected 'satellite' foci. These demonstrated the mode of origin of the tumour. In the vast majority of the tissue, the tumour arose as a mesenchymal neoplasm affecting *the specialized connective tissue of the lobules* and was restricted to this tissue without affecting the ordinary interlobular stroma. The incipient neoplastic tissue separated and diluted out the epithelial constituents of the lobule. In the earliest stages the epithelial tissue showed little or no evidence of hyperplasia, suggesting that *the mesenchymal change might precede the epithelial alteration.* An additional somewhat unexpected finding was the involvement of ducts as well as lobules, albeit on a much more limited scale. These ducts, identifiable by virtue of their elastic tissue coats, were cuffed by neoplastic mesenchyme restricted to the specialized connective tissue of the ductal wall. They were not involved simply by entrapment between expanding neoplastic lobules; there was, rather, a selective involvement of their walls by neoplastic tissue. It is possible that the primary change was all lobular and that the ductal wall involvement was caused by secondary spread of tumour from the lobules via the ductules to involve ducts. The appearances are, however, more suggestive of a field change with the sarcomatous change involving the ductal walls pari passu with the involvement of the lobules. One way to settle this question would be to reconstruct such tumours in order to determine whether the stromal changes are always in continuity and diminish in quantity as the distance from the lobules increases. Such a finding might support the concept of secondary spread along the ductal wall. If, on the other hand, ductal involvement could be shown to be independent of neoplastic change in the lobules served by them, the concept of a field change would be strongly supported. Whichever view is correct, *the involvement of ductal walls* by neoplastic mesenchyme adds another dimension to the distinction between cystosarcoma phyllodes and fibroadenoma.

The Epithelial Component

The epithelial changes in cystosarcoma are similar to those seen in fibroadenoma (Figures 14–1 and 14–2). The usual two cell types line the spaces, crevices and cysts except where the epithelial cells become so markedly flattened and attenuated by the sarcomatous component as to become nondescript. Varying degrees of hyperplasia frequently affect both cell types so that there is often quite a florid degree of epithelial proliferation with stratification of the cell layers and formation of epithelial buds. The epithelial efflorescence is often rather more striking than that of most fibroadenomas. With rare exceptions considered below, the epithelial hyperplasia remains benign. When the epithelial component becomes malignant it usually takes the form of lobular neoplasia. Before one considers the diagnosis of carcinoma of ductal type in cystosarcoma, the evidence must be overwhelming. If one excludes lobular neoplasia, a worrisome but not overtly malignant epithelial proliferation in cystosarcoma should be regarded as benign and can be safely ignored.

There is a point about the epithelial proliferation in cystosarcoma which requires further study. Occasionally there is a proliferation of cells which takes the form of budding towards the connective tissue, instead of the much more common hyperplasia taking the form of a largely epithelial proliferation which, insofar as it projects, does so in the direction of the lumina. This budding is similar structurally and cytologically to that described on page 52 in fibroadenomas and fibroadenoma variants. The search for argyrophilic cells in these cell buds is currently in progress.

Epithelial Metaplasia. Some types of metaplasia affecting the epithelial component are more common, others much less common, in cystosarcoma than in fibroadenoma. Squamous metaplasia can occur focally and may rarely be extensive (Bader and Isaacson, 1960). Norris and Taylor (1967) found evidence of squamous metaplasia in eight of their 94 cases. Haagensen (1971) reported that it was present in several of their cases and that it was especially prominent in one of their four fatal cases. There is evidently a much higher incidence of squamous metaplasia in cystosarcoma than in fibroadenoma. Apocrine metaplasia, on the other hand, is distinctly unusual in cystosarcoma, especially considering its comparative frequency in fibroadenoma. McDivitt, Urban and Farrow (1967) merely mentioned it and other authors do not refer to it; the writer has not seen it. There is no mention of it in the McDivitt fascicle (1968). If it is noted in future work, it should be fully documented. The changes of sclerosing adenosis which are comparatively common in fibroadenoma have not, to my knowledge, been recorded in cystosarcoma, though I have seen it in a solitary instance of benign cystosarcoma phyllodes.

THE DIFFERENTIATION OF BENIGN FROM MALIGNANT CYSTOSARCOMA

It is *the connective tissue element which dictates whether a CSP should be classified as a benign or a malignant tumour* just as, in the first place, the character of this component separates CSP from fibroadenoma. In benign CSP the connective tissue proliferation usually assumes the guise of a very cellular fibroma (Figure 14–1) or at worst of a very well differentiated low-grade fibrosarcoma. The malignant CSP usually has the appearance of a less well differentiated fibrosarcoma (Figure 14–2) with plumper cells with plumper nuclei. The appearances are, however, often very variable in different parts of the same tumour and very extensive sampling is frequently necessary to establish as precisely as possible the category into which an individual case falls. If generous sampling is required in an average-sized tumour, it is that much more essential in the very large tumours. Blocks should be taken from softer parts especially, but the colour or presence of cysts offers no guide to the parts requiring sampling. It is particularly important to sample generously the margins of the tumour, for reasons which will become apparent.

In general, mitoses are more numerous in the malignant CSP than in the benign form. The same applies to cellular atypia (Figures 14–1 and 14–2) but when Lester and Stout (1954) made a very determined attempt to separate the benign from the malignant tumours on the basis of these two criteria they met with only very limited success.

There are four criteria which taken together offer a reasonable but certainly not infallible guide to whether CSP should be classed as benign or malignant:

1. A 'pushing' or well-demarcated edge at the *microscopic level* is a good prognostic indicator, and conversely for an infiltrative tumour margin (Figures 14–2 and 14–6).
2. If growth of the connective tissue component outstrips the epithelial tissue so that parts of the tumour are devoid of epithelial structures, the lesion should be regarded as malignant (Figure 14–6). The more

definite the outstripping of one component by the other, the more certain one can be of the malignancy of the tumour. In the most extreme form of this, a nodule or nodules of pure fibrosarcoma form within the cystosarcoma, i.e. there is tumour-within-tumour formation. The importance of 'sarcomatous overgrowth' relative to the epithelial component was stressed originally by Oberman (1965) and more recently by Hart, Bauer and Oberman (1978). It is a feature deserving of greater emphasis than is currently accorded to it.

3. Three or more mitoses/10 HPF are *potential* indicators of malignancy since two of the 15 fatal cases of Norris and Taylor (1967) had fewer than five mitotic figures/10 HPF.
4. Cellular atypia, if pronounced, indicates a malignant tumour (Figures 14–3 and 14–4) but only five of the 15 fatal cases of Norris and Taylor (1967) showed marked atypia that would of itself justify a diagnosis of malignancy. In other words the absence of severe atypia does not indicate that the tumour is benign (Figure 14–2).

Most cases of malignant CSP have a fibrosarcomatous structure without marked atypia but generally with three or more mitoses/10 HPF and often considerably more than that. Severe atypia is important only as a positive finding. The degree of mitotic activity is probably the most important single cytological, as opposed to structural, feature in assessing the status of a particular tumour and its potential to metastasize. In the series of Norris and Taylor (1967) mitotic activity was best correlated with this potential. But by adopting such a low cut-off point, one is necessarily placing a larger number of tumours in the malignant bracket.

These four factors considered together constitute the most reliable criteria currently available for distinguishing between benign CSP and malignant CSP. But even then, according to the majority of workers, the distinction is not easy and exceptions will occur. In an important study Pietruszka and Barnes (1978) analysed the features of prognostic importance in the assessment of cystosarcoma phyllodes. In the main they confirmed the findings of Norris and Taylor (1967). One important difference is that they regarded 10 or more mitoses/10 HPF as

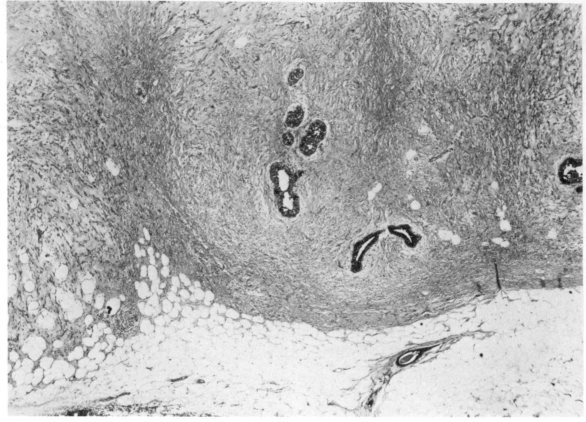

Figure 14–6   Cystosarcoma phyllodes with lack of microscopic circumscription in one focus where there is extension of the sarcomatous component into adjacent adipose tissue. The glandular component of the tumour was very sparse or altogether deficient in neighbouring fields of tissue. On these two grounds the tumour should be regarded as potentially malignant. H and E. ×45. (By courtesy of Dr M. G. Cook.)

indicative of a malignant tumour, 0 to 4 as a characteristic of a benign tumour while 5 to 9 were found in their borderline group. Their cut-off point for mitotic activity is thus set at a higher level than Norris and Taylor (1967) and they make a very reasonable case for adopting this level. There are other possible indicators of behaviour and valuable information in this work.

On the other hand, McDivitt, Urban and Farrow (1967) found classification into benign and malignant types relatively easy and state that unlike other authors they found it unnecessary to include a borderline category *'believing the histology to be sufficiently distinct in each case to permit classification as benign or malignant'*. The patterns found in their benign CSP were the same fibrous, myxoid and fatty ones observed in malignant CSP, 'the difference being that the degree of pleomorphism was significantly less'. This statement is difficult to reconcile with Norris

and Taylor's (1967) observation that cell atypia by itself was not a reliable criterion. The malignant patterns illustrated by McDivitt, Stewart and Berg (1968) are easy to recognize as such but Norris and Taylor stated that in the final analysis *'a clearcut separation of benign from malignant tumours could not be made'*. There is a serious discrepancy here. The writer can find no total explanation for such a discrepancy between distinguished authors and suspects, as with most such situations, that the truth must lie somewhere between these extremes. It is characteristic of CSP that it can generate disagreement of this order of magnitude. The tumour has the final laugh in continuing to baffle pathologists!

Not unexpectedly in view of what has been said, extremely wide ranges are given in the literature of the percentage of all CSP which are malignant. Figures cited vary between 8 and 40 per cent (Oberman, 1965). Kessinger et al (1972) concluded that the accepted incidence of *histologically* malignant tumours appears to be around 25 per cent of all cases; even this conclusion has to be hedged by the observation that the series of Lee and Pack (1931) is usually disregarded when calculating this figure as it contains an exceptionally small percentage of malignant cases compared with other large series (only a single malignant case among 111 tumours). Metastases are said to occur in between 2.8 and 12 per cent of all cases, and between 6.6 and 37.5 per cent of the malignant variety of CSP (Kessinger et al, 1972). These ranges are so wide that they are not very meaningful and they are included here because they serve the purpose of highlighting the problems which surround most aspects of this tumour.

Causes of the Widely Discrepant Figures

In looking for causes of these widely discrepant figures the possible factors involved can be divided into *those which involve selection* and *those which do not*. The former include a consideration of the geographical origin of the reported series, with a cancer hospital or other highly specialized centre more likely to be dealing with a high proportion of the more malignant cases. But even when this is taken into account many of the discrepancies still persist. One is forced to the conclusion that the major problem is *the inherent difficulty of classifying these tumours* and that the difficulties experienced by Lester and Stout (1954) are still largely with us today.

There are two main problems:

1. *When is a tumour a cystosarcoma as opposed to certain variants of a fibroadenoma?* Giant fibroadenoma is not a CSP and should not be so classified. Corrections for this have to be made especially when considering some of the older reports in the literature. Thus, three of the tumours occurring in adolescent girls in Lester and Stout's series (1954) were reclassified by Haagensen (1971) with the 'massive adenofibromas of youth'. And similar corrections are needed for some other series as noted later. Just as important, a proportion of the tumours labelled 'fibroadenoma variant' in Chapter Four are sufficiently cellular as to be difficult to classify with any precision. The writer suspects that some of these cases are called benign CSP by certain workers, a reasonable enough diagnosis but one which is bound to alter the balance between benign and malignant CSP and also allow for more categorical recognition of some CSP as *definitely* benign. Pertinently the youngest patient in Haagensen's (1971) series of 84 cases was a 14-year-old Negro girl. Her fibroadenoma, illustrated in his Figure 13–13, suggests the tumour called 'fibroadenoma variant' here and is also similar to the 'juvenile fibroadenoma' of Ashikari, Farrow and O'Hara (1971). These *two varieties of fibroadenoma* occur dominantly in younger age groups as with the more conventional fibroadenoma. If they were accounting for a significantly large number of tumours called benign CSP by some workers, the average age of their patients with benign CSP, or with all types of CSP, should be lower than in other series, but this does not appear to be the case. The explanation offered can, therefore, at most, only partially explain the existing discrepancies.

2. *The second major problem is the separation of benign from malignant CSP.* McDivitt, Urban and Farrow (1967) found this reasonably straightforward; Norris and Taylor (1967) did not. Evans (1966) also experienced considerable difficulty. The writer aligns himself with the latter. He is further handicapped by the fact that many of the patients with CSP seen at this hospital have been referred for recurrent or even metastatic disease. Much of my experience has been with referred pathological material and this is naturally not only selected but inherently likely to be problematical. Study of referred cases is of course very unsatisfactory from the point of view of the natural history of the disease because the clinical facts and details of treatment are usually not accurately known, as so rightly stressed by Haagensen (1971).

Some workers give a very high incidence of malignant cases among their CSP, with a high incidence of metastatic disease at the time of presentation or subsequently (Blichert-Toft et al, 1975). These figures are partly attributable to *selection*, the truly malignant sarcomatous cases receiving the label CSP while less aggressive tumours may be diagnosed as giant fibroadenoma instead of the benign CSP category of other workers. Indeed, it may well be the designation of 'cystosarcoma' which is responsible, for some workers are reluctant to use the term 'sarcoma' for the less aggressive and quasi-benign tumours and do not recognize a 'benign cystosarcoma' category, a view with which one sympathizes because the latter is such an unsatisfactory and even contradictory name. While the reasons for it are understandable, this approach is bound to result in CSP, as defined by these workers, including a much higher proportion of aggressive and metastasizing tumours than in most other series (Blichert-Toft et al, 1975).

Norris and Taylor (1967) suggested that some authors' contention that the distinction between benign and malignant cases can be drawn with relative ease is based on *the placing of all borderline cases in the malignant group.* If this is the explanation it should lead to a lower benign/malignant ratio of CSP in the figures of those who follow this practice. Yet the B/M ratio of McDivitt, Urban and Farrow (1967) is 4/1, which is slightly higher than the B/M ratio of 3/1 which Kessinger et al (1972) found to be the generally accepted figure (Notley and Griffiths, 1965). In fact McDivitt, Stewart and Berg (1968) made the point that 'we found that the yearly incidence of benign and malignant cystosarcoma had varied but little' during the 35 years spanned by the two reviews from the Memorial Sloan-Kettering Centre. However, because of differences in the duration of symptoms between patients covered by their first and second reviews, as well as the differences in the clinical stories of patients with malignant as opposed to benign CSP, these workers were *anticipating a possible rise in the B/M ratio* during the second period, but this did not materialize. This anticipated rise may have occurred but been completely masked by the anticipated fall that would result if Norris and Taylor's (1967) contention were correct. Thus *two factors acting in opposite directions could have maintained an apparent status quo.*

If one divides CSP into benign and malignant categories along the McDivitt lines, then *about 20 per cent of all tumours are malignant.* If the individual pathologist cannot identify the distinct subdivisions after careful study of these various papers, it might be better to regard all CSP as one rather than two entities but encompassing a wide range of appearances (Figures 14–1 to 14–4) and behaviour. At one end of the spectrum there is the quasi-benign, well-delimited, 'pushing' tumour, with appearances of a cellular fibroma in the connective tissue component but with little or no atypia and fewer than 3 mitoses/10 HPF (Figure 14–1). At the other end of the spectrum is the tumour with an infiltrative edge, marked atypia (Figures 14–3

and 14–4) and numerous mitoses in which the diagnosis of malignancy is relatively obvious. Between the two ends there is a whole range of tumours in which clear categorization is not easy and in which the criteria of Oberman (1965) and of Norris and Taylor (1967) are valuable for separating the more aggressive from the less aggressive.

RECURRENCE

Norris and Taylor (1967) recorded a 30 per cent recurrence rate, with most recurrences occurring within two years of the initial surgery. Haagensen (1971) recorded a recurrence of 28 per cent (12/43) among patients with CSP treated by local excision. In 11 of the 12 patients the recurrence appeared within six years. In the twelfth remarkable case, local recurrence took 17 years to develop and this was deemed to be 'beyond question genuine local recurrence'. Hajdu, Espinosa and Robbins (1976) found a recurrence rate of 16 per cent (32 of 199 patients). This important study is devoted specifically to the subject of recurrence. Recurrence developed in 28 of 150 women with benign CSP (18 per cent) while only 4 of 49 patients (8 per cent) with malignant CSP developed recurrences. Patients with histologically benign lesions had had surgical excision of the tumour usually with some adjacent, normal-appearing breast tissue of variable amount. On the other hand, most patients with malignant CSP were treated by mastectomy, accounting for the lower recurrence rate. Three of the four patients with recurrent malignant CSP had been treated by surgery short of mastectomy; recurrence with malignant CSP is probably a sign of a grave prognosis since two of the three patients with adequate follow-up died with disseminated disease. That exceptions occur is indicated by Hart, Bauer and Oberman (1978): two patients with recurrent malignant CSP fared badly while two apparently fared well, though the follow-up period in one of these two was very short.

Benign CSP recurred a second time in 11 of 28 women and even a third time in three patients (Hajdu, Espinosa and Robbins, 1976). Recurrent tumours tend in general to be similar histologically to the primary neoplasms. *Occasionally a benign CSP recurs as a malignant CSP*, a transformation which took place in two of the 28 recurrent benign CSP in this series. The 'malignant transformation' may take place at the first or a subsequent recurrence. That the histology of the recurrence is usually the same is illustrated by a patient of McDivitt, Urban and Farrow (1967), in whom the tumour remained unchanged throughout five recurrences, an occurrence which these authors regarded as discrediting the concept that cystosarcoma, when recurrent, will invariably appear more aggressive. The latter concept is clearly erroneous but it is also true that a malignant transformation can occur, as exemplified by the two cases of Hajdu, Espinosa and Robbins (1976), by two cases noted by Haagensen (1971), by four cases of Rix, Tredwell and Forward (1971) and by a personal case of the writer. The frequency of recurrence in benign CSP, and the rarer more sinister developments in recurrences, underline the need to excise these lesions with a generous portion of adjacent mammary tissue.

METASTASES

Metastases are said to occur in 3 to 12 per cent of cystosarcomas. This is a wide range and both lower and higher figures are also found in the literature. Figures of less than 3 per cent in the older literature tend to be less reliable mainly because giant fibroadenoma was frequently confused with cystosarcoma. Treves and Sunderland (1951) in an important study found that 13 per cent of their cystosarcomas metastasized. However, they pointed out that their series of cystosarcomas may have been overweighted with referred malignant tumours. Norris and Taylor (1967) found that 17 per cent of patients in their series died of metastatic disease. In the series of Hart et al (1978), three of 13 patients with malignant CSP and follow-up information developed metastases. This represents 23 per cent of the patients with malignant tumours and only 12 per cent of the entire series of their 25 patients with follow-up information. As Hart et al (1978) emphasized, their series included a large proportion of cases judged to be histologically malignant, probably reflecting the fact that many of their cases were expressly referred for consultation. This selection of material is inherent in many of the larger series reported on from the most famous institutions, a point so aptly stressed by Haagensen (1971). Thus, again, there is an

incidence of metastases of 4 cases among 36 with follow-up information in the series of Pietruszka and Barnes (1978), an incidence of 11 per cent. But no fewer than 14 cases in their total of 42 were submitted as consultations from community hospitals. The incidence of metastasizing lesions in the series of Haagensen (1971) was only 6.2 per cent and there is reason to believe that this figure is not far from the true figure in an unselected series. It is likely that this figure will eventually be found to lie somewhere between about 6 and 9 per cent, a figure based on the most reliable data of the last few years with some allowance for the factor of selection. A point of considerable practical importance is that there is a distinct suggestion that earlier and more appropriate treatment than that received by patients in former years has succeeded in some centres in reducing a substantial mortality rate of 10 to 15 per cent to a very much lower figure (McDivitt, Urban and Farrow, 1967).

Kessinger et al (1972) reviewed 67 cases of metastatic cystosarcoma. They considered that 53 of the 67 had an adequate description of the metastatic lesions. One half of these 53 patients had local recurrence in addition to metastatic disease. *All metastatic lesions are devoid of malignant epithelial elements*; it is the sarcomatous component which metastasizes. Spread is mainly by the blood rather than the lymphatic system although the latter may also be involved. An apparent exception to the rule that the epithelial element does not metastasize is recorded by West, Weiland and Clagett (1971). The pulmonary metastasis contained sarcomatous tissue as well as an epithelial component, which, however, appeared to be benign. In a site like the lung, it is not easy to be certain that epithelial structures of this type are not the result of entrapment of altered pulmonary parenchyma. If this explanation could be excluded with any conviction, an interesting possibility is that the non-malignant epithelium could be carried passively to its destination by the sarcomatous tissue. But the first explanation offered remains the more likely.

The *lungs* are far and away the most common site of metastases; they are involved in 66 per cent of cases with metastatic disease (Kessinger et al, 1972). The *skeleton* is involved in 28 per cent of cases. After the lungs and bones, there is a sharp drop in the incidence of involvement of individual organs with the heart affected in 9.4 per cent and the liver in only 5.6 per cent of cases. Too much significance should not be attached to these last figures as they are based on only five and three cases respectively. Also, cases with cardiac metastases are inherently more likely to be reported as single cases (McCullough and Lynch, 1960); nevertheless four of the five cases with cardiac metastases are derived from two major series (Lester and Stout, 1954; Norris and Taylor, 1967) so that this element of selection would not appear to be an important factor, except insofar as unusual cases might be more likely to be referred to centres like the Armed Forces Institute of Pathology. It is true to say that liver involvement is distinctly rare and, when present, accompanied by extensive metastatic disease in other organs. Cardiac involvement is generally also accompanied by extensive metastases elsewhere, with the exception of Case 2 of Lester and Stout (1954), who developed a solitary metastasis in the myocardium. *No organ is spared* and metastases have been recorded in the stomach, pancreas, ileum and its mesentery, omentum, larynx, kidney, thyroid, adrenal, spleen, gum, mediastinum, pleura, abdominal wall, vulva, scalp and the sole of the foot (see Kessinger et al, 1972, for references). The writer has seen metastasis over the bridge of the nose. Rhodes et al (1978) documented metastases in the spinal cord and brain, as well as metastases to a uterine leiomyoma and to an area of hepatic adenomatous hyperplasia.

Metastases usually become manifest within 12 to 24 months of treatment but there is a very wide variation. They may be already present at the time of diagnosis and treatment or may appear as late as 12 years after the initial therapy (Treves and Sunderland, 1951). In a personally studied case, the tumour was initially removed in 1957, there were multiple local recurrences starting in 1958 and distant metastases, initially a solitary one to the calvarium, were delayed until 1967, 10 years after the first surgical treatment (Figure 14–2). Delays of the order of 10 to 12 years between first surgical treatment and the appearance of distant metastases are, nevertheless, distinctly rare. They are possibly more common if persistent recurrences are inadequately treated. In the series of Norris and Taylor (1967) all 15 patients who died of their tumour did so within six years. In the collected series of Kessinger at al (1972), 58 patients were reported dead of metastases at an average of 30 months after initial treatment.

Lymph Node Metastases

Regional Lymph Node Metastases. Regional lymph node metastases are uncommon even among cases with metastatic disease, but they are apparently not quite as rare as was at one time thought. Fernandez, Hernandez and Spindler (1976) added another case to the eight cases collected from the literature by Kessinger et al (1972), making a total of nine cases with axillary node metastases. Kessinger et al (1972) found that eight of 53 or 15 per cent of the adequately described metastatic cases had nodal metastases. If one considers the whole 67 patients reviewed, nodal metastasis occurred in 12 per cent of patients and, if the two cases of Norris and Taylor (1967) without histological proof are excluded, this percentage drops to 9 per cent. Although axillary nodes were enlarged in 15 of 94 patients in the Norris and Taylor (1967) series, metastasis to them occurred in not more than three instances and only one of these was histologically proven. Thus, axillary node metastases were potentially present in three of their 15 patients who died of metastatic cystosarcoma. It can justifiably be concluded that, in the reported cases of patients dying of metastatic cystosarcoma, there is a maximum incidence of nodal involvement of about 20 per cent and a minimum incidence of about 8 to 9 per cent. It should be remembered, moreover, that cases reported tend to be selected either by virtue of their unusual features constituting the main reason for publication or because they are reported from institutions which by their nature tend to accumulate unusual cases. The lower figure of about 10 per cent probably reflects the real behaviour of the tumour more accurately.

Number of Nodes Involved. In the case of Minkowitz et al (1968) only a single lymph node was involved, in that of Cooper and Ackerman (1943) three of 14 nodes were involved, while in the case of Fernandez, Hernandez and Spindler (1976) four of 19 axillary nodes were affected.

Other Nodal Metastases. Very rarely other lymph node groups have been involved, cervical as well as axillary in one case, and periaortic nodes in another (Norris and Taylor, 1967); cervical, axillary, periaortic and suprapancreatic nodes were involved in Case 1 of Rhodes et al (1978).

Bearing on Treatment. Because three patients at most out of 94 had axillary node metastases in the series of Norris and Taylor (1967), which included 15 patients who died of their disease, i.e. 3 per cent or less in a series with a relatively high mortality rate, neither radical mastectomy nor routine axillary node dissection is indicated.

More Recent Studies on Metastatic Disease

Rhodes et al (1978) *found that there are now 84 cases of metastatic cystosarcoma phyllodes in the English-language literature.* This represents an increase of 17 over the 67 compiled by Kessinger et al (1972). This increase includes the five cases of Lubin and Rywlin (1972), Hoover, Trestioreanu and Ketcham (1975), Hines et al (1976) and Fernandez, Hernandez and Spindler (1976), the five cases with metastatic disease among the 17 in the series of Blichert-Toft et al (1975) and the six cases with metastases among the 16 patients in the series of Halverson and Hori-Rubaina (1974). It is not entirely clear, however, whether all of the cases in the last series are newly reported ones or included some already reported by Long, Hesker and Johnson (1962).

Rhodes et al (1978) found only 10 cases with well-documented metastases to axillary lymph nodes. In addition to the nine up to the time of the report of Fernandez, Hernandez and Spindler (1976), they included also a case in the series of Halverson and Hori-Rubaina (1974) but, again, the writer is not clear whether this had already been reported on. Lymph node metastases at necropsy were present in Case 1 of Rhodes et al (1978), *bringing the number with nodal metastases to at least 10, and possibly 11.*

Rhodes et al (1978) reported on two patients who presented with neurological symptoms as a manifestation of metastatic cystosarcoma phyllodes. Symptoms of metastases were delayed in both cases for two years after mastectomy. There were a number of unusual features in both patients.

Histopathology of Metastatic Tumour

Metastatic tumour is usually similar to the primary tumour; the usual appearance is that of a fibrosarcoma. Liposarcomatous differentiation may be seen, especially when it is also present in the primary lesion (Jackson, 1962). Even cartilaginous and osseous differentiation was present in the lymph node metastases in Case 2 of Fernandez, Hernandez and Spindler (1976). Both liposarcoma and chondrosarcoma were present in the distant metastases, as they were in the primary tumour, in Case 37 of Pietruszka and Barnes (1978).

SPECIAL FEATURES OF CYSTOSARCOMA

Multifocality. In the patient of Minkowitz et al (1968), the breast contained two distinct fibroadenomas in addition to two distinct cystosarcomas. This case is unique in being associated also with metastasis to an axillary lymph node.

Bilaterality. Cystosarcoma phyllodes is usually unilateral. There was only a single patient with bilateral tumours among the 94 patients studied by Norris and Taylor (1967) and in this patient the tumours appeared simultaneously. There was again only a single patient with bilateral tumours among 84 patients in the Columbia series (Haagensen, 1971) and in this patient there was an interval of one year before the development of the contralateral tumour. *Series showing a high incidence of bilaterality must be scrutinized with care* since in many cases, especially in the older literature, the authors were referring to giant fibroadenomas and not to genuine cystosarcomas. Thus, in the series of McDonald and Harrington (1950) under the heading of 'giant fibroadenoma of the breast — cystosarcoma phyllodes', there are four bilateral cases in a total of 13. It is interesting that three of the four bilateral cases are in children aged 13, 13 and 15 years. This contrasts with the nine unilateral cases, only one of which occurred in a patient below the age of 20 years. This underlines the clinical distinction between giant fibroadenoma and cystosarcoma phyllodes. *Giant fibroadenoma is not infrequently bilateral and is seen not uncommonly in adolescent girls. Cystosarcoma is rarely bilateral and is rare in adolescence.* The differences between giant fibroadenoma and cystosarcoma are both clinical and pathological and have prognostic and therapeutic implications. It is not a mere matter of semantics. This is why a sharp distinction between the two entities is essential.

Bilateral Malignant Cystosarcoma. Nevertheless, there are rare reports of bilateral
cystosarcoma phyllodes even of the malignant
variety, the first reported by Reich and
Solomon (1958). Their patient, aged 23 years,
developed the contralateral tumour eight
years later and, after three local recurrences,
died with extensive metastases six years after
removal of the second tumour. The total
course in this patient was 14 years from the
time of excision of the first tumour. The case
of Bader and Isaacson (1960) was similar with
a six-year interval before involvement of the
second breast. The second tumour recurred
as a cluster of three nodules, two with the
structure of cystosarcoma phyllodes while the
third showed frank fibrosarcoma. The patient
was well at the time of reporting, eight and
one-half years after the occurrence of the first
tumour but only six months after the second
simple mastectomy. This case illustrates well
the potential of this tumour to undergo frank
fibrosarcomatous change in space or time.
Such changes were present initially in parts of
the tumour in the first breast and were
demonstrated in the recurrence in the case of
the second breast. Another example of
bilateral malignant cystosarcoma was reported by Notley and Griffiths (1965); a
woman of 68 years developed the second
tumour only four months after the first simple
mastectomy and the whole course of the
disease was rapid, the patient dying ten
months after initial presentation for treatment.

*Malignant Cystosarcoma with Contralateral
Stromal Sarcoma.* The unique case of
Seemayer, Tremblay and Shibata (1975) had a
stromal sarcoma in one breast associated with
a malignant cystosarcoma in the other breast.
Although this patient did not have bilateral
cystosarcomas, the pathogenesis of the
sarcomatous lesions in the two breasts may be
related.

CYSTOSARCOMA IN UNUSUAL HOSTS

Children are very rarely affected by
cystosarcoma phyllodes. There were only
three patients younger than 20 years among
the 94 patients studied by Norris and Taylor
(1967); the youngest patient was 15 years old.
A further three cases were included in the
series of McDivitt, Urban and Farrow (1967).
There were four patients among 84 in the

series of Haagensen (1971) but the youngest, a
14-year-old, had a tumour which would
probably be classified by the writer as a
fibroadenoma rather than a CSP, as previously noted. The writer suspects that some of
the cystosarcomas reported in childhood are
more properly regarded as special variants of
fibroadenoma. Cystosarcomas in this age
group are almost always benign, both
histologically and in their behaviour. What is
more, they may well be less aggressive in
children than tumours of the corresponding
appearance in adults (Amerson, 1970).

*Malignant cystosarcoma phyllodes is extremely
rare in childhood,* only a single case having been
reported of a 14-year-old girl who died of the
disease with distant metastases (Hoover,
Trestioreanu and Ketcham, 1975). The writer
has studied another histologically malignant
cystosarcoma in a girl of the same age by
courtesy of Dr Dorothy Lewis of Johannesburg, South Africa. This 14-year-old girl had a
history of only six weeks' duration and a
tumour of 7 cm maximum diameter was
excised. Despite the evil appearance of this
tumour, which was only locally resected, on
the 8th September 1978, three and one-half
years later, Dr Lewis reported that 'this girl is
now an attractive 18-year-old who has
remained completely well'. A 17-year-old girl
in the series of Long, Hesker and Johnson
(1962) had axillary node metastases but was
free of disease at eight years after a radical
mastectomy.

A further case of malignant cystosarcoma in
a 12-year-old Filipino girl is the first known
occurrence of this tumour in a prepubertal
female (Gibbs, Roe and Thomas, 1968). The
diagnosis was confirmed at the Armed Forces
Institute of Pathology, Washington, D.C.
Following radical mastectomy, the girl was
well, without recurrence, one year after
operation. Another malignant tumour in an
18-year-old was locally excised at the age of 21
years and recurred at six months: the patient
refused simple mastectomy and, after a
further local excision, she married, became
pregnant and was delivered of a baby. She
remained well 42 months after her initial
presentation (Naryshkin and Redfield, 1964).
Pertinent also in this regard is the 16-year-old
girl with malignant CSP in the series of
Pietruszka and Barnes (1978). This girl had a
7.5 cm tumour with a 3+ degree of atypia (the
highest grade given). Histologically the
sarcomatous component consisted of fibrosarcoma, liposarcoma and chondrosarcoma.

Despite two recurrences in nine months, both treated by wide excision only, this girl came to no harm and was free of disease 37 months after initial diagnosis. A very strong plea is made for the separate identification of these tumours in adolescent girls. There is an overwhelming case against aggressive surgery in this age group. The behaviour of the tumour in the occasional patient who has refused the recommended surgery and opted for limited excision has taught us this lesson and it is one which must be taken to heart.

Cystosarcoma in Men. Lee and Pack (1931) mentioned three cases of cystosarcoma occurring in the male breast but McDivitt, Stewart and Berg (1968) had never seen it, and the writer has been able to trace only two acceptable more recent cases. In the case recorded by Reingold and Ascher (1970), a 64-year-old man had a mobile 6×4 cm mass in his breast for some 20 months. Excision revealed a tumour with the characteristics of cystosarcoma as well as pronounced gynaecomastia, including lobule formation, in the adjacent tissue. A testicular biopsy revealed atrophy and fibrosis but buccal smears were negative for sex chromatin and chromosome analysis revealed a normal male karyotype. Pantoja, Llobet and Lopez (1976) reported on a man with a gigantic cystosarcoma phyllodes; the tumour measured 30×30 cm and weighed 8.6 kg. It had been present for about 50 years and the patient was aged 70 years when he presented for treatment. The opposite breast showed gynaecomastia, of which the patient had been aware for many years, though its precise duration was not known. The gynaecomastia progressed in the 31 months following surgery for the cystosarcoma. Pantoja, Llobet and Lopez (1976) pointed out that while the normal male breast is probably incapable of developing a cystosarcoma, this does not apply to the gynaecomastic gland, a conclusion justified by the evidence.

Potential Resectability of Metastases

One of Long's (1962) cases, mentioned above, represents cystosarcoma phyllodes with metastasis to axillary nodes which was probably cured. Distant metastases are rarely potentially resectable as in Case 1 of Fernandez, Hernandez and Spindler (1976); in this patient a total of three lung metastases were resected six and eight years after a simple mastectomy for cystosarcoma phyllodes. The final outcome is not known. Most remarkable is the woman who had a solitary pulmonary metastasis resected by lobectomy two years after mastectomy for a 10 cm cystosarcoma. She was alive and well 16 years later, having had no further metastasis or recurrence (Hart et al, 1978).

Fatality without Metastatic Disease

At the opposite end of the spectrum from the rare metastasizing tumours which are curable, or potentially so, are the equally interesting unusual tumours which prove fatal by direct extension without exhibiting their metastatic potential. Two such cases were reported recently. A 'borderline' tumour recurred 14 times and proved fatal 23.5 years after presentation, as a result of direct invasion of the lungs (Pietruszka and Barnes, 1978). A similar case is the malignant CSP of Hart et al (1978) which killed the patient by direct invasion of recurrent tumour into the pleura and lung four years after simple mastectomy for the primary tumour. These events continue to illustrate the seemingly endless vagaries of this tumour.

CONCLUSIONS

The pathologist and surgeon should have a healthy respect for cystosarcoma phyllodes. These tumours should not be regarded and treated merely as 'overgrown' fibroadenomas. The cystosarcomas of adolescence are usually an exception and can be treated by local excision only (Amerson, 1970). *Cystosarcomas in adults need to be resected with a wide margin of healthy tissue.* Resection with a couple of centimetres of healthy tissue is recommended by Haagensen (1971) and is the treatment of choice in most cases. With very large tumours, adequate surgery will sometimes entail a total simple mastectomy or even extended mastectomy but *radical mastectomy is an unnecessary and a mutilating procedure* in the treatment of patients with this tumour. There are a few selected patients in whom low axillary dissection has been considered desirable by some workers (Norris and Taylor, 1967) but Haagensen (1971) did not consider this justified.

Haagensen (1971) recommended total excision together with a zone of surrounding breast tissue. He defended wide local excision because, despite the incidence of local recurrence, re-excision succeeded in all the non-metastasizing cystosarcomas in which it was performed and, above all, because the women did not lose their breasts. He advocated the same treatment even for recurrent tumour when this has the same microscopical appearance as the original lesion. On the other hand, in the relatively rare cases in which the connective tissue component becomes more malignant-looking with successive recurrences, he advised total mastectomy but without an axillary dissection. The case for preserving the breast, while adequately excising the tumour so as to minimize the chance of local recurrence, was precisely put by Haagensen (1971).

At the other end of the scale, it is equally bad to underestimate the aggressive potential of some of these tumours, especially the 20 per cent or so which belong to the histologically more malignant categories. *Excision of cystosarcoma of adults by enucleation or with a rim of only 1 to 2 mm of apparently healthy tissue is a recipe for further trouble* and, less frequently, for disaster. Treated inadequately, these tumours may recur locally many times and some eventually infiltrate the chest wall and give rise to inoperable thoracic and axillary masses. This type of case is preferentially seen in specialized cancer institutes and no doubt explains why some pathologists, including the writer, have seen more than their fair share of these cases. In such cases, haematogenous metastases may develop sooner or later. This sequence of events is seen in up to 15 per cent of patients who are treated inadequately. This is a regrettable and an unnecessary sequence, for, with proper treatment, the mortality can be reduced from 15 to 20 per cent to no more than 2 to 3 per cent. McDivitt, Urban and Farrow (1967) gave an excellent account of how this was achieved by tailoring the extent of the operative procedure to individual needs. On the other hand, six out of 20 patients studied by Rix, Tredwell and Forward (1971) died from their disease, a mortality rate of no less than 30 per cent.

The pathologist has the duty of *making the correct diagnosis,* of *educating himself and his colleagues if necessary in the behaviour of this quixotic lesion* and of *ensuring that there is generous clearance of the tumour.* Only in this way can preventable recurrences and deaths be avoided on the one hand, while mutilating surgery is avoided on the other.

BREAST CARCINOMA AND CYSTOSARCOMA PHYLLODES

This subject was thoroughly reviewed by Rosen and Urban (1975). Norris and Taylor (1967) found infiltrating ductal carcinoma in 2/94 cystosarcomas. Haagensen (1971) described seven patients with carcinoma associated with cystosarcoma, among whom there were two patients with lobular carcinoma limited to the tumour. A third patient with CLIS limited to the tumour was described by Treves (1964) and a fourth was reported by Rosen and Urban (1975). Of a total of six tumours with carcinoma restricted to the lesion, four had the lobular form (Rosen and Urban, 1975), a finding which agrees neatly with the type of carcinoma usually found restricted to the interior of an ordinary fibroadenoma. Of seven carcinomas found exclusively in the breast tissue *outside* the cystosarcoma, only two were of lobular type. Rosen and Urban (1975) reported a total of five cases with simultaneous carcinoma and cystosarcoma: four ipsilateral and one contralateral, of which two were infiltrating ductal and three lobular carcinomas in situ (one within the lesion, two in the surrounding breast). Four of their five cases were identified during a period in which 18 patients with cystosarcoma phyllodes were treated. The authors considered that this high incidence of associated carcinoma could represent the result of a chance clustering of cases, but rightly drew attention to the need for further study of this unusual combination. It should be pointed out that no patient had died as a result of the carcinomas which were associated with cystosarcomas.

Haagensen (1971) found lobular neoplasia closely associated with four of 84 cases of cystosarcoma: two were limited to the tumour, one was found within and without it and the fourth was present only in breast tissue adjacent to the tumour. Three additional patients in the Columbia series had concurrent infiltrating carcinoma detected pathologically in the resected breast tissue: these conventional carcinomas, as opposed to lobular neoplasia, were all outside the cystosarcoma. An additional two patients developed cancer subsequently, one on the same side and one contralaterally. Haagensen believes that patients who have had cystosarcoma should be followed with special care, a view which is shared by Rosen and Urban (1975).

Lobular neoplasia is the tumour type most frequently associated with cystosarcoma phyllodes. Infiltrating ductal carcinoma when associated with CSP usually involves the breast tissue outside the tumour. However, this is not meant to indicate that carcinoma of 'ductal' type never affects CSP to the exclusion of the surrounding tissue. Ductal type carcinoma may rarely be limited to CSP just as it may very rarely be limited to the interior of a fibroadenoma. We should not draw a completely rigid division between the sites of origin of lobular and ductal carcinoma. Indeed in the consideration of the extremely rare carcinosarcomas (page 374) it will be seen that five of the more acceptable 15 are believed to have originated in cystosarcomas or related tumours (Harris and Persaud, 1974). The carcinomatous component in these is of ductal type, taking the form of adenocarcinoma, squamous carcinoma or a mixture of the two. If complex carcinosarcomas can very rarely arise in a CSP, presumably the epithelial component of CSP can give rise to 'ductal type' carcinoma, in situ or infiltrating, without an overtly malignant alteration in the connective tissue component. This type of alteration affected the CSP described by Philip (1976); the infiltrating ductal carcinoma in this case had metastasized to lymph nodes. Cornog et al (1971) identified a squamous carcinoma originating in cystosarcoma and a similar personal case is referred to on page 298. But in fact it should be stated that carcinomatous change of ductal type restricted to a CSP, in the absence of frankly malignant change in the connective tissue element, is extremely rare.

OTHER SARCOMAS

STROMAL SARCOMA

The term 'stromal sarcoma' is applied to breast tumours which are composed of the same sarcomatous elements found in malignant cystosarcoma phyllodes but which lack the epithelial element which is essential for diagnosis of the latter (Berg et al, 1962). Thus fibrosarcomatous and liposarcomatous patterns are found as well as areas of giant-cell and spindle-cell sarcoma which are not further identifiable. Norris and Taylor (1968) considered the 'sarcomas and related mesenchymal tumors of the breast' together, excluding only haemangiosarcoma and malignant lymphoma. While fibroblastic differentiation was the most common, liposarcomatous foci were present in three of their 32 cases. Osteoid and cartilage were found in five tumours, and bone without cartilage in a sixth case. Heterologous elements were present in eight out of the total 32 cases. Two desmoid-like tumours were found, as well as a tumour in the breast indistinguishable from dermatofibrosarcoma protuberans but without skin involvement. The writer has seen another case in the last category.

Tumours with Rhabdomyosarcomatous Differentiation. Norris and Taylor (1968) included in their series a tumour with rhabdomyosarcomatous differentiation. A case could be made for segregating primary tumours of the breast with rhabdomyosarcomatous differentiation in a category of their own, if only because of their great rarity. Only seven fully acceptable examples had been recorded by 1970 (Bird tabulated five acceptable cases and added a sixth; the seventh case is that of Norris and Taylor, 1968). An eighth case was added recently by Barnes and Pietruszka (1977). But the relationship to other types of sarcoma is indicated by Bird's case, in which there was cartilaginous and osteoid differentiation in addition to striated muscle.

While it is accepted that breast sarcomas can show metaplastic chondroid, osseous and even muscular metaplasia, *the admonition of Stewart (1950) that many apparent cases of sarcoma probably in fact represent carcinoma with osseous and cartilaginous metaplasia remains valid* today and great care must be exercised in attempting to make this important distinction.

Tumours Resembling Osteogenic Sarcoma and Giant-cell Tumour of Bone. Among the most difficult groups of breast tumour to identify are those which resemble osteogenic sarcoma and especially those that resemble giant-cell tumours of soft tissue or of bone. Much more needs to be learnt about these tumours before definite conclusions can be drawn and they deserve intensive study. Some apparently may even represent metaplastic carcinomas with epulis-type giant cells (McDivitt, Stewart and

Berg, 1968). The writer has seen a case in which osteoclast-like cells were inextricably mixed with a type of mammary adenocarcinoma.

Osteogenic Sarcoma, Osteoclastoma and Chondrosarcoma. True osteogenic sarcomas of the breast do, however, occur (Rottino and Howley, 1945). The rare polymorphic and giant-cell tumours are also referred to in the literature as 'osteoclastomas of the breast', 'osteoclastoma-like tumour' or 'giant-cell tumour'. Rottino and Howley (1945), probably rightly, considered that these 'giant-cell' tumours should be classified together with those that show osseous or chondroid differentiation. These tumours occur in the older age groups. Of the 25 tumours reviewed by these authors, only 10 contained osteoid or bone. Giant-cell sarcomas of the breast are *highly malignant* and, in the 16 cases with follow-up, rapid local recurrence within weeks or months was usual and all the patients were dead, usually with metastatic disease, within twelve months of treatment irrespective of its type. Haematogenous metastases are the rule and even a case with axillary node metastases has been recorded.

That *exceptions to this generally sinister behaviour do occur* is suggested by Kennedy and Biggart (1967), in whose series of 18 'pure' sarcomas there were no fewer than four with osseous or chondroid differentiation. Inexplicably two patients with chondrosarcoma and osteochondrosarcoma had no recurrence of tumour at $9\frac{1}{2}$ and 11 years respectively. Another case of osteosarcoma had not recurred at nine months.

Tumours in which Cartilaginous and Osseous Tissue is a Minor Component. At present, it seems essential to separate giant-cell and osteogenic sarcomas from the types of sarcoma discussed by Norris and Taylor (1968) in which 'heterologous' elements constituted only a minor component of the tumours. In the latter group the prognosis appears to be substantially better. Pertinently, the tumour of the patient reported on by Jernstrom, Lindberg and Meland (1963), contained only 'occasional' areas of chondroid and osteoid elements, and she is reported to have died several years later apparently of some unrelated disease. Similarly, the case of leiomyosarcoma with osseous and cartilaginous metaplasia (Barnes and Pietruszka, 1977)

died at 52 months without evidence of tumour.

Histogenesis of the Two Groups of Sarcoma. The histogenesis of the two groups of breast sarcomas may also be different. The 'stromal sarcomas', with or without focal heterologous elements, seem to arise de novo. On the other hand, there is reasonably convincing evidence that about 40 per cent of the giant-cell and pleomorphic sarcomas, of the type reviewed by Rottino and Howley (1945), arise in a pre-existing fibroadenoma. Rottino and Howley (1945) suggested that, with more thorough study, the proportion arising in fibroadenomas may prove to be even greater. It would be an understatement to say that the last word has not been written on this complex group of tumours. Since some, perhaps most, of these sarcomas probably arise in pre-existing fibroadenomas or cystosarcomas, the problem is referred to also on page 328.

Barnes and Pietruszka (1977), in a report on 10 cases of breast sarcoma, criticized the use of the term 'stromal sarcoma' as meaningless. What their report does show, and most other authors would agree, is that *the osteogenic sarcomas should be segregated.* Two of their three fatal cases were osteogenic sarcomas and, conversely, both cases of osteogenic sarcoma were fatal. Of the five fibrosarcomas only one proved fatal, the patient having multiple local recurrences before developing pulmonary and osseous metastases.

These workers collected *100 cases of 'stromal sarcoma'* from the literature starting with the paper of Berg et al (1962) and including their own 10 cases. The average age of the patients was 52 years, the median size of the tumours was 5.3 cm, while the number of tumour-related deaths was 29 per cent. Virtually all of the deaths occurred within five years of diagnosis and treatment.

Prognosis, Nodal Involvement and Treatment. Norris and Taylor (1968) stressed the better behaviour of the tumours with a 'pushing' as opposed to an infiltrative edge. The actuarial survival was 73 per cent at five years in the whole group, a somewhat better prognostic outlook than in the patients studied by Berg et al (1962). A slight cautionary note should be introduced here since, in a later paper (Smith and Taylor, 1969), patients with 'stromal sarcomas' with cartilaginous and osseous differentiation did not fare so well. Four out of nine had died of metastases and a fifth was alive with metastases. It would appear that cases with pure osteogenic sarcoma were also included in the later report and these are known to have a poor prognosis, which may account for the discrepancy in survival rates. Wide local excision for small lesions and simple mastectomy for larger lesions is recommended. With local excision, McDivitt, Stewart and Berg (1968) found local recurrence in nine of 13 patients, compared with only one local recurrence among seven patients treated by simple mastectomy. If local excision is practised for small lesions, it must be a genuinely wide excision. In addition, low axillary dissection is advised in selected cases by Norris and Taylor (1968), but radical mastectomy should be avoided. Axillary node metastases are rare with these tumour types and there is need for better documentation of cases with such metastases. In none of Berg's (1962) cases were lymph nodes involved by tumour.

Barnes and Pietruszka (1977) found that of five patients with initial axillary node dissection, only one had a solitary lymph node which contained tumour, and they regarded this as direct tumour extension rather than metastasis.

The Significance of Mitotic Counts. Barnes and Pietruszka (1977) confirmed the significance of infiltrating as opposed to 'pushing' margins pointed out by Norris and Taylor (1968). They concluded that sarcomas with eight or more mitoses/10 HPF may behave in an aggressive fashion, analogous to the finding of Norris and Taylor (1968), who, in a larger series, determined that tumours with five or six mitoses/10 HPF have the potential to metastasize. It should, however, be pointed out that four tumours in Barnes' series had five or more mitoses/10 HPF but did not behave aggressively (three fibrosarcomas and one leiomyosarcoma with a 'pushing' margin).

LIPOSARCOMA

The extremely rare pure liposarcoma of the breast is best categorized separately but extensive sampling is necessary to prove that it is genuinely pure. Cystosarcomas with a liposarcomatous component must be excluded (Figures 14–3 to 14–5) (Qizilbash, 1976). When this was done Haagensen (1971) was able to find only eight cases of liposarcoma

culled from the literature and his own material. If haemangiosarcoma is among the deadliest of malignant tumours of the breast, pure liposarcoma must be among the rarest.

According to McDivitt, Stewart and Berg (1968) this tumour may metastasize to the axilla like a carcinoma, a view not shared by Haagensen (1971); this is a point in need of clarification. There was an adequate follow-up study in five of the eight cases reviewed by Haagensen (1971). Four patients were alive and well at six, seven, seven and 12 years respectively, the last only to be extinguished dramatically in a tornado. Only one patient was known to have died of her disease. A further case of liposarcoma was reported by Menon and van Velthoven (1974). A patient with myxoid liposarcoma in the series of Barnes and Pietruszka (1977) was living and well at 20 years.

Liposarcomatous Differentiation in Cystosarcoma Phyllodes. Hummer and Burkart (1967) reviewed and tabulated 22 liposarcomas of the breast and added another of their own, making a total of 23 cases. One of the problems in assessing many of these cases is in determining whether they represent pure liposarcomas or dominantly liposarcomatous differentiation in a cystosarcoma phyllodes (Figures 14–3 to 14–5). Thus the case of Jackson (1962), Case 21 in the Table of Hummer and Burkart (1967), was a 'metastasizing liposarcoma arising in a fibroadenoma'. The same applies to the tumours reported by Stout and Bernanke (1946) and De Navasquez and Horton (1947). Even the more recent case of Anderson and Kafrouni (1972), widely cited as an instance of liposarcoma, was clearly described as arising in a cystosarcoma phyllodes. Qizilbash (1976) rightly concluded that the vast majority of reported cases of liposarcoma of the breast represent examples of malignant cystosarcoma phyllodes; he was struck by the distinctive pattern of 'periductal' localization of the malignant lipomatous tissue. In fact Oberman, Nosanchuk and Finger (1969), in reporting on two tumours, referred to this variant of malignant cystosarcoma phyllodes as a 'periductal liposarcoma' (Figures 14–3 to 14–5).

Liposarcomatous Differentiation in Stromal Sarcoma. Liposarcoma also occurs admixed with other mesenchymal elements in the specialized soft tissue sarcoma of the breast, which Berg and colleagues (1962) named 'stromal sarcoma'. Berg et al (1962) reported six predominantly liposarcomatous tumours in their review of 25 stromal sarcomas. Norris and Taylor (1968) encountered three similar cases in their study of 32 stromal sarcomas.

LEIOMYOSARCOMA

Leiomyosarcoma of the breast is *an exceptionally rare tumour*. Only six previous cases were identified in the literature by Pardo-Mindan, Garcia-Julian and Altuna (1974), who reported a seventh thoroughly studied case. Three of the previously re- corded six tumours were in men, indicating, if this finding is confirmed in future studies, that pure leiomyosarcoma is relatively more common in the male breast. This might perhaps mean that this tumour is not closely related to stromal sarcomas or cystosarcomas.

ANGIOSARCOMA

Angiosarcoma is *perhaps the most devastat- ingly deadly* of all malignant breast tumours (Figures 14–7 and 14–9). *The deceptively benign appearance of some of these tumours* is analogous to some of the cutaneous angiosarcomas and those seen in other sites but the prognosis is much gloomier (Figures 14–7 and 14–8). That rare exceptions to this bad prognosis do occur even with this vicious tumour is illustrated by two patients who survived seven and 14 years postoperatively; these are the first reported examples of probable cures (Steingaszner, Enzinger and Taylor, 1965).

These two long-term survivors of Steingasz- ner, Enzinger and Taylor (1965) both had small tumours; one was treated by radical mastectomy and the other by wide local excision. Gulesserian and Lawton (1969) collected 42 haemangiosarcomas of the breast reported since 1907. Twenty of these are in the series of Steingaszner, Enzinger and Taylor (1965) (10 cases), McClanahan and

Hogg (1954) (six cases) and Edward and Kellett (1968) (four cases). In different series the time from the onset of symptoms to death had averaged 1.6 to 2.6 years with variation between two and 39 months.

Tumours With Less Fulminant Behaviour. There have been some more recent reports of unusual behaviour by this tumour. Kessler and Kozenitzky (1971) reported on a patient who survived three years without metastases, despite two local recurrences in the breast following local excision and a subtotal mastectomy. Following wide excision of recurrent tumour in the scar, in her fourth postoperative year the patient developed metastases in the subcutaneous tissues, the contralateral breast and later the liver, spleen and lungs. She died four and one-half years after the initial operation from rupture of splenic metastases into the peritoneal cavity. The liver and spleen had a honeycombed 'Swiss cheese' appearance caused by angiosar- comatous metastases.

Tumours With Less Aggressive Behaviour. Still more remarkable is the patient of Horne and Percival (1975). The original excision speci- men contained a lesion diagnosed as 'organiz- ing haematoma'. It recurred during the following two years and then presented as a nodular tumour 15 cm in diameter. It was treated by modified radical mastectomy after simple excision had established the correct diagnosis of haemangiosarcoma. Despite the two-year delay before definitive surgery and the massive size of the tumour on second presentation, the patient remained well seven years after the initial operation and five years after the definitive surgery. Horne and Percival (1975) found nothing in the path- ology to explain the innocuous behaviour of the tumour; solid areas of the tumour showed nuclear atypia and many mitoses. Both Kessler and Kozenitzky (1971) and Horne and Percival (1975) stress the fact that *misdiagnosis of these sarcomas as benign conditions is still common*, the former having been diagnosed as

Figure 14–7   (*Opposite, above.*)   Deceptively benign appearance of the vascular spaces in a haemangiosarcoma of the breast. H and E. ×150. (By courtesy of Dr S. Rao.)

Figure 14–8   (*Opposite, below.*)   Intercommunicating vascular channels have ramified in and dissected the adipose and fibrous tissue in the characteristic style of a haemangiosarcoma. Individual channels have a deceptively innocuous appearance. H and E. ×150. (By courtesy of Dr M. D. Lagios.)

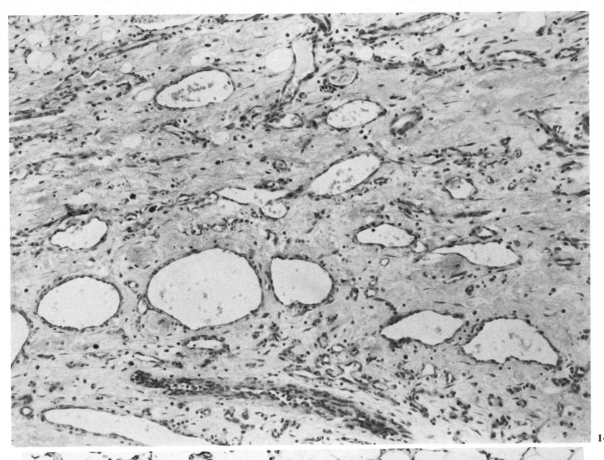

14–7

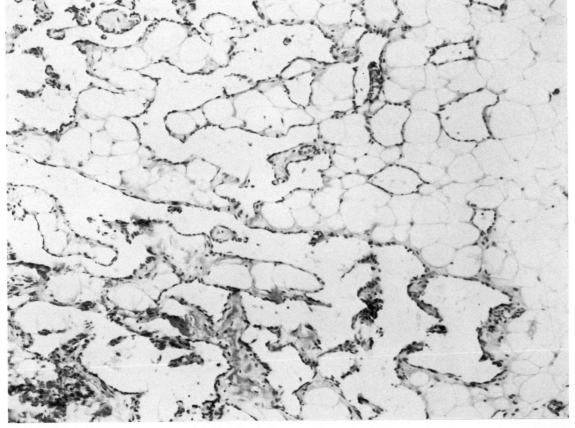

14–8

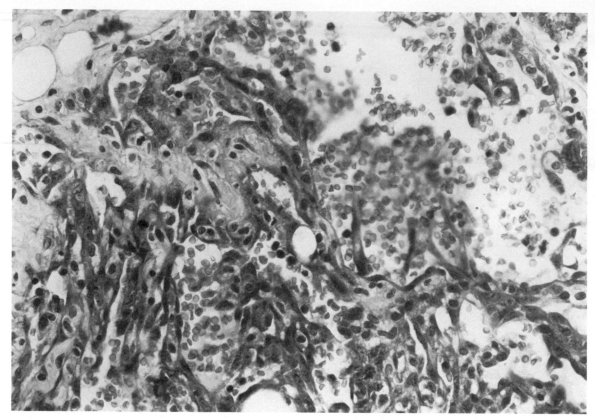

Figure 14–9 From same tumour as Figure 14–7. More obviously angiosarcomatous area. The patient died of metastases within 12 months. H and E. ×400.

a benign haemangioma on at least two occasions and the latter as an organizing haematoma. Rarity of the condition and lack of familiarity with its appearance combine to maintain this tendency to misdiagnosis. In many tumours there are well-differentiated parts which resemble benign haemangioma closely (Figures 14–7 and 14–8).

A case with similarities to that of Horne and Percival (1975) is one reported by Massé, Mongeau and Rioux (1977). The tumour recurred locally eight and 14 months after initial treatment. Despite this 14-month delay before definitive therapy, the patient was alive and free of disease more than seven years after the tumour was first noted and six years after a simple mastectomy. This represents the fourth recorded case to survive five years or more after definitive therapy and the second such case in the Canadian literature. Massé, Mongeau and Rioux (1977) recommended total (simple) mastectomy in order to eradicate the local disease. They stressed the

fact that infiltration by tumour tends to extend beyond the limits defined by gross palpation. Axillary dissection is unnecessary. In this case, as in so many others, the original biopsy was interpreted as benign; *the diagnosis was 'mammary dysplasia', a remarkable example of the way this term can be abused.* Massé, Mongeau and Rioux (1977) collected another nine cases, including their own, since the 42 collected by Gulesserian and Lawton (1969), making a total of 51 documented cases at the time of their report. They are a good source of references.

The author has seen a case similar to the two Canadian ones by courtesy of Dr M. Lagios of San Francisco. The original biopsy was interpreted as a benign lesion at another hospital and locally recurrent tumour was excised 22 months later (Figure 14–8): both specimens in fact showed angiosarcoma and there was residual tumour in the mastectomy specimen. Despite this delay of 22 months in instituting definitive treatment, the patient has no signs of recurrence or metastatic disease 12 months after definitive surgery.

Role of Radiotherapy and Chemotherapy. Gogas and Kotsianos (1977) reported on a 15-year-old girl with angiosarcoma of the breast. They document beneficial effects with radiotherapy as ancillary treatment but found chemotherapy ineffective. Myerowitz, Pietruszka and Barnes (1978) adduced some evidence to suggest that chemotherapy may have a role in the treatment of this condition though the evidence is inconclusive.

Of considerable interest is the behaviour of the tumours in the three patients with haemangiosarcoma treated by Myerowitz, Pietruszka and Barnes (1978). One patient with a 'lemon-size' tumour was treated by radical mastectomy and has remained well without recurrence after 22 years. This patient represents the longest recorded survival to date. A second patient with a 3 cm mass was treated by modified radical mastectomy and she has no evidence of disease at five years. Thus there are, as of January 1978, *six documented patients with haemangiosarcoma of the breast who have survived at least five years after definitive surgery without recurrence.* It is noteworthy that four of these six patients have been reported on since 1975. The third patient of Myerowitz, Pietruszka and Barnes (1978) succumbed to her disease four years after presentation, with metastatic disease in the intervening period. This is the patient, already mentioned, in whom chemotherapy was regarded as having played a useful role in controlling the disease. The fact that two of the three patients treated by these workers had such a good outcome is rightly regarded by them as a happy but chance occurrence. The overall prognosis of haemangiosarcoma of the breast is very poor, though the more recent literature does throw a ray of light into the gloom which has enshrouded this tumour until very recently.

Differential Diagnosis Between Haemangioma and Haemangiosarcoma. In the differential diagnosis it is important to stress that *a benign angioma has never to date constituted a palpable or symptom-producing breast tumour.* Hence an angiomatous tumour of the breast which has presented clinically is sarcomatous until proved otherwise (Dunegan, Tobon and Watson, 1976).

MALIGNANT LYMPHOMA OF THE BREAST

Incidence. Primary malignant lymphoma of the breast is extremely rare, especially if one is strict in defining what is apparently 'primary' (DeCosse et al, 1962; McDivitt, Stewart and Berg, 1968). The first group of workers found 14 patients with this tumour among 8000 with operable breast cancer between 1930 and 1955, while the second group (Fred Stewart specifically) identified only 10 cases among 11 000 breast cancers at the same institute, *an incidence of only 1 in 1000 cancers,* and even then Stewart had reservations about the 'primary' nature of some of these (there was some overlap between the cases in these two series).

Clinicopathological Features

In the series of DeCosse et al (1962) a second mass was palpated in four of their 14 patients and they consider that such a finding might suggest the possibility of lymphosarcoma clinically, but otherwise there were no real distinguishing clinical features. Pathologically the tumours can be usefully separated into reticulosarcoma (seven), lymphoblastic lymphosarcoma (five) (diffuse four, and follicular one), and lymphocytic lymphosarcoma (two), both of which were of the follicular variety. The main prognostic indicator was the histological type, 'small cell' tumours correlating well with longer survival though the ultimate outcome was not any better. Axillary node involvement was frequent but of no prognostic value. Their results (64 per cent five-year survival and 54 per cent 10-year survival) are more encouraging than other workers have indicated. Excisional surgery and radiotherapy can result in at least a temporary 'cure' of these localized lymphomas. Nevertheless, a number of patients die of recurrent disease at the 10 to 20 year interval.

Other Workers' Experience. The experience of other workers has been different. Lattes (1967) reviewed 38 cases of apparently primary lymphoma of the breast. Fourteen patients were below 40 years of age. Bilateral involvement occurred nine times and six of these were detected during pregnancy or the puerperium. Twenty-one patients died of their disease, mostly within a year of diagnosis. Only six patients were living and apparently free of disease one to 10 years after treatment. Lattes' (1967) study suggests that radiation therapy alone is probably adequate to control the local disease.

The prognosis is also regarded as evil by Wiseman and Liao (1972). Of 14 of their 16 patients with follow-up study, only three survived five years or more; two with lymphocytic tumours were alive and well at 11 and 14 years respectively, and one patient survived 17 years with disease in multiple organs in the intervening period, from which she eventually succumbed. But most of their patients ran a rapidly fatal course. Bilateral breast involvement was present in four of their 16 patients.

The report of Lawler and Richie (1967) is a useful source of the earliest references and that of Ross and Eley (1975) of the more recent ones.

Literature Survey. Jernstrom and Sether (1967) reviewed the world literature up to 1966 and discovered only 10 cases to add to the 58 found acceptable by DeCosse et al in 1962. To these 68 cases Jernstrom and Sether (1967) added three of their own, making a total of 71 cases to the end of 1966. Their three cases were found in a review of 6300 mammary malignancies, an incidence of only 1 in 2000 breast cancers. Ross and Eley (1975) found 50 more cases in nine papers in the world literature since 1966, making a total of 121 cases. Freeman, Berg and Cutler (1972) reported on 1467 patients with extranodal lymphomas collected from 100 hospitals in the USA. There were 33 cases of breast lymphoma and another nine were found by Haagensen (1971), making a grand total of 164 (including the case report of Ross and Eley, 1975). The 38 cases reported on by Lattes (1967) were missed by the review of Ross and Eley (1975); it is likely that there is an overlap between these cases and the nine mentioned by Haagensen (1971). It would, however, appear that *the total number of cases of apparently primary lymphoma of the breast* up to the time of the review by Ross and Eley (1975) *is not far short of 200.*

Comparison with Carcinoma. The age incidence is the same as for carcinoma except in the series of Lattes (1967) with 14 of 38 patients below 40 years of age. There is a predilection for the right breast according to Ross and Eley (1975), a point in need of verification. The incidence is given as 1 in 500 of malignant breast tumours in the female by Ross and Eley (1975) but an incidence of 1 in 1000 or even 1 in 2000 is given by most authors. The lower incidence of about 1 in 1000 is obtained if one adopts strict criteria of what is truly primary in the breast (McDivitt, Stewart and Berg, 1968).

Bilaterality. While DeCosse et al (1962) stressed the finding of multiple nodules in one breast in four of their 14 patients as a possibly significant feature of this disease, bilaterality has been stressed in some more recent reports. Lattes (1967) found bilateral tumours in nine of 38 patients, although one might have some reservation about the primary nature of the lesions in some of the cases in Lattes' (1967) series. Wiseman and Liao (1972) found bilateral involvement in four of 16 patients. Freedman, Kagan and Friedman (1971) dealt specifically with bilaterality in primary lymphosarcoma of the breast. They had two such patients among six personal cases. These authors calculated that the incidence of bilaterality is of the order of 6 to 7 per cent and they were unaware of the Lattes (1967) series. Bilaterality could be nearer 10 per cent. Freedman, Kagan and Friedman (1971) found three previous cases of bilaterality in the English literature, with the contralateral tumour developing five and six years later in the cases of DeCosse et al (1962) and Stringer (1959) respectively. In the two patients of Freedman, Kagan and Friedman (1971) there were intervals of eight years and 10 years before the appearance of tumour in the contralateral breast. Pseudolymphoma is considered in the diagnosis and effectively ruled out in Case 1 by the involvement of the axillary nodes at the same time as the first breast lesion. At necropsy there was no evidence of lymphoma elsewhere in the body eight years after treatment of the original lesion. The patient died of lung infection superimposed on chronic lung disease. Their second case is a remarkable one in that, in addition to the breast tumours, separated by a 10-year interval, there were bilateral pulmonary lesions and an inguinal mass, which were presumed to be neoplastic although there was no biopsy proof of this; these lesions responded to small doses of radiotherapy. The patient was well six years after the appearance of the second breast lump and 16 years after resection of the first tumour. These authors stressed the fact that bilaterality does not appear to worsen the chances of survival.

Prognosis. Ross and Eley (1975) stressed that prognosis is essentially related to the histological type, being best with lymphocytic tumours and worst with reticulum cell sarcomas. Cure, or at any rate survival for 10 years or more without disease, is commoner with the well-differentiated tumours. In the series of Freeman, Berg and Cutler (1972) there were no deaths from disease at the five to 10 year interval but the case of Ross and Eley (1975) with death at seven years 10 months is an exception. Perhaps pertinently the patient of Ross and Eley (1975), who presented with a well-differentiated lymphosarcoma of the breast followed by a tumour of the same type in the subcutaneous tissue two years later, remained well for almost three more years, when an inguinal node was found replaced by tumour which was then classified as a reticulum cell sarcoma. At this time, the tempo of the disease appeared to accelerate despite chemotherapy and she died three years after the change from well-differentiated lymphosarcoma to reticulum cell sarcoma.

PLASMACYTOMA

Extramedullary plasmacytoma of the breast is extremely rare. The patient of Proctor et al (1975) was alive and well at 46 months at the time of reporting.* Only two cases were discovered in the literature in which plasmacytoma of the breast proved to be the first manifestation of systemic disease.

CARCINOSARCOMA

Spindle-cell Carcinoma. Carcinosarcoma is one of the most contentious tumour types in pathology, especially as it affects the breast. Carcinomas can undergo marked spindle-cell and other metaplasias, thereby closely simulating fibrosarcomas and other types of sarcoma (Willis, 1958). In this context, it is important to stress that reticulin silver impregnations are virtually valueless in the differentiation of certain sarcomatoid carcinomas from true sarcomas. A spindle-cell carcinoma with desmoplastic reaction can

* A personal communication from Dr Cynthia Cohen (1976) stated that the patient died, almost six years after presentation, in diabetic ketosis without evidence of recurrence or systemic tumour.

have an abundant reticulin and collagen framework which may even surround individual tumour cells in the manner classically associated with sarcomas. Indeed, reticulin impregnations may be deceptive and merely serve to 'confirm' an erroneous diagnosis of sarcoma. Were it otherwise, the diagnostic problems would be very greatly minimized. A sarcomatoid appearance is especially frequent with squamous carcinomas in certain sites (Willis, 1958; Jones, 1969). The curious polypoid squamous carcinomas of the upper alimentary and respiratory tracts are notorious in this regard. That a sarcomatoid appearance can be assumed also by mammary carcinoma needs fuller recognition.

Easily Recognizable Carcinoma May Be a Very Minor Component. The second point of importance is that the obviously carcinomatous component may be a very minor one and may appear, on inadequate sampling, to be entirely in situ. If the carcinomatous elements are missed entirely, an erroneous diagnosis of sarcoma is likely to be made. If in situ carcinoma is detected but no infiltrating carcinoma is found, the pathologist may be comforted in his belief that the carcinomatous component is quite distinct from the bulky, apparently sarcomatous component and thus his impression that he is dealing with a true carcinosarcoma may be reinforced.

Heterologous Elements. Thirdly, the finding of 'heterologous' elements, like osteoid, bone or cartilage, is often regarded as unequivocal proof that one is dealing with a sarcoma. This is perhaps the most difficult problem of all, since there is no absolute way as yet of settling this complex issue. The identification of osteoid is by no means easy, and *even the presence of neoplastic bone or cartilage is probably not unequivocal proof that one is dealing with a sarcoma, at any rate in the conventional sense* of a tumour of mesenchymal derivation. As already cited, Stewart (1950) warned that breast carcinomas can show chondroid and osseous metaplasia, and Smith and Taylor (1969) demonstrated that cartilage may arise in breast tumours by epithelial metaplasia. Kahn et al (1978) demonstrated very convincing transitions between the carcinomatous and chondrosarcomatous areas in two such tumours at both light microscopic and ultrastructural levels. These are in a sense 'carcinosarcomas' but not in the histogenetic sense in which the term is usually used.

However, the presence of *elements such as malignant striated muscle can reasonably be regarded as definitive proof of a sarcomatous tumour* (Bird, 1970), and the fact that the tumour reported by Bird contained, in addition, chondroid and osseous foci can be regarded as acceptable evidence that chondro- and osteosarcomas of mesenchymal derivation undoubtedly do occur in the human breast. However, as striated muscle fibres are only very rarely demonstrable in these debatable tumours, these exceptionally rare tumours shed little light on the classification of the tumours which constitute the more common diagnostic problem.

The Metaplastic Potential of the Myoepithelial Cell. The fourth problem, which is related to the third, is the metaplastic potential of the myoepithelial cell, for it is known that myoepithelial cells can undergo metaplasia to chondrocytes and that the neoplastic cartilage can in turn undergo endochondral ossification. This is seen in chondroid syringomas ('mixed' salivary-type hidradenomas) and extremely rarely even in 'mixed' tumours of the salivary glands. A similar phenomenon is seen not infrequently in the case of the malignant mammary tumours of bitches, in which chondroid elements are regarded as being of myoepithelial derivation (von Bomhard and von Sandersleben, 1974). A similar derivation of neoplastic cartilage may apply to the human breast also, as in the tumours studied by Kahn et al (1978), although further confirmation of their findings is desirable. It has yet to be proven that the conversion of carcinomatous to chondrosarcomatous tissue which they demonstrated is dependent on an element of myoepithelial differentiation: but studies of salivary gland tumours and comparative studies of tumours of the breast in bitches make this a distinct and intriguing possibility. Even *a leiomyosarcoma of the breast has been traced to a myoepithelial origin* (Cameron, Hamperl and Warambo, 1974) and the evidence in this unique and fascinating case, which the writer was enabled to study through the kindness of the late Professor H. Hamperl, is convincing. Indeed, Hamperl (1970) implied that many, if not all, carcinosarcomas of the breast may be interpreted as having an epithelial/myoepithelial derivation, thus making it unnecessary to postulate a dual origin from mesenchymal as well as from epithelial tissue. While the writer agrees that certain special cases can be explained on this basis, he is not convinced that all carcinosarcomas can be interpreted in this way.

Magnitude of the Problem. The purpose of the foregoing discussion is by way of a warning against a too ready acceptance of cases of carcinosarcoma, and even of certain sarcomas of the breast. The magnitude of the diagnostic problems and the multiplicity of the pitfalls must be appreciated by all those with an interest in this field. In future these tumours should be studied far more extensively than in the past, and attempts at reconstruction of such complex tumours by serial slicing and by mapping out of tissue elements may help in determining their precise nature.

THE MORE CREDIBLE CARCINOSARCOMAS

Taking all these objections into account, there is some *a priori reason to believe that carcinosarcomas of the breast do exist.* Fibroadenoma and cystosarcoma phyllodes are both diploblastic tumours, and it is now generally accepted that malignant change can affect both the epithelial and the connective tissue elements of these tumours. It might therefore be expected that on very rare occasions a true carcinosarcoma may take origin in one of these tumours. *The more credible and best-documented carcinosarcomas reported since 1937 have been tabulated by Harris and Persaud (1974), who listed only 16 cases,* including two of their own. Interestingly, six of the 16 cases were regarded as probably originating in a pre-existing fibroadenoma or cystosarcoma and this histogenesis is regarded by many workers as true also of many of the more exotic breast sarcomas (Rottino and Howley, 1945; see page 366). Case 1 of Harris and Persaud (1974) is a good illustration of the second and third problems mentioned at the start of this section. In their Case 2 the apparently sarcomatous component could represent metaplastic carcinoma, though perhaps the origin in a cystosarcoma makes their diagnosis of carcinosarcoma more acceptable than it might otherwise be. In Case 2, and possibly also in their Case 1, the carcinomatous component was a squamous carcinoma.

Osseous, Cartilaginous and Squamous Differentiation. Of the 16 carcinosarcomas accepted by Harris and Persaud (1974), no fewer than eight showed bony or cartilaginous differentiation. Squamous differentiation of the epithelial element is also disproportionately frequent since six of the 16 showed squamous differentiation. This was malignant in five and apparently benign in the sixth case (Wayte, Stewart and McKenzie, 1970).

Imperfect Documentation. The documentation of a few of these 16 cases leaves something to be desired. Thus the case of Smithy and Charleston (1944) is clearly identifiable now as a cystosarcoma phyllodes. The authors found no evidence of malignancy in the epithelial element but interpreted some glandular structures in a lymph node as metastatic from a presumed primary carcinoma in the cystosarcoma. This is clearly not acceptable to document a great rarity and *exclusion of this case reduces the number of acceptable cases to 15.* Even among more recent reports the data presented lead one to suspect that the authors have not always been fully aware of the potential pitfalls.

Carcinosarcomas with a Rhabdomyosarcomatous Component. Govan (1945) described two cases in which the sarcomatous component consisted of rhabdomyosarcoma. Only very partial cross striations were demonstrated but the evidence that these two tumours were genuine carcinosarcomas is in general convincing.

Very Well Documented Carcinosarcoma. Wayte, Stewart and McKenzie (1970) described a carcinosarcoma of the breast in which there was no evidence of pre-existing fibroadenoma. The tense cystic tumour contained a unilocular cyst into which projected two polypoid nodules and five smaller papillary lesions. The cyst was lined by non-keratinizing squamous epithelium, which was thrown into papillary projections in the five smaller projecting lesions. Squamous epithelium lined the bases of the two larger polyps. The interior of one of these consisted entirely of osteosarcomatous tissue. The larger polyp contained mature bone with adenocarcinomatous tissue embedded in it, and osteosarcoma at the apex of the protuberance. This case report is one of the best-documented and credible instances of carcinosarcoma recorded to date.

Though squamous carcinoma with metaplasia is the type of breast carcinoma which most frequently assumes a sarcomatoid aspect, this should not be taken to mean that adenocarcinomas cannot also exhibit sarcomatoid features. By courtesy of Dr R. Pisa of Verona, the writer recently studied a papillary carcinoma of the breast in which the stroma of the fronds contained pleomorphic pseudosarcoma which could be traced to the carcinomatous covering of the fronds.

CONCLUSION

In summary, it is fair to state that true carcinosarcoma of the breast represents a genuine but extremely rare entity which is still being overdiagnosed. In the presence of striated muscle elements and carcinoma, as in the two tumours of Govan (1945), the diagnosis must be accepted. In the presence of apparent osteo- and chondrosarcoma, the distinction from a metaplastic carcinoma is often difficult and not always objectively possible. The most debatable cases are those in which the 'sarcomatous' component is 'fibrosarcoma' and the carcinomatous component is a squamous carcinoma. Many such tumours probably represent spindle-cell carcinomas with a desmoplastic reaction. Some true carcinosarcomas almost certainly arise in pre-existing fibroadenomas or cystosarcomas. But very rarely carcinosarcomas arise in the absence of any evidence of a pre-existing tumour.

Need for Further Study. There is a need for further study of carcinosarcomas, especially any very small ones, in which it is technically easier to study the tumour completely, if necessary by serial section. In this way it will be possible to determine what proportion of these tumours arises in a pre-existing tumour and what proportion arises de novo. It should also be possible to determine the origin of any rhabdomyoblastic tissue, whether found in a sarcoma of the breast, as in the case of Bird (1970), or in carcinosarcomas, as in the two cases of Govan (1945). From what is already known of the versatility of the specialized connective tissue of the breast — the ability to show chondrogenic, osteogenic and especially lipoblastic differentiation — it would not be very surprising if it were found to have rhabdomyoblastic potency also, as indeed appears to be the case from the study of these unusual tumours. What is not known at the moment is whether this unusual degree of versatility is limited mostly or even entirely to the specialized connective tissue of the breast or whether even the ordinary interlobular connective tissue participates in the process.

A Special Type of Carcinosarcoma

A very special type of associated carcinoma and sarcoma of the breast is that described by Seemayer, Tremblay and Shibata (1975). In this unique case stromal sarcoma was associated with intraductal carcinoma. This case report is a model of how a tumour of great complexity should be documented to achieve credibility.

CARCINOMA AND SARCOMA SITUATED CONTIGUOUSLY

The presence within the same breast of both carcinoma and sarcoma should be distinguished from carcinosarcoma. This subject is discussed by Wester and Finlay-Jones (1960). They cite nine cases in the old and four cases in the more recent literature. In their own patient, a 35-year-old Papuan woman, carcinoma and osteogenic sarcoma were contiguous but distinct, and separated by a fairly well-defined fibrous barrier; there was no intermingling of the sarcomatous and carcinomatous elements. A very similar case of osteosarcoma and chondrosarcoma occurring contiguously with infiltrating carcinoma is Case 1 of Robb and MacFarlane (1958).

References

Amerson, J. R. (1970) Cystosarcoma phyllodes in adolescent females. A report of seven patients. *Annals of Surgery,* **171,** 849–858.

Anderson, D. K. and Kafrouni, G. I. (1972) Mammary liposarcoma. *International Surgery,* **57,** 67–69.

Ashikari, R., Farrow, J. H. and O'Hara, J. (1971) Fibroadenomas in the breast of juveniles. *Surgery, Gynecology and Obstetrics,* **132,** 259–262.

Bader, E. and Isaacson, C. (1960) Bilateral malignant cystosarcoma phyllodes. *British Journal of Surgery,* **48,** 519–521.

Barnes, L. and Pietruszka, M. (1977) Sarcomas of the breast. A clinicopathologic analysis of ten cases. *Cancer,* **40,** 1577–1585.

Berg, J. W., Decosse, J. J., Fracchia, A. A. and Farrow, J. (1962) Stromal sarcomas of the breast. *Cancer,* **15,** 418–424.

Bird, C. C. (1970) A breast sarcoma containing rhabdomyosarcomatous and other metaplastic elements. *Journal of Pathology,* **101,** 286–288.

Blichert-Toft, M., Hansen, J. P. H., Hansen, O. H. and Schiødt, T. (1975) Clinical course of cystosarcoma phyllodes related to histologic appearance. *Surgery, Gynecology and Obstetrics,* **140,** 929–932.

Cameron, H. M., Hamperl, H. and Warambo, W. (1974) Leiomyosarcoma of the breast originating from myothelium (myoepithelium). *Journal of Pathology,* **114,** 89–92.

Cooper, W. G., Jr and Ackerman, L. V. (1943) Cystosarcoma phyllodes with a consideration of its more malignant variant. *Surgery, Gynecology and Obstetrics,* **77,** 279–283.

Cornog, J. L., Mobini, J., Steiger, E. and Enterline, H. T. (1971) Squamous carcinoma of the breast. *American Journal of Clinical Pathology,* **55,** 410–417.

DeCosse, J. J., Berg, J. W., Fracchia, A. A. and Farrow, J. H. (1962) Primary lymphosarcoma of the breast. A review of 14 cases. *Cancer,* **15,** 1264–1268.

De Navasquez, S. and Horton, R. E. (1947) Liposarcoma of the breast. *Guy's Hospital Reports,* **96,** 57–59.

Dunegan, L. J., Tobon, H. and Watson, C. G. (1976) Angiosarcoma of the breast: a report of two cases and a review of the literature. *Surgery,* **79,** 57–59.

Edwards, A. T. and Kellett, H. S. (1968) Haemangiosarcoma of breast. *Journal of Pathology and Bacteriology,* **95,** 457–459.

Evans, R. W. (1966) *Histological Appearances of Tumours.* Second edition. p. 810. London: E. & S. Livingstone.

Fernandez, B. B., Hernandez, F. J. and Spindler, W. (1976) Metastatic cystosarcoma phyllodes. A light and electron microscopic study. *Cancer,* **37,** 1737–1746.

Freedman, S. I., Kagan, A. R. and Friedman, N. B. (1971) Bilaterality in primary lymphosarcoma of the breast. *American Journal of Clinical Pathology,* **55,** 82–87.

Freeman, C., Berg, J. W. and Cutler, S. J. (1972) Occurrence and prognosis of extranodal lymphomas. *Cancer,* **29,** 252–260.

Gibbs, B. F., Jr, Roe, R. D. and Thomas, D. F. (1968) Malignant cystosarcoma phyllodes in a pre-pubertal female. *Annals of Surgery,* **167,** 229–231.

Gogas, J. G. and Kotsianos, G. (1977) Angiosarcoma of the breast. *International Surgery,* **62,** 144–145.

Govan, A. D. T. (1945) Two cases of mixed malignant tumour of the breast. *Journal of Pathology and Bacteriology,* **56,** 397–404.

Gulesserian, H. P. and Lawton, R. L. (1969) Angiosarcoma of the breast. *Cancer,* **24,** 1021–1026.

Haagensen, C. D. (1971) *Diseases of the Breast.* Second edition — revised reprint. pp. 235, 236, 238, 244–249. Philadelphia, London, Toronto: W. B. Saunders.

Hafner, C. D., Mezcer, E. and Wylie, J. H., Jr (1962) Cystosarcoma phyllodes of the breast. *Surgery, Gynecology and Obstetrics,* **115,** 29–34.

Hajdu, S. I., Espinosa, M. H. and Robbins, G. F. (1976) Recurrent cystosarcoma phyllodes. A clinicopathologic study of 32 cases. *Cancer,* **38,** 1402–1406.

Halverson, J. D. and Hori-Rubaina, J. M. (1974) Cystosarcoma phyllodes of the breast. *American Surgeon,* **40,** 295–301.

Hamperl, H. (1970) The myothelia (myoepithelial cells). In *Current Topics in Pathology,* Vol. 53. Berlin: Springer-Verlag.

Harris, M. and Persaud, V. (1974) Carcinosarcoma of the breast. *Journal of Pathology,* **112,** 99–105.

Hart, W. R., Bauer, R. C. and Oberman, H. A. (1978) Cystosarcoma phyllodes. A clinicopathologic study of twenty-six hypercellular periductal stromal tumors of the breast. *American Journal of Clinical Pathology,* **70,** 211–216.

Hines, J. R., Gordon, R. T., Widger, C. and Kolb, T. (1976) Cystosarcoma phyllodes metastatic to a Brenner tumor of the ovary. *Archives of Surgery,* **111,** 299–300.

Hoover, H. C., Trestioreanu, A. and Ketcham, A. S. (1975) Metastatic cystosarcoma phylloides in an adolescent girl: an unusually malignant tumor. *Annals of Surgery,* **181,** 279–282.

Horne, W. I. and Percival, W. L. (1975) Hemangiosarcoma of the breast. *Canadian Journal of Surgery,* **18,** 81–84.

Hummer, C. D., Jr and Burkart, T. J. (1967) Liposarcoma of the breast. A case of bilateral involvement. *American Journal of Surgery,* **113,** 558–561.

Jackson, A. V. (1962) Metastasising liposarcoma of the breast arising in a fibro-adenoma. *Journal of Pathology and Bacteriology,* **83,** 582–584.

Jernstrom, P. and Sether, J. M. (1967) Primary lymphosarcoma of the mammary gland. *Journal of the American Medical Association,* **201,** 93–96.

Jernstrom, P., Lindberg, A. L. and Meland, O. N. (1963) Osteogenic sarcoma of the mammary gland. *American Journal of Clinical Pathology,* **40,** 521–526.

Jones, E. L. (1969) Primary squamous-cell carcinoma of breast with pseudosarcomatous stroma. *Journal of Pathology,* **97,** 383–385.

Kahn, L. B., Uys, C. J., Dale, J. and Rutherfoord, F. (1978) Carcinoma of the breast with metaplasia to chondrosarcoma: a light and electron microscopic study. *Histopathology,* **2,** 93–106.

Kennedy, T. and Biggart, J. D. (1967) Sarcoma of the breast. *British Journal of Cancer,* **21,** 635–644.

Kessinger, A., Folcy, J. F., Lemon, H. M. and Miller, D. D. (1972) Metastatic cystosarcoma phyllodes. a case report and review of the literature. *Journal of Surgical Oncology,* **4,** 131–147.

Kessler, E. and Kozenitzky, I. L. (1971) Haemangiosarcoma of breast. *Journal of Clinical Pathology,* **24,** 530–532.

Lattes, R. (1967) Sarcomas of the breast. *Journal of the American Medical Association,* **201,** 531–532.

Lawler, M. R. and Richie, R. E. (1967) Reticulum-cell sarcoma of the breast. *Cancer,* **20,** 1438–1446.

Lee, B. J. and Pack, G. T. (1931) Giant intracanalicular myxoma of the breast. *Annals of Surgery,* **93,** 250–286.

Lester, J. and Stout, A. P. (1954) Cystosarcoma phyllodes. *Cancer,* **7,** 335–353.

Long, R. T. L., Hesker, A. E. and Johnson, R. E. (1962) Surgical management of cystosarcoma phyllodes: with a report of eight cases. *Missouri Medicine,* **59,** 1179–1181.

Lubin, J. and Rywlin, A. M. (1972) Cystosarcoma phyllodes metastasizing as a mixed mesenchymal sarcoma. *Southern Medical Journal,* **65,** 636–637.

Massé. W. R., Mongeau, C. J. and Rioux, A. (1977) Angiosarcoma of the breast. *Canadian Journal of Surgery,* **20,** 341–343.

McClanahan, B. J. and Hogg, L. Jr (1954) Angiosarcoma of the breast. *Cancer,* **7,** 586–594.

McCullough, K. and Lynch, J. M. (1960) Metastatic sarcoma of heart from cystosarcoma phyllodes of the breast. *Maryland State Medical Journal,* **9,** 66–68.

McDivitt, R. W., Stewart, F. W. and Berg, J. W. (1968) *Tumors of the Breast.* Atlas of Tumor Pathology,

Second series, Fascicle 2. Washington, D.C.: Armed Forces Institute of Pathology.

McDivitt, R. W., Urban, J. A. and Farrow, J. H. (1967) Cystosarcoma phyllodes. *Johns Hopkins Medical Journal,* **120,** 33–45.

McDonald, J. R. and Harrington, S. W. (1950) Giant fibro-adenoma of the breast — 'cystosarcoma phyllodes'. *Annals of Surgery,* **131,** 243–251.

Menon, M. and van Velthoven, P. C. M. (1974) Liposarcoma of the breast. A case report. *Archives of Pathology,* **98,** 370–372.

Minkowitz, S., Zeichner, M., Di Maio, V. and Nicastri, A. D. (1968) Cystosarcoma phyllodes: a unique case with multiple unilateral lesions and ipsilateral axillary metastasis. *Journal of Pathology and Bacteriology,* **96,** 514–517.

Myerowitz, R. L., Pietruszka, M. and Barnes, E. L. (1978) Primary angiosarcoma of the breast. (Letter.) *Journal of the American Medical Association,* **239,** 403.

Naryshkin, G. and Redfield, E. S. (1964) Malignant cystosarcoma phyllodes of the breast in adolescence, with subsequent pregnancy. Report of a case with endocrinologic studies. *Obstetrics and Gynecology,* **23,** 140–142.

Norris, H. J. and Taylor, H. B. (1967) Relationship of histologic features to behavior of cystosarcoma phyllodes. Analysis of ninety-four cases. *Cancer,* **20,** 2090–2099.

Norris, H. J. and Taylor, H. B. (1968) Sarcomas and related mesenchymal tumors of the breast. *Cancer,* **22,** 22–28.

Notley, R. G. and Griffiths, H. J. L. (1965) Bilateral malignant cystosarcoma phyllodes. *British Journal of Surgery,* **52,** 360–362.

Oberman, H. A. (1965) Cystosarcoma phyllodes. A clinicopathologic study of hypercellular periductal stromal neoplasms of breast. *Cancer,* **18,** 697–710.

Oberman, H. A., Nosanchuk, J. S. and Finger, J. E. (1969) Periductal stromal tumors of breast with adipose metaplasia. *Archives of Surgery,* **98,** 384–387.

Pantoja, E., Llobet, R. E. and Lopez, E. (1976) Gigantic cystosarcoma phyllodes in a man with gynaecomastia. *Archives of Surgery,* **111,** 611.

Pardo-Mindan, J., Garcia-Julian, G. and Altuna, M. E. (1974) Leiomyosarcoma of the breast. Report of a case. *American Journal of Clinical Pathology,* **62,** 477–480.

Philip, P. J. (1976) Carcinosarcoma of the breast. *Proceedings of the Royal College of Surgeons of Edinburgh,* **21,** 229–232.

Pietruszka, M. and Barnes, L. (1978) Cystosarcoma phyllodes. A Clinicopathologic analysis of 42 cases. *Cancer,* **41,** 1974–1983.

Proctor, N. S. F., Rippey, J. J., Shulman, G. and Cohen, C. (1975) Extramedullary plasmacytoma of the breast. *Journal of Pathology,* **116,** 97–100.

Qizilbash, A. H. (1976) Cystosarcoma phyllodes with liposarcomatous stroma. *American Journal of Clinical Pathology,* **65,** 321–327.

Reich, T. and Solomon, C. (1958) Bilateral cystosarcoma phyllodes, malignant variant, with a 14-year followup. A case report. *Annals of Surgery,* **147,** 39–43.

Reingold, I. M. and Ascher, G. S. (1970) Cystosarcoma phyllodes in a man with gynecomastia. *American Journal of Clinical Pathology,* **53,** 852–856.

Rhodes, R. H., Frankel, K. A., Davis, L. and Tatter, D. (1978) Metastatic cystosarcoma phyllodes. A report of 2 cases presenting with neurological symptoms. *Cancer,* **41,** 1179–1187.

Rix, D. B., Tredwell, S. J. and Forward, A. D. (1971) Cystosarcoma phylloides (cellular intracanalicular fibroadenoma): clinical-pathological relationships. *Canadian Journal of Surgery,* **14,** 31–37.

Robb, P. M. and McFarlane, A. (1958) Two rare breast tumours. *Journal of Pathology and Bacteriology,* **75,** 293–298.

Rosen, P. P. and Urban, J. A. (1975) Coexistent mammary carcinoma and cystosarcoma phyllodes. *Breast,* **1,** 9–15.

Ross, C. F. and Eley, A. (1975) Lymphosarcoma of the breast. *British Journal of Surgery,* **62,** 651–652.

Rottino, A. and Howley, C. P. (1945) Osteoid sarcoma of the breast: a complication of fibroadenoma. *Archives of Pathology,* **40,** 44–50.

Scarff, R. W. and Torloni, H. (1968) *Histological Typing of Breast Tumours.* International Histological Classification of Tumours No. 2. Geneva: World Health Organization.

Seemayer, T. A., Tremblay, G. and Shibata, H. (1975) The unique association of mammary stromal sarcoma with intraductal carcinoma. *Cancer,* **36,** 599–605.

Smith, B. G. and Taylor, H. B. (1969) The occurrence of bone and cartilage in mammary tumors. *American Journal of Clinical Pathology,* **51,** 610–618.

Smithy, H. G. and Charleston, S. C. (1944) Mixed malignancy of the breast. Case report of a combined carcinoma and sarcoma in a child, with review of the literature. *Surgery,* **16,** 854–864.

Steingaszner, L. C., Enzinger, F. M. and Taylor, H. B. (1965) Hemangiosarcoma of the breast. *Cancer,* **18,** 352–361.

Stewart, F. W. (1950) *Tumors of the Breast.* Atlas of Tumor Pathology, Section 9, Fascicle 34. pp. 75–87. Washinton, D.C.: Armed Forces Institute of Pathology.

Stout, A. P. and Bernanke, M. (1946) Liposarcoma of the female mammary gland. *Surgery, Gynecology and Obstetrics,* **83,** 216.

Stringer, P. (1959) Reticulosarcoma of both breasts. *British Journal of Surgery,* **47,** 51–52.

Treves, N. (1964) A study of cystosarcoma phyllodes. *Annals of the New York Academy of Sciences,* **114,** 922–936.

Treves, N. and Sunderland, D. A. (1951) Cystosarcoma phyllodes of the breast: a malignant and a benign tumor. A clinicopathological study of seventy-seven cases. *Cancer,* **4,** 1286–1332.

von Bomhard, D. and von Sandersleben, J. (1974) Über die Feinstruktur von Mammamischtumoren der Hündin. II. Das Vorkommen von Myoepithelzellen in chondroiden Arealen. *Virchows Archiv A: Pathological Anatomy and Histology,* **362,** 157–167.

Wayte, D. M., Stewart, J. B. and McKenzie, C. G. (1970) A composite malignant tumour of the elderly female breast. *Journal of Clinical Pathology,* **23,** 414–422.

West, T. L., Weiland, L. H. and Clagett, O. T. (1971) Cystosarcoma phyllodes. *Annals of Surgery,* **173,** 520–528.

Wester, J. G. and Finlay-Jones, L. R. (1960) Osteogenic sarcoma of the breast. *Tropical and Geographical Medicine,* **12,** 222–228.

Willis, R. A. (1958) Squamous-cell mammary carcinoma of predominantly fibrosarcoma-like structure. *Journal of Pathology and Bacteriology,* **76,** 511–515.

Wiseman, C. and Liao, K. T. (1972) Primary lymphoma of the breast. *Cancer,* **29,** 1705–1712.

Chapter Fifteen

Elastosis and Other Connective Tissue Changes

HISTORICAL DEVELOPMENT OF IDEAS

The story of elastosis is a fascinating one. The 'scirrhous' carcinoma has long been known to have yellow streaks and dots on its cut face and its appearance and consistency have been likened to an unripe pear. In much of the modern literature this yellow streaking has been attributed to foci of *necrosis* in the tumour, and the yellow streaks have also been called '*chalky streaks*'. This is puzzling, as the presence of *elastosis* in carcinoma of the breast was known to Cheatle and Cutler (1931) and to Muir and Aitkenhead (1934). However, in the later edition of Cutler's book (1962) all reference to elastic tissue had been deleted, an unfortunate omission as it turned out. Elastic tissue in breast cancer, which has been the source of so much confusion, has even been mistaken for *amyloid*, because of the affinity of the material for Congo red (Bernath, 1952). In the older literature the streaks were attributed to '*fatty degeneration*' (Beattie and Dickson, 1926).

ELASTOSIS AND THE CONCEPT OF DUCTAL 'COLLAPSE'

Jackson and Orr (1957) studied over 400 consecutive breasts removed for carcinoma, including five cases of Paget's disease of the nipple, and they extended their observation to a further three cases of Paget's disease. They showed unequivocally that the '*flecks and streaks of yellow material' consist of elastic tissue* and are not, as often stated, attributable to necrosis. These workers also stressed the frequency of 'subepithelial collagenosis' affecting the ducts. Unfortunately, Jackson and Orr (1957) went further and claimed that the collagenosis and elastosis were not a reaction to the neoplastic epithelium but 'changes developing pari passu with the malignant change in the epithelium and sometimes preceding it'. They also concluded that breast carcinoma usually occupies a volume less, and sometimes considerably less, than that occupied by the normal breast tissue which it has replaced. Whilst this last conclusion is true, and their concept of *a collapse of the mammary duct system to account for ductal crowding* in 'scirrhous'

379

carcinoma is a valid one, few pathologists will agree with their contention that cancer cells do not stimulate a fibrous reaction. By overstating their case Jackson and Orr (1957) would appear to have spoiled their argument. They believed that the ductal stromal changes, when combined with epithelial hyperplasia, represented a precancerous lesion. They were uncertain of the significance of the stromal changes when not associated with epithelial hyperplasia but felt that, even then, the possibility of a precancerous lesion had to be considered.

Jackson and Orr's (1957) factual observations on the stromal changes in the ductal walls were largely correct, though the writer is unaware of any work that confirms or refutes their observation of differences in these changes between different sectors of the breast. Their concept of 'ductal crowding' is both a valid and an important one; on the other hand, their denial that desmoplasia can be a response to cancer is unacceptable. Their weakest argument is their conclusion that the stromal changes are an accompaniment or even a harbinger of malignancy rather than a response to it. Partly perhaps because of the far-reaching practical implications of this last conclusion, which I believe to be erroneous, the valuable observations of Jackson and Orr (1957) have received little attention.

AMYLOID

Meanwhile, in 1952, Bernath had drawn attention to the presence in breast carcinoma of a substance she thought was amyloid on the basis of an affinity for Congo red. It was not at that time widely recognized that Congo red is a tolerably good stain for elastic tissue and that, without the additional use of polaroids, it is not by any means a specific method for amyloid.

Elastosis and 'Amyloid-like Substance'

Lundmark (1972) realized that far too little attention had been paid to elastosis in the breast and he therefore studied the elastic tissue content of a large series of breast cancers. He confirmed the findings of Jackson and Orr (1957) but wisely refrained from drawing any conclusions about the possible significance of the stromal changes as a

precursor of cancer. He found that no elastin was demonstrable after treatment with elastase, though he noted the presence of a faintly visible residual material 'resembling amyloid'. Lundmark (1972) appears to have been influenced by the work of Sümegi and Rajka (1972), who described an 'amyloid-like substance surrounding mammary cancer and basal cell carcinoma'. These workers unfortunately lumped together two very different tumours in their study. Basal cell carcinomas of the skin frequently contain amyloid, and we have found small amyloid deposits in 50 per cent of basal cell carcinomas, and larger amounts of amyloid in 10 per cent of these skin tumours (Sloane and Azzopardi, 1977). On the other hand, the 'hyaline' material in breast cancers is not amyloid and the coining of the term 'elastic amyloid' by Sümegi and Rajka (1972) has not clarified the subject. *The spectre of amyloid in breast cancer* had raised its head again. Carstens et al (1972), in an otherwise excellent study of tubular carcinoma of the breast, claimed to have found amyloid in the stroma of 21 of their 35 cases. They used Congo red staining and detected apple-green anomalous colours with polarized light, a finding which the writer has been unable to confirm. Tremblay (1974) also refuted the suggestion that amyloid is present in breast cancer and confirmed that the material is elastic tissue by means of elastase digestion and by ultrastructural studies. The latter showed electron-lucent amorphous cores fringed by microfibrils. Schiødt et al (1972), in a detailed tinctorial, enzymatic and ultrastructural study, reached the same conclusion. Tobon and Salazar (1977) found no amyloid in tubular carcinoma of the breast.

CHALKY STREAKS

In the past the writer, like most others, had been led to believe that the yellow streaks of the common 'scirrhous' represented either foci of necrosis or 'chalky streaks'. The latter term was curious because there appeared to be no reason for calcium deposits to appear yellow to the naked eye. Staining showed that in fact the yellow streaks were devoid of calcium in the vast majority of cases, a conclusion also reached by Levitan, Witten and Harrison (1964), who, while correlating a microscopical study of breast calcification with mammographic studies, noted that calcium was absent in the zone which they termed periductal 'hyalinized fibrosis' and which is now known to consist of elastic tissue.

NECROSIS

Superficially the notion that the yellow streaks represented necrosis had a little more to commend it, since necrotic tissues often have a yellowish tinge. However, close inspection of the yellow flecks and streaks shows that they are smooth rather than granular, are always sharply delineated and are thus unlike necrotic tissue in appearance; furthermore, they are centred on a smooth-lined cavity which appears as a circular or elliptical ring, or as a linear slit, depending on the plane of sectioning. Most of these observations had already been made by Jackson and Orr (1957) though, for various reasons, they were forgotten or ignored. The view that the yellow streaks represent amyloid does not stand up to even superficial scrutiny.

Amyloid is translucent and 'waxy', and not opaque and yellow.

CORRELATION OF ELASTOSIS WITH DURATION OF SURVIVAL

Shivas and Douglas (1972) devised a very simple and easily reproducible 'elastica index' and related it to duration of survival in patients treated by local mastectomy and radiotherapy, all of whom had died from metastatic disease. The mean survival in their 0, +, ++ and +++ groups (defined and illustrated) was 33.5, 70.7, 75.0 and 93.7 months respectively. The Pearson correlation ratio was 0.2395 with a significance level of 0.8 per cent. The same trend was found in patients with metastatic disease at the time of presentation who were treated by simple mastectomy and adrenalectomy. Shivas and Douglas (1972) did not regard the focal elastosis as corresponding to pre-existing

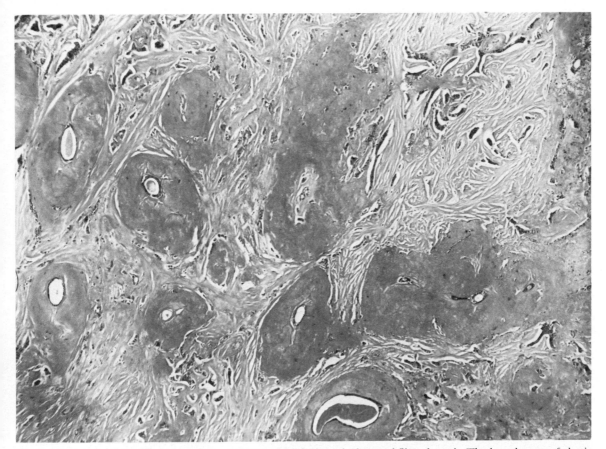

Figure 15–1   A typical infiltrating ductal carcinoma which had marked central fibroelastosis. The broad zones of elastic tissue cuffing otherwise normal ducts are clearly visible. The ducts are closely congregated because of 'collapse' caused by preceding necrosis. H and E. ×60.

structures because of the very close aggregation of the elastic foci in tumours with a high
elastica index. However, they did not allow for
the 'collapse of the duct system' as described
by Jackson and Orr (1957) nor for the fact that
elastic tissue survives when necrosis and its
consequences have caused other tissues to
disappear. Shivas and Douglas (1972) also
postulated that the elastica is probably directly
produced by the malignant cells.

ELASTOSIS OF MAJOR DUCTS IN CARCINOMATOUS AND NON-CARCINOMATOUS BREASTS

Davies (1973), in a detailed and careful
study, found that *the incidence of elastosis and
fibrosis in the major ducts of the nipple does not
differ significantly between carcinomatous breasts,
on the one hand, and both normal, as well as
pathological but non-malignant, breasts on the
other.* This constitutes a convincing rebuttal of
one of the more sweeping conclusions of
Jackson and Orr (1957).

ELASTOSIS IN PRIMARY BREAST CARCINOMA

We investigated a consecutive series of 115
cases of infiltrating breast carcinoma (Azzopardi and Laurini, 1974) and fully confirmed

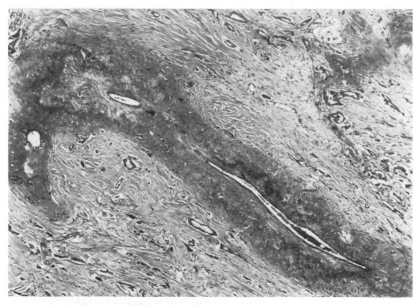

Figure 15–2 A dense zone of
elastosis around a duct containing
non-neoplastic epithelium. H and
E. ×55.

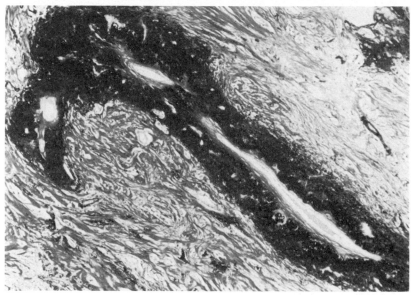

Figure 15–3 The same tissue as
shown in Figure 15–2 stained for
elastica. Weigert elastic and HVG.
×55.

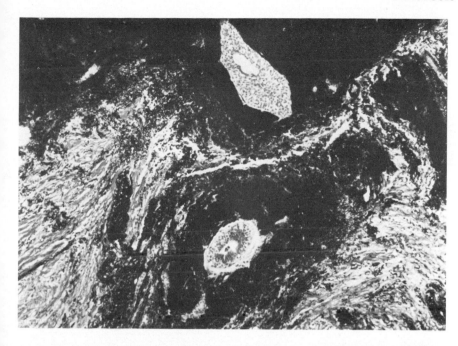

Figure 15–4 Gross elastosis in an invasive carcinoma. There is massive elastosis surrounding ducts containing neoplastic epithelium. Weigert elastic and HVG. ×105.

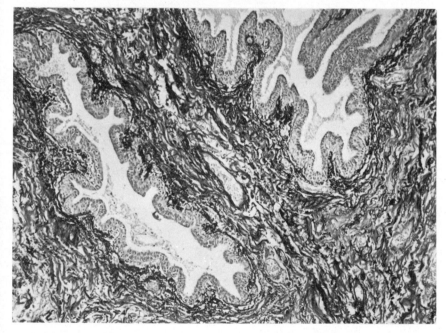

Figure 15–5 Normal lactiferous sinuses from the breast of a 54-year-old postmenopausal woman. Weigert elastic and HVG. ×105.

the findings of Jackson and Orr (1957) regarding the elastic nature of the yellow streaks of 'scirrhous' cancer (Figures 15–1 to 15–4). *Elastosis was found in about 90 per cent of infiltrating ductal and infiltrating lobular carcinomas,* an identical figure to that obtained by Shivas and Douglas (1972), and somewhat higher than that recorded by Lundmark (1972). Like Lundmark (1972), we found no difference in the incidence of elastosis between infiltrating ductal and infiltrating

lobular carcinoma. It should be stressed that *elastosis is much less marked in medullary carcinoma* and some other circumscribed carcinomas.

FOCAL ELASTOSIS

Elastosis takes two main forms, focal and diffuse. The focal form is mainly in a *periductal* location (Figures 15–1 to 15–6), and the rounded, ovoid or linear slits identifiable

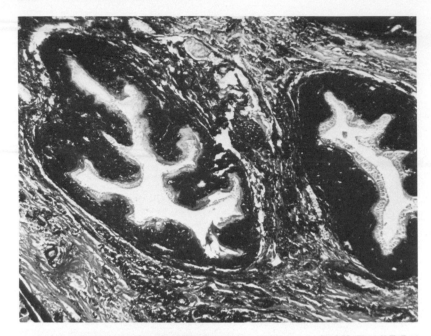

Figure 15–6 Lactiferous sinuses with marked elastosis from the breast of a 52-year-old postmenopausal woman with an infiltrating carcinoma involving this area. Weigert elastic and HVG. ×105.

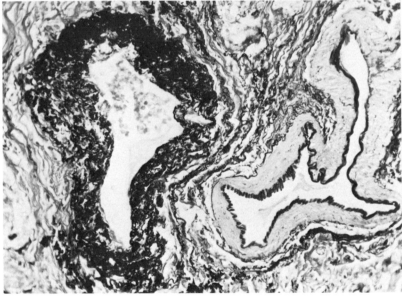

Figure 15–7 Venous elastosis compared with an unaffected artery in an infiltrating carcinoma. Weigert elastic and HVG. ×230.

macroscopically correspond most frequently to ductal lumina. We amply confirmed Jackson and Orr's (1957) findings in this regard and disagree with Shivas and Douglas (1972), who maintained that the dense aggregates of focal elastosis do not correspond to pre-existing structures. The confusion has arisen because the pre-existing structures are brought much closer together by the pathological process itself, as already described (Figure 15–1). Focal elastosis also affects *blood vessels,* both arteries and veins being involved and *venous elastosis occurring more often than arterial* (Figure 15–7). Venous elastosis can be so gross that the lumen of the vessel is reduced to a narrow slit and may be invisible in a given plane of sectioning; in such cases step sections may be necessary to demonstrate the vascular lumen (Figure 15–9). This explains why venous elastosis has been missed in the past, not because it was insignificant, but, on the contrary, because it was frequently so massive that the observer remained unaware that he was dealing with the wall of a blood vessel (Figures 15–9 and 15–10). Venous elastosis is more marked than arterial elastosis probably because of the flow differences that obtain both in the walls and in the lumina of the two types of vessel. While most of the slits seen with the naked eye within the elastotic streaks represent ductal lumina, some of the smaller ones represent vascular lumina. *Focal elastosis*, therefore, *affects mainly if not exclusively pre-existing structures* already endowed with elastic tissue. These findings have been confirmed by Adnet et al (1976).

DIFFUSE ELASTOSIS

In addition to focal elastosis, we also found a diffuse type of elastic tissue increase in the stroma (Azzopardi and Laurini, 1974). While some of this might be due to the disruption of pre-existing structures, the profusion of the elastic fibres seen in some cases with diffuse elastosis strongly suggests that elastic fibre is also produced at sites where previously little or none had been present.

ORIGIN OF ELASTIC TISSUE

Infiltrating cancer cells stimulate periductal fibroblasts, and smooth muscle cells and possibly other cells in vascular walls, to synthesize elastic fibre resulting in focal elastosis. The origin of the more diffuse deposits of elastic tissue is debatable. They are probably produced by stromal fibroblasts, which, in normal circumstances, are not engaged in elastic fibre production but which are potentially capable of doing so given the right stimulus. Alternatively, some of these elastic fibres may be produced by myofibroblasts which have been demonstrated in the stroma of infiltrating carcinomas (Ahmed, 1974). The suggestion by Shivas and Douglas (1972) that elastica is produced directly by the neoplastic cells themselves is an intriguing one which has yet to be substantiated.

ULTRASTRUCTURE OF ELASTOSIS

Tremblay (1976) investigated the ultra-structure of elastosis in breast carcinoma. He dissected out the yellowish streaks and flecks of tissue apparent on the cut surface and confirmed that they were composed predominantly of material which stained intensely with elastic tissue stains. He thus established a method for providing fresh material for ultrastructural study. Tremblay (1976) found that the dissected fragments were composed of elastic fibres that varied markedly in size. The fibres consisted of a core of amorphous material and a peripheral mantle of micro-fibrils, the two characteristic constituents of elastic fibres, and the variations in the relative proportions of the two constituents suggested that the elastic fibres were at different stages of maturation.

Active Fibroblasts. Tremblay (1976) further found cells with the features of 'active fibroblasts' interspersed among the elastic fibres. The striking features were the abundant rough endoplasmic reticulum, often with distended cisternae, large and often multiple Golgi complexes and, frequently, numerous cytoplasmic filaments. These are known features of fibroblasts engaged in the synthesis of both collagen and elastic fibres. These and other findings collectively suggested that, in periductal elastosis, the cells responsible for the synthesis of elastic fibres are fibroblasts, supporting the view of Azzopardi and Laurini (1974).

On the other hand, while not excluding entirely the possibility that the neoplastic cells are *directly* involved in the formation of elastic fibres, as suggested by Douglas and Shivas (1974), Tremblay (1976) regarded this suggestion as unlikely in view of the general paucity of rough endoplasmic reticulum found in the tumour cells present in the elastotic zones.

Tremblay (1976), in agreement with Azzopardi and Laurini (1974), maintained that the hypothesis that breast carcinoma tumour cells induce periductal fibroblasts to overproduce elastic tissue can be extended to explain a similar effect on smooth muscle cells and fibroblasts in vascular walls.

Cells Responsible for Synthesis of Elastic Tissue. This study by Tremblay demonstrated unequivocally that at the ultrastructural level the yellow streaks are composed chiefly of elastic fibres. More importantly, perhaps, it provided *independent evidence that the elasto-genesis in these tumours is probably the result of synthesis of elastic tissue by the two types of mesenchymal cell which are normally capable of forming elastic fibres*, viz. fibroblasts and smooth muscle cells, and that the role of the cancer cells is probably an indirect one.

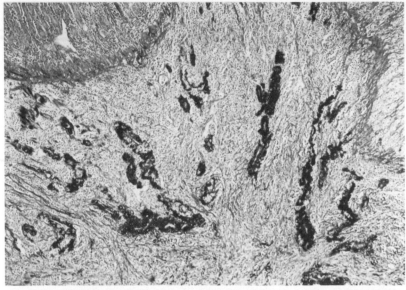

Figure 15–8 A metastasis in the jejunum from a primary breast carcinoma. The muscularis mucosae is visible as a curved narrow band. There is marked vascular elastosis in the submucosa. This patient had a mastectomy for carcinoma 13 years previously without evidence of recurrence in the interval. Weigert elastic and HVG. ×55.

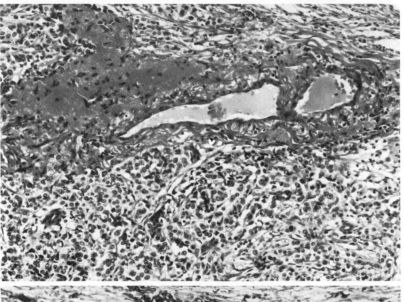

Figure 15–9 From the same case illustrated in Figure 15–8. There is arterial elastosis but the most striking elastosis, producing a sausage-shaped mass adjacent to the artery, is in the accompanying vein. The venous lumen is reduced to a minute chink. H and E. ×120.

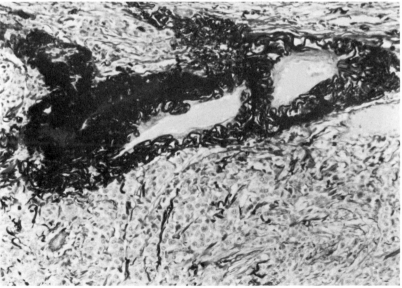

Figure 15–10 From the same tissue as Figure 15–9. The venous elastosis is so marked that identification of the structure as a vein is less easy than in the preceding figure. Weigert elastic and HVG. ×120.

ELASTOSIS IN METASTATIC DEPOSITS OF BREAST
CARCINOMA

To date, elastosis has been described only in
primary breast carcinomas. In preliminary
studies Masters et al (1976) found that little or
no elastosis is present in metastatic deposits.
Our own studies indicate that metastatic
deposits from breast carcinoma do show
elastosis (Figures 15–8 to 15–10), though
rarely in very large amounts, and certainly
never in the massive amounts found in 23 per
cent of primary lesions by Shivas and Douglas
(1972) and in 17 per cent by us (Azzopardi and
Laurini, 1974). We observed that *metastases in
such sites as the gut and the pancreas show
elastosis more frequently* than hepatic and
osseous secondaries (Azzopardi and Laurini,
1975). The elastosis in metastatic deposits
occurs almost exclusively in sites and
structures already endowed with elastic fibres
(Figures 15–8 to 15–10). Vascular and
predominantly venous elastosis is seen quite
frequently (Figures 15–9 and 15–10). Lymphatic elastosis is uncommon and inconspicuous, but we have identified it adjacent to
axillary lymph nodes on rare occasions. In
addition, we observed hyperplasia of the fine
elastic network associated with the muscularis
mucosae in the gastrointestinal tract, as well as
an increase of elastic tissue in the wall of
pancreatic ducts. The last two observations
partly explain why elastosis is commoner with
metastases in the gut and the pancreas than in,
say, the liver. But the apparently greater
frequency of vascular elastosis in the gut
compared with other organs requires some
other explanation.

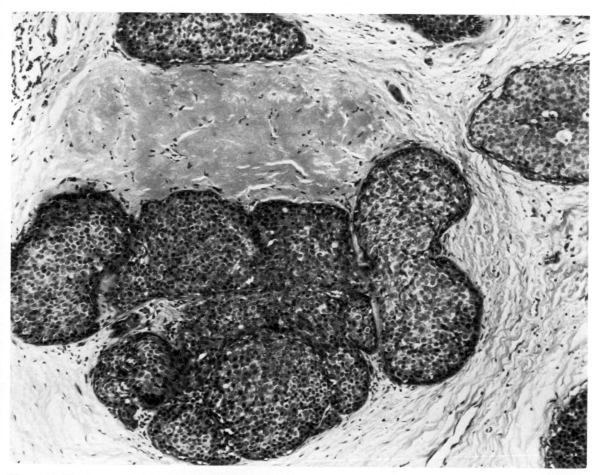

Figure 15–11 A cancerized lobule and small parts of others. A broad column of elastosis lies alongside the cancerized
lobule. It proved to be venous elastosis on deeper sectioning. Such a localized zone of elastosis in the presence of in situ
carcinoma is suspicious and warrants a search for a cause. Deeper levels of an adjacent field of tissue revealed the changes
shown in Figures 15–12 and 15–13. H and E. ×150.

ELASTOSIS IN OTHER PRIMARY CARCINOMAS

Preliminary observations of 20 colonic carcinomas by the writer indicate that venous elastosis does occur to some degree in primary cancer of the large bowel. *Elastosis as a phenomenon is, therefore, not specific to mammary malignancies.* Its prominence in primary breast cancer is attributable to the specialized anatomical structure of the ductal system and to certain characteristics of the mode of development and growth pattern of 'scirrhous' carcinoma.

THE SIGNIFICANCE OF ELASTOSIS

ELASTOSIS WITH INFILTRATING CARCINOMA

The views of other workers on the significance of elastosis in breast cancer have been summarized elsewhere (Azzopardi and Laurini, 1974). We are in agreement with Bonser, Dossett and Jull (1961) that ductal elastosis in malignant disease is most frequently the result of infiltrating carcinoma acting from without; thus, ducts showing marked elastosis contain epithelium which may be normal, hyperplastic but benign, or malignant (Figures 15–1 to 15–4 and 15–6). The localization of the ducts involved is generally related to the proximity of infiltrating cancer cells around them and we would extend this interpretation to explain the histogenesis of venous elastosis.

ELASTOSIS WITH PURE OR APPARENTLY PURE DUCTAL CARCINOMA IN SITU

Because of these findings, Bonser, Dossett and Jull (1961) interpreted elastosis accompanying intraductal carcinoma as an indication of infiltration by tumour. The writer only partially shares this view because studies of a few adequately sampled in situ ductal carcinomas with a cuff of surrounding increased elastica failed to reveal any signs of tumour

invasion. Martinez-Hernandez, Francis and Silverberg (1977) confirmed this finding at the ultrastructural level. The high microfibril content suggested that the elastic tissue was recently secreted. To this extent the writer is in agreement with the findings of Muir and Aitkenhead (1934) and of Jackson and Orr (1957) that *elastosis does not, therefore, always signify infiltration.* On the other hand, elastosis, and especially *a focus of localized elastosis, may well be an indicator that infiltration by malignant cells has occurred* (Figures 15–11 to 15–13). To this extent the writer is in agreement with Bonser, Dossett and Jull (1961). I have now seen nine cases in which a localized focus of elastosis accompanying in situ carcinoma drew attention to the presence of microscopic infiltration, identifiable either in the original sections or on step-sectioning of the block (Figures 15–11 to 15–13). When it is realized that these nine cases have been collected over approximately 12 years, it will be appreciated that this is not a frequent occurrence. Nevertheless, localized elastosis is definitely useful as *a potential indicator of invasion* in a lesion which might otherwise be regarded as an exclusively in situ malignancy.

ELASTOSIS IN THE ABSENCE OF MALIGNANCY

The next problem to be considered is the circumstances in which elastosis occurs in the absence of malignancy. The work of Jackson and Orr (1957) gave rise to the view that elastosis combined with epithelial hyperplasia was a precancerous lesion. As already mentioned, they went so far as to suggest that elastosis and 'subepithelial collagenosis' of ducts might be precancerous even in the absence of epithelial hyperplasia. When the scope of their study and its thoroughness was taken into account, their views obviously deserved serious consideration. The writer therefore felt obliged to study the elastic content and distribution in several hundred breast specimens. The contention of Jackson and Orr (1957) that elastosis can be equated with malignancy or, at any rate, with a precancerous state must be categorically

Figure 15–12 (*Opposite, above.*) Parts of cancerized lobules with both solid and comedo patterns. The elastosis visible centrally is accompanied by spikes of infiltrating carcinoma cells. H and E. ×150.

Figure 15–13 (*Opposite, below.*) From the same tissue as Figure 15–12. There is severe elastosis in the infiltrating zone. Weigert elastic and HVG. ×150.

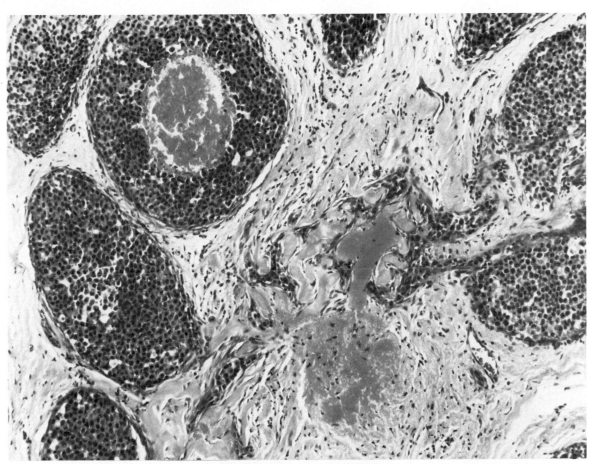

15-12

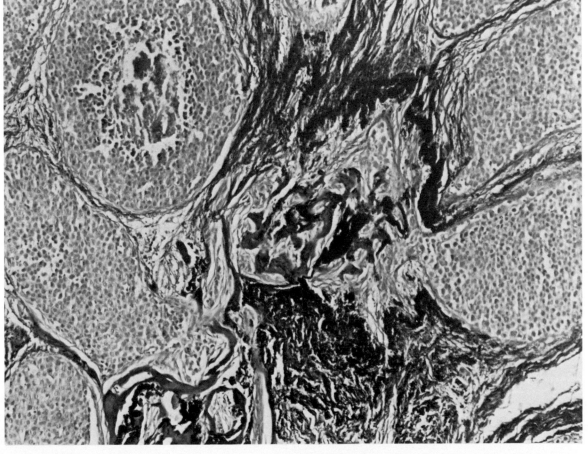

15-13

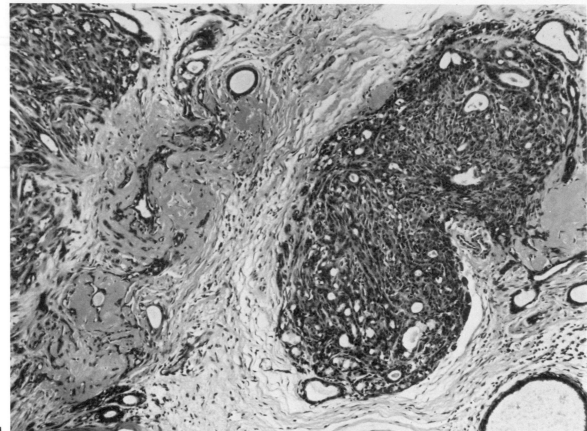

15–14

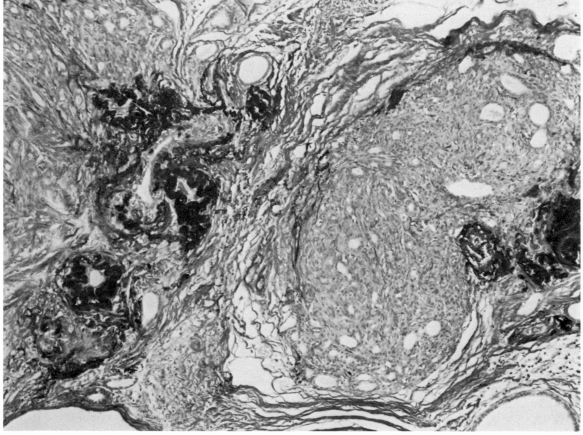

15–15

rejected. It has already been indicated that Davies (1973) showed this to be quite untrue as far as the large ducts of the nipple are concerned. The writer has found that *elastosis may be present in a variety of benign breast diseases and that its presence, with or without collagenosis, cannot be equated with malignancy.* Nor is there any concrete evidence that it is, in any sense, precancerous.

ELASTOSIS IN BENIGN DISEASES

In most purely lobular diseases, e.g. fibroadenoma and pure cystic disease, there is little or no elastic tissue, a finding in keeping with the normal anatomy of the lobule. With ruptured tension cysts, a trivial or small amount of elastic tissue may accompany the fibrous stromal response which is usually present. In classical *sclerosing adenosis* there may be little or no elastic tissue, but in some cases moderate amounts of elastic tissue are discernible (Figures 15–14 and 15–15). *Epitheliosis* is usually not accompanied by significant fibrosis or elastosis, but there are exceptions in which both fibrosis and elastosis may be found. Moreover, in the type of disease related to sclerosing adenosis and described earlier under the heading of '*infiltrating epitheliosis*', moderate or even severe elastosis is frequently present and this is accompanied by varying amounts of fibrosis. The conclusion of Martinez-Hernandez, Francis and Silverberg (1977) that sclerosing adenosis is not accompanied by elastosis was based on a study of a single case and is not acceptable. Cases of epitheliosis with marked fibroelastosis deserve segregation for further study (page 167) but, on present evidence, there is nothing to suggest that the stromal changes alter the behaviour of the epithelial hyperplasia.

In *duct ectasia*, inflammatory changes, when severe, lead to patchy or even subtotal destruction of elastica with periductal fibrosis and ductal dilatation, with loss of the elastic recoil of the duct. In other cases, or in other parts of the same breast, lesser degrees of inflammatory change lead to ductal fibrosis and an actual increase of elastic tissue. For this reason, Davies (1973) found that hyper-elastosis and fibrous obliterative changes in the ducts were closely associated with each other. Thus, while one of the major conclusions of Jackson and Orr (1957) must be refuted, the value of their work lay in the revival of interest in the elastic tissue of the breast which they stimulated; had it not been for their studies, the pathology of breast diseases might now be far less well understood than it is.

'*Early Elastic Cancer*'

There is another possible application of the study of elastic tissue in relation to breast cancer. Dossett (1976) has described what he calls 'early elastic cancer', meaning a ductal cancer with marked elastosis and sparse infiltrating cancer cells limited to the elastic zone; according to Dossett (1976), metastasis from this type of lesion at this stage has not been observed, an important observation in need of further documentation and study.

Association with High-affinity Oestrogen Receptors

Another remarkable observation has been recorded more recently. Masters et al (1976) demonstrated a definite association between elastosis and high-affinity oestrogen receptors in human primary breast carcinomas. This was particularly striking in the 19 tumours accompanied by a gross degree of elastosis (grade 2), 18 of which were receptor-positive. The results of further studies by this group of workers are eagerly awaited.

SUMMARY

Our present knowledge about elastosis can be summarized as follows:

1. *The yellow streaks of breast cancer consist of elastic tissue.* They are not necrotic foci, they are not calcific streaks, and they are not amyloid. Calcification *may* rarely be present in the elastic tissue, as it may occur

---

Figure 15–14 (*Opposite, above.*) Sclerosing adenosis. The presence of significant elastosis can usually be suspected in routine preparations. H and E. ×120.

Figure 15–15 (*Opposite, below.*) From the same tissue as Figure 15–14. Weigert elastic and HVG. ×120.

in pathological elastic tissue in a variety of conditions. The yellow streaks of breast cancer are mainly due to periductal elastosis. Elastosis also affects blood vessels, with veins being affected preferentially. Apart from these varieties of focal elastosis, there is frequently also a diffuse type of elastosis.

2. *The hypothesis that periductal fibrosis and elastosis is precancerous is rejected.* The interpretation that elastosis accompanying an intraductal carcinoma is an indication of invasion has more substance but must be treated with great caution. Elastosis may accompany intraductal carcinoma even in the absence of invasion. Nevertheless, in the presence of ductal carcinoma, localized elastosis should draw attention to the possibility of invasion at that point, meriting further detailed examination for the presence of extraductal spread.

3. *Elastosis is usually conspicuous by its absence in most lobular diseases.* Thus in fibroadenoma and pure cystic disease, as exemplified by apocrine cysts, elastic tissue is usually absent or present in only negligible quantities. Even in malignant disease as it affects the lobule, e.g. in CLIS or with cancerization, there is usually no significant elastic increase. This follows from what is known of the structure of the normal tissues. Elastosis is, in general, more frequent in sites like the ducts and the blood vessels, which normally have a complement of elastic tissue. *In sclerosing adenosis a modest or even a considerable degree of elastosis is often encountered* and this is particularly true of the infiltrative varieties, e.g. infiltrating epitheliosis. Even in conventional epitheliosis, especially when affecting the ducts, elastosis may be present and there is a case for segregating cases with marked elastosis for further study. *On the present evidence, however, fibroelastosis accompanying epitheliosis or sclerosing adenosis does not alter the significance or the behaviour of the proliferative epithelial lesions.*

CONNECTIVE TISSUE CHANGES OTHER THAN ELASTOSIS

PERIDUCTAL FIBROSIS

The concept of a diffuse periductal stromal change as a precancerous phenomenon in the breast was put forward by Jackson and Orr as long ago as 1957. They concluded, from their extensive data, that periductal fibrosis and elastosis in a segment of breast accompanied or even preceded neoplastic change in the mammary epithelium of that segment. This was a novel, almost revolutionary, idea with widespread implications at both the practical and theoretical level. This concept influenced workers in the field of experimental carcinogenesis. Jackson and Orr (1957) claimed that the stromal changes affected the whole sector or segment of the breast affected by the carcinomatous process. Davies (1973) refuted this notion emphatically, as far as the major ducts of the nipple are concerned at least. My own observations are in agreement with Davies (1973).

Recently this concept has been revived in a modified and more extended form. Gallager and Martin (1969), in their correlation of mammographic and histopathological findings, stated categorically that 'the periductal connective tissue in *all* of the breasts containing primary carcinomas is increased'. They found these changes throughout the breast tissue and not confined to the region of the invasive carcinoma. Furthermore the 'severe periductal collagenosis' they noted did not show any correlation with the presence or absence of invasive tumour, the size of the invasive mass present, or the localization of the carcinoma in the breast. Somewhat remarkably these important findings are not referred to in their discussion, but in the summary they concluded that 'the supportive connective tissue of the breast is also affected by the carcinogenic agent'. In their 1969 work, Gallager and Martin mentioned collagenosis only. In 1974 Gallager again stressed that these changes in the mammary connective tissue occur regularly. He described them as consisting of a sleeve-like thickening of periductal fibrous and elastic tissue which is mammographically reflected as 'a peculiar ropy density radiating outward from the subareolar region'. Gallager (1974) concluded that the connective tissue changes described occur 'early in the development process'. Radiologically these changes are said to lead to the 'developing density' sign which is attributed to Martin.

In effect, Gallager and Martin (1969) and Gallager (1974) appear to be describing the same histological changes observed by Jackson and Orr (1957). It is very difficult to assess accurately the findings of Gallager (1974) in this respect. In view of the conclusions of

Davies (1973), these findings must be treated with great caution. It should be emphasized that periductal fibrosis of the type described by Gallager (1974) is very common in late stage 'periductal mastitis' and that the latter disease is extremely common at the histopathological level in the later decades of life. The writer suspects that most of the stromal changes described by Gallager and Martin (1969) can be explained in this way and that they are not specific to the cancer-containing breasts. Late stage 'periductal mastitis' and carcinoma of the breast will often be associated by serendipity. *Mammoth studies, with giant sections, as detailed by Gallager and Martin (1969), may well have laid stress on a fortuitous relationship between these diffuse stromal changes and breast cancer.* Only identical studies with control non-cancerous material can establish this point with certainty. Meanwhile, it would be wise to accept the more conventional belief that there is *no known stromal change in the breast which can be regarded as precancerous and, indeed, that there is no stromal change which invariably accompanies breast cancer at a distance from the cancerous sites.* The value of the work of Gallager and Martin (1969) lies in other directions.

THE ORIGIN OF THE COLLAGEN IN BREAST CANCER

Desmoplastic Response to Cancer. The fibrous stroma of scirrhous carcinomas of the breast is generally regarded as a host reaction to the carcinoma by the connective tissue of the breast, the so-called desmoplastic response to cancer. Jackson and Orr (1957) postulated that most of the fibrous tissue was not in fact newly formed but resulted from condensation of pre-existing collagen as a result of a 'collapse' of the breast tissues, brought about by destruction caused by the presence of the cancer. The concept of 'collapse' bringing close together pre-existing structures is a valid one and can be invoked to explain the concentration of elastotic ducts in a given area seen in scirrhous carcinoma. Probably it explains also some of the fibrous tissue content, but the postulate of Jackson and Orr (1957) that it can all be explained in this way cannot be accepted. A fibrous reaction accompanying breast cancer is sometimes seen even in lymph node metastases and is more frequently seen in metastases in the gastrointestinal tract and in the pancreas. In sites like the lymph nodes the question of condensation of pre-existing collagenous tissue barely arises, and, in the gut, the fact that actual fibrous strictures can develop indicates that there is a production of new collagenous stroma.

It is accepted by most authors that breast carcinoma elicits a collagenous response in its neighbourhood. This is seen classically in the 'scirrhous' carcinoma of the breast. It is also seen to some extent in the so-called 'knobby carcinoma' described by Gallager and Martin (1969) and Gallager (1974). In the 'scirrhous' carcinoma the fibrosis usually has the same stellate distribution as the actual cancer. In the knobby carcinoma, fibrosis, if present to a significant extent, tends to occupy a central position without the radiating tentacles which are more characteristic of the stellate type of cancer of Gallager and Martin (1969).

Types of Fibrosis. The fibrous stroma of breast cancer, apart from periductal collagenosis or 'subepithelial collagenosis', has at least two origins: fibrosis secondary to tumour necrosis, as may be seen in any type of malignancy, and fibrosis not associated with preceding necrosis. The first is a *post-necrotic fibrosis*; the second is a *productive fibrosis*, in which collagen production accompanies the presence of live tumour. It is the productive fibrosis which has understandably given rise to the greater interest, especially in terms of pathogenesis.

Origin of Productive Fibrosis. The traditional and conventional view is that the cancer cells induce productive fibrosis by stimulating the stroma of the host. The assumption to date has been that the fibroblasts and possibly other stromal cells are responsible for the laying down of new collagenous tissue around the infiltrating cancer cells. This traditional view has been challenged by Al-Adnani, Kirrane and McGee (1975), who concluded that the collagen was produced directly by the breast cancer cells. They disagreed with the view that scirrhous reactions in human breast tumours represent a host reaction to tumour invasion. These workers studied 32 'scirrhous' cancers of the breast and, employing immunohistochemical techniques, demonstrated that *the carcinoma cells in 30 of these tumours contain not only collagen but also prolyl hydroxylase,* a key enzyme in collagen biosynthesis. Neither this enzyme nor collagen was detected in the spindle cells of the stroma. Negative results were also obtained with the epithelium of normal breast, that of fibrocystic disease and of fibroadenomas. The carcinoma cells of the two medullary cancers examined contained neither collagen nor prolyl hydroxylase. These workers concluded that the results strongly suggest that scirrhous carcinoma cells produce their own collagen stroma rather than inducing its production by stromal fibroblasts. They drew an analogy with the well-established phenomena of inappropriate hormone production by tumours and the inappropriate production of foetal antigens and enzymes. They suggested that synthesis of collagen by breast cancer cells could be regarded as another example of inappropriate protein production by malignant epithelial cells. Al-Adnani, Kirrane and McGee (1975) receive indirect support for their view from the work of Douglas and Shivas (1974), who concluded, on the basis of electron microscopic evidence, that breast cancer cells also produce one other connective tissue protein, elastin, inappropriately. As previously pointed out, however, the evidence that elastin can be produced by the cancer cells themselves is not yet proven. *The suggestion of Al-Adnani, Kirrane and McGee (1975) that breast cancer cells synthesize collagen is a fascinating one* and, should it be confirmed, will open a new chapter in the biology and metabolic activity of breast cancer cells.

References

Adnet, J.-J., Pinteaux, A., Caulet, T., Hibon, E., Petit, J., Pluot, M. and Roth, A. (1976) L'élastose dans les cancers du sein. Étude anatomo-clinique, histochimique et ultrastructurale. *Annales de Médicine de Reims,* **13,** 147–153.

Ahmed, A. (1974) The myoepithelium in human breast carcinoma. *Journal of Pathology,* **113,** 129–135.

Al-Adnani, M. S., Kirrane, J. A. and McGee, J. O'D. (1975) Inappropriate production of collagen and prolyl hydroxylase by human breast cancer cells in vivo. *British Journal of Cancer,* **31,** 653–660.

Azzopardi, J. G. and Laurini, R. N. (1974) Elastosis in breast cancer. *Cancer,* **33,** 174–183.

Azzopardi, J. G. and Laurini, R. N. (1975) Unpublished observations.

Beattie, J. M. and Dickson, W. E. C. (1926) *A Textbook of Special Pathology.* Third edition. London: Heinemann Medical.

Bernath, G. (1952) Amyloidosis in malignant tumors. *Acta Morphologica Academiae Scientiarum Hungaricae,* **2,** 137–144.

Bonser, G. M., Dossett, J. A. and Jull, J. W. (1961) *Human and Experimental Breast Cancer.* London: Pitman Medical.

Carstens, P. H. B., Huvos, A. G., Foote, F. W., Jr and Ashikari, R. (1972) Tubular carcinoma of the breast: a clinicopathologic study of 35 cases. *American Journal of Clinical Pathology,* **58,** 231–238.

Cheatle, Sir, G. L. and Cutler, M. (1931) *Tumours of the Breast — Their Pathology, Symptoms, Diagnosis and Treatment.* London: Edward Arnold.

Cutler, M. (1962) *Tumors of the Breast — Their Pathology, Symptoms, Diagnosis and Treatment.* London: Pitman Medical. Philadelphia: J. B. Lippincott.

Davies, J. D. (1973) Hyperelastosis, obliteration and fibrous plaques in major ducts of the human breast. *Journal of Pathology,* **110,** 13–26.

Dossett, J. A. (1976) Malignant potential of breast lesions. In *Risk Factors in Breast Cancer* (Ed.) Stoll, B. A. Chapter 3, pp. 54–66. London: Heinemann Medical.

Douglas, J. G. and Shivas, A. A. (1974) The origins of elastica in breast carcinoma. *Journal of the Royal College of Surgeons of Edinburgh,* **19,** 89–93.

Gallager, H. S. (1974) Current concepts in breast cancer and tumor immunology. In *Newer Understanding of Pathology of Breast Cancer,* p. 27. New York: Medical Examination.

Gallager, H. S. and Martin, J. E. (1969) Early phases in the development of breast cancer. *Cancer,* **24,** 1170–1178.

Jackson, J. G. and Orr, J. W. (1957) The ducts of carcinomatous breasts, with particular reference to connective-tissue changes. *Journal of Pathology and Bacteriology,* **74,** 265–273.

Levitan, L. H., Witten, D. M. and Harrison, E. G., Jr (1964) Calcification in breast disease. Mammographic-pathologic correlation. *American Journal of Roentgenology,* **92,** 29–39.

Lundmark, C. (1972) Breast cancer and elastosis. *Cancer,* **30,** 1195–1201.

Martinez-Hernandez, A., Francis, D. J. and Silverberg, S. G. (1977) Elastosis and other stromal reactions in benign and malignant breast tissue. An ultrastructural study. *Cancer,* **40,** 700–706.

Masters, J. R. W., Sangster, K., Hawkins, R. A. and Shivas, A. A. (1976) Elastosis and oestrogen receptors in human breast cancer. *British Journal of Cancer,* **33,** 342–343.

Muir, R. and Aitkenhead, A. C. (1934) The healing of intra-duct carcinoma of the mamma. *Journal of Pathology and Bacteriology,* **38,** 117–127.

Schiødt, T., Jensen, H., Nielsen, M. and Ranløv, P. (1972) On the nature of amyloid-like duct wall changes in carcinoma of the breast. *Acta Pathologica et Microbiologica Scandinavica,* Section A (Supplement 233), **80,** 151–157.

Shivas, A. A. and Douglas, J. G. (1972) The prognostic significance of elastosis in breast carcinoma. *Journal of the Royal College of Surgeons of Edinburgh,* **17,** 315–320.

Sloane, J. P. and Azzopardi, J. G. (1977) Personal observations.

Sümegi, I. and Rajka, G. (1972) Amyloid-like substance surrounding mammary cancer and basal cell carcinoma. *Acta Pathologica et Microbiologica,* Section A, **80,** 185–192.

Tobon, H. and Salazar, H. (1977) Tubular carcinoma of the breast. Clinical, histological, and ultrastructural observations. *Archives of Pathology and Laboratory Medicine,* **101,** 310–316.

Tremblay, G. (1974) Elastosis in tubular carcinoma of the breast. *Archives of Pathology,* **98,** 302–307.

Tremblay, G. (1976) Ultrastructure of elastosis in scirrhous carcinoma of the breast. *Cancer,* **37,** 307–316.

Chapter Sixteen

Miscellaneous Entities

FIBROMATOSIS

Rosen, Papasozomenos and Gardner (1978) collected 15 cases of fibromatosis of the breast reported in the world literature, mostly within the last 10 years. They added a case of their own in a 37-year-old Egyptian woman. In five of the 15 reported cases there was additional involvement of the underlying pectoral muscles, raising the possibility that some of these may have been of pectoral musculoaponeurotic origin. Two cases occurred in patients with Gardner's syndrome and one in a patient with 'familial multicentric fibromatosis'. Fibromatosis of the breast probably requires wide local excision to avoid the high incidence of local recurrence otherwise found with extra-abdominal desmoids. Metastases do not occur. In the remarkable case of Zayid and Dihmis (1969), the patient suffered multiple postmastectomy chest wall recurrences, which resulted in her death five years later.

LEIOMYOMA

Leiomyomas of the breast are very rare, if tumours of the nipple region are excluded. A case was reported by Craig (1947), who accepted and tabulated only four other cases in the literature. They were all large, slow-growing tumours. In two cases an origin in blood vessel walls was suggested but the histogenesis is still a matter for speculation.

Libcke (1969) described a 5 mm leiomyoma in association with cystic disease. Haagensen (1971) had seen only two leiomyomas within the substance of the breast parenchyma. He regarded one of the two cases as an adenoleiomyoma, unique in his experience, since it contained epithelial structures which were considered to be an integral part of the lesion. The evidence is not entirely convincing since the epithelial structures could have been residua of incorporated tissue. Riddell and Davies (1973) described two smooth muscle tumours which they regarded as hamartomat-

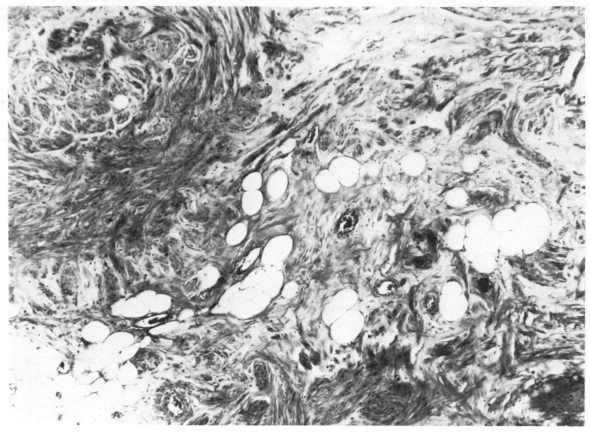

Figure 16–1   A circumscribed breast mass consisting largely of interlacing bundles of smooth muscle with a little interspersed adipose tissue. Epithelial elements are conspicuous by their absence. H and E. ×60.

ous. The writer has seen a leiomyomatous tumour of the breast containing some adipose tissue but no epithelial structures (Figure 16–1). Such pure leiomyomas and other benign mesenchymal neoplasms of the breast must be distinguished from fibroadenomas with an unusual muscular metaplasia.

LIPOMA AND SO-CALLED 'ADENOLIPOMA'

This is, as might be expected, a not uncommon lesion. It does not differ pathologically from lipomas as seen in other parts of the body, notably the subcutaneous fat. Lipomas of the breast tend to occur in older rather than younger women, with a mean age of 45 years in the large series of Haagensen (1971). The so-called 'adenolipoma' of the breast is probably merely a lipoma which has incorporated lobular epithelial elements.

'CHONDROMA' AND 'CHONDROLIPOMA'

Kaplan and Walts (1977) discussed benign cartilage-containing tumours of the breast other than fibroadenomas. They found a total of only seven cases in the world literature to which they added an eighth. Three are known to have contained adipose tissue also and three contained included breast ducts. They regarded their case as having an origin in metaplasia in the stroma; this benign chondrolipomatous type of tumour, if such it be, is excessively rare.

Kaplan and Walts (1977) stated that the presence of cartilage in benign human mammary tumours was last reported in 1909 but they appear to have excluded the ductal papillomas containing cartilage reported on by Smith and Taylor (1969), though they referred to this work. Also omitted was the curious case of 'benign fibroma' with cartilaginous metaplasia reported by Lawler

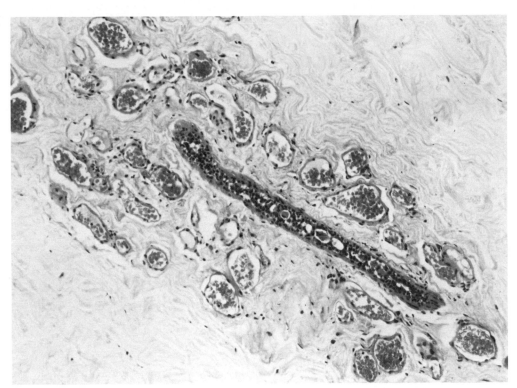

Figure 16–2 A periductal haemangioma, merely an incidental microscopic finding. H and E. ×150.

(1969). As Kaplan and Walts (1977) rightly stated, human cartilage-containing mammary tumours are more frequently malignant tumours, either carcinomas or sarcomas.

HAEMANGIOMA

Incidence. Benign haemangiomas of the breast parenchyma do occur but they are relatively rare and virtually always, if not always, *incidental microscopic findings* (Figure 16–2). Rosen and Ridolfi (1977), in a specific search, found seven so-called 'perilobular' haemangiomas in 555 mastectomy specimens for mammary carcinoma, *an incidence of 1.2 per cent.* These were found only with extensive sampling of the normal-appearing breast parenchyma and a careful search for these lesions. Similar haemangiomas were observed as frequently in a series of breast biopsies performed for benign conditions. These haemangiomas were all microscopic lesions which had not been apparent to the prosector.

Localization. Three of the seven lesions involved the specialized lobular stroma only,

two involved specialized lobular as well as interlobular stroma, while in two cases the haemangiomas were restricted to the ordinary interlobular stroma. While the term 'perilobular' may not be a completely accurate description of the location of all these lesions, there is certainly no reason to displace it with any new names, in the absence of a practical reason for any subclassification on the basis of anatomical localization (Rosen and Ridolfi, 1977).

Differentiation from Haemangiosarcoma. Microscopic haemangiomas of the breast are easily overlooked. It is highly unlikely that one of these lesions would be mistaken for an angiosarcoma. *It is the reverse error which is common enough, viz. the diagnosis of an angiosarcoma as a benign haemangioma.* Gulesserian and Lawton (1969) found that 14 out of 39 cases of angiosarcoma were originally misdiagnosed as benign haemangiomas. From a diagnostic point of view it must be stressed that *benign angiomas of the breast parenchyma never constitute a palpable or symptom-producing tumour.* Indeed, all seven described by Rosen and Ridolfi (1977) were microscopic findings only. This applies also to those described by Stewart (1950) and apparently to those of

McDivitt, Stewart and Berg (1968). The three seen by the writer were all incidental microscopic findings (Figure 16–2).

If a vascular tumour of the breast substance is producing a palpable lump or other symptoms, it must be regarded as angiosarcoma unless otherwise proven. *Of course this rule applies only* when one is sure that the angiomatous tumour in question is situated *within the breast parenchyma.* A lesion which can create problems is an *angiolipoma of the subcutaneous tissue* which happens to be situated over the mamma. This can be confused with an angiosarcoma of the breast infiltrating adipose tissue. This mistake will not be made if the surgeon describes accurately the position of the tumour and the pathologist confirms this by demonstrating either an absence of breast tissue or, alternatively, breast tissue distinctly limited to one side of the tumour and not involved by it. In addition there are subtle microscopic findings which will specifically identify the angiolipoma as it occurs in any part of the subcutaneous tissues.

Pathology. These haemangiomas consist of delicate, mainly cavernous vascular channels (Figure 16–2). There is no hint whatever of pleomorphism or anaplasia in the endothelial cells. There is usually a little connective tissue between the vascular spaces but there is an absence of the 'dissection' between both collagen fibres and adipose cells which is so characteristic a feature of angiosarcoma (contrast Figure 16–2 with Figure 14–8). According to Rosen and Ridolfi (1977), haemosiderin pigment is not present within or adjacent to these benign lesions.

The distinction on the basis of size is an important one to emphasize. Benign haemangiomas are generally limited to less than a low-power microscopic field in diameter. Because angiosarcomas may have in part an almost equally bland appearance, any larger lesion must be evaluated carefully after generous sampling (Rosen and Ridolfi, 1977).

AMYLOID 'TUMOUR'

A unique case of amyloid pseudotumour of the breast was reported by Fernandez and Hernandez (1973). This presented clinically as a firm, movable 3 cm mass in the breast of a 62-year-old woman. Mammograms suggested a malignant tumour. In view of the typical staining reactions for amyloid and the ultrastructural confirmation, this is regarded as a genuine case of amyloid pseudotumour. This interpretation is also borne out by the association of the deposits with lymphocytes, plasma cells and multinucleated giant cells. This remarkable case must be distinguished from the rare instances in which a breast carcinoma consists very largely of elastic tissue with very sparse carcinomatous areas. This distinction is important in view of the frequency with which the elastosis of breast cancer has been mistaken for amyloid. For this reason it is not possible to accept as authentic the reputed amyloid deposition in a breast carcinoma reported on by Patil, Joshi and Datar (1970).

In a different category is the case of Sadeghee and Moore (1974). Their 60-year-old patient had bilateral massive amyloid tumours of the breasts probably secondary to her rheumatoid arthritis. The only other known site of amyloid deposition took the form of cutaneous plaques in the abdominal wall, a combination of sites which is quite bizarre, as these authors emphasized.

GRANULAR-CELL 'MYOBLASTOMA'

Possibility of Confusion with Cancer. This lesion, when it occurs in the breast, can easily be confused with cancer both clinically and on macroscopic examination. It may be fixed to the pectoral fascia and can be attached to skin with evidence of skin retraction on clinical examination (Mulcare, 1968). It is firm to hard, may lack mobility and frequently even circumscription. The usually off-white or yellowish colour and solid fibrous consistency make clear differentiation from a carcinoma virtually impossible without using the microscope.

Incidence. It is a distinctly uncommon lesion. Mulcare (1968) found a total of only 15 granular-cell 'myoblastomas' of the breast parenchyma, as opposed to the overlying skin, in a review of the world literature, and added another 15 of his own to make a total of 30 cases.

Umansky and Bullock (1968) reported on a large series of 19 cases involving either the breast or the skin of the breast. Mulcare (1968) carefully excluded cases not primarily involving the breast parenchyma: this is desirable in order to appreciate the characteristics of this lesion as it affects the breast proper. Von Toth (1972) tabulated exactly 100 cases from the world literature, including two of his own: 93 were in female and seven in male patients. This total includes, however, cases which are more properly classified as cutaneous lesions.

Localization. Of the 15 personal cases studied by Mulcare (1968), 11 were situated in the *upper inner quadrant* of the breast.

Pathology. The breast lesions are identical with 'myoblastomas', better known to pathologists in sites like the skin, subcutis, tongue and larynx. They are benign and require only local excision.

Malignant 'Myoblastoma'. Even malignant granular-cell 'myoblastoma' has been described and von Toth (1972) cites three cases. One is the case of Crawford and De Bakey (1953), the second is in a German journal I have been unable to acquire and the third, though attributed by von Toth (1972) to Vidyarthi in the American literature, is actually attributable to an Italian author, whose work I have also been unable to obtain. Malignant granular-cell 'myoblastoma' of the breast is a vanishingly rare lesion. The important point to remember is that the *common or garden variety of this lesion can easily be mistaken for a carcinoma or some other malignant tumour on frozen section,* as happened in three of the patients reported on by Umansky and Bullock (1968).

TUBERCULOSIS

Incidence and Mode of Presentation. Tuberculosis of the breast is nowadays a rare disease in most countries. Most of the reports come from countries like South Africa with a relatively high incidence and a reasonably abundant scientific literature. Gottschalk, Decker and Schmaman (1976) reported on 28 cases of tuberculosis of the breast treated at Baragwanath Hospital since 1956, an incidence of approximately one case per year. All patients were female, with the majority aged between 20 and 35 years, though the oldest

patient was aged 64 years. Ten of the 28 patients were either pregnant or lactating. The disease presented as an abscess (10 cases) or with a firm breast mass (18 cases). In 10 of the latter group, a clinical diagnosis of carcinoma had been made. Axillary lymphadenopathy was present in half the patients but in none was it a striking feature. According to Symmers (1966a) the regional lymph nodes are rarely enlarged. He emphasized particularly that *caseous lymphadenitis in association with tuberculosis of the breast is rare* and that a breaking-down tuberculoid axillary lymphadenitis is in fact generally due to extramammary causes, often non-tuberculous in nature — for example, cat-scratch disease.

Ikard and Perkins (1977) calculated that the incidence of tuberculous mastitis was 0.025 per cent of surgically treated breast disease in economically developed parts of the world. These workers reviewed all aspects of the disease, including the incidence in different countries during different decades, and provided a valuable bibliography.

Histopathology. The histopathological picture in the lesions reported by Gottschalk, Decker and Schmaman (1976) was typical of tuberculosis, but acid-fast bacilli could be demonstrated in only two cases. It is worth remembering the cautionary note sounded by Symmers (1966a) about the necessity of identifying tubercle bacilli in the lesions before interpreting mammary granulomatous disease as tuberculous.

Signs of Disease Elsewhere. Two of the patients of Gottschalk, Decker and Schmaman (1976) had active pulmonary tuberculosis and an additional four patients had extrapulmonary tuberculosis in areas other than the breast.

Mode of Spread of Disease to the Breast. There was no evidence of tuberculous cervical lymphadenopathy in any of their patients. Retrograde lymphatic spread has been regarded traditionally as the mode of spread to the breast, axillary or other lymph node groups being considered the source of the disease. Gottschalk, Decker and Schmaman (1976) challenged this view and thought it *more likely that blood-spread infection occurred, from an active or occult pulmonary or other focus in most cases.* The increased vascularity of the breast in pregnant and lactating women may favour blood-spread infection. It is likely that both haematogenous and lymphatic routes play a part in causation of this disease. The infection may also reach the breast by lymphatic spread from the internal mammary lymph nodes or by direct spread from the pleura.

Coexistent Carcinoma. Tuberculosis of the breast and mammary carcinoma may co-exist on rare occasions (Miller, Salomon and West, 1971); the association is fortuitous.

Distinction from 'Granulomatous Mastitis'. Tuberculosis of the breast has to be distinguished from the curious condition labelled 'granulomatous mastitis' by Kessler and Wolloch (1972). The latter condition differs in not showing caseation and in containing neutrophils in the granulomas. This lesion has been described as characteristically confined to the lobules. The relationship of 'granulomatous mastitis' of Kessler and Wolloch (1972) to other breast diseases is not yet clear and is in need of clarification.

MYCOTIC PSEUDOTUMOURS AND OTHER RARE INFECTIONS AND INFESTATIONS

Salfelder and Schwarz (1975) reported on four patients with mycotic mastitis seen over a nine-year period in a single laboratory. Only three reports of similar type were traced in the literature but these workers regarded only one as acceptable as a deep mycosis of the breast.

Cryptococcus. Salfelder and Schwarz (1975) found one patient with cryptococcosis in both breasts. She was a woman with systemic lupus erythematosus on cortisone treatment. The breast lesions were unsuspected clinically and detected only at necropsy. Disseminated cryptococcosis was found in several organs. Apart from a mild meningitis, there was no inflammatory response in the breasts and other organs affected, a well-known negative finding in cryptococcosis. Only one other reported case of cryptococcal mastitis was found, also detected at necropsy (Symmers, 1966b).

Blastomycosis. One patient with unilateral blastomycosis presented with an abscess, which was diagnosed preoperatively as an infected para-areolar cyst. *Blastomyces dermatitidis* was identified in the breast tissue associated with a characteristic tissue reaction. After excision and topical anti-fungal treatment, healing took place. After eight years, the patient was well with no signs of disease in the breast or elsewhere.

Histoplasmosis. The remaining two patients of Salfelder and Schwarz (1975) presented with breast tumours. Both had masses caused by *Histoplasma capsulatum*. One mass was genuinely in the breast while the other turned out to be situated in axillary lymph nodes. Histoplasmic mastitis had not been reported previously.

Possible Relationship of Other Entities. Salfelder and Schwarz (1975) found it difficult to understand why mycotic mastitis had hardly ever been described in the literature. Only one other case, an instance of cryptococcic mastitis, was regarded as authentic. They attributed this paucity of reports to a lack of suspicion or a failure to recognize the causative agents in tissue sections or on culture; they stressed the value of the Grocott staining method for the detection of fungi in tissue. These workers suggested that some of the lesions of the type described by Kessler and Wolloch (1972) and by Murthy (1973) might be attributable to mycotic infections.

Deep Mycosis in Britain: Actinomycosis. All mycotic infections of the breast are rare but probably not quite as rare as the literature would indicate. In Great Britain actinomycosis is the only deep-seated fungal infection to occur in the breast with any frequency, and it is very rare (Symmers, 1966a). Its manifestations are comparable with those of the infection when it involves other sites.

Rarer Infections. Rarer infections and even metazoan infestations of the breast, including hydatid disease and cysticerosis, are referred to by Symmers (1966a).

SARCOIDOSIS

The breast parenchyma is very rarely involved in sarcoidosis. The writer has seen only a single case and, as the patient had evidence of sarcoidosis in other organs, this did not present a diagnostic problem.

SPONTANEOUS INFARCTION

Spontaneous infarction of normal mammary tissue in pregnant and lactating women is considered on page 44, since it has to be distinguished from infarction occurring in a fibroadenoma.

BREAST LUMPS CAUSED BY ARTERIAL DISEASE

Giant-cell Arteritis. Waugh (1950) reported on a remarkable case of a 64-year-old woman who presented with an asymptomatic lump in her right breast. She had an unexplained high erythrocyte sedimentation rate. Because of the clinical probability that the lesion was malignant, a simple mastectomy was carried out, despite a report on frozen section that there was no evidence of malignancy and that the tissue excised contained a thickened thrombosed artery. Approximately two months later, the patient presented complaining of pain in the left breast. A tender firm lump with skin fixation was found. Clinically it also appeared to be a carcinoma. Frozen sections revealed a lesion similar to that found in the other breast, i.e. an arteritis probably involving one of the penetrating branches of the internal mammary artery. The histopathological changes in the blood vessels in both breast lumps corresponded to those seen in giant-cell arteritis.

The patient remained well up to 16 months following her second operation without evidence of systemic symptoms. The high sedimentation rate persisted and it was considered possible that this indicated the presence of more generalized arterial disease, but no evidence of this became manifest.

Focal Arteritis of the Polyarteritis Type. McCarty, Imbrigia and Hung (1968) described bilateral focal arteritis in the breasts of a 66-year-old woman. The patient complained of multiple indurated and tender masses in her breasts. The histopathology was typical of polyarteritis nodosa. The breast lumps and

symptoms, persisting after biopsies had been carried out, responded to treatment with prednisone. There was no clinical or laboratory evidence of visceral involvement and no clinical evidence of giant-cell arteritis. Despite some differences from the case reported by Waugh (1950), there were also distinct similarities.

McCarty, Imbrigia and Hung (1968) concluded that this case probably represented a focal arteritis, having the pathological features of polyarteritis nodosa, with one organ involvement only, as in the cases of focal arteritis which involve the vermiform appendix and those more recently described in the cervix uteri.

Wegener's Granulomatosis. Pambakian and Tighe (1971) described two patients with Wegener's granulomatosis in whom the early and predominant lesions were situated in the breast. Elsner and Harper (1969) were the first workers to report breast involvement in Wegener's granulomatosis.

Arteritis affecting the breasts may be only a localized phenomenon or part of a systemic disorder as in the patients of Pambakian and Tighe (1971).

HAEMORRHAGIC NECROSIS COMPLICATING ANTICOAGULANT THERAPY

Haemorrhagic necrosis of the breast following anticoagulation with coumarin and indanedione derivatives is rare. It was first reported by Flood et al (1943) and rare reports have appeared since in the Dutch, German, Scandinavian, English and Italian as well as the North American literature (see Tong, 1971, for references). Haemorrhagic necrosis supervenes a few days after starting treatment with the drug. The patient of Tong (1971) is only the third recorded case of gangrene of the breast occurring during phenindione therapy. The pathogenesis of this form of total or subtotal mammary necrosis is obscure. The final picture is one of aseptic ischaemic necrosis, which is difficult to reconcile with the extensive collateral circulation of the breast (Tong, 1971).

The process of infarction is apparently irreversible. It remains localized and the process does not appear to be aggravated by continuing with the same anticoagulant if this is indicated for the treatment of any systemic disease.

OTHER CAUSES OF INFARCTION

Mammary necrosis has been recorded very rarely in association with other conditions or diseases, in the absence of anticoagulant therapy. Its association with pregnancy has already been noted. Very rarely it has been recorded with diabetes mellitus and carbon monoxide poisoning (Tong, 1971).

Clinicopathological Division of Causes of Breast Infarction. Robitaille et al (1974) reviewed the literature on breast infarction and divided the lesions into two broad categories, depending on whether or not they mimicked carcinoma. A number of common features emerged in each group, prompting them to consider the two categories as clinicopathological entities. These two categories and their main characteristics are summarized in Tables 16–1 and 16–2.

FOCAL PREGNANCY-LIKE CHANGES: FOCAL SECRETORY LOBULAR CHANGES

Microscopic Appearance. Kiaer and Andersen (1977) examined and discussed very critically the vexed question of 'focal pregnancy-like changes' in the breast. These are lobular epithelial changes with a morphology which is indistinguishable from the more diffuse changes seen in the breast during pregnancy or lactation. In isolated lobules, which may be hypertrophic, the epithelial cells have a copious, pale, vacuolated cytoplasm and a nucleus which is large, deeply staining and variable in location (Figures 16–3 and 16–4). Appearances simulating the Arias–Stella reaction are frequently present, with a characteristic hobnail epithelium. An individual lobule is partially or totally involved; when the involvement is partial or subtotal,

Table 16–1   Classification of cases of mammary infarction[a]

Breast infarcts mimicking carcinoma	Breast infarcts not mimicking carcinoma
Fibroadenomas (associated with pregnancy or lactation; or not so associated)	Anticoagulant therapy
Adenomas or 'lactation adenomas' (associated with pregnancy or lactation)	So-called 'thrombophlebitis migrans disseminata' (possibly anticoagulant treatment played a part)
Hyperplastic but non-neoplastic breast tissue in pregnancy or during lactation	Complicating postpartum abscess
	Postpartum gangrene of skin and breast
Wegener's granulomatosis Giant-cell arteritis Focal arteritis	Haemolytic streptococcal gangrene of breast (no histology)
Case of Robitaille et al (1974)	Mitral stenosis and congestive heart failure
Intraductal papilloma	

[a] Modified from Robitaille et al (1974).

It should be emphasized that some of the conditions listed in the left-hand column of this table are extremely rare causes of mammary infarction and most of those in the right-hand column are also extremely rare as causes of this disorder. These rarities are by no means all well documented.

Intraductal papilloma undergoing infarction is relatively common and is a well-known and important cause of symptoms which mimic those of cancer. It is listed only at the bottom of the column because it more properly belongs in Chapter Eight.

Table 16–2 Main clinicopathological characteristics of the two groups of mammary infarction

Mimicking carcinoma	Not mimicking carcinoma
Mostly in younger women	Mostly in women over 40 years of age
Low incidence of associated skin necrosis overlying breast	High incidence of associated mammary skin necrosis
Usually a pale infarct	Usually a haemorrhagic infarct
When blood vessels are involved, the lesions affect arteries predominantly	Blood vessels, especially veins, are involved
High incidence of underlying benign tumours or hyperplastic tissue as seen in pregnancy	No underlying tumours or physiological hyperplasia
Low incidence of associated diseases with high morbidity	Higher incidence of associated diseases with high morbidity (e.g. thrombophlebitis, cardiovascular diseases)

This is a useful working classification of breast infarction, and all the relevant references are supplied by Robitaille et al (1974).

the peripheral or marginal acini of the lobule are the ones which are not involved. These workers found no transition to apocrine epithelium in the affected lobules, though such a transitional appearance has been claimed by some other workers. The writer agrees with Kiaer and Andersen (1977) in that he has been unable to find any evidence of such transition in many personally studied cases.

Incidence. Kiaer and Andersen (1977) found these changes in 3 per cent of all breast tissue examined. They collected 31 cases in just over 1000 specimens from two hospitals. An average of seven sections was examined in each case. This incidence is remarkably similar to the 3.1 per cent recorded by Frantz et al (1951) and the 3.7 per cent of Sandison (1962) in necropsy series. The focal pregnancy-like changes were found by Kiaer and Andersen (1977) in from one to 12 isolated foci, depending to some extent on the size of the tissue specimen.

There is *no association between the pregnancy-like changes and other breast pathology* (Kiaer and Andersen, 1977).

Aetiology. Kiaer and Andersen (1977) applied themselves especially to the problem of whether the focal pregnancy-like changes

could represent a persistence of alterations induced by a previous pregnancy or whether they could be caused by the previous or current administration of exogenous hormones. They considered also the possibility of the interaction of both of these factors. Their conclusions can be summarized thus:

1. The changes could be explained as '*residual lactational acini*' in those patients who had completed their last pregnancy or lactation within a year of the biopsy. It seems highly unlikely, however, that pregnancy changes can persist for up to 36 years, the longest interval in their series. Frantz et al (1951) had a 48-year interval in one patient. In addition, three of the patients studied by Kiaer and Andersen (1977) had never been pregnant.
2. All patients in the literature in whom benign epithelial changes, including 'focal pregnancy-like change', have been related to *oestrogen therapy or contraceptive pills* had been receiving hormone therapy at the time of the biopsy. In their material, only four patients were on contraceptive medication at the time of biopsy, and all these had previously been pregnant (intervals ranging from six months to 20 years). In a few cases, therefore, they could not rule out a relationship between

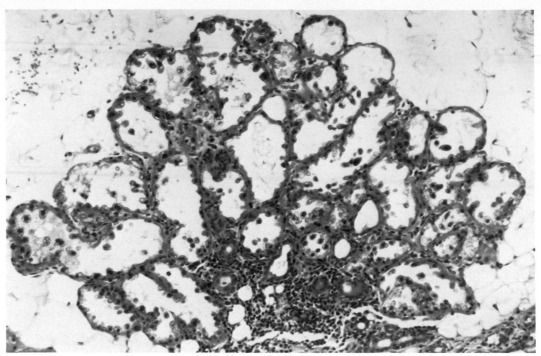

Figure 16–3 A secretory lobule unassociated with preceding lactation, pregnancy or hormone therapy. H and E. ×180.

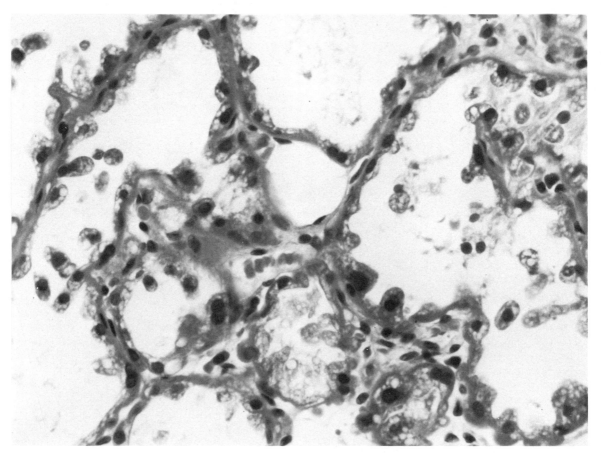

Figure 16–4 Pregnancy-like change in the isolated lobule shown in Figure 16–3. It is probably attributable to an individual lobular susceptibility to endogenous hormones or, in other cases, to exogenous hormone treatment. H and E. ×600.

contraceptive pills and the breast changes, or even perhaps a combined effect of contraceptive pills and a fairly recent pregnancy.

3. In their series, the breast changes were present in 25 women who were *not receiving hormone therapy* at the time of biopsy. The intervals between discontinuation of the hormone therapy and the biopsy extended to 20 years. Two of these patients had never been pregnant, and in one of these no hormones had been administered for nine years. In addition, one patient had never been pregnant and had never received hormone therapy.

Lobular Selective Susceptibility. The authors concluded that these results support the 'selective susceptibility' hypothesis of Foote and Stewart (1945) and of Taylor (1971). They believe that focal pregnancy-like breast changes probably have an oestrogenic aetiology and usually indicate a selective susceptibility of individual breast lobules rather than a dose-related response to endogenous or exogenous hormones. Accordingly, they interpret the changes as *a normal, non-pathological variation in the histology of the female breast.*

Similar Changes in Men. Schwartz and Wilens (1963) observed that in two of eight breasts with gynaecomastia, which showed acinar differentiation in addition to the usual changes, there was also focal pregnancy-like change akin to that seen in women. These changes were identified in men on oestrogen therapy for prostatic cancer. Apart from confirming that pregnancy is not a prerequisite for the development of this breast change, these findings also suggest that exogenous hormones can play an aetiological role.

The report of Kiaer and Andersen (1977) is invaluable because of its critical analysis of the pertinent literature and the very thorough way they conducted their study. Their conclusions are very convincingly stated and appear to be thoroughly validated by their data and their analysis of other workers' findings.

Hamperl (1975) had previously described what is essentially the same phenomenon. He also concluded that the secretory lobular changes observed appeared to be the result of unduly susceptible lobules in the 'mastopathic'

breast. His choice of the term 'mastopathic breast' did, however, suggest that he regarded the change as a pathological one, unlike the conclusion of Kiaer and Andersen (1977).

References

Craig, J. M. (1947) Leiomyoma of the female breast. *Archives of Pathology,* **44,** 314–317.

Crawford, E. S. and De Bakey, M. E. (1953) Granular-cell myoblastoma. Two unusual cases. *Cancer,* **6,** 786–789.

Elsner, B. and Harper, F. B. (1969) Disseminated Wegener's granulomatosis with breast involvement. Report of a case. *Archives of Pathology,* **87,** 544–547.

Fernandez, B. B. and Hernandez, F. J. (1973) Amyloid tumor of the breast. *Archives of Pathology,* **95,** 102–105.

Flood, E. P., Redish, M. H., Bociek, S. J. and Shapiro, S. (1943) Thrombophlebitis migrans disseminata: report of a case in which gangrene of a breast occurred. *New York State Journal of Medicine,* **43,** 1121–1124.

Foote, F. W. and Stewart, F. W. (1945) Comparative studies of cancerous versus noncancerous breast. I. Basic morphologic characteristics. *Annals of Surgery,* **121,** 6–53.

Frantz, V. K., Pickren, J. W., Melcher, G. W. and Auchincloss, H., Jr (1951) Incidence of chronic cystic disease in so-called 'normal breasts'. A study based on 225 postmortem examinations. *Cancer,* **4,** 762–783.

Gottschalk, F. A. B., Decker, G. A. G. and Schmaman, A. (1976) Tuberculosis of the breast. *South African Journal of Surgery,* **14,** 19–22.

Gulesserian, H. P. and Lawton, R. L. (1969) Angiosarcoma of the breast. *Cancer,* **24,** 1021–1026.

Haagensen, C. D. (1971) *Diseases of the Breast.* Second edition — revised reprint. pp. 297–299. Philadelphia, London, Toronto: W. B. Saunders.

Hamperl, H. (1975) Sekretionserscheinungen in der mastopathischen Brustdrüse. Beiträge zur pathologischen Histologie der Mamma. *Virchows Archiv B: Cell Pathology,* **18,** 73–81.

Ikard, R. W. and Perkins, D. (1977) Mammary tuberculosis: a rare modern disease. *Southern Medical Journal,* **70,** 208–212.

Kaplan, L. and Walts, E. (1977) Benign chondrolipomatous tumor of the human female breast. *Archives of Pathology and Laboratory Medicine,* **101,** 149–151.

Kessler, E. and Wolloch, Y. (1972) Granulomatous mastitis: a lesion clinically simulating carcinoma. *American Journal of Clinical Pathology,* **58,** 642–646.

Kiaer, H. W. and Andersen, J. A. (1977) Focal pregnancy-like changes in the breast. *Acta Pathologica et Microbiologica Scandinavica,* Section A, **85,** 931–941.

Lawler, R. G. (1969) Cartilaginous metaplasia in a breast tumour. *Journal of Pathology,* **97,** 385–387.

Libcke, J. H. (1969) Leiomyoma of the breast. *Journal of Pathology,* **98,** 89–90.

McCarty, D. J., Imbrigia, J. and Hung, J. K. (1968) Vasculitis of the breasts. *Arthritis and Rheumatism,* **11,** 796–801.

McDivitt, R. W., Stewart, F. W. and Berg, J. W. (1968) *Tumors of the Breast.* Atlas of Tumor Pathology, Second series, Fascicle 2. Washington, D.C.: Armed Forces Institute of Pathology.

Miller, R. E., Salomon, P. F. and West, J. P. (1971) The coexistence of carcinoma and tuberculosis of the breast and axillary lymph nodes. *American Journal of Surgery,* **121,** 338–340.

Mulcare, R. (1968) Granular cell myoblastoma of the breast. *Annals of Surgery,* **168,** 262–268.

Murthy, M. S. N. (1973) Granulomatous mastitis and lipogranuloma of the breast. *American Journal of Clinical Pathology,* **60,** 432–433.

Pambakian, H. and Tighe, J. R. (1971) Breast involvement in Wegener's granulomatosis. *Journal of Clinical Pathology,* **24,** 343–347.

Patil, S. D., Joshi, B. G. and Datar, K. G. (1970) Amyloid deposit in the carcinoma of breast. *Indian Journal of Cancer,* **7,** 60–62.

Riddell, R. H. and Davies, J. D. (1973) Muscular hamartomas of the breast. *Journal of Pathology,* **111,** 209–211.

Robitaille, Y., Seemayer, T. A., Thelmo, W. L. and Cumberlidge, M. C. (1974) Infarction of the mammary region mimicking carcinoma of the breast. *Cancer,* **33,** 1183–1189.

Rosen, P. P. and Ridolfi, R. L. (1977) The perilobular hemangioma. A benign microscopic vascular lesion of the breast. *American Journal of Clinical Pathology,* **68,** 21–23.

Rosen, Y., Papasozomenos, S. Ch. and Gardner, B. (1978) Fibromatosis of the breast. *Cancer,* **41,** 1409–1413.

Sadeghee, S. A. and Moore, S. W. (1974) Rheumatoid arthritis, bilateral amyloid tumors of the breast, and multiple cutaneous amyloid nodules. *American Journal of Clinical Pathology,* **62,** 472–476.

Salfelder, K. and Schwarz, J. (1975) Mycotic 'pseudotumors' of the breast. Report of four cases. *Archives of Surgery,* **110,** 751–754.

Sandison, A. T. (1962) *An Autopsy Study of the Adult Human Breast.* National Cancer Institute Monograph No. 8, pp. 1–145. Washington, D.C.: U.S. Department of Health, Education and Welfare.

Schwartz, I. S. and Wilens, S. L. (1963) The formation of acinar tissue in gynecomastia. *American Journal of Pathology,* **43,** 797–807.

Smith, B. G. and Taylor, H. B. (1969) The occurrence of bone and cartilage in mammary tumors. *American Journal of Clinical Pathology,* **51,** 610–618.

Stewart, F. W. (1950) *Tumors of the Breast.* Atlas of Tumor Pathology, Section 9, Fascicle 34, p. 107. Washington D.C.: Armed Forces Institute of Pathology.

Symmers, W. St. C. (1966a) The breasts. In *Systemic Pathology* (Ed.) Payling Wright, G. and Symmers, W. St. C. Ch. 28, Vol. 1, pp. 953–955. London: Longmans, Green.

Symmers, W. St. C. (1966b) Deep-seated fungal infections currently seen in the histopathologic service of a medical school laboratory in Britain. *American Journal of Clinical Pathology,* **46,** 515–537.

Taylor, H. B. (1971) Oral contraceptives and pathologic changes in the breast. *Cancer,* **28,** 1388–1390.

Tong, D. (1971) Haemorrhagic necrosis of the breast complicating anticoagulant therapy and mitral stenosis. *British Journal of Surgery,* **58,** 624–628.

Umansky, C. and Bullock, W. K. (1968) Granular cell myoblastoma of the breast. *Annals of Surgery,* **168,** 810–817.

von Toth, J. (1972) Das granulärzellige Myoblastom der Mamma. *Zentralblatt für allgemeine Pathologie und pathologische Anatomie,* **115,** 366–371.

Waugh, T. R. (1950) Bilateral mammary arteritis. Report of a case. *American Journal of Pathology,* **26,** 851–861.

Zayid, I. and Dihmis, C. (1969) Familial multicentric fibromatosis-desmoids. *Cancer,* **24,** 786–795.

Chapter Seventeen

Ultrastructural Aspects of Human Breast Disease

NORMAL MAMMARY DUCTS AND DUCTULES

The mammary ducts and ductules are lined by luminal epithelial cells (E) and peripheral myoepithelial cells (M) (Figure 17–1). The epithelial cell nucleus is round or oval with a smooth nuclear membrane and shows peripheral condensation of the chromatin. The myoepithelial cell nucleus is irregular in shape with indentation of the nuclear envelope and the cytoplasm contains basally located characteristic filaments (f) with dense bodies. Desmosomes (D) are present between the epithelial and myoepithelial cells. The myoepithelial cell basal plasma membrane forms club-like processes capped by hemidesmosomes (H). Occasional pinocytotic vesicles (arrowhead) are seen along the basal plasma membrane. Basal lamina (arrows) follows the contours of the myoepithelial cell. The adjacent connective tissue contains collagen bundles.

EPITHELIOSIS

Epitheliosis (so-called 'papillomatosis') represents the proliferation of epithelial elements within the lumina of ducts or ductules. Myoepithelial cells, which are alkaline phosphatase positive, are present among these proliferating cells (Figure 17–2).

At ultrastructural level, myoepithelial cells (M) are seen at the periphery of the duct as well as among the proliferating epithelial cells (E) (Figures 17–3 and 17–4). Such myoepithelial cells may reach almost up to the lumen (L) and are differentiated from the adjacent epithelial cells (E) by the presence of cytoplasmic filaments (f) with dense bodies and of pinocytotic vesicles (arrowhead). Desmosomes (D) are present between the epithelial and myoepithelial cells.

The identification of myoepithelial cells in epitheliosis is of considerable value in its differentiation from an intraductal carcinoma, in which, apart from the persisting

Text continues on page 412

407

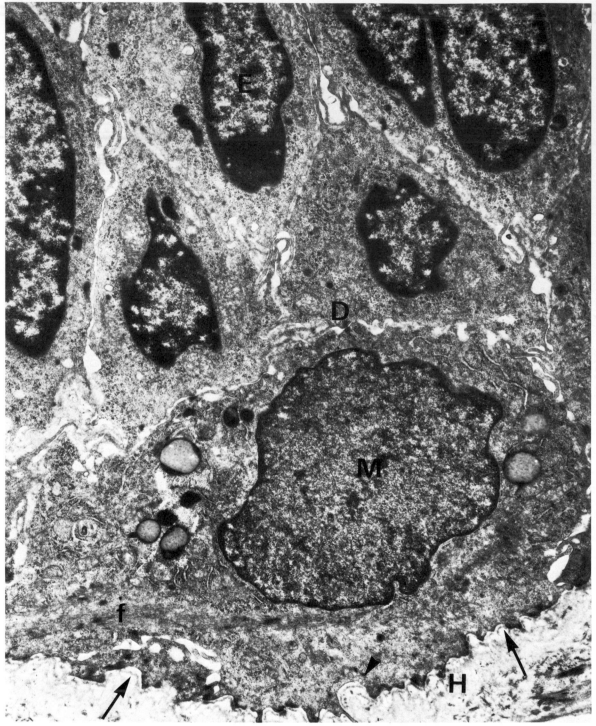

Figure 17–1   Mammary duct and ductules. ×12 500. (All electron micrographs are stained with lead citrate and uranyl acetate except for Figures 17–18 and 17–19, which are stained with uranyl acetate only.)

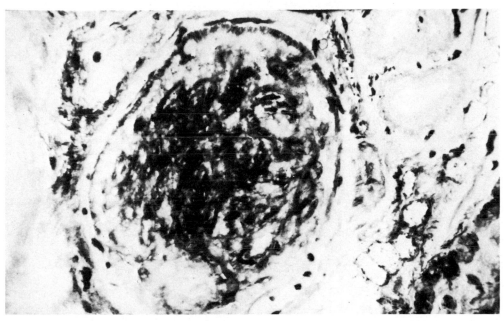

Figure 17–2 Epitheliosis. Alkaline phosphatase reaction. ×135. From Ahmed (1974c) with kind permission of the editor of *Journal of Pathology.*

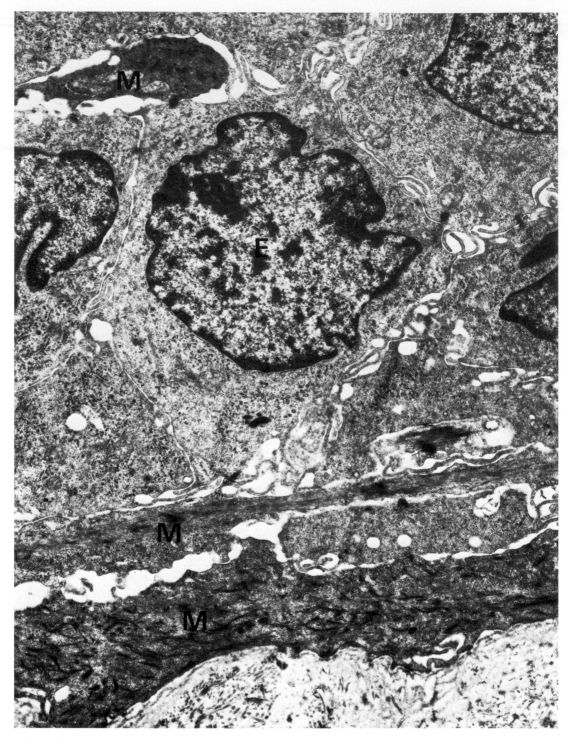

Figure 17–3   Epitheliosis. ×12 500.

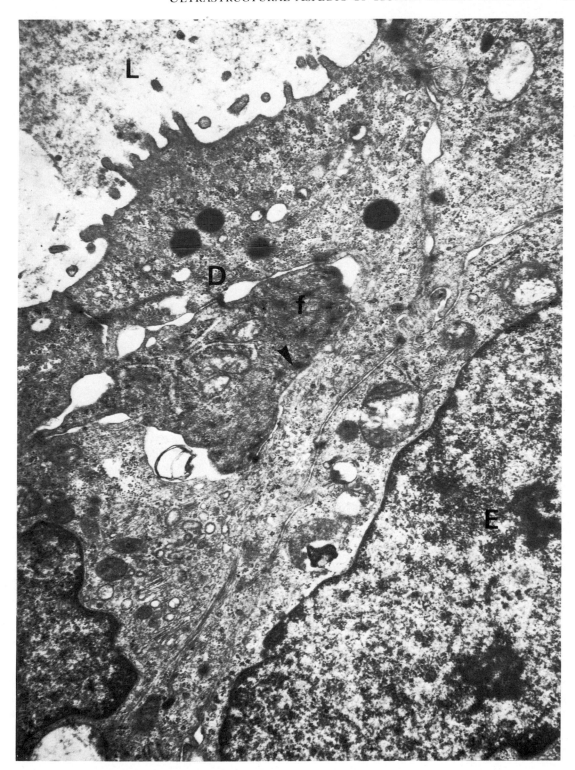

Figure 17–4   Epitheliosis. ×18 750.

peripheral myoepithelial cell layer, no myoepithelial cells are present among the carcinoma cells (Ahmed, 1974c).

SCLEROSING ADENOSIS

In sclerosing adenosis there is epithelial cell hyperplasia accompanied by a varying degree of myoepithelial cell proliferation (Figure 17–5, inset).

The progressive myoepithelial cell proliferation results in the distortion of the epithelial elements with resultant loss of glandular lumina (Figure 17–5). The remaining epithelial elements sometimes consist almost entirely of proliferating myoepithelial cells (M), which contain the characteristic cytoplasmic filaments with dense bodies.

The myoepithelial cell processes may eventually become markedly elongated (Figure 17–6) but they retain the cytoplasmic filaments (f) and hemidesmosomes (H). The basal lamina persists and may be multilayered. The adjacent stroma contains bundles of collagen (co) and elastic tissue.

The involvement of myoepithelial cell proliferation in the process of sclerosing adenosis has been shown in previous ultrastructural studies (Murad and von Haam, 1968a; Ahmed, 1974c).

Electron microscopy may prove to be of value in differentiating more complex cases of sclerosing adenosis from an infiltrating carcinoma.

APOCRINE METAPLASIA

Apocrine metaplasia is a common histological manifestation of cystic hyperplastic mastopathy. The luminal apocrine-type cells contain round, basally located nuclei (n) and are characterized by the presence of numerous mitochondria and collections of osmiophilic bodies (ob) (Figure 17–7). Myoepithelial cells (M) are present at the periphery.

The mitochondria (mi) have an electrondense matrix and contain a few, thin cristae, which extend to the centre of the mitochondria and are incomplete (Figure 17–8). The basal plasma membrane forms elaborate infoldings (arrow) resulting in wide intercellular spaces between the myoepithelial cells. The presence of numerous mitochondria and the multifolding of the basal plasma membrane have been described in the normal apocrine gland epithelium of the skin (Munger, 1965).

The increased number of mitochondria in apocrine-type cells of the breast was noted by Murad and von Haam (1968b) and by Pier, Garancis and Kuzma (1970). This presence of large numbers of mitochondria led Archer and Omar (1969) to compare these cells with oncocytes. However, unlike the apocrine-type cells, in the oncocyte the mitochondrial cristae are increased in number and the basal plasma membrane is rudimentary and lacks elaborate infoldings (Tandler, 1966).

The metaplastic derivation of apocrine cells from normal breast epithelium is suggested by recent ultrastructural and histochemical observations (Ahmed, 1975).

INTRADUCTAL PAPILLOMA

The papillary processes are lined by luminal epithelial and peripheral myoepithelial cells and possess a well-formed connective tissue stalk (Figure 17–9).

The epithelial cell nuclei (n) are round with smooth nuclear membranes. The apical cytoplasm displays well-formed microvilli (mv). Some of the epithelial cells may show morphological features of apocrine-type cells.

Myoepithelial cells (M) are often elongated and are a prominent feature of intraductal papillomas (Ahmed, 1974c). A basal lamina is always present along the basal plasma membranes of the myoepithelial cells.

The intrapapillary connective tissue consists of compressed bundles of collagen (co) and may contain prominent blood vessels.

PAPILLARY CARCINOMA

A papillary carcinoma of the breast often presents as a diagnostic problem in its differentiation from a benign intraductal papilloma. In contrast to an intraductal papilloma, the processes of a papillary carcinoma are lined by cells of one type and usually lack well-developed fibrovascular cores (Figure 17–10, inset).

Text continues on page 418

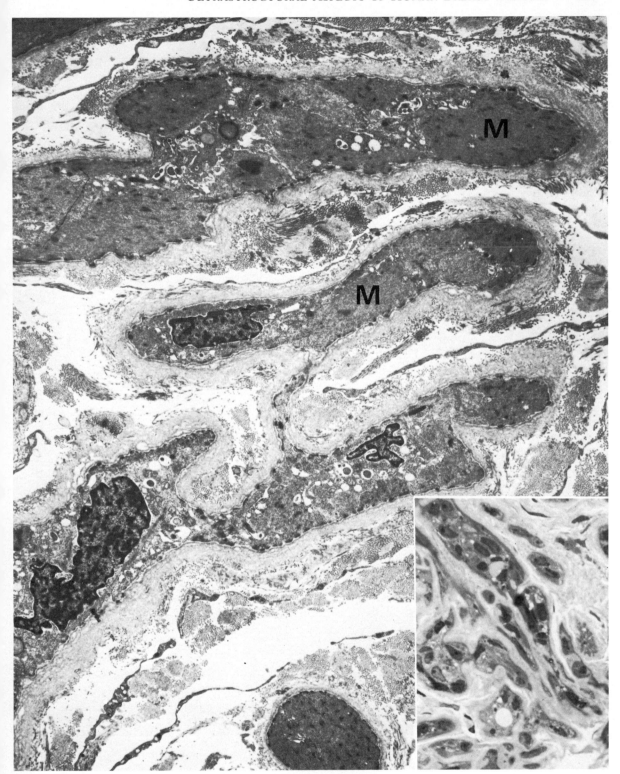

Figure 17–5   Sclerosing adenosis. ×10 000. Inset, toluidine blue. ×300.

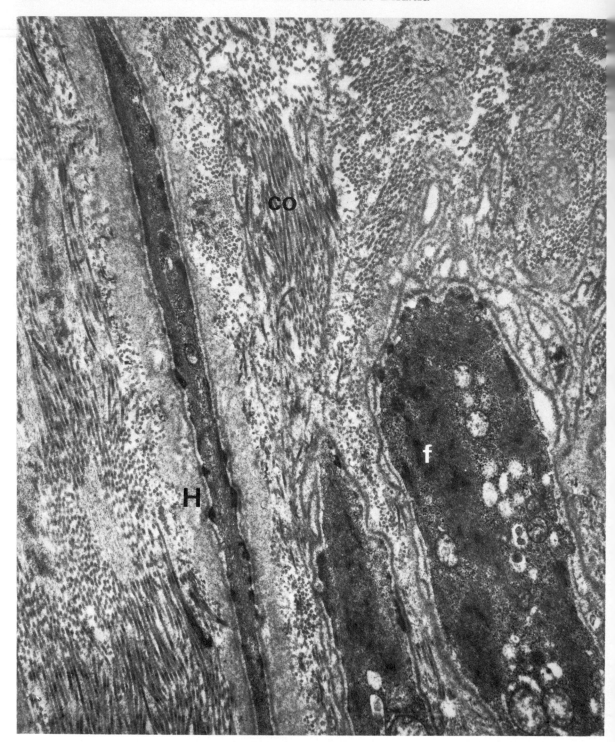

Figure 17–6   Sclerosing adenosis. ×18 750.

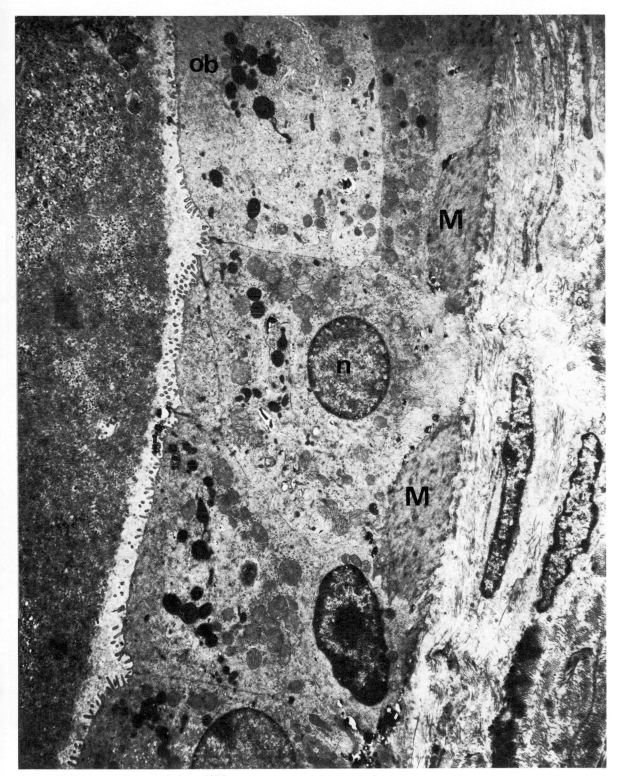

Figure 17–7   Apocrine metaplasia. ×6250.

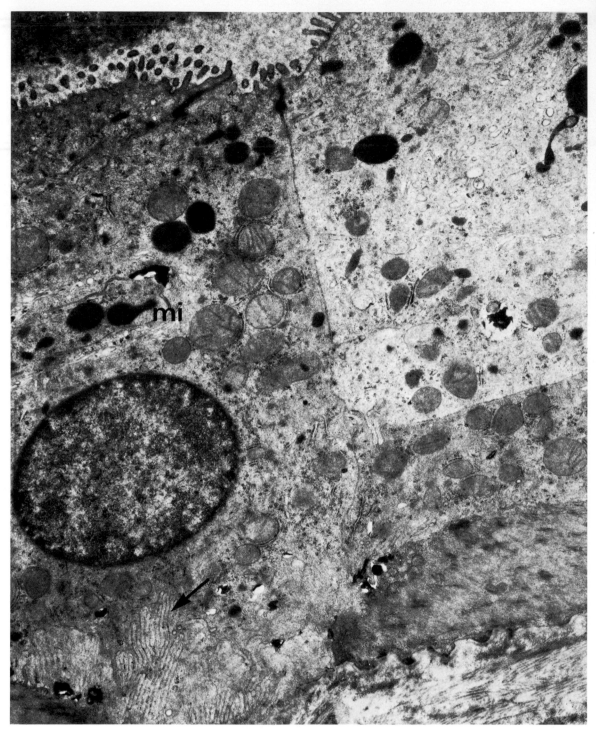

Figure 17–8 Apocrine metaplasia. ×12 500.

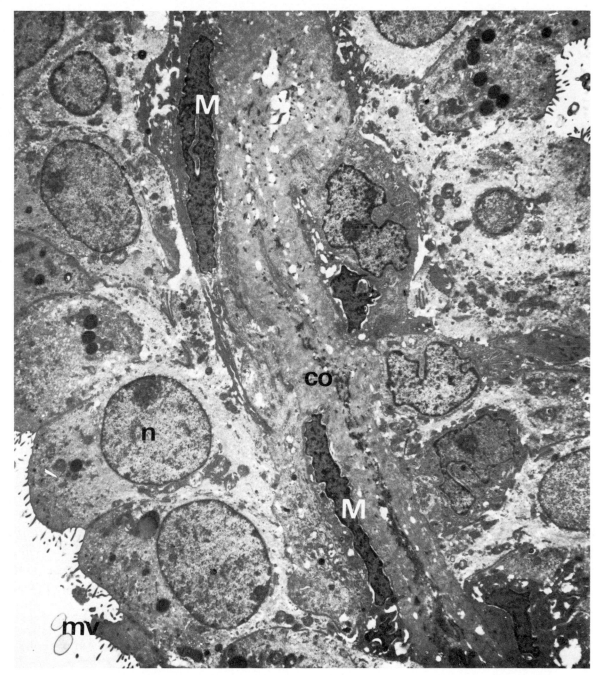

Figure 17–9   Intraductal papilloma. ×5625.

Ultrastructurally, the tumour cells of relatively uniform size are arranged in single or multiple layers to form papillary processes (Figure 17–10). The apical surface projecting towards the lumen (L) is usually covered by short, extremely stunted microvilli. The papillae lack peripheral myoepithelial cells and exhibit a defective or completely absent basal lamina (arrow). The connective tissue core contains loosely arranged collagen bundles (co) and occasional blood vessels (B).

The tumour cell nuclei (n) show a moderate degree of pleomorphism (Figure 17–11). The luminal surface exhibits tight junctions (Tj) and very occasional short microvilli (mv). Along the basal surface, cytoplasmic processes (arrowhead) project towards the stroma and a basal lamina is absent.

The lack of myoepithelial cells in the carcinomatous papillary processes and the defective or absent basal lamina represent important differentiating features from an intraductal papilloma.

INTRADUCTAL CARCINOMA

The tumour cells are confined to the ducts (Figure 17–12) and have large, irregular nuclei (n) with usually prominent nucleoli. Occasional interepithelial lymphocytes (IEL) may be present among the tumour cells, but their functional significance is uncertain. An important diagnostic feature of an intraductal carcinoma is the persistence of myoepithelial cells (M) with associated basal lamina (arrows).

The myoepithelial cells (M) contain spindle-shaped nuclei and are often flattened with the loss of their club-like processes (Figures 17–13 and 17–14). The cytoplasmic filaments (f) are confined to the basal zone and Golgi complexes (G) are prominent. No myoepithelial cells are present among the intraductal carcinoma cells, a feature which is of considerable value in the differentiation of an intraductal carcinoma from epitheliosis, in which myoepithelial cells are frequently seen among the proliferating cells (Ahmed, 1974c).

The basal lamina may vary in thickness and, rarely, it can be multilayered. Focal defects of variable size may also be seen in the basal lamina (arrow). Ozzello (1971) demonstrated the protrusion of carcinoma cells through such defects and suggested that this possibly represents the earliest evidence of invasion.

INTRACYTOPLASMIC LUMINA IN BREAST CANCER CELLS

Intracytoplasmic lumina (I) are encountered among carcinoma cells in both ductal and infiltrating lobular carcinomas, in which they are a common occurrence (Figure 17–15).

Intracytoplasmic lumina are lined by microvilli and may contain central deposits of an amorphous material which almost certainly represents the intracytoplasmic mucin globules described by Gad and Azzopardi (1975) as characterizing the cells of lobular carcinomas.

Intracytoplasmic lumina may very occasionally be seen in benign proliferating lesions of the breast but they are a more frequent feature of mammary carcinomas. The identification of intracytoplasmic lumina has been utilized to denote a primary breast origin of lymph node metastases (Battifora, 1975) and of neoplastic cells in serous fluids (Spriggs and Jerrome, 1975). The finding of intracytoplasmic lumina may also be of value in the differential diagnosis between undifferentiated breast carcinomas and malignant lymphomas, the latter lacking intracytoplasmic lumina as well as desmosomes.

Text continues on page 425

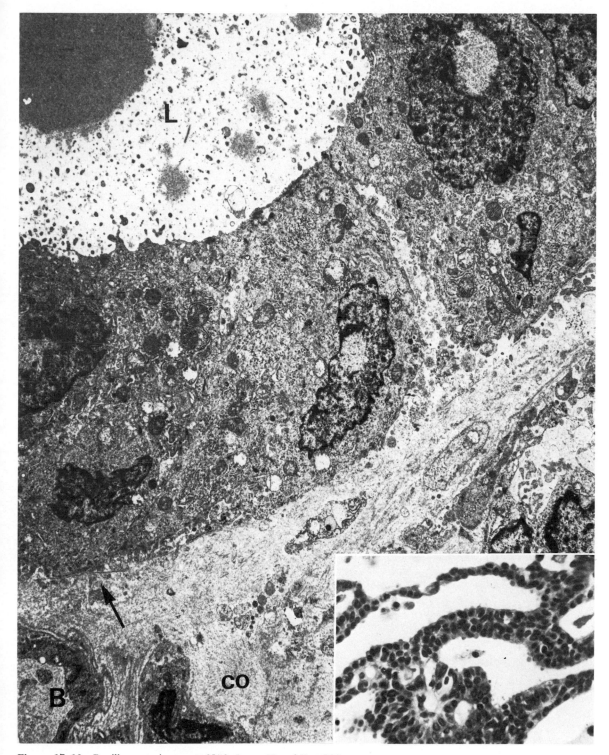

Figure 17–10   Papillary carcinoma. ×6250. Inset, H and E. ×300.

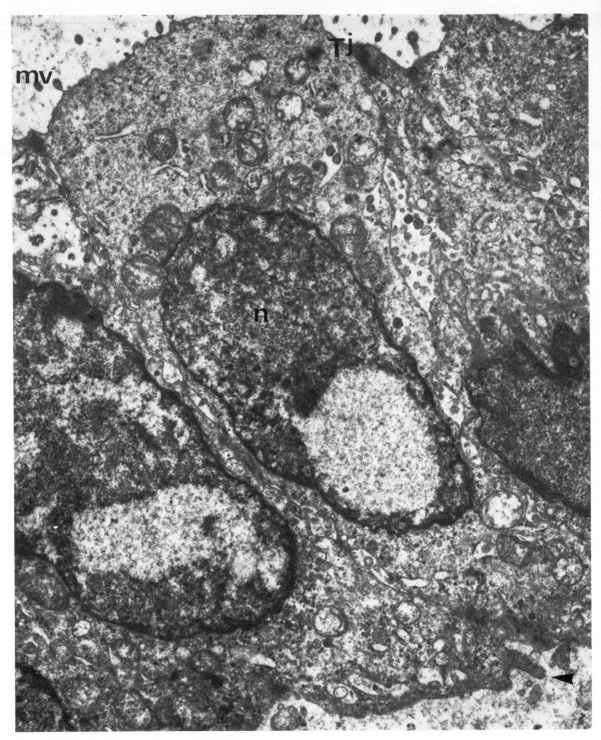

Figure 17–11 Papillary carcinoma. ×12 500.

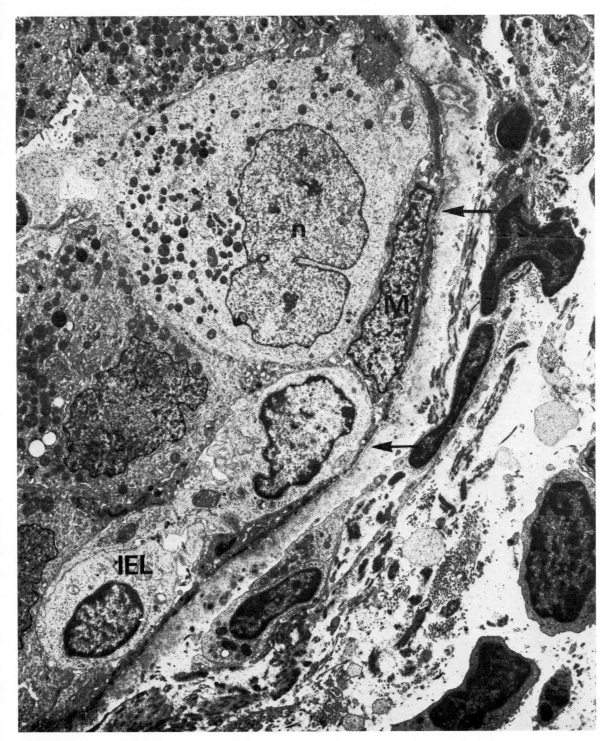

Figure 17–12 Intraductal carcinoma. ×6250.

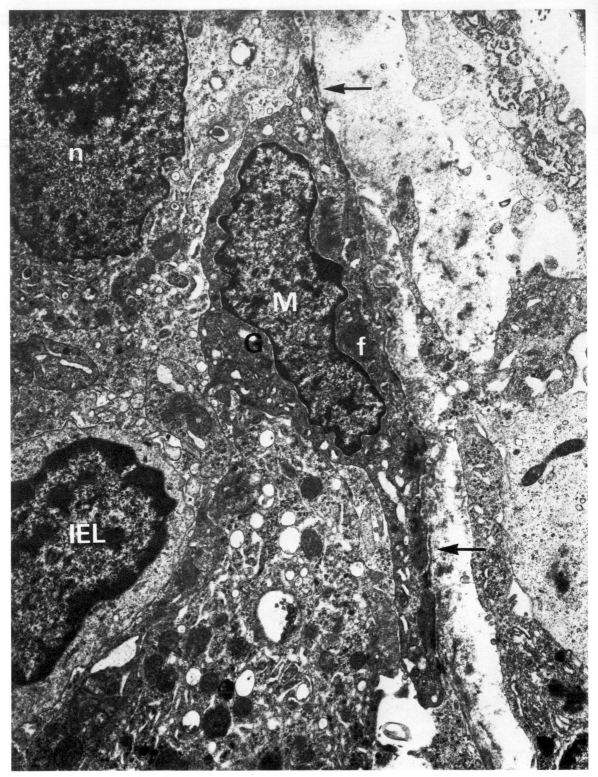

Figure 17–13   Intraductal carcinoma.   ×12 500.

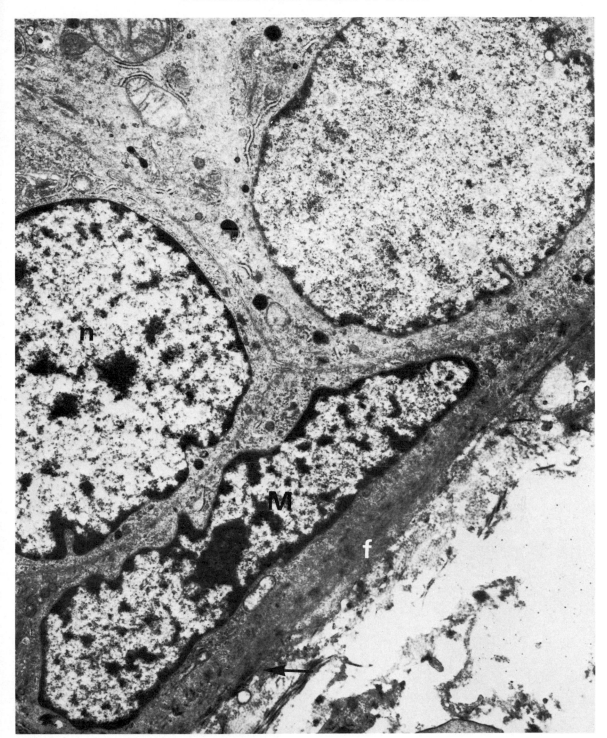

Figure 17–14   Intraductal carcinoma. ×12 500.

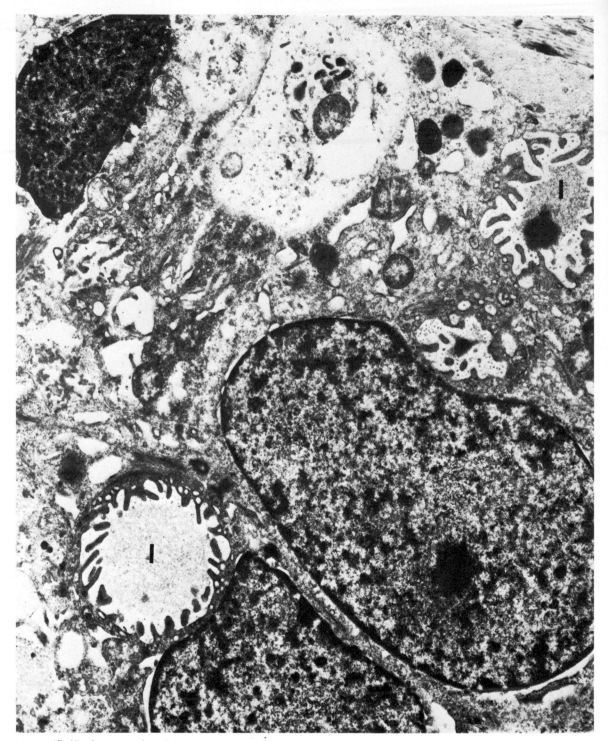

Figure 17–15   Intracytoplasmic lumina. ×12 500.

MYOFIBROBLASTS IN THE STROMA OF BREAST CARCINOMAS

Myofibroblasts exhibiting the morphological features of both fibroblasts and smooth muscle cells have been described in various types of lesion including Dupuytren's contracture (Gabbiani and Majno, 1972) and granulation tissue (Ryan et al, 1974).

Occasional groups of myofibroblasts (MF) may be seen among the tumour cells of an infiltrating ductal carcinoma (TC) (Figures 17–16 and 17–17). Myofibroblasts are characterized by the presence of cytoplasmic filaments (f) with dense bodies (arrowheads) and by well-developed rough-surfaced endoplasmic reticulum (er). Desmosome-like contacts (D) between myofibroblasts have been described.

Stromal cells, previously described in the literature as myoepithelial cells (Ahmed, 1974b) and as active smooth muscle cells (Busch, 1969), probably also represent myofibroblasts.

Myofibroblasts have recently been described in the stroma of tubular carcinoma of the breast and are considered to be a constant feature of this histological variant (Harris and Ahmed, 1977).

The origin of myofibroblasts is still speculative but such cells may represent modified, reactive fibroblasts or may possibly be derived from myoepithelial cells.

ADENOSINE TRIPHOSPHATASE (ATPase) IN BREAST CARCINOMAS

ATPase activity seen as a black deposit (arrow) is located predominantly on the plasma membranes of non-neoplastic myoepithelial cells (Figure 17–18).

Murad (1971) suggested that the presence of strong ATPase activity in certain breast carcinomas implies a myoepithelial cell origin. However, ATPase activity has been observed in mucin-producing carcinoma cells (Ahmed, 1974b), an observation confirmed by Buell, Tremblay and Rowden (1976). In ductal carcinoma cells, ATPase activity is present along the plasma membranes of a cell containing secretory vesicles (sv) (Figure 17–19).

The cytohistochemical localization of ATPase cannot be considered to be a specific indication of a myoepithelial cell origin but may simply reflect the metabolic status of the carcinoma cell plasma membrane.

MUCIN-PRODUCING CARCINOMA

Mucin-producing carcinoma cells are characterized by the presence of fairly prominent cytoplasmic organelles and especially well developed Golgi complexes (G) (Figure 17–20). The cytoplasm contains collections of secretory vesicles (sv), which are said to be formed by synthesizing activity in the rough-surfaced endoplasmic reticulum (er).

The progressive accumulation of the secretory material is said to result in the compression and degeneration of the cytoplasmic organelles and may account for the low-grade malignancy of 'pure' mucin-producing (colloid) carcinomas (Tellem et al, 1966; Ahmed, 1974a). Norris and Taylor (1965) reported the longest survival period in patients with tumours producing copious amounts of mucin.

Text continues on page 431

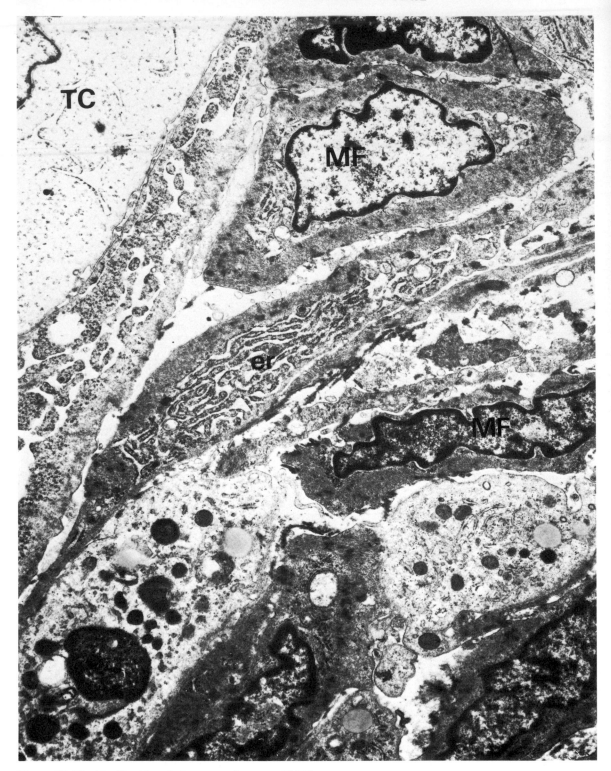

Figure 17–16   Myofibroblasts in breast carcinoma. ×12 500.

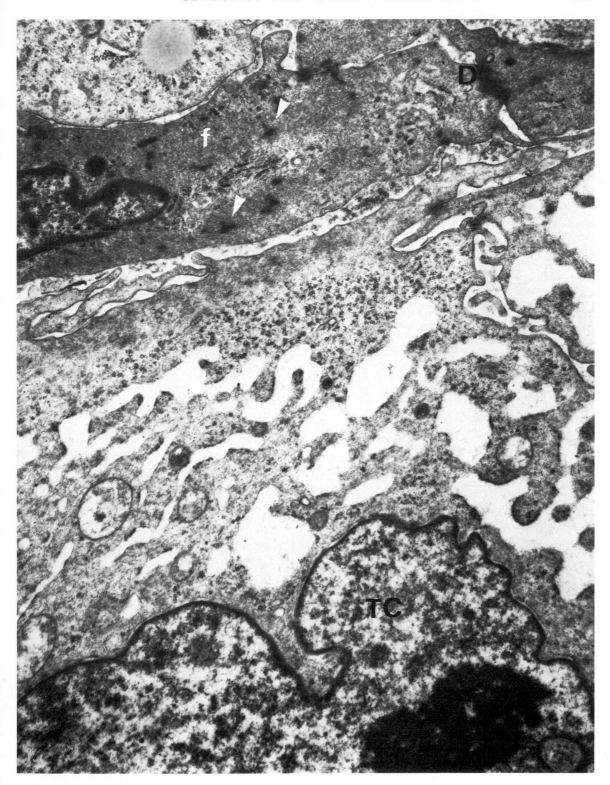

Figure 17–17   Myofibroblasts in breast carcinoma. ×18 750.

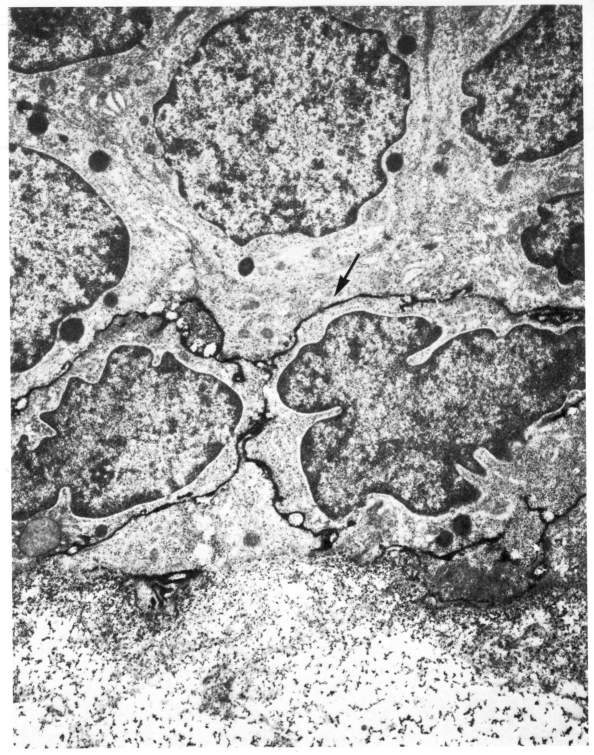

Figure 17–18 ATPase in myoepithelial cells. ×12 500.

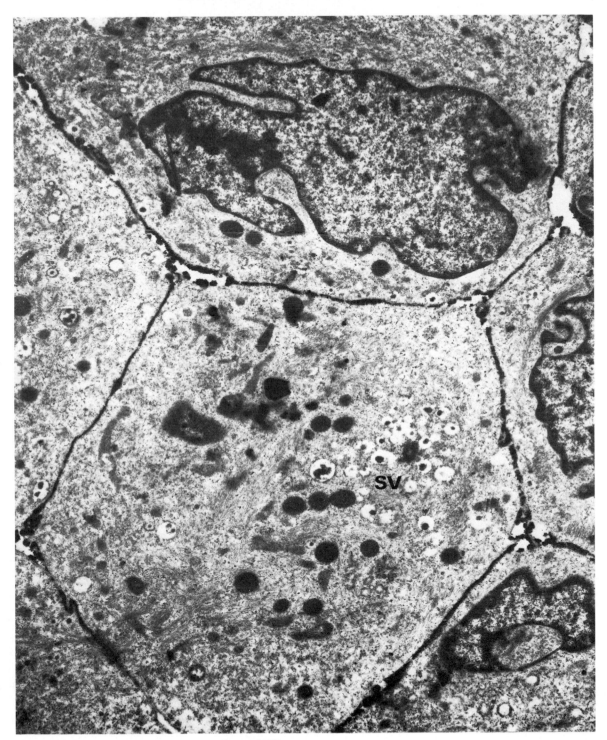

Figure 17–19   ATPase in breast cancer cells. ×12 500.

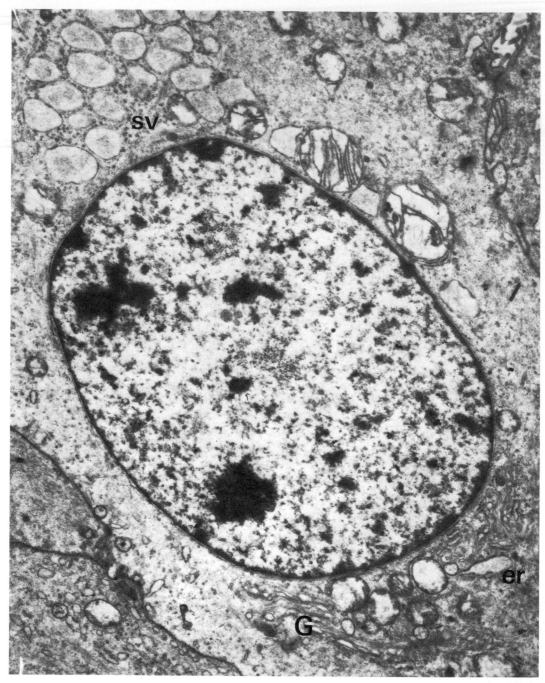

Figure 17–20   Mucin-producing carcinoma. ×12 500. From Ahmed (1974a) with kind permission of the editor of *Journal of Pathology.*

TUBULAR CARCINOMA AND ELASTOSIS

Tubular carcinomas are composed of glandular structures with distinct patent lumina (Figure 17–21) and they are clinically associated with a good prognosis (Taylor and Norris, 1970).

The tumour cells contain large nuclei (n), which sometimes have prominent nucleoli. The glandular structures lack a peripheral myoepithelial cell layer and a basal lamina. The latter features help to distinguish tubular carcinoma from sclerosing adenosis, in which the glandular elements retain the myoepithelial layer and a basal lamina (Jao, Recant and Swerdlow, 1976).

The luminal surface is often covered by a profusion of microvilli and the cytoplasm forms apical snouts (arrow).

The adjacent stroma contains numerous elastic fibres (el). The prominence of elastic tissue in tubular carcinomas of the breast has been stressed by Tremblay (1974). Stromal myofibroblasts (MF) are also commonly seen in tubular carcinomas, and they are considered to be an important feature of this tumour type (Harris and Ahmed, 1977).

APOCRINE CARCINOMA

Tumours of the breast consisting of large, eosinophilic cells often arranged in glandular and tubular formations have been called apocrine carcinomas (Figure 17–22). Such tumours have been considered to be derived from metaplastic apocrine epithelium but an origin de novo is not excluded.

Ultrastructurally the tumour cells are characterized by the presence of numerous round or elongated mitochondria (mi) and scattered osmiophilic granules. Both of these features are seen in cells of apocrine metaplasia and in normal apocrine gland cells (Munger, 1965). The large irregular nuclei (n) contain prominent nucleoli.

Although apocrine carcinoma cells possess distinct morphological features, these tumours do not differ in their behaviour when compared with the commoner infiltrating ductal carcinoma.

PAGET'S DISEASE OF THE NIPPLE

The nipple shows intraepidermal nests of Paget cells, which are larger than adjacent epidermal cells and are characterized by a usually pale cytoplasm and large nuclei with prominent nucleoli (Figure 17–23, inset).

At the ultrastructural level, Paget cells (PC) show widely dispersed cytoplasmic organelles consisting of endoplasmic reticulum, mitochondria, Golgi complexes and secretory granules but lacking tonofilaments (Figure 17–23). The adjacent epidermal cells (EC) are characterized by electron dense cytoplasm containing bundles of tonofilaments (arrowhead).

The large nuclei (n) of Paget cells show prominent nucleoli (Figure 17–24). The plasma membranes possess microvilli (arrow) and desmosomes (D), which are located between Paget cells and occasionally even between Paget cells and adjacent epidermal cells (EC).

The origin of Paget cells remains controversial. Toker (1967) and Gros and Girardie (1971), in common with most workers, considered Paget cells to be the neoplastic counterparts of mammary duct epithelium, a suggestion strongly supported by the absence of tonofilaments and the presence of secretory vesicles and of microvillous differentiation in Paget cells. The presence of desmosomes linking Paget cells and keratinocytes, however, raises the possibility of an additional element of in situ transformation of epidermal cells to Paget cells, as suggested by Sagebiel (1969), although such a derivation cannot be regarded as proven.

Text continues on page 436

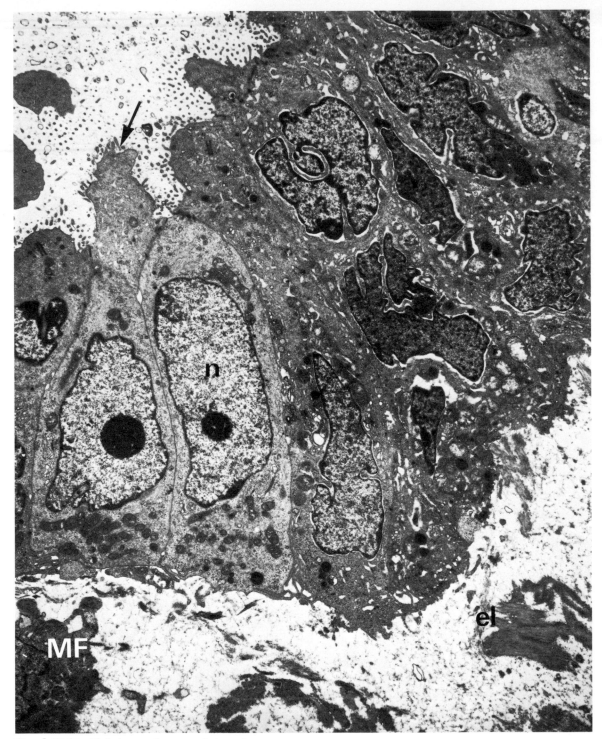

Figure 17–21   Tubular carcinoma and elastosis. ×6250.

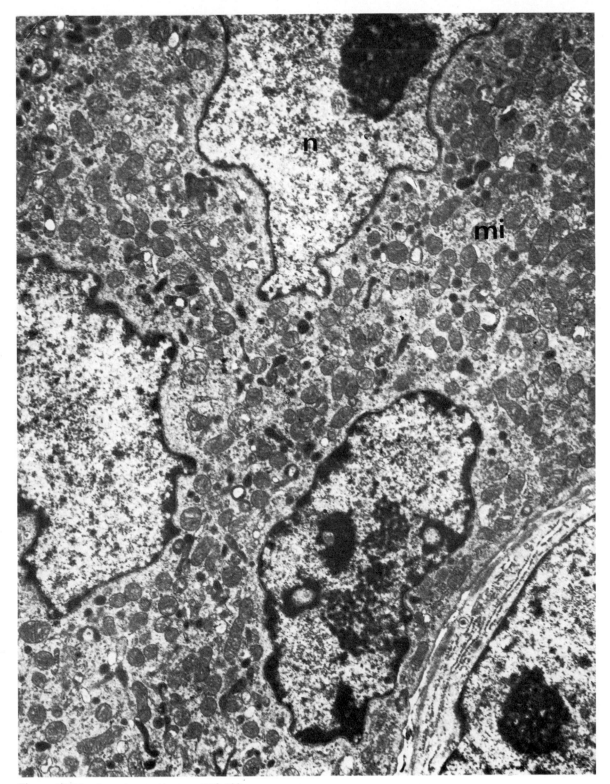

Figure 17–22   Apocrine carcinoma. ×12 500.

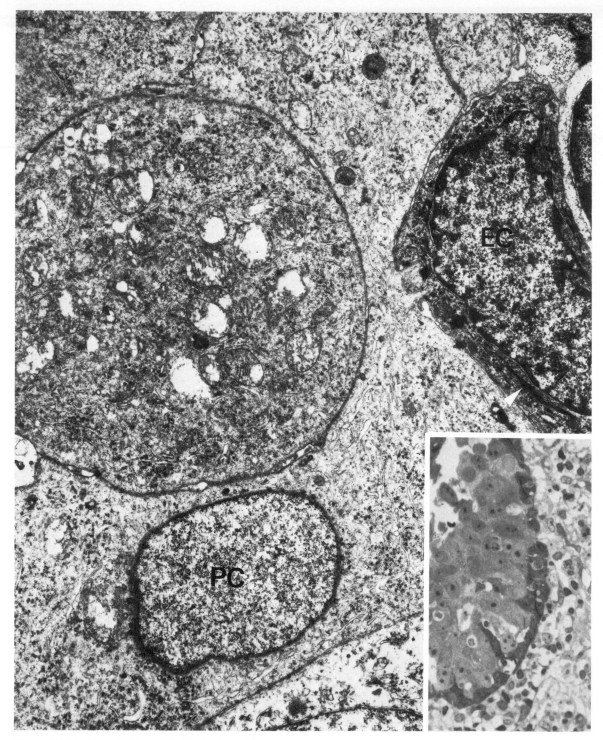

Figure 17–23   Paget's disease of the nipple. ×12 500. Inset, toluidine blue. ×300.

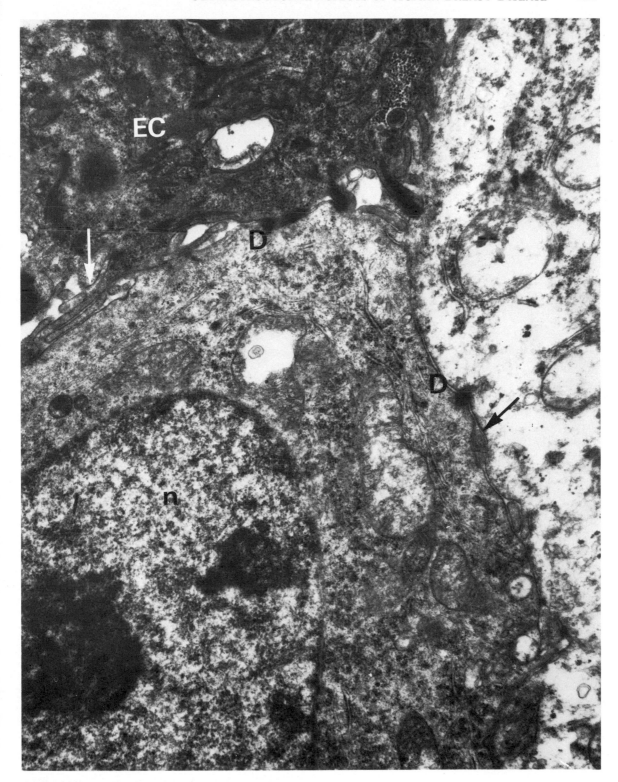

Figure 17–24   Paget's disease of the nipple. ×25 000.

References

Ahmed, A. (1974a) Electron microscopic observations of scirrhous and mucin-producing carcinomas of the breast. *Journal of Pathology,* **112,** 177–181.

Ahmed, A. (1974b) The myoepithelium in human breast carcinoma. *Journal of Pathology,* **113,** 129–135.

Ahmed, A. (1974c) The myoepithelium in cystic hyperplastic mastopathy. *Journal of Pathology,* **113,** 209–215.

Ahmed, A. (1975) Apocrine metaplasia in cystic hyperplastic mastopathy: histochemical and ultrastructural observations. *Journal of Pathology,* **115,** 211–214.

Archer, F. and Omar, M. (1969) Pink cell (oncocytic) metaplasia in a fibroadenoma of the human breast: electron microscopic observations. *Journal of Pathology,* **99,** 119–124.

Battifora, H. (1975) Intracytoplasmic lumina in breast carcinoma. *Archives of Pathology,* **99,** 614–617.

Buell, R. H., Tremblay, G. and Rowden, G. (1976) Distribution of adenosine triphosphatase in infiltrating ductal carcinoma and non-neoplastic breast. *Cancer,* **38,** 875–887.

Busch, W. (1969) Elektronenmikroskopische Untersuchungen an der Tumor-Bindegewebsgrenze beim Mammacarcinom der Frau. *Virchows Archiv A: Pathologische Anatomie,* **346,** 15–28.

Gabbiani, G. and Majno, G. (1972) Dupuytren's contracture: fibroblast contraction? An ultrastructural study. *American Journal of Pathology,* **66,** 131–146.

Gad, A. and Azzopardi, J. G. (1975) Lobular carcinoma of the breast: a special variant of mucin-secreting carcinoma. *Journal of Clinical Pathology,* **28,** 711–716.

Gros, C. and Girardie, J. (1971) Données ultrastructurales concernant l'origine des cellules de Paget du mamelon. *Annales de Dermatologie et de Syphiligraphie (Paris),* **98,** 57–62.

Harris, M. and Ahmed, A. (1977) The ultrastructure of tubular carcinoma of the breast. *Journal of Pathology,* **123,** 79–83.

Jao, W., Recant, W. and Swerdlow, M. A. (1976) Comparative ultrastructure of tubular carcinoma and sclerosing adenosis of the breast. *Cancer,* **38,** 180–186.

Munger, B. L. (1965) The cytology of apocrine sweat glands. II. Human. *Zeitschrift für Zellforschung,* **68,** 837–851.

Murad, T. M. (1971) A proposed histochemical and electron microscopic classification of human breast cancer according to cell of origin. *Cancer,* **27,** 288–299.

Murad, T. M. and von Haam, E. (1968a) Ultrastructure of myoepithelial cells in human mammary gland tumors. *Cancer,* **21,** 1137–1149.

Murad, T. M. and von Haam, E. (1968b) The ultrastructure of fibrocystic disease of the breast. *Cancer,* **22,** 587–600.

Norris, H. J. and Taylor, H. B. (1965) Prognosis of mucinous (gelatinous) carcinoma of the breast. *Cancer,* **18,** 879–885.

Ozzello, L. (1971) Ultrastructure of the human mammary gland. In *Pathology Annual* (Ed.) Sommers, S. C. pp. 1–59. New York: Appleton-Century-Crofts.

Pier, W. J., Garancis, J. C. and Kuzma, J. F. (1970) The ultrastructure of apocrine cells. In intracystic papilloma and fibrocystic disease of the breast. *Archives of Pathology,* **89,** 446–452.

Ryan, G. B., Cliff, W. J., Gabbiani, G., Irle, C., Montandon, D., Statkov, P. R. and Majno, G. (1974) Myofibroblasts in human granulation tissue. *Human Pathology,* **5,** 55–67.

Sagebiel, R. W. (1969) Ultrastructural observations on epidermal cells in Paget's disease of the breast. *American Journal of Pathology,* **57,** 49–64.

Spriggs, A. I. and Jerrome, D. W. (1975) Intracellular mucous inclusions — a feature of malignant cells in effusions in the serous cavities, particularly due to carcinoma of the breast. *Journal of Clinical Pathology,* **28,** 929–936.

Tandler, B. (1966) Fine structure of oncocytes in human salivary gland. *Virchows Archiv für pathologische Anatomie und Physiologie und für klinische Medizin,* **341,** 317–326.

Taylor, H. B. and Norris, H. J. (1970) Well-differentiated carcinoma of the breast. *Cancer,* **25,** 687–692.

Tellem, M., Nedwich, A., Amenta, P. S. and Imbriglia, J. E. (1966) Mucin-producing carcinoma of the breast: tissue culture, histochemical and electron microscopic study. *Cancer,* **19,** 573–584.

Toker, C. (1967) Further observations in Paget's disease of the nipple. *Journal of the National Cancer Institute,* **38,** 79–92.

Tremblay, G. (1974) Elastosis in tubular carcinoma of the breast. *Archives of Pathology,* **98,** 302–307.

Chapter Eighteen

Mammography

It has been claimed that mammography is the most useful diagnostic aid in the earlier detection of malignant disease of the breast and that it has done more to stimulate interest in breast cancer than any single procedure since Halstead introduced radical mastectomy (Scott, 1967). Certainly the evolution of mammography has led to a more co-operative approach to breast cancer between surgeon, pathologist and radiologist (Egan, 1975). The increasing use of radiological examination of tissue specimens in recent years, as part of routine and research procedures in many pathology departments, has been due largely to the increasing use of mammographic techniques.

HISTORY AND DEVELOPMENT OF MAMMOGRAPHY

Mammography is the radiological examination of the tissues of the breast, relying on differential absorption within the tissues to produce a detailed outline of the internal structure. Additional techniques such as injection of contrast media into ducts, or air into cysts, can be employed where appropriate.

The radiological appearance of the breast was first described in 1913 by Salomon, a German surgeon who studied mastectomy specimens. Clinical radiological examination of the breast was used as early as 1930 by Warren in the United States and numerous articles were published in the following years as the diagnostic potential of mammography became apparent. Technical difficulties and indifferent radiographs led to a wane in the initial enthusiasm, but a few pioneers persisted. Notable amongst these were Gershon-Cohen (1937) in the United States, Leborgne (1949) of Uruguay and Gros and Sigrist (1952) in France. In 1960 a major step forward occurred when Egan published a paper in the United States claiming a high degree of accuracy in the identification of malignant disease by mammography. Since then the technique has become widely employed in centres throughout the world. Subsequent improvements have included the use of molybdenum anodes (rather than the conventional tungsten), giving a softer radiation energy which is especially suited to discriminate between fat, muscle and fibrous tissue. More recently, the combination of vacuum-packed film backed by an intensifying screen such as Agfa Gevaert Medichrome, Dupont Lo-dose and Kodak Min-R has considerably reduced the necessary patient dose.

Concurrent with these developments in conventional film mammography was the introduction of xeromammography. In this process the recording medium is an electro-statically charged selenium-coated plate. Exposure to radiation causes the charge to leak away through the plate leaving a latent charge image. When a cloud of powder is sprayed towards the plate, particles adhere to the latent charge, producing a visible image. The picture is then transferred for permanent record onto special plastic-coated paper. The development and popularization of xero-radiography is due mainly to the work of Wolfe (1968) in the United States. Proponents of xeroradiography claim that the pictures obtained provide greater detail and are easier to interpret (Martin, 1973; Frankl and Rosenfeld, 1975; Malone et al, 1975), but the method requires slightly higher dosage than some of the latest film–screen combinations.

MAMMOGRAPHIC TECHNIQUES

Comparative studies of the different methods used in mammography have often reached different conclusions and trials comparing all methods are difficult to organize. The selection of a particular technique will depend on various factors. In a screening centre it is important that the radiation dose is as low as possible and the technical process of producing pictures is fast, so that an efficient rate of patient flow can be maintained. Comparison of different methods has suggested that lower-dose systems produce some loss in discrimination (Tonge, Davis and Millis, 1976) and therefore in symptomatic patients other techniques such as xeroradiography, with slightly higher dosage but very good discrimination, may be the method of choice.

The use of different recording devices does not influence the positioning of the patient during radiological examination. In most centres two views of the breast are taken, the cranio-caudal and lateral. In some institutes an axillary view is also routine. Other additional views can be taken where necessary — for example, when a lesion is felt in a part of the breast which may not be shown to the best advantage in the conventional views.

Single view mammography, which obviously cuts down radiation dose and increases patient flow, has been practised in some centres, and some workers report a high degree of diagnostic accuracy (Lundgren and Jakobsson, 1976; Buchanan and Jager, 1977; Cukier, Lopez and Maravilla, 1977). Others, however, are less enthusiastic and claim that there is a loss of sensitivity and increase in the number of false negative findings when only one view is used (Libshitz et al, 1976; Andersson et al, 1978).

The cranio-caudal view is usually taken with the patient standing or sitting. The lateral view may also be taken in the upright position, but many radiologists feel that a better picture is obtained with the patient lying down. The amount of compression employed depends on individual preferences. Compression produces thinner more uniformly distributed tissue over the whole area of the breast, at the same time bringing the tissue closer to the recording media. This reduces the dose of radiation necessary and produces a clearer and more uniform image.

It is not within the scope of this chapter to discuss mammographic technique and radiological appearances in any detail, but a number of books have been devoted to this subject to which the reader is referred for further information (Gershon-Cohen, 1970; Egan, 1972; Wolfe, 1972, 1977).

MAMMOGRAPHIC APPEARANCES AND THEIR CORRELATION WITH HISTOLOGICAL FINDINGS

NORMAL APPEARANCES

Radiological examination of the normal breast in young women shows a cone of mainly dense glandular tissue extending from the nipple. With maturity there is a greatly increased amount of fat within the breast with regression of glandular tissue. This is most marked after the menopause. With the increase in the amount of fat the suspensory ligaments and connective tissue trabeculae running through the breast become more easily visible.

Detection of pathological lesions in the breast depends on changes in the normal picture. Most important of these are:

1. Changes in the lesion itself: an opacity and/or calcified particles.
2. Changes in adjacent structures: distortion of trabeculae and changes in skin, nipple, vessels or ducts.

CHANGES IN MALIGNANT DISEASE

Primary Signs. Carcinoma of the breast classically produces a dense opacity with an irregular outline, and prominent tentacles often extend from the main tumour opacity. The surrounding structures are infiltrated rather than compressed, resulting in distortion and destruction of the normal trabecular pattern (Figure 18–1).

Tumours with abundant dense collagenous stroma, even when very small, produce a stellate distortion of the breast architecture due to thickening and shortening of surrounding trabeculae (Figure 18–1).

The more cellular carcinomas, particularly those in which the stroma is less densely collagenous, may have a scalloped or almost rounded outline, but usually there are some areas of irregularity (Figure 18–2).

Less common histological types of carcinoma such as medullary, mucoid or intracystic carcinomas often have a very smooth round outline indistinguishable from a benign tumour (Figure 18–3).

Diffusely infiltrating carcinomas, particularly those with an 'Indian file' or 'single cell' pattern of infiltration, may show very little abnormality, as the change in tissue density of the tumour is minimal in comparison with the surrounding breast tissue. A slight increase in density in a particular area of the breast when compared with the contralateral side, or a previous mammogram, is often the only abnormality detectable.

Leborgne's Law. A malignant tumour usually feels considerably larger on palpation than on radiological examination, whereas a benign lesion has a similar clinical and radiological size. This discrepancy between the clinical and radiological size is sometimes known as Leborgne's Law.

Calcification. This occurs in both malignant and benign lesions of the breast and is seen in

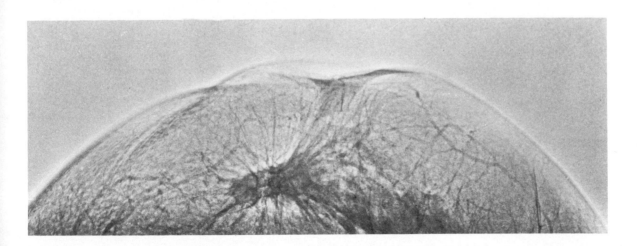

Figure 18–1 Xeroradiograph showing a typical carcinoma with an irregular stellate edge and nipple retraction. Cranio-caudal view. (Courtesy of Dr C. A. Parsons.)

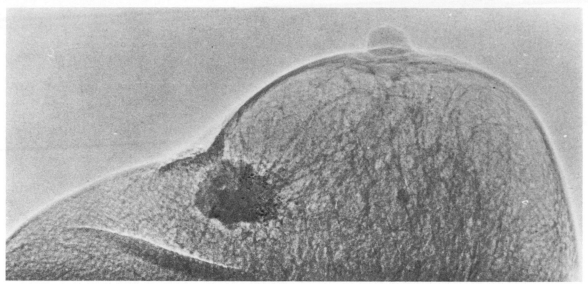

Figure 18–2 Xeroradiograph demonstrating a carcinoma with a partly lobulated and partly stellate edge and fine calcification within and around the tumour density. The overlying skin is thickened and retracted. Lateral view. (Courtesy of Dr C. A. Parsons.)

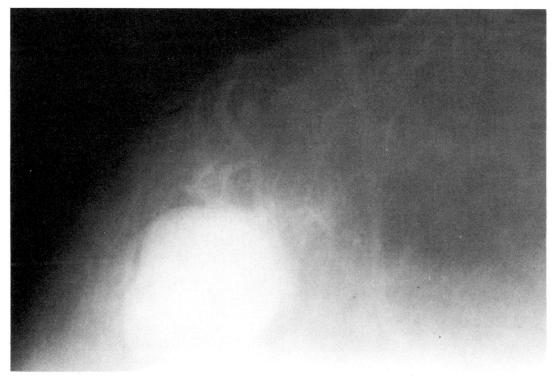

Figure 18–3 Film mammogram showing a well-circumscribed medullary carcinoma with an adjacent dilated vein. Cranio-caudal view. (Courtesy of Dr B. E. Nathan.)

mammograms in 30 to 55 per cent of mammary carcinomas (Table 18–1). It is a most important sign of carcinoma and is the most frequent indicator of clinically occult carcinomas. The significance of different patterns of calcification will be discussed more fully below.

Secondary Signs. The changes seen in the tissues adjacent to a carcinoma are frequently

and Ackerman, 1977). An asymmetrical duct pattern or any abnormally prominent ducts should also be regarded as suspicious. Enlarged axillary lymph nodes can occasionally be detected radiographically before they are clinically palpable (Kalisher, Chu and Peyster, 1976). Calcification has been seen in nodes containing metastases, but is not necessarily significant as it can also occur in normal lymph nodes.

Table 18–1   Incidence of calcification in carcinoma of breast

Report	Calcification	
Preoperative mammography		
Levitan, Witten and Harrison (1964)	29.0%	
Black and Young (1965)	39.0%	
Friedman et al (1966)	24.0%	Film
James and Irvine (1969)	32.0%	
Nathan, Burn and Doyle (1972)	26.0%	
Price, Davies and Butler (1976)	35.5%	
Wolfe (1974)	51.0%	
Millis, Davis and Stacey (1976)	48.5%	Xeromammography
Frankl and Ackerman (1977)	54.7%	
Specimen radiology		
Shepard, Crile and Strittmatter (1962)	75.0%	
Black and Young (1965)	42.0%	
Koehl et al (1970)	62.0%	
Rosen et al (1970)	54.0%	
Fisher, Posada and Ramos (1974)	86.0%	
Histology		
Levitan, Witten and Harrison (1964)	58.0%	
Koehl et al (1970)	39.0%	
Fisher, Gregorio and Fisher (1975)	59.7%	
Millis, Davis and Stacey (1976)	63.0%	

referred to as secondary signs of malignancy. Skin thickening may be recognized on a mammogram long before it can be appreciated clinically (Figure 18–2). Skin retraction (Figure 18–2), nipple retraction (Figure 18–1) and distortion of the normal trabecular pattern have all been described as secondary signs of malignant disease. Increased vascularity, either in the number or size of the veins (Figure 18–3), has been found useful by some authorities (Dodd and Wallace, 1968; Raskin and Poole, 1973), but others have found this an unreliable sign of malignancy (James and Irvine, 1969; Frankl

CHANGES IN BENIGN DISEASE

Fibroadenomas as well as the so-called benign cystosarcoma phyllodes produce a homogeneous opacity with a sharp outline which is usually round, ovoid or lobulated and sometimes surrounded by a translucent zone of compressed fat. Large irregular calcifications are occasionally present, particularly in older women (Figure 18–4).

Fibrocystic disease usually produces a bilateral and symmetrical increase in density, which is most marked in the upper outer quadrant. This may obscure other details of

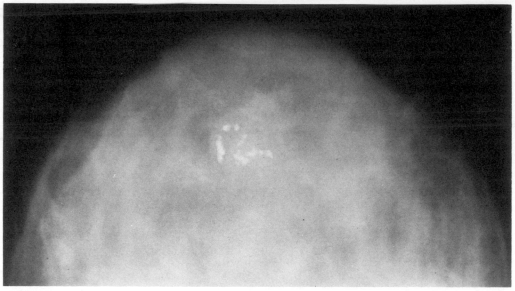

Figure 18–4   Film mammogram of a fibroadenoma containing coarse calcification. The sharp outline of the neoplasm is partly obscured by the density of the surrounding breast structures. Cranio-caudal view. (Courtesy of Dr B. E. Nathan.)

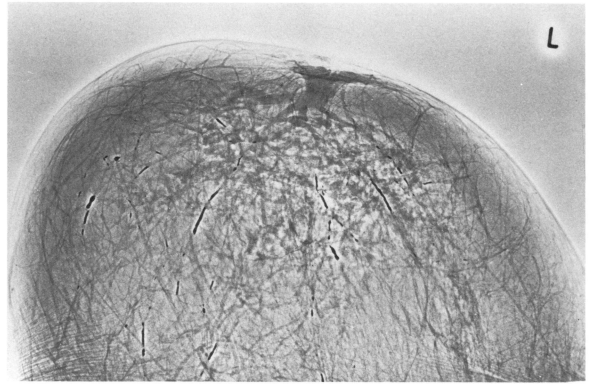

Figure 18–5   Xeroradiograph showing a breast with duct ectasia containing tubular calcification. Cranio-caudal view. (Courtesy of Dr C. A. Parsons.)

the breast architecture including the presence of a neoplasm. Characteristically the density is not homogeneous; multiple overlying cysts with intervening, more translucent areas may be present, as well as sparse, diffusely scattered calcifications. In cases with dominant cysts these are seen as well circumscribed, round or ovoid opacities, often similar to fibroadenomas but more frequently multiple.

In *duct ectasia*, dilated ducts are outlined beneath the nipple, often with characteristic annular or tubular calcifications (Figure 18–5).

negative reports in order to avoid an unnecessarily large number of biopsies. The incidence of false positive reports is unfortunately usually highest in those series in which there is a high degree of accuracy in correctly identifying malignant lesions.

False Positive Reports. Benign lesions which can be misinterpreted as carcinoma include (1) the cystic disease complex, in particular sclerosing adenosis, (2) duct ectasia, (3) postoperative scarring, (4) skin lesions, (5) breast abscess and (6) fat necrosis.

Table 18–2   Reported accuracy of mammography in detecting breast cancer

Report	True positive	False positive
Clark et al (1965)	79.0%	10.0%
Friedman et al (1966)	68.0%	9.0%
James and Irvine (1969)	82.0%	
Stewart, Gravelle and Apsimon (1969)	93.0%	7.0%
Nathan, Burn and Doyle (1972)	88.0%	9.7%
McClow and Williams (1973)	89.0%	
Block and Reynolds (1974)	66.0%	14.8%
Wolfe (1974)	95.3%	
Frankl and Rosenfeld (1975)	98.0%	16.0%
Egan (1977)	87.0%	
Feig et al (1977)	78.0%	
Manoliu and Ooms (1977)	86.6%	19.3%

Lipomas produce a circumscribed area of translucency with compression of the surrounding structures.

ACCURACY OF MAMMOGRAPHY

The reported accuracy of mammography ranges from 66 to 98 per cent (Table 18–2). The interpretation of mammograms is by no means infallible and in all the series there are false positive and false negative reports. The degree of accuracy that can be achieved depends on the method of selection of the population studied, the type of breast examined, the procedure used and the experience of the individual observer. It is important to strike a reasonable balance between the number of false positive and false

Sclerosing adenosis and focal sclerotic scars (see Chapter Nine) in particular may mimic the appearance of 'scirrhous' carcinoma, both on mammographic and gross appearance, even to the presence of fine calcification (MacErlean and Nathan, 1972; Eusebi, Grassigli and Grosso, 1976) (Figure 18–6).

Duct ectasia can produce nipple retraction as well as calcification, although the latter is usually of a characteristic type (Figure 18–5).

Postoperative changes following a biopsy can produce irregular fibrosis, skin thickening and puckering. This emphasizes the need for close communication between clinician and radiologist. Surgical scars and other skin lesions such as a mole must always be noted and clearly marked by the clinician and radiographer so that the radiologist is not misled on examining the mammogram.

The presence of inflammation in the breast

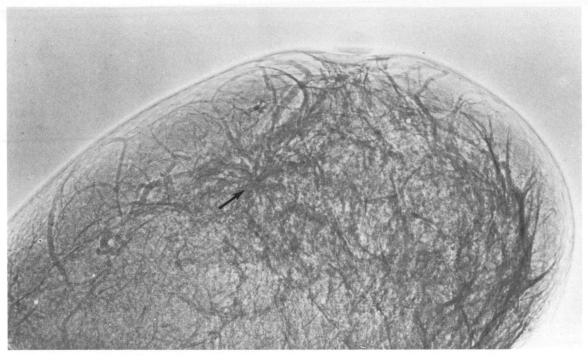

Figure 18–6 Xeroradiograph demonstrating an area of sclerosing adenosis producing a stellate distortion of the breast architecture resembling a carcinoma. Lateral view. (Courtesy of Dr C. A. Parsons.)

may obviously produce distortion in the architecture as well as skin changes.

Fat necrosis has been reported to produce a spectrum of changes within the breast ranging from an appearance indistinguishable from that of a carcinoma to the presence of cystic spaces sometimes with calcified walls (Bassett, Gold and Cove, 1978).

False Negative Reports. Failure to identify a malignant tumour may occur because the lesion is (1) not visualized or (2) mistaken for a benign lesion.

A carcinoma may be obscured by the density of the surrounding breast. This happens most frequently in young women with small dense breasts or in the presence of extensive fibrocystic disease. Occasionally a peripheral lesion or one close to the chest wall may not be included for technical reasons in routine mammographic views.

Diffusely infiltrating tumours may produce very little change in density and may therefore be missed. In situ carcinomas often do not produce a localized density and will not be visualized unless there is associated calcification.

Very well circumscribed malignant tumours may easily be mistaken for benign lesions. In many of these situations the secondary signs of malignancy can be helpful (Figure 18–3).

BREAST PARENCHYMAL PATTERNS AS AN INDEX OF CANCER RISK

Differences in the radiographic pattern of the breast parenchyma have been related to the subsequent risk of developing breast cancer, a finding of considerable importance if it is reproducible. In a retrospective study using xeroradiography, Wolfe (1976) found that women with a prominent duct pattern and those with severe 'dysplasia' had a greater incidence of breast cancer than those with predominantly fatty breasts. Some subsequent studies have tended to confirm these findings (Peyster, Kalisher and Cole, 1977; Wilkinson et al, 1977; Krook et al, 1978) and in one series a correlation was found between age at

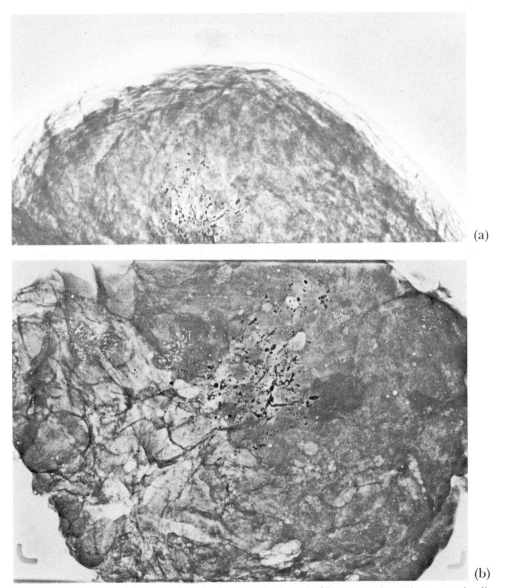

(a)

(b)

Figure 18–7   Xeroradiograph of (a) breast — lateral view — and (b) surgical biopsy specimen demonstrating linear and branching calcifications in an infiltrating ductal carcinoma with a large in situ component. From Millis, Davis and Stacey (1976) with kind permission of the authors and the editor of *British Journal of Radiology.*

first pregnancy and parenchymal pattern (Andersson, Andren and Pettersson, 1978). However, other experienced workers have failed to confirm Wolfe's (1976) findings and have challenged their validity on the basis of an inherent bias in his study (Egan and Mosteller, 1977; Mendell, Rosenbloom and Naimark, 1977). While even very small carcinomas are easily detectable in radiolucent breasts, dense fibroglandular tissue may have delayed detection of carcinomas in the

highest-risk group defined by Wolfe (1976). This would result in an *apparent* subsequent increase in cancer incidence in this group.

In a recent histopathological study, Fisher et al (1978) failed to show any consistent correlation with the parenchymal patterns described by Wolfe (1976) apart from a significantly greater incidence of 'fibrous mazoplasia' in his highest-risk group. Conversely another correlative study found histopathological grading of 'precancerous lesions' corresponded closely with xeroradiographic risk classes (Wellings and Wolfe, 1978).

CALCIFICATION

Radiography is the only method of detecting calcification within the breast prior to surgery. Calcification occurs in both malignant and benign disease. Its significance was first documented by Leborgne in 1949 and since then much has been written concerning the pattern associated with malignant and benign breast disease (Black and Young, 1965; Gershon-Cohen, Berger and Curcio, 1966; Hassler, 1969; Koehl et al, 1970). Attempts have been made to devise computer pattern-recognition programmes to evaluate calcification seen on mammograms (Ackerman and Gose, 1972; Wee et al, 1975). The characteristic radiological appearance of calcification associated with malignancy has been described as clusters of numerous small particles, irregular in density and shape. These are sometimes linear or spiculated and frequently so fine that they can be seen only with the aid of a hand lens. They are usually closely packed together on both the mammographic views and may occur alone, although, more frequently, they are located within or around a tumour density (Figure 18–2). Calcifications associated with benign disease are said to be larger, more uniform in shape and size, fewer in number and more diffusely scattered within the breast.

TYPES OF CALCIFICATION

Radiological types of calcification can be broadly subdivided into the following groups.

1. A cluster of small irregular particles is strongly suggestive of malignancy, although it may be seen also in benign disease, especially in sclerosing adenosis (Figure 18–2).
2. Larger linear or branching calcifications are seen in intraductal carcinomas, but can also occur in duct ectasia (Figure 18–7).
3. A few widely scattered and more uniform particles are often seen in cystic disease. These are usually rather larger than those typically seen in malignant disease.
4. Coarse irregular deposits may be seen in fibroadenomas and more rarely in irradiated carcinomas (Figure 18–4).
5. Annular or tubular calcifications occur classically in duct ectasia but can also be seen rarely in intraductal carcinomas (Figure 18–5).
6. Tortuous streaks as a result of calcification in the walls of arteriosclerotic vessels are sometimes seen.

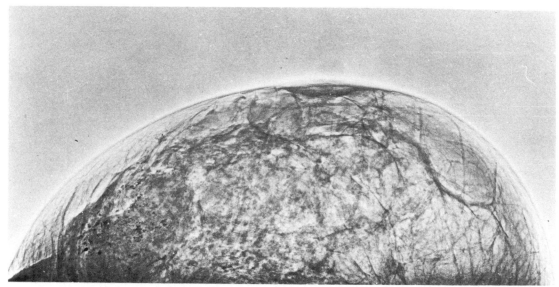

Figure 18–8   Xeroradiograph of a breast containing calcifications in an area of fibrocystic disease resembling those seen in a carcinoma. Cranio-caudal view. From Millis, Davis and Stacey (1976) with kind permission of the authors and the editor of *British Journal of Radiology.*

Is there a Pathognomonic 'Malignant Calcification'? In the past the problem of distinguishing between the calcifications associated with benign and malignant disease was usually minimized and many leading authorities felt that certain appearances were pathognomonic of malignancy. However, with increasing use of mammography there has been growing awareness that patterns of calcification are not always as specific as originally claimed and that identical appearances may be seen in malignant and benign conditions (Fisher, Posada and Ramos, 1974; Millis, Davis and Stacey, 1976; Murphy and DeSchryver-Kecskemeti, 1978) (compare Figures 18–7 and 18–8).

CALCIFICATION AS AN INDICATION FOR BIOPSY

A cluster of calcifications, particularly when including fine particles, should be considered an indication for biopsy. The detection of calcification of this type is of great importance. In some patients the presence of calcification is the only indicator of malignancy and is the most important single factor in the diagnosis of clinically occult carcinomas (Kieraldo et al, 1976; Frankl and Ackerman, 1977). Most centres find that between 20 and 40 per cent of biopsies performed because of mammographic calcification contain malignant disease (Rogers and Powell, 1972; Bauermeister and Hall, 1973; Rosen, Snyder and Robbins, 1974; Murphy and DeSchryver-Kecskemeti, 1978).

Tumour Types Detected when Calcification is the Only Indication for Biopsy. A relatively high proportion of malignancies detected by virtue of the presence of calcification *alone* are found to be 'early' carcinomas, often of the non-invasive type. In addition histological examination of benign biopsies performed because of abnormal mammographic findings, particularly those associated with calcifications, are often said to show marked epithelial proliferation and atypia (Moskowitz et al, 1976a; Owen et al, 1977). It has even been suggested that benign lesions showing microcalcification may represent a high-risk

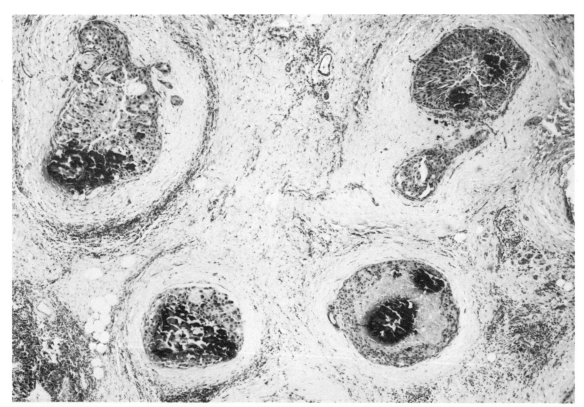

Figure 18–9   In situ ductal carcinoma with calcification in the necrotic debris in the centre of the ducts. H and E. ×50. (Courtesy of Professor N. F. C. Gowing.)

group (Gibbs et al, 1975). An alternative explanation is that some of these cases of severe epithelial proliferation with atypia actually represent 'early' in situ malignancies.

INCIDENCE OF CALCIFICATION IN CARCINOMAS

The reported incidence of calcification in carcinomas seen on preoperative mammograms using conventional film ranges from 30 to 40 per cent (Table 18–1). When tissue blocks or thin slices of tissue are examined a higher percentage is found, ranging from 40 to 60 per cent, and, in one series, as many as 86 per cent of carcinomas were found to contain calcifications when 3 to 5 mm tissue slices were examined radiologically (Fisher, Posada and Ramos, 1974). Many of the calcified particles are too fine to be seen on preoperative mammograms unless they are very closely clustered together. Although very fine particles not visible mammographically can be seen on histological examination, with the practical limitations of tissue sampling the regions containing calcification may be missed. In centres using xeroradiography, calcification is noted in a slightly higher number of preoperative mammograms, mainly due to the increased discrimination of this technique (Martin, 1973; Wolfe, 1974; Malone et al, 1975; Millis, Davis and Stacey, 1976). Quantitative methods of evaluating the discriminating ability of different mammographic techniques, using phantoms and samples of breast tissue, have shown that there is a difference in the capability of the various recording media to detect fine particles of calcification (Tonge, Davis and Millis, 1976).

SIZE OF CALCIFIED PARTICLES

The size of particles of calcification seen on mammograms varies from approximately 100 to 1500 μm with occasional larger particles. In carcinomas the range of size is particularly wide and usually includes some very fine particles. When calcifications are measured in histological sections they are found on average to be smaller, ranging from approximately 10 to 500 μm with aggregates up to 1500 μm. This discrepancy in size is due to a number of factors, including the irregular shape of the calcifications, which are only occasionally sectioned across their greatest diameter, and

the frequency of shattering on sectioning. In addition several small particles in close proximity, either two- or three-dimensionally, appear as a single particle radiologically.

HISTOLOGICAL APPEARANCES

The histological appearances of calcification have not been studied so extensively (Levitan, Witten and Harrison, 1964; Patton, Poznanski and Zylak, 1966; Hassler, 1969; Koehl et al, 1970; Millis, Davis and Stacey, 1976). Calcification has been noted in virtually all types of carcinoma, but occurs most frequently in ductal carcinoma in situ and in infiltrating ductal carcinoma with a large in situ component. Calcification is also present in a high percentage of tubular and papillary carcinomas. On the whole it tends to be seen more frequently in well-differentiated carcinomas than in poorly differentiated carcinomas and this may in part account for the fact that it is rarely if ever seen in medullary carcinoma with lymphoid stroma (see also Chapter Twelve for other possible explanations). The incidence of calcification in lobular carcinomas is variable and it is said to be present frequently in the adjacent benign breast tissue rather than amongst the malignant cells (Koehl et al, 1970; Rosen, Snyder and Robbins, 1974).

Calcification in Necrotic In Situ Tumour. In ductal carcinoma in situ, calcification is frequently found in the necrotic debris in the lumen of the ducts (Figure 18–9). In infiltrating carcinomas, the in situ component may also be present outside the confines of the main tumour mass and thus, on the mammogram, calcification may be seen within and around the tumour density (Figure 18–2). The calcification within the ducts consists of granular aggregates of numerous particles which vary in size and are irregular and angular in shape. The texture of the calcification resembles that of the granular necrotic material in which it is deposited. This irregular appearance is exaggerated by the shattering of the calcium particles on section. It is this type of calcification that may give rise to the linear or branching pattern on mammography (Figure 18–7). The calcification may occur in the centre of the necrotic material or be deposited around the periphery and, in the latter situation, it may

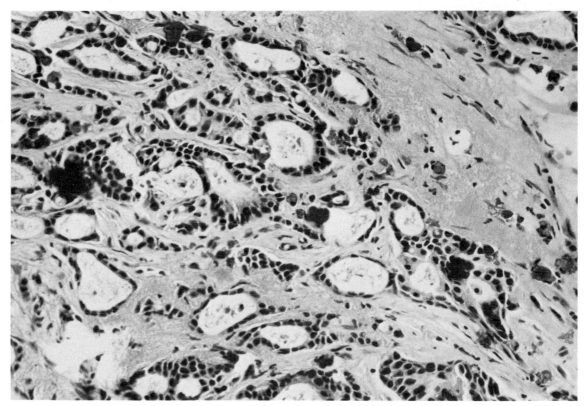

Figure 18–10   Well-differentiated infiltrating carcinoma of breast containing small round homogeneous and laminated calcifications. H and E. ×235. (Courtesy of Professor N. F. C. Gowing.)

mimic radiologically the pattern of calcification more typical of duct ectasia.

Calcification in Areas of Viable In Situ and Infiltrating Carcinoma. In ductal carcinoma with a cribriform pattern and in areas of infiltrating carcinoma the calcium most frequently takes the form of small, sharply defined, round, homogeneous or laminated bodies which occur either singly or in small aggregates. These bodies may be present within tubules, among solid islands of malignant cells or in the stroma (Figure 18–10). When located in the latter position calcification has presumably remained after the epithelial cells have degenerated and disappeared.

Granular and Laminated Calcification. The granular calcification typically seen in the centre of malignant ducts appears to be deposited in degenerating necrotic tissue. The rounded or laminated bodies are more often deposited among mucinous and proteinaceous secretion.

Ultrastructure. Electron microscopic studies of calcification in breast carcinomas have shown needle-like crystals associated with electron-dense material, identical in appearance, among tumour cells, in intracytoplasmic lumina and in the adjacent stroma (Ahmed, 1975). In this study the calcified material was found to be hydroxyapatite. Previous studies using x-ray diffraction demonstrated hydroxyapatite and tricalcium phosphate in the calcifications associated with carcinomas (Hassler, 1969).

Calcium in Benign Disease. Calcium deposits in benign disease are sometimes of the psammomatous type, especially when present in areas of sclerosing adenosis (Figure 18–11) and apocrine cysts. However, larger, more homogeneous particles are also seen. In fibroadenomas very large coarse areas of

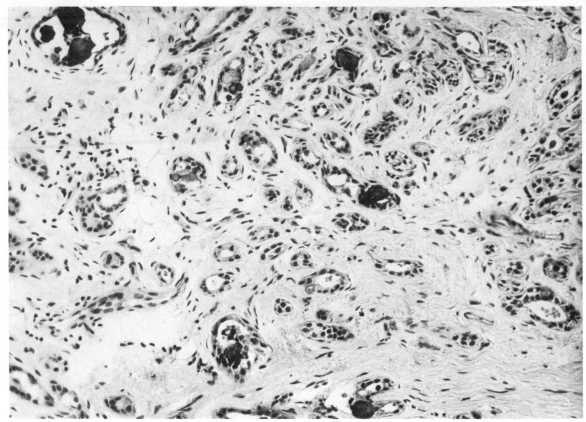

Figure 18–11   Sclerosing adenosis containing small round homogeneous and laminated calcifications. H and E. ×235. (Courtesy of Professor N. F. C. Gowing.)

calcification are sometimes present, usually in densely hyaline stroma. Similar types of calcification have been noted occasionally in the stroma of an irradiated carcinoma. The calcification seen in duct ectasia consists of relatively large, homogeneous deposits which may be situated within the ductal lumen but are more usually located in the collagenous wall of the ducts.

EFFECT OF RADIATION ON CALCIFICATION

Following irradiation, calcifications seen on mammography within a carcinoma may persist unchanged, increase in number, or alter in appearance. Even the disappearance of calcification has been reported. The persistence of calcification or a change in the pattern or even the appearance of calcification for the first time following irradiation does not necessarily indicate recurrent or persistent malignant disease (D'Orsi, 1977; Libshitz, Montague and Paulus, 1977).

SPECIMEN RADIOGRAPHY

Value in Occult Carcinomas. The greatest value of specimen radiography is in the management of specimens from patients with clinically occult carcinoma, when a breast biopsy is performed entirely on the basis of an abnormal mammogram. Close co-operation between surgeon, radiologist and pathologist is essential to ensure that the mammographic abnormality is included in the tissue which is excised and to localize the area of the specimen from which tissue blocks should be taken for section. The surgeon has to remove an impalpable lesion and the pathologist has to section an area of abnormality that frequently cannot be differentiated from the adjacent tissue either by palpation or visual examination.

Surgical Localization of a Suspicious Area. An attempt must be made to 'pin-point' the exact area of suspicion in the breast to avoid massive distorting biopsies. In practice this can usually be done by using the two standard mammographic views, aided when necessary by further special views (Berger et al, 1966; Stevens and Jamplis, 1971). Occasionally, however, a more precise method is required.

Special Localizing Techniques. Various localizing techniques have been described including the use of skin markers, the injection of radio-opaque material with or without visible dye or the insertion of needles into the breast. These can then be related to the area under suspicion after further mammographic views are taken with the marker in situ (Simon et al, 1972; Rosato, Thomas and Rosato, 1973; Frankl and Rosenfeld, 1975; Frank, Hall and Steer, 1976; Millis et al, 1976; Bigongiari et al, 1977; Owen et al, 1977; Preece et al, 1977). Devices for needle biopsy of the breast under radiographical monitoring have also been described (Mühlow, 1974; Bolmgren, Jacobson and Nordenström, 1977).

Radiography of Biopsy Specimens. Regardless of the localizing method used, radiological examination of the specimen for accurate comparison with the preoperative mammogram is essential in order to confirm that the tissue under suspicion has been removed. This is particularly important when locating calcifications. Specimen radiography is often less helpful in identifying a mammographically suspicious area that does not contain calcifications. If the surgeon labels the biopsy with a radio-opaque marker the specimen can be orientated in relation to the radiograph and, if the suspicious area is found to have been incompletely removed, the region in which excision is incomplete can be identified. The specimen radiograph also helps the pathologist to localize the area of tissue to section. Unless there is an obvious tumour it is *best to forgo frozen section examination* and to take multiple blocks of tissue for permanent paraffin sections. If the tissue is sliced and further radiographs are made, blocks can be taken accurately from the areas containing calcification or showing other mammographic abnormalities.

Matching the Number of Calcified Particles. Examination of sections from a biopsy removed because of calcification must reveal a similar number of particles to that seen on the mammogram. If not, then deeper sections and if necessary more tissue must be examined. A radiograph should be taken of the spare tissue and the blocks. If calcification is seen in the blocks, further radiographic examination at right angles to the cut surface will help the technician cutting deeper sections to establish its depth within the block. It should be remembered, however, that not all opacities seen in paraffin blocks represent calcifications; some are found to be artefacts (Black and Young, 1965; Koehl et al, 1970). Only when all the tissue containing calcification has been examined can the possibility of a carcinoma be reasonably excluded.

Calcification Adjacent to Carcinoma. It must be appreciated, moreover, that a carcinoma may be found adjacent to an area of benign tissue containing calcification. Although it has been suggested that this occurs particularly frequently with lobular carcinoma in situ, the association may well be entirely fortuitous (Fisher and Fisher, 1977).

Postoperative Management. If there is any serious doubt about the removal of the suspicious area, a repeat mammogram should be performed a few weeks postoperatively.

Other Indications for Specimen Radiography. In the early days of mammography carcinomas were sometimes detected by specimen radiography, even when the tissue had been pronounced benign following routine gross and microscopic examination (Rosen et al, 1970). Many of these occult carcinomas were located by the presence of fine calcifications which were not always seen on the preoperative mammogram. However, with improvements in the quality of mammography, patient mammograms now have clarity approaching that of specimen radiographs, thus reducing the yield of carcinomas unsuspected on clinical mammography. Routine specimen radiography, however, is still rewarding, particularly in biopsies (a) from patients in a high-risk category, e.g. with a contralateral breast carcinoma, (b) where preliminary sections have shown carcinoma in situ or atypia, and possibly (c) where the large size of the specimen may warrant it (Snyder and Rosen, 1971; Gallager, 1975). However, some workers have suggested that thorough examination of specimens utilizing whole mount histopathological preparations or step sections or serial blocks may yield more information than radiological techniques (Patchefsky et al, 1973).

Technique of Specimen Radiography. Although specimen radiography may be carried out in the routine x-ray department, it is quicker and more convenient if units designed for radiographic examination of tissue specimens are sited in the laboratory. Recording media of the highest resolution may be employed as levels of radiation exposure are obviously unimportant. Fine grain radiographic films or xeroradiography are suitable. Polaroid film has also been used, but, although convenient, lacks the high degree of resolution necessary for demonstrating fine calcifications (Rosen, Snyder and Robbins, 1974; Gallager, 1975). Compression of specimens is claimed to improve the image obtained (Frankl, 1978).

Radiography of Mastectomy Specimens. The application of radiographic examination to the study of mastectomy specimens has led to renewed interest and understanding of the extent and evolution of mammary carcinomas. Techniques have been described in which mastectomy specimens are sliced at 5 to 10 mm intervals and then arranged on a radiolucent background for specimen radiology (Egan, Ellis and Powell, 1969; Gallager and Martin, 1969; Hutter and Kim, 1971; Davies, Roberts and Richardson, 1973). It may be helpful if the tissue is chilled first, as the inflexible material can then be readily cut on a meat slicer. When using xeroradiography as a recording medium the specimen must be x-rayed prior to fixation in order to obtain the full benefit of increased architectural detail demonstrated by this technique. The slices of tissue can also be examined using a dissecting microscope and large sections prepared and areas of abnormality seen on the radiographs matched up with their gross counterpart. Tissue for paraffin blocks should be selected on the basis of both gross and radiological findings to identify the non-palpable lesions. The method is somewhat time consuming and is not suitable for small laboratories, but is useful as a research technique in evaluating the full extent of mammary disease. Lymph nodes can also be demonstrated on specimen mammograms and this may be helpful in locating and enumerating the number of nodes present. However, small or fatty nodes can be missed and careful gross examination is also necessary. Differentiation between uninvolved lymph nodes and those containing metastatic tumour is usually possible only when large or irregular nodes are obviously replaced by tumour.

OTHER MALIGNANT NEOPLASMS

The radiological appearances of the less common mammary neoplasms of the breast are less well studied.

Sarcomas, including Malignant Cystosarcoma Phyllodes. These tumours are usually seen as well-demarcated, rounded or lobulated lesions similar to, but generally larger than, fibroadenomas (Berger and Gershon-Cohen, 1962; Millis, Atkinson and Tonge, 1976). Areas of coarse calcification are occasionally present. Sometimes there is blurring and irregularity of part of the tumour margin. As a rule the diagnosis of sarcoma can be suspected only in the case of very large tumours, particularly if there is evidence of rapid growth.

Lymphoma. Lymphomatous deposits within the breast may be unilateral or bilateral and usually appear as discrete, circumscribed densities very similar to cysts. However, lymphomatous involvement can also be diffuse, producing skin thickening, oedema and a disturbed trabecular pattern with increased and coarse trabeculae most noticeable in the subdermal region (Millis, Atkinson and Tonge, 1976).

Leukaemia. Involvement of the breast by leukaemic infiltration is more often bilateral and may take the form of either a discrete lump or diffuse involvement. The former usually has an irregular outline and may resemble a primary carcinoma of the breast both clinically and radiologically. When the breasts are diffusely involved, dense granularity with multiple ill-defined homogeneous densities has been described. After successful chemotherapy the mammographic appearance of the breast may return to normal (Millis, Atkinson and Tonge, 1976).

Metastatic Carcinoma. Metastatic carcinoma in the breast, although uncommon, does occur and correct diagnosis may save the patient from an unnecessary mastectomy. The metastatic lesion can then be treated by chemotherapy appropriate for the type of malignancy concerned. On mammography the lesions are usually represented by well-defined rounded densities which may be single or multiple. The appearances may be confused with a benign breast lesion, such as a fibroadenoma (Jochimsen and Brown, 1976; McIntosh et al, 1976; Toombs and Kalisher, 1977). Metastatic spread from a contralateral breast carcinoma has been described as producing diffuse skin thickening, increased stromal density and blurring of the trabeculae and vein margins, without a mass or calcifications (Egan, 1976).

SCREENING FOR BREAST CANCER

Screening for breast cancer was introduced in an attempt to detect 'early' carcinomas and reduce breast cancer death rates. Regular clinical examination long preceded the widespread use of mammography, but it was hoped that mammographic examination would detect some clinically occult carcinomas. Mammography as a screening procedure is of value only if its use increases the detection of small and clinically occult carcinomas.

The Value of Screening. The successful results of screening of well women are perhaps best illustrated by the well-known controlled trial carried out by the Health Insurance Plan of Greater New York, in which a group of women was screened annually for five years and compared with a control group which was not screened (Strax et al, 1967; Strax, Venet and Shapiro, 1973). Results have shown a 35 per cent reduction in the number of deaths from breast cancer in the group offered annual screening, the decreased mortality being mainly restricted to women aged over 50 years. This decrease persisted over an eight-year follow-up period (Shapiro, 1977). The value of multiple modes of examination is evident in that one-third of the cancers were detected *only* by mammography while two-fifths were detected by clinical examination *alone* (Strax, Venet and Shapiro, 1973). With improvement of mammographic techniques, the proportion of cancers detected by mammography has increased. Nevertheless suspicious clinical findings should never be disregarded in the presence of normal mammographic findings, just as a suspicious mammogram should always be investigated even in the presence of normal clinical findings.

Cancer Detection Rates. Screening clinics are now to be found all over the USA and in several centres in Europe. Cancer detection rates reported have varied between 1.6 and 19.3 per 1000 women, depending on whether truly asymptomatic women are examined, whether there is an element of selection by the women themselves or whether there is deliberate selection of groups of women at high risk (Table 18–3). The pick-up rate is always highest in the first year. Most cancer screening programmes find the highest pick-up rate in women over the age of 50 years and a comparatively high rate in the fifth decade. This is due to the prevalence of cancer in older women and to the ease of interpreting mammograms of fatty postmenopausal breasts, compared with the difficulty of interpretation of the small, dense, glandular breasts of younger women. In all these studies a small proportion of cancers appeared between the annual screening visits. Education of women in self-examination of the breast is important in the detection of these '*interval cancers*' (Strax, 1976).

Tumour Types Detected by Screening. Tumours detected by screening are usually relatively small and relatively frequently in situ. The number of stage one carcinomas of the breast found in screening clinics is striking. The percentage of tumours with negative axillary nodes is highest in those detected by mammography alone (Table 18–4 and see Chapter Twelve).

Value Questioned. Despite the apparent benefits of screening, the value of detecting cancer at an 'early' stage has been questioned. If a disease is merely detected two years sooner and the patient lives two years longer from diagnosis to death no actual benefit from an earlier diagnosis has resulted: it could in fact be argued that harm has been done. Attempts are made to allow for this '*lead time*' bias when evaluating the benefits of screening. It has also been suggested that the end results of treatment are dependent more on the biological activity of the tumour and on the host than on the time at which treatment is started. Some studies have shown an overall

Table 18-3   Cancer detection rates reported in screening programmes

Report	Detection rate per 1000 women	Selection of women	Screening method
Witten and Thurber (1964)	1.60	Asymptomatic. No clinical evidence of breast disease. Over 40 years	Mammography only
Wolfe (1965)	4.10	Normal physical examination. Over 46 years	Mammography only
Stevens and Weigen (1966)	6.50	Asymptomatic. Clinically normal. Over 40 years	Mammography only
Davey, Greening and McKinna (1970)	8.50	Asymptomatic but some had palpable lumps	Clinical examination Mammography Thermography
Dowdy et al (1971)	13.20	Mostly asymptomatic. Over 40 years	Clinical examination Mammography Thermography
Gilbertsen and Kjelsberg (1971)	1.32	Asymptomatic. Over 45 years	Clinical examination only
Strax, Venet and Shapiro (1973)	2.72	Invited women. 40 to 64 years	Clinical examination Mammography
Stark and Way (1974)	19.30	Asymptomatic high - risk group. Over 35 years	Clinical examination Mammography Thermography
Chamberlain et al (1975)	14.00	Self-referred. Over 40 years	Clinical examination Mammography
Lewis et al (1975)	6.70	Asymptomatic. Over 35 years	Clinical examination Mammography Thermography
Bailey et al (1976)	6.86	Self-referred. Mostly asymptomatic	Clinical examination Thermography Mammography on selected women
George et al (1976)	8.40	Invited, referred and self-referred	Clinical examination Mammography
Kieraldo et al (1976)	7.70	Negative clinical examination	Mammography only
Lundgren and Jakobsson (1976)	6.70	Self-referred. Over 34 years	Single view mammography only
Moskowitz et al (1976b)	9.20	Self-referred. 35 years and over	Clinical examination Mammography Thermography
Egan (1977)	11.50	Asymptomatic. 35 years or over	Mammography only
Sayler et al (1977)	9.70	Asymptomatic. Self-selected. 35 years and over	Clinical examination Mammography Thermography
Owen et al (1977)	3.00	Invited. 40 to 60 years	Clinical examination Mammography Thermography
Patchefsky et al (1977)	8.90	Asymptomatic. 45 to 65 years	Clinical examination Mammography Thermography

lack of association between treatment failure and duration of symptoms. Patients with slowly growing tumours before treatment frequently show slow progression after treatment and survive longer when compared with patients who have rapidly growing tumours before treatment (Charlson and Feinstein, 1974; Fisher, Redmond and Fisher, 1977). Slowly progressive tumours will remain in the preclinical phase longer, increasing the time during which they can be detected by screening. Thus screening may not be

use. The need for information relating risk to benefit and cost to benefit, attendant on the increased use of mammography, is paramount.

Radiation Hazards. There is no *direct* evidence that the low dose of radiation currently used in mammography increases the incidence of breast cancer. Current fears are largely based on extrapolations from data on the carcinogenic effects of high doses of radiation. These are mainly derived from

Table 18–4   Reported incidence of positive axillary lymph nodes in clinically occult carcinomas detected by mammography

Report	Positive axillary lymph nodes
Strax, Venet and Shapiro (1973)	23.0%
McClow and Williams (1973)	36.7%
Malone et al (1975)	32.0%
Kalisher and Schaffer (1975)	35.0%
Moskowitz et al (1976b)	10.9%
Egan (1977)	8.0%
Frankl and Ackerman (1977)	23.0%
Letton, Wilson and Mason (1977)	12.5%
Patchefsky et al (1977)	8.0%
Sayler et al (1977)	7.0%

detecting cancers at a more curable stage but merely finding slow-growing tumours which would have a better prognosis in any event (Feinleib and Zelen, 1969).

Value and Dangers of Mammography. The place of mammography in screening centres in particular has been questioned, both with regard to the radiation hazard and to the real value of the detection of occult tumours (Bailar, 1976, 1977; Moskowitz et al, 1977; Upton et al, 1977; Mole, 1978). The evidence for the role of mammography in the reduction of breast cancer mortality has been challenged. The question of radiation hazard to the breast during mammography is an emotive one and currently the topic of considerable discussion. Although much work has been done to determine the patient dose, the issue is a very complex and controversial one because there are many variables in the wide range of mammographic systems in

studies showing an increased incidence of breast carcinoma in women who received repeated chest fluoroscopies in tuberculosis clinics (Mackenzie, 1965; Myrden and Hiltz, 1969; Boice and Monson, 1977), those treated by radiation for acute postpartum mastitis (Mettler et al, 1969; Shore et al, 1977) and other non-neoplastic conditions of the breast (Baral, Larsson and Mattsson, 1977), and from atomic bomb survival data (Wanebo et al, 1968; McGregor et al, 1977). The validity of extrapolating known risks from high doses of radiation to lower doses is not known. Nor is there information available on whether there is any interreaction between radiation and other known risk factors.

CONCLUSIONS ON SCREENING

The value of mammography as a diagnostic technique in helping to evaluate patients with signs and symptoms of breast disease is well established and not in question. At present there is more or less general agreement that there is a net benefit from screening by mammography and clinical examination in women over the age of 50, but the value of screening particularly by mammography in younger women is much more controversial (Lesnick, 1977; Lester, 1977; Letton, Wilson and Mason, 1977; Sayler et al, 1977; Shapiro, 1977). Fewer occult carcinomas are detected in younger age groups (but see page 275 for a different point of view) and the radiation dose required to obtain a good image is somewhat greater. In addition the sensitivity of the breast to radiation may well be greater in young women (Mole, 1978). A case can however be made for selecting younger women for screening who are at a higher risk of developing breast cancer on the basis of certain known aetiological factors; these include a history of carcinoma in the contralateral breast and a family history of breast carcinoma. When screening high-risk groups, however, one must not forget the possibility already mentioned that these may be the very women who are most sensitive to radiation.

It is important that continued attention should be directed towards assessing the actual carcinogenic risks of mammography and to improving radiological techniques so that the radiation dose required may be further reduced.

References

Ackerman, L. V. and Gose, E. E. (1972) Breast lesion classification by computer and xeroradiograph. *Cancer*, **30**, 1025–1035.

Ahmed, A. (1975) Calcification in human breast carcinomas: ultrastructural observations. *Journal of Pathology*, **117**, 247–251.

Andersson, I., Andren, L. and Pettersson, H. (1978) Influence of age at first pregnancy on breast parenchymal pattern: a preliminary report. *Radiology*, **126**, 675–676.

Andersson, I., Hildell, J., Mühlow, A. and Pettersson, H. (1978) Number of projections in mammography: influence on detection of breast disease. *American Journal of Roentgenology*, **130**, 349–351.

Bailar, J. C., III (1976) Mammography: a contrary view. *Annals of Internal Medicine*, **84**, 77–84.

Bailar, J. C., III (1977) Screening for early breast cancer: pros and cons. *Cancer*, **39**, 2783–2795.

Bailey, A., Davey, J., Pentney, H., Tucker, A. and Wright, H. B. (1976) Screening for breast cancer: a report of 11 654 examinations. *Clinical Oncology*, **2**, 317–322.

Baral, E., Larsson, L.-E. and Mattsson, B. (1977) Breast cancer following irradiation of the breast. *Cancer*, **40**, 2905–2910.

Bassett, L. W., Gold, R. H. and Cove, H. C. (1978) Mammographic spectrum of traumatic fat necrosis: the fallibility of 'pathognomic' signs of carcinoma. *American Journal of Roentgenology*, **130**, 119–122.

Bauermeister, D. E. and Hall, M. H. (1973) Specimen radiography: a mandatory adjunct to mammography. *American Journal of Clinical Pathology*, **59**, 782–789.

Berger, S. M. and Gershon-Cohen, J. (1962) Mammography of breast sarcoma. *American Journal of Roentgenology*, **87**, 76–81.

Berger, S. M., Curcio, B. M., Gershon-Cohen, J. and Isard, H. J. (1966) Mammographic localization of unsuspected breast cancer. *American Journal of Roentgenology*, **96**, 1046–1052.

Bigongiari, L. R., Fidler, W., Skerker, L. B., Comstock, C. and Threatt, B. (1977) Percutaneous needle localisation of breast lesions prior to biopsy: analysis of failures. *Clinical Radiology*, **28**, 419–425.

Black, J. W. and Young, B. (1965) A radiological and pathological study of the incidence of calcification in diseases of the breast and neoplasms of other tissues. *British Journal of Radiology*, **38**, 596–598.

Block, M. A. and Reynolds, W. (1974) How vital is mammography in the diagnosis and management of breast carcinoma. *Archives of Surgery*, **108**, 588–591.

Boice, J. D., Jr and Monson, R. R. (1977) Breast cancer in women after repeated fluoroscopic examinations of the chest. *Journal of the National Cancer Institute*, **59**, 823–832.

Bolmgren, J., Jacobson, B. and Nordenström, B. (1977) Stereotaxic instrument for needle biopsy of the mamma. *American Journal of Roentgenology*, **129**, 121–125.

Buchanan, J. B. and Jager, R. M. (1977) Single view negative mode xeromammography: an approach to reduce radiation exposure in breast cancer screening. *Radiology*, **123**, 63–68.

Chamberlain, J., Ginks, S., Rogers, P., Nathan, B. E., Price, J. L. and Burn, I. (1975) Validity of clinical examination and mammography as screening tests for breast cancer. *Lancet*, **ii**, 1026–1030.

Charlson, M. E. and Feinstein, A. R. (1974) The auxometric dimension. *Journal of the American Medical Association*, **228**, 180–185.

Clark, R. L., Copeland, M. M., Egan, R. L., Gallager, H. S., Geller, H., Lindsay, J. P., Robbins, L. C. and White, E. C. (1965) Reproducibility of the technic of mammography (Egan) for cancer of the breast. *American Journal of Surgery*, **109**, 127–133.

Cukier, D. S., Lopez, F. A. and Maravilla, R. B., Jr (1977) One-view follow-up mammogram. *Journal of the American Medical Association*, **237**, 661–662.

Davey, J. B., Greening, W. P. and McKinna, J. A. (1970) Is screening for cancer worth while? Results from a well-woman clinic for cancer detection. *British Medical Journal*, **iii**, 696–699.

Davies, J. D., Roberts, G. and Richardson, P. J. (1973) Technical methods: a serial whole-organ slicing technique for examining surgically resected breasts. *Journal of Clinical Pathology*, **26**, 891–892.

Dodd, G. D. and Wallace, J. D. (1968) The venous diameter ratio in the radiographic diagnosis of breast cancer. *Radiology*, **90**, 900–904.

D'Orsi, C. J. (1977) Effects of therapy on breast calcification. *British Journal of Radiology*, **50**, 66–67.

Dowdy, A. H., Barker, W. F., Lagasse, L. D., Sperling, L., Zeldis, L. J. and Longmire, W. P., Jr (1971) Mammography as a screening method for the examination of large populations. *Cancer*, **28**, 1558–1562.

Egan, R. L. (1960) Experience with mammography in a tumor institution. *Radiology*, **75**, 894–900.

Egan, R. L. (1972) *Mammography*. 2nd Edition. Springfield, Illinois: Charles C. Thomas.

Egan, R. L. (1975) Evolution of the team approach in breast cancer. *Cancer*, **36**, 1815–1822.

Egan, R. L. (1976) Bilateral breast carcinomas. *Cancer*, **38**, 931–938.

Egan, R. L. (1977) Mammographic detection of early breast cancer. *International Journal of Radiation Oncology, Biology and Physics*, **2**, 743–746.

Egan, R. L. and Mosteller, R. C. (1977) Breast cancer mammography patterns. *Cancer*, **40**, 2087–2090.

Egan, R. L., Ellis, J. T. and Powell, R. W. (1969) Team approach to the study of diseases of the breast. *Cancer*, **23**, 847–854.

Eusebi, V., Grassigli, A. and Grosso, F. (1976) Lesioni focali sclero-elastotiche mammarie simulanti il carcinoma infiltrante. *Pathologica*, **68**, 507–518.

Feig, S. A., Shaber, G. S., Schwartz, G. F., Patchefsky, A., Libshitz, H. I., Edeiken, J., Nerlinger, R., Curley, R. F. and Wallace, J. D. (1977) Thermography, mammography and clinical examination in breast cancer screening. *Radiology*, **122**, 123–127.

Feinleib, M. and Zelen, M. (1969) Some pitfalls in the evaluation of screening programs. *Archives of Environmental Health*, **19**, 412–415.

Fisher, E. R. and Fisher, B. (1977) Lobular carcinoma of the breast. An overview. *Annals of Surgery*, **185**, 377–385.

Fisher, E. R., Gregorio, R. M. and Fisher, B. (1975) The pathology of invasive breast cancer. *Cancer*, **36**, 1–85.

Fisher, E. R., Posada, H. and Ramos, H. (1974) Evaluation of mammography based upon correlation of specimen mammograms and histopathologic findings. *American Journal of Clinical Pathology*, **62**, 60–72.

Fisher, E. R., Redmond, C. and Fisher, B. (1977) A perspective concerning the relation of duration of symptoms to treatment failure in patients with breast cancer. *Cancer*, **40**, 3160–3167.

Fisher, E. R., Palekar, A., Kim, W. S. and Redmond, C. (1978) The histopathology of mammographic patterns. *American Journal of Clinical Pathology*, **69**, 421–426.

Frank, H. A., Hall, F. M. and Steer, M. L. (1976) Pre-operative localization of nonpalpable breast lesions demonstrated by mammography. *New England Journal of Medicine*, **295**, 259–260.

Frankl, G. (1978) Compression in specimen xeromammography. *American Journal of Roentgenology*, **130**, 377–378.

Frankl, G. and Ackerman, M. (1977) Xeromammography: five years and 559 carcinomas. *American Journal of Obstetrics and Gynecology*, **129**, 61–64.

Frankl, G. and Rosenfeld, D. D. (1975) Xeroradiographic detection of occult breast cancer. *Cancer*, **35**, 542–548.

Friedman, A. K., Askovitz, S. I., Berger, S. M., Dodd, G. D., Fisher, M. S., Lapayowker, M. S., Moore, J. P., Parlee, D. E., Stein, G. N. and Pendergrass, E. P. (1966) A co-operative evaluation of mammography in seven teaching hospitals. *Radiology*, **86**, 886–891.

Gallager, H. S. (1975) Breast specimen radiography. *American Journal of Clinical Pathology*, **64**, 749–755.

Gallager, H. S. and Martin, J. E. (1969) The study of mammary carcinoma by mammography and whole organ sectioning. *Cancer*, **23**, 855–873.

George, W. D., Gleave, E. N., England, P. C., Wilson, M. C., Sellwood, R. A., Asbury, D., Hartley, G., Barker, P. G., Hobbs, P. and Wakefield, J. (1976) Screening for breast cancer. *British Medical Journal*, **ii**, 858–860.

Gershon-Cohen, J. (1937) A chest cradle for the roentgen examination of the female breast. *Radiology*, **28**, 234–236.

Gershon-Cohen, J. (1970) *Atlas of Mammography*. Berlin, Heidelberg, New York: Springer-Verlag.

Gershon-Cohen, J., Berger, S. M. and Curcio, B. M. (1966) Breast cancer with microcalcifications: diagnostic difficulties. *Radiology*, **87**, 613–622.

Gibbs, N. M., Price, J. L., Ainsworth, R. W. and Korpal, K. (1975) A radiological and histological study of prostatic calcification associated with primary carcinoma: a comparison with mammary microcalcification. *Clinical Oncology*, **1**, 305–313.

Gilbertsen, V. A. and Kjelsberg, M. (1971) Detection of breast cancer by periodic utilization of methods of physical diagnosis. *Cancer*, **28**, 1552–1554.

Gros, C. M. and Sigrist, R. (1952) La radiographie de la glande mammaire. *Journal Belge de Radiologie*, **35** 226–268.

Hassler, O. (1969) Microradiographic investigations of calcifications of the female breast. *Cancer*, **23**, 1103–1109.

Hutter, R. V. P. and Kim, D. U. (1971) The problem of multiple lesions of the breast. *Cancer*, **28**, 1593–1607.

James, W. B. and Irvine, R. W. (1969) Mammography in management of breast lesions. *British Medical Journal*, **iv**, 655–657.

Jochimsen, P. R. and Brown, R. C. (1976) Metastatic melanoma in the breast masquerading as fibroadenoma. *Journal of the American Medical Association*, **236**, 2779–2780.

Kalisher, L. and Schaffer, D. L. (1975) Xeromammography in early detection of breast cancer. *Journal of the American Medical Association*, **234**, 60–63.

Kalisher, L., Chu, A. M. and Peyster, R. G. (1976) Clinicopathological correlation of xeroradiography in determining involvement of metastatic axillary nodes in female breast cancer. *Radiology*, **121**, 333–335.

Kieraldo, J. H., Bearc, J., Jamplis, R. W., Lee, R. H. and Mackenzie, A. S. (1976) Mammographically detectable breast cancer. *American Journal of Surgery*, **132**, 150–155.

Koehl, R. H., Snyder, R. E., Hutter, R. V. P. and Foote, F. W., Jr (1970) The incidence and significance of calcifications within operative breast specimens. *American Journal of Clinical Pathology*, **53**, 3–14.

Krook, P. M., Carlile, T., Bush, W. and Hall, M. H. (1978) Mammographic parenchymal patterns as a risk indicator for prevalent and incident cancer. *Cancer*, **41**, 1093–1097.

Leborgne, R. (1949) Diagnostico de los tumores de la mama por la radiografia simple. *Boletin de la Sociedad de Cirugia del Uruguay*, **20**, 407–422.

Lesnick, G. J. (1977) Detection of breast cancer in young women. *Journal of the American Medical Association*, **237**, 967–969.

Lester, R. G. (1977) Risk versus benefit in mammography. *Radiology*, **124**, 1–6.

Letton, A. H., Wilson, J. P. and Mason, E. M. (1977) The

value of breast screening in women less than fifty years of age. *Cancer,* **40,** 1–3.

Levitan, L. H., Witten, D. M. and Harrison, E. G., Jr (1964) Calcification in breast disease mammographic-pathologic correlation. *American Journal of Roentgenology,* **92,** 29–39.

Lewis, J. D., Milbrath, J. R., Shaffer, K. A. and DeCosse, J. J. (1975) Implications of suspicious findings in breast cancer screening. *Archives of Surgery,* **110,** 903–907.

Libshitz, H. I., Montague, E. D. and Paulus, D. D. (1977) Calcifications and therapeutically irradiated breast. *American Journal of Roentgenology,* **128,** 1021–1025.

Libshitz, H. I., Fetouh, S., Isley, J. and Lester, R. G. (1976) One-view mammographic screening? *Radiology,* **120,** 719–722.

Lundgren, B. and Jakobsson, S. (1976) Single view mammography. *Cancer,* **38,** 1124–1129.

MacErlean, D. P. and Nathan, B. E. (1972) Calcification in sclerosing adenosis simulating malignant breast calcification. *British Journal of Radiology,* **45,** 944–945.

Mackenzie, I. (1965) Breast cancer following multiple fluoroscopies. *British Journal of Cancer,* **19,** 1–8.

Malone, L. J., Frankl, G., Dorazio, R. A. and Winkley, J. H. (1975) Occult breast carcinomas detected by xeroradiography. *Annals of Surgery,* **181,** 133–136.

Manoliu, R. A. and Ooms, G. H. (1977) The accuracy of mammography. *Radiologia Clinica,* **46,** 422–429.

Martin, J. E. (1973) Xeromammography — an improved diagnostic method. *American Journal of Roentgenology,* **117,** 90–96.

McClow, M. V. and Williams, A. C. (1973) Mammographic examinations (4030). *Annals of Surgery,* **177,** 616–619.

McGregor, D. H., Land, C. E., Choi, K., Tokuoka, S., Liu, P., Wakabayashi, T. and Beebe, G. W. (1977) Breast cancer incidence among atomic bomb survivors, Hiroshima and Nagasaki, 1950–69. *Journal of the National Cancer Institute,* **59,** 799–811.

McIntosh, I. H., Hooper, A. A., Millis, R. R. and Greening, W. P. (1976) Metastatic carcinoma within the breast. *Clinical Oncology,* **2,** 393–401.

Mendell, L., Rosenbloom, M. and Naimark, A. (1977) Are breast patterns a risk index for breast cancer? A reappraisal. *American Journal of Roentgenology,* **128,** 547.

Mettler, F. A. Jr, Hempelmann, L. H., Dutton, A. M., Pifer, J. W., Toyooka, E. T. and Ames, W. R. (1969) Breast neoplasms in women treated with x-rays for acute postpartum mastitis. A pilot study. *Journal of the National Cancer Institute,* **43,** 803–811.

Millis, R. R., Atkinson, M. K. and Tonge, K. A. (1976) The xeroradiographic appearances of some uncommon malignant mammary neoplasms. *Clinical Radiology,* **27,** 463–471.

Millis, R. R., Davis, R. and Stacey, A. J. (1976) The detection and significance of calcifications in the breast: a radiological and pathological study. *British Journal of Radiology,* **49,** 12–26.

Millis, R. R., McKinna, J. A., Hamlin, I. M. E. and Greening, W. P. (1976) Biopsy of the impalpable breast lesion detected by mammography. *British Journal of Surgery,* **63,** 346–348.

Mole, R. H. (1978) The sensitivity of the human breast to cancer induction by ionizing radiation. *British Journal of Radiology,* **51,** 401–405.

Moskowitz, M., Pemmaraju, S., Fidler, J. A., Sutorius, D. J., Russell, P., Scheinok, P. and Holle, J. (1976a) On the diagnosis of minimal breast cancer in a screenee population. *Cancer,* **37,** 2543–2552.

Moskowitz, M., Keriakes, J., Saenger, E. L., Pemmaraju, S., Kurnar, A. and Tafel, G. (1976b) Breast cancer screening. *Radiology,* **120,** 431–432.

Moskowitz, M., Gartside, P., Gardella, L., de Groot, I. and Guenther, D. (1977) The breast cancer screening controversy: a perspective. *American Journal of Roentgenology,* **129,** 537–543.

Mühlow, A. (1974) A device for precision needle biopsy of the breast at mammography. *American Journal of Roentgenology,* **121,** 843–845.

Murphy, W. A. and DeSchryver-Kecskemeti, K. (1978) Isolated clustered microcalcifications in the breast: radiologic-pathologic correlation. *Radiology,* **127,** 335–341.

Myrden, J. A. and Hiltz, J. E. (1969) Breast cancer following multiple fluoroscopies during artificial pneumothorax treatment of pulmonary tuberculosis. *Canadian Medical Association Journal,* **100,** 1032–1034.

Nathan, B. E., Burn, J. I. and Doyle, F. H. (1972) An evaluation of mammography in a breast clinic. *Clinical Radiology,* **23,** 87–92.

Owen, A. W. M. C., Forrest, A. P. M., Anderson, T. J., Samuel, E., Young, G. B. and Scott, A. M. (1977) Breast screening and surgical problems. *British Journal of Surgery,* **64,** 725–728.

Patchefsky, A. S., Potok, J., Hoch, W. S. and Libshitz, H. I. (1973) Increased detection of occult breast carcinoma after more thorough histologic examination of breast biopsies. *American Journal of Clinical Pathology,* **60,** 799–804.

Patchefsky, A. S., Shaber, G. S., Schwartz, G. F., Feig, S. A. and Nerlinger, R. E. (1977) The pathology of breast cancer detected by mass population screening. *Cancer,* **40,** 1659–1670.

Patton, R. B., Poznanski, A. K. and Zylak, C. J. (1966) Pathologic examination of specimens containing nonpalpable breast cancers discovered by radiography. *American Journal of Clinical Pathology,* **46,** 330–334.

Peyster, R. G., Kalisher, L. and Cole, P. (1977) Mammographic parenchymal patterns and the prevalence of breast cancer. *Radiology,* **125,** 387–391.

Preece, P. E., Gravelle, I. H., Hughes, L. E., Baum, M., Fortt, R. W. and Leopold, J. G. (1977) The operative management of subclinical breast cancer. *Clinical Oncology,* **3,** 165–169.

Price, J. L., Davies, P. M. and Butler, P. D. (1976) Mammograms on medichrome film. *Clinical Radiology,* **27,** 371–373.

Raskin, M. M. and Poole, D. O. (1973) The venous diameter ratio revisited — its significance in mammographic interpretation. *Cancer,* **32,** 1357–1359.

Rogers, J. V., Jr and Powell, R. W. (1972) Mammographic indications for biopsy of clinically normal breasts: correlation with pathologic findings in 72 cases. *American Journal of Roentgenology,* **115,** 794–800.

Rosato, F. E., Thomas, J. and Rosato, E. F. (1973) Operative management of nonpalpable lesions detected by mammography. *Surgery, Gynecology and Obstetrics,* **137,** 491–493.

Rosen, P. P., Snyder, R. E. and Robbins, G. (1974) Specimen radiography for nonpalpable breast lesions found by mammography: procedures and results. *Cancer,* **34,** 2028–2033.

Rosen, P. P., Snyder, R. E., Foote, F. W. and Wallace, T.

(1970) Detection of occult carcinoma in the apparently benign breast biopsy through specimen radiography. *Cancer,* **26,** 944–952.

Salomon, A. (1913) Beiträge zur Pathologie und Klinik der Mammacarcinome. *Archiv für klinische Chirurgie,* **101,** 573–668.

Sayler, C., Egan, J. F., Raines, J. R. and Goodman, M. J. (1977) Mammographic screening. *Journal of the American Medical Association,* **238,** 872–873.

Scott, W. G. (1967) Mammography and the training program of the American College of Radiology. *American Journal of Roentgenology,* **99,** 1002–1008.

Shapiro, S. (1977) Evidence on screening for breast cancer from a randomized trial. *Cancer,* **39,** 2772–2782.

Shepard, T. J., Crile, G., Jr and Strittmatter, W. C. (1962) Roentgenographic evaluation of calcifications seen in paraffin block specimens of mammary tumours. *Radiology,* **78,** 967–968.

Shore, R. E., Hempelmann, L. H., Kowaluk, E., Mansur, P. S., Pasternac, B. S., Albert, R. E. and Haughie, G. E. (1977) Breast neoplasms in women treated with x-rays for acute postpartum mastitis. *Journal of the National Cancer Institute,* **59,** 813–822.

Simon, N., Lesnick, G. J., Lerer, W. N. and Bachman, A. L. (1972) Roentgenographic localization of small lesions of the breast by the spot method. *Surgery, Gynecology and Obstetrics,* **134,** 572–574.

Snyder, R. E. and Rosen, P. (1971) Radiography of breast specimens. *Cancer,* **28,** 1608–1611.

Stark, A. M. and Way, S. (1974) The screening of well women for the early detection of breast cancer using clinical examination with thermography and mammography. *Cancer,* **33,** 1671–1679.

Stevens, G. M. and Jamplis, R. W. (1971) Mammographically directed biopsy of nonpalpable breast lesions. *Archives of Surgery,* **102,** 292–295.

Stevens, G. M. and Weigen, J. F. (1966) Mammography survey for breast cancer detection. *Cancer,* **19,** 51–59.

Stewart, H. J., Gravelle, I. H. and Apsimon, H. T. (1969) Five years' experience with mammography. *British Journal of Surgery,* **56,** 341–344.

Strax, P. (1976) Results of mass screening for breast cancer in 50 000 examinations. *Cancer,* **37,** 30–35.

Strax, P., Venet, L. and Shapiro, S. (1973) Value of mammography in reduction of mortality from breast cancer in mass screening. *American Journal of Roentgenology,* **117,** 686–689.

Strax, P., Venet, L., Shapiro, S. and Gross, S. (1967) Mammography and clinical examination in mass screening for cancer of the breast. *Cancer,* **20,** 2184–2188.

Tonge, K. A., Davis, R. and Millis, R. R. (1976) The problem of discrimination in mammography. Arguments for using a biological test object. *British Journal of Radiology,* **49,** 678–685.

Toombs, B. D. and Kalisher, L. (1977) Metastatic disease to the breast: clinical, pathologic, and radiographic features. *American Journal of Roentgenology,* **129,** 673–676.

Upton, A. C., Beebe, G. W., Brown, J. M., Quimby, E. H. and Shellabarger, C. (1977) Report of NCI Ad Hoc Working Group on the risks associated with mammography in mass screening for the detection of breast cancer. *Journal of the National Cancer Institute,* **59,** 479–493.

Wanebo, C. K., Johnson, K. G., Sato, K. and Thorslund, T. W. (1968) Breast cancer after exposure to the atomic bombings of Hiroshima and Nagasaki. *New England Journal of Medicine,* **279,** 667–671.

Warren, S. L. (1930) A roentgenologic study of the breast. *American Journal of Roentgenology,* **24,** 113–124.

Wee, W. G., Moskowitz, M., Chang, N.-C., Ting, Y.-C. and Pemmaraju, S. (1975) Evaluation of mammographic calcifications using a computer program. *Radiology,* **116,** 717–720.

Wellings, S. R. and Wolfe, J. N. (1978) Correlative studies of the histologic and radiographic appearance of the breast parenchyma. *Radiology,* **129,** 299–306.

Wilkinson, E., Clopton, C., Gordonson, J., Green, R., Hill, A. and Pike, M. C. (1977) Mammographic parenchymal pattern and the risk of breast cancer. *Journal of the National Cancer Institute,* **59,** 1397–1400.

Witten, D. M. and Thurber, D. L. (1964) Mammography as a routine screening examination for detecting breast cancer. *American Journal of Roentgenology,* **92,** 14–20.

Wolfe, J. N. (1965) Mammography as a screening examination in breast cancer. *Radiology,* **84,** 703–708.

Wolfe, J. N. (1968) Xerography of the breast. *Radiology,* **91,** 231–240.

Wolfe, J. N. (1972) *Xeroradiography of the Breast.* Springfield, Illinois: Charles C. Thomas.

Wolfe, J. N. (1974) Analysis of 462 breast carcinomas. *American Journal of Roentgenology,* **121,** 846–853.

Wolfe, J. N. (1976) Breast patterns as an index of risk for developing breast cancer. *American Journal of Roentgenology,* **126,** 1130–1139.

Wolfe, J. N. (1977) *Xeroradiography: Uncalcified Breast Masses.* Springfield, Illinois: Charles C. Thomas.

INDEX